Nursing Education
&
Educational Technology

About the Authors

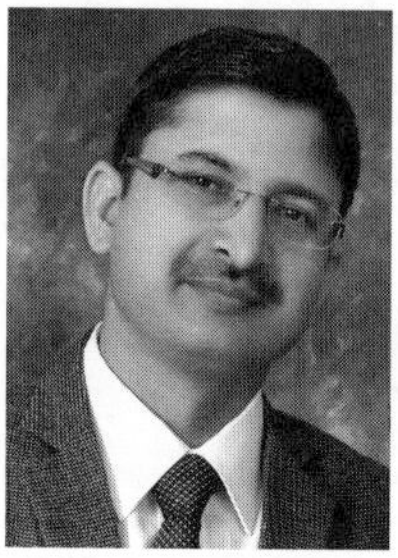

Dr Suresh K. Sharma is Professor cum Principal, College of Nursing, All India Institute of Medical Sciences (AIIMS), Jodhpur. He received his master's degree in Medical-Surgical Nursing from the Postgraduate Institute of Medical Education and Research (PGIMER), Chandigarh, and PhD in administration with a specialization in patient satisfaction with nursing care from Panjab University, Chandigarh.

He has been a GNLI-2020 Scholar at Global Nursing Leadership Institute, Geneva, Switzerland (2020 Aug – 2021 Sep) and has obtained a Post-Doctoral Fellowship from the Nursing Research Society of India (2017 – 2018, awarded in 2019 Nov). He also did his observership in Clinical Nursing Research at the University of York, Yorkshire, UK (2019, Aug) and hospital management and leadership at National University Hospitals, Singapore (2014 Sep), and Post-Doctoral Fellowship at the University of California, USA (2011 Sep – 2012 Aug).

He has more than 20 years of experience as a nurse academician, researcher, and leader while working as Lecturer, Reader, and Professor of Nursing at Dayanand Medical College & Hospitals, Ludhiana (Jun 2005 – Mar 2013); Professor & Principal and Dean, College of Nursing at AIIMS, Rishikesh (2013 Mar – 2020 Dec) and currently serving as Professor & Principal, College of Nursing, AIIMS Jodhpur (w.e.f. 2020 Dec) He was also a visiting professor at Sri Ramachandra Institute of Higher Education & Research, Chennai (2020 Dec to 2022 Dec) and Adjunct Faculty at School of Public Health, AIIMS Jodhpur and Adjunct Faculty at Datta Meghe Institute of Medical Sciences, Wardha. Besides being an examiner of UG/PG and PhD examiner at several universities/institutions in India also served as a postgraduate/doctoral nursing examiner at Sultan Qaboos University Muscat, Oman, and the University of Brunei Darussalam, Brunei.

He is a prolific writer. He has authored 6 and edited 5 textbooks, in addition to more than 200 research papers contributed to indexed journals. He also served as editor and member of the editorial team in national and international journals of repute. He is the founder and President, Society of Perioperative Nursing, India and Society for Critical Care Nursing, India. He has also served as a board member of the International Federation of Preoperative Nurses (IFPN). He has delivered 20 international and more than 200 national keynote/plenary/invited talks at conferences. He has been conferred with many prestigious awards including 'Florence Nightingale Award-2001'. His areas of research include nursing education, critical care nursing, and diabetes.

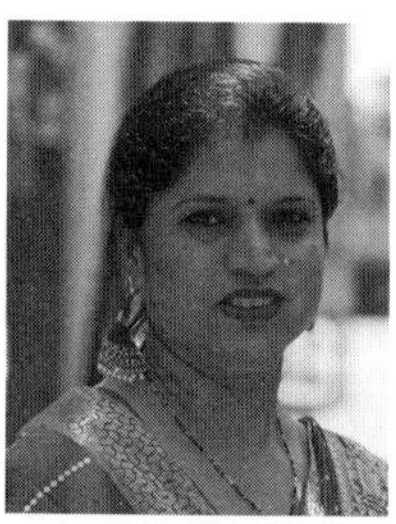

Ms Reena Sharma is an educationist and educational researcher. She received her bachelor degree in arts from Rajasthan University, Jaipur; her master degree in political science from Rajasthan University, Jaipur; and her M.Phil. in Gandhian Thought from Gandhian Study Centre, Rajasthan University, Jaipur. She received her B.Ed. from Rajasthan University, Jaipur, and M.Ed. (Educational Technology) from the Department of Education, Rajasthan University, Jaipur.

Ms Sharma has taught economics and political science in school education at Jaipur for several years. She has also taught *Educational Technology* to undergraduate education students at Baba Kundan College of Education, Ludhiana, Punjab, and Sambal College of Education, Sikar, Rajasthan, for a significant tenure.

She can be considered as a wordsmith or poignant writer, who has published research papers and articles in the field of education, in national and international journals. She is active in participating in and contributing to the academic developments among the educational fraternity.

She is practising as an educationist and educational researcher with a philosophy of *considering education a right of every child and being an educationist with difference, devoting self towards this social cause.* She is devoted to generating the evidence to provide the quality of education to each stratum of society at an affordable cost and maintaining standards of education at par with international standards.

Nursing Education & Educational Technology

THIRD EDITION

Suresh K. Sharma PhD, MScN, RN (USA)
Professor-cum-Principal
College of Nursing
All India Institute of Medical Sciences
Jodhpur, Rajasthan, India

Reena Sharma MPhil, MEd, BEd, MA
Department of Education, Rajasthan University,
Jaipur, Rajasthan, India

ELSEVIER

ELSEVIER
RELX India Pvt. Ltd.
Registered Office: 818, 8th Floor, Indraprakash Building, 21, Barakhamba Road, New Delhi 110001
Corporate Office: 14th Floor, Building No. 10B, DLF Cyber City, Phase II, Gurgaon-122002, Haryana, India

Nursing Education and Educational Technology, 3e
Suresh K. Sharma and Reena Sharma

First Edition 2012.

ISBN: 978-81-312-6156-9
e-ISBN: 978-81-312-6157-6
ISBN: 978-81-312-6723-3 (Set)
e-Book ISBN: 978-81-312-6724-0 (Set)
This book is part of the set ISBN: 978-81-312-6723-3. Not to be sold separately.

First Printed in India 2024, Reprinted 2024

Content Strategist: Deepti Damodaran
Content Project Manager: Subodh Kumar
Sr Production Executive: Dhan Singh Rana
Sr Cover Designer: Gopalakrishnan Venkatraman

Typeset by GW India

Printed in India by Rajkamal Electric Press, Kundli, Haryana.

Dedicated to Parents

Late Smt. Bhagwati Devi Sharma
and
Sh. Badri Narayan Sharma

whose unconditional love and belief in our capabilities provided us with the power and energy to complete this book

—Authors

Contributors

Shiv Kumar Mudgal, PhD, MScN, RN
Associate Professor, College of Nursing
All India Institute of Medical Sciences (AIIMS)
Deoghar, Jharkhand, India
Email: shiv.nur@aiimsdeoghar.edu.in

Dinesh K. Sharma, MSc (N), RPN (Ireland)
Mental Health Nursing Consultant, St. Brendans Mental Health Hospital, Dublin, Ireland
Email ID: dineshrajrolia@yahoo.com

Manjulata Evatt, RN, MSc (N), DNP
Clinical Associate Professor at Duquesne University School of Nursing, Pittsburgh, Pennsylvania, USA
Email ID: manjulata-evatt@yahoo.com

Dimple Madan, RN, MSc (N), PhD
Professor & Principal, SGRD College of Nursing, Hoshiarpur, Punjab, India
Email ID: principal@sgrdnursingcollege.com

Manpreet Kaur, RN, MSc (N)
Professor & Principal, SGRD College of Nursing, SGRDIMSR, Vallah, Amritsar, Punjab, India
Email ID: manpreet-arora001@rediffmail.com

Nidhi Sagar, RN, MSc (N)
Professor, College of Nursing, Dayanand Medical College and Hospital, Ludhiana, Punjab, India
Email ID: nidhisagar24@yahoo.com

Prabhjot Kaur, RN, MSc (N)
Clinical Instructor, National Institute of Nursing Education, PGIMER, Chandigarh, India
Email ID: prab.pgi@gmail.com

Parmees Kaur, RN, MSc (N)
Lecturer, College of Nursing, Govt. Medical College & Hospital, Chandigarh
Email ID: parmeeskaur@yahoo.com

Harshpunit, RN, MSc (N)
Associate Professor, Guru Nanak College of Nursing, Dahanklera, SBS Nagar, Punjab, India
Email ID: pariharsh.kauro@gmail.com

Ruchika Rani, RN, MSc (N)
Assistant Professor, College of Nursing, All India Institute of Medical Sciences, Rishikesh, Uttarakhand, India
Email ID: ruchikaheera@gmail.com

Khushveer Kaur, RN, MSc (N)
Child Development Project Officer, Department of Social Security and Women & Child Development, Govt. of Punjab, Kotkapura, District Faridkot, Punjab, India
Email ID: khushveer767@gmail.com

Bidisha Basu, RN, MSc (N)
Cardiac Nurse Tutor, UN Mehta Institute of Cardiology and Research Center, Ahmadabad, Gujrat, India
Email ID: basubidisha@ymail.com

Jaison Joseph, MScN, RN
Assistant Lecturer, College of Nursing, Pt BD Sharma University of Health Sciences, Rohtak, Haryana
Email: jaisonjsph@yahoo.com

International advisors

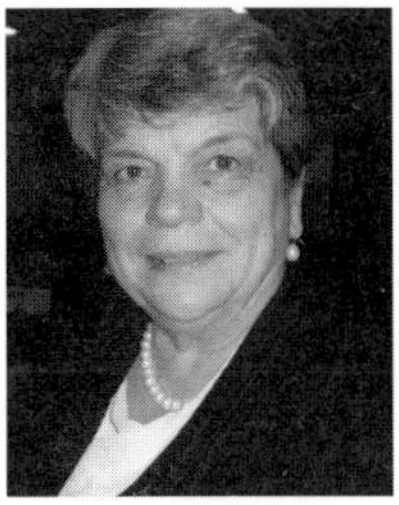

Carol R. Taylor, RN, PhD
Professor in Medicine and Nursing
Georgetown University
Washington DC 20057, USA
Email: taylorcr@georgetown.edu

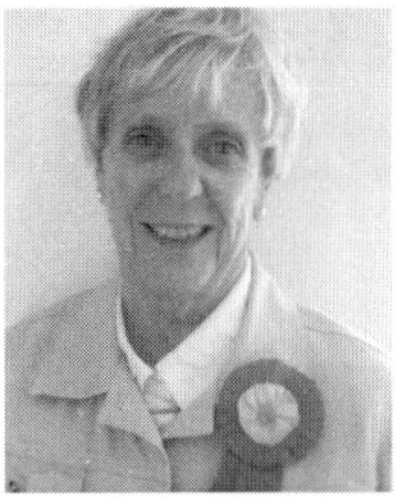

Marylou K. McHugh, RN, EdD, CNE
Professor in Nursing
College of Nursing and Health Professionals
Drexel University, 245 N 15th Street, Bellet Building,
Philadelphia, PA 19102, USA
Email: mm64@drexel.edu

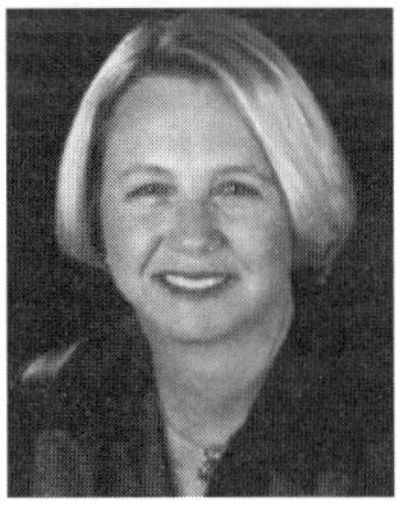

Joan T. Bickes, RN, MSN, PHCNS-BC
Assistant Professor
Wayne State University College of Nursing
262 Cohn Building, 5557 Cass Avenue
Detroit, MI 48202, USA
Email: jbickes@wayne.edu

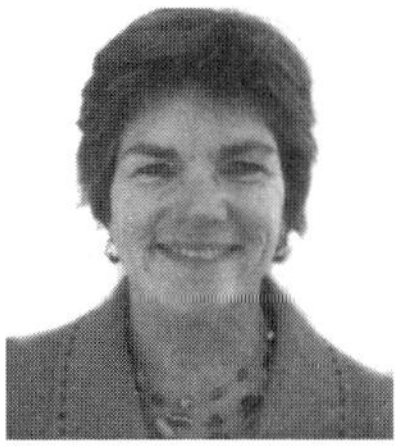

Margaret L. Falahee, APRN, FNP
Assistant Professor
Wayne State University College of Nursing
261 Cohn Building, 5557 Cass Avenue
Detroit, MI 48324, USA
Email: Ab2479@wayne.edu

National advisors

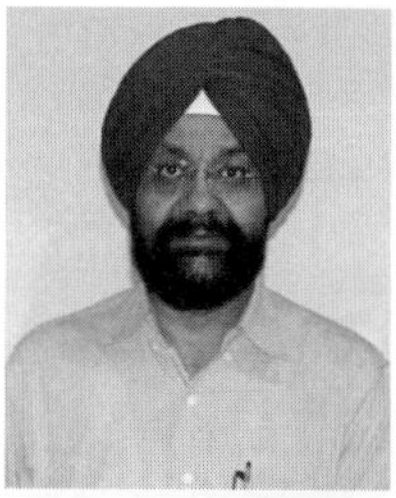

Daljit Singh, MD
Former Principal
Dayanand Medical College and Hospital
Ludhiana, Punjab
Email: dr-daljit-singh@dmch.edu

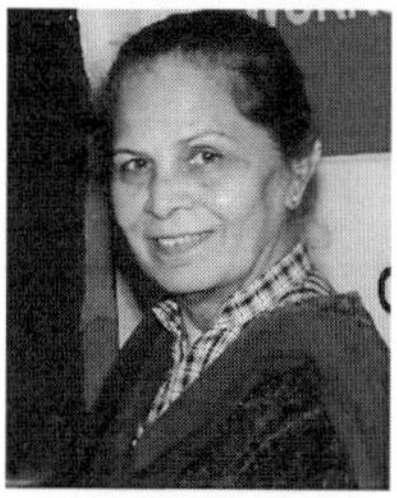

Indarjit Walia, PhD
Former Principal
National Institute of Nursing Education
PGIMER, Chandigarh
Email: indrajitwalia@yahoo.com

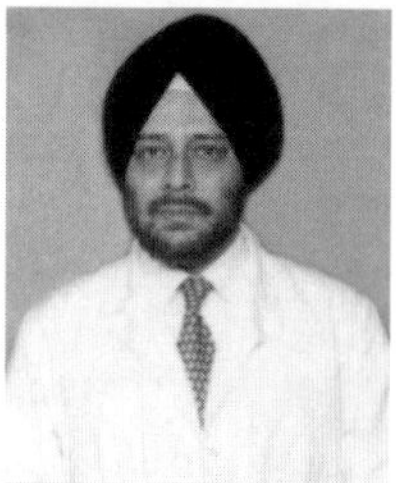

Rajoo Singh Chhina, MD, DM
Former Dean (Academics)
Dayanand Medical College and Hospital
Ludhiana, Punjab
Email: drrajoosingh@rediffmail.com

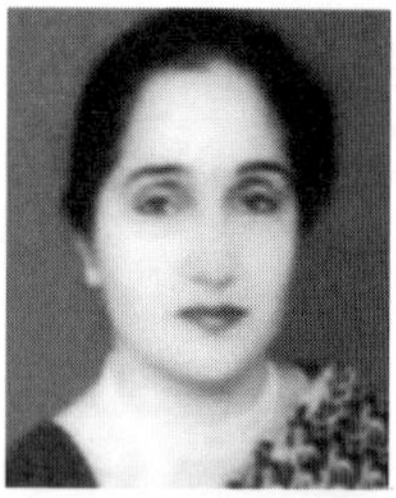

Sandhya Ghai, PhD
Former Principal
National Institute of Nursing Education
PGIMER, Chandigarh
Email: sandhya.ghai@yahoo.com

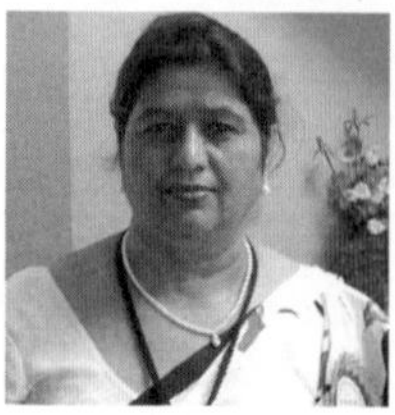

Jasbir Kaur, PhD
Former Principal
College of Nursing
Dayanand Medical College and Hospital
Ludhiana, Punjab
Email: jksaini1952@yahoo.com

Reviewers

Vimla Kapoor, Former Director, School of Health Sciences, Indira Gandhi National Open University, New Delhi, India

Deepika Khaka, Nursing Advisor, Ministry of Health & Family Welfare, Nirman Bhawan, New Delhi, India

Asha P. Shetty, Professor-cum-Principal, College of Nursing, AIIMS, Bhubaneswar, Odisha, India

M.J. Kumari, Professor & Principal (Actg), College of Nursing, JIPMER, Puducherry, India

Judith Angelitta Noronha, Dean, Manipal College of Nursing Manipal, Manipal Academy of Higher Education, Manipal, Udupi, Karnataka, India

Filiz OGCE, Professor, Nursing Department, Faculty of Health Science, Izmir University of Economics, Izmir, Turkey

Khadizah Haji Abdul Mumin, Assistant Professor, Programme Leader for Nursing & Midwifery, Institute of Health Sciences, Universiti Brunei Darussalam (UBD), Jalan Tungku, Brunei Darussalam

Michael Joseph S. Dino, Director, Research, Development and Innovation, Our Lady of Fatima University, Manila, Philippines

Binda Ghimire, Associate Professor, National Academy of Medical Sciences, Kathmandu, Nepal

Deki Pem, Associate Professor, Faculty of Nursing & Public Health, Khesar Gyalpo University of Medical Sciences, Bhutan

Foreword

In the last few decades, nursing education in India has undergone tremendous change, from informal bedside hospital-based training to university-based graduate, postgraduate and doctoral nursing education. Furthermore, the rapid growth and development in science and technology has largely influenced the need as well as method of teaching–learning process for nurses in India. Nurses are actively involved in teaching the patients, family and community as well as educating and training the new budding nurses. India has observed a rapid growth and development in nursing education and the Indian nursing faculty has increasing responsibility to educate future nurses using basic and advanced concepts and principles of communication and educational technology. Further, they need to equip the budding nurses, nurse educators and nursing faculty with the basic concepts, principles and methods of communication and educational technology so that they efficiently handle the communication, patient teaching and nursing education and training. However, there was scarcity of literature encompassing the Indian perspective with regard to communication and educational technology in nursing. A sound knowledge of communication and educational technology is essential for the present as well as future nurses that make them capable of offering efficient and effective communication and teaching to their patients.

Therefore, I feel that this textbook, titled *Communication and Educational Technology in Nursing*, will fill the gap in the literature on pedagogy that is tailored to the peculiar needs of teaching–learning process in nursing among developing countries, especially India. This book is a modest attempt to present the content related to communication and educational technology in a lucid manner and includes most of the basic and essential concepts of the communication, interpersonal relationship, educational media and teaching–learning process. I, therefore, commend its author, Dr Suresh K. Sharma, as well as other contributors and advisors for this unique contribution with an Indian background in the area of communication and educational technology. I further commend that this book caters to the needs of the graduate nursing students and their faculty; it may even be used by postgraduate nursing students and other health care professionals.

Dr S.S. Gill
Former Vice Chancellor
Baba Farid University of Health Sciences
Faridkot, Punjab, India

Preface to the Third Edition

Welcome to the fascinating intersection of Nursing Education and Educational Technology! This textbook aims to provide a comprehensive and contemporary overview of how the dynamic realm of educational technology is transforming the landscape of nursing education. As we delve into this exciting field, we invite educators, students, and healthcare professionals to embark on a transformative journey together.

Nursing education has always been at the heart of producing competent, compassionate, and skilled healthcare providers. However, in recent years, the rapid advancements in technology have brought about profound changes in various industries, including healthcare and education. Integrating educational technology into nursing education has the potential to enhance the learning experience, improve patient outcomes, and prepare nursing graduates for the complex challenges of the modern healthcare landscape.

Since the release of the first edition, the healthcare industry has undergone significant transformations, driven by advances in medical technology, new treatment modalities, a deeper understanding of patient-centered care and significant changes in the curriculum of nursing education by Indian Nursing Council. These changes have brought forth both challenges and opportunities for nursing professionals, making the role of educators even more critical. This textbook has been thoughtfully updated to address these shifts and align with the current needs of nursing education.

This textbook seeks to bridge the gap between the ever-evolving world of educational technology and the unique demands of nursing education. From traditional classroom settings to cutting-edge virtual simulations, we explore a diverse range of educational tools and techniques that hold the promise of revolutionizing the nursing education process. Key features of the third edition of Nursing Education and Educational Technology textbook are:

Comprehensive Coverage: This edition continues to provide a comprehensive overview of nursing education, catering to the needs of both novice and experienced educators. From fundamental principles to advanced teaching methodologies, the textbook covers the entire spectrum of nursing education.

Innovative Teaching Strategies: We recognize the importance of engaging and effective teaching methods to enhance the learning experience for students. Therefore, this edition incorporates innovative strategies and technologies to foster a dynamic and interactive learning environment.

Integration of Evidence-Based Practice: As nursing education increasingly emphasizes evidence-based practice, this edition ensures that the latest research findings and evidence are integrated into the content. By doing so, we aim to help educators bridge the gap between theory and practice in nursing education.

Emphasis on Cultural Competence: In today's diverse and multicultural world, cultural competence is paramount in healthcare settings. This edition dedicates a substantial portion to this topic, helping educators instill cultural sensitivity in their students, leading to more effective and compassionate care.

Interprofessional Collaboration: With the growing importance of collaborative care models, nursing professionals must work seamlessly with other healthcare providers. This edition delves into the significance of interprofessional education and collaboration, promoting a team-oriented approach to healthcare delivery.

Real-World Case Studies: To facilitate a deeper understanding of nursing concepts and their practical application, we have included real-world case studies that encourage critical thinking and problem-solving skills among students.

Online Resources: Complementing the printed text, this edition offers access to online resources, including supplementary materials, interactive exercises, and further readings, to enrich the learning experience beyond the classroom.

Pedagogical Strategies for the Digital Age: To harness the full potential of educational technology, it is essential to adapt and optimize pedagogical strategies. We discuss evidence-based teaching methods tailored to the digital age, emphasizing learner-centered approaches that promote critical thinking, problem-solving, and clinical reasoning skills.

Throughout this journey, we draw insights from pioneering educators, researchers, and practitioners who have embraced the fusion of nursing education and educational technology. Their experiences serve as beacons, illuminating the path for others to follow in their pursuit of innovative and effective nursing education.

As we embark on this venture together, we hope that this textbook serves as a valuable resource, inspiring educators and learners to reimagine the possibilities of nursing education through the lens of educational technology. The transformation begins here, and we are thrilled to have you join us on this exciting expedition.

—Authors

Preface to the First Edition

Most ideas about teaching are not new, but not everyone knows the old ideas.

—Euclid, Circa 300 BC

Nursing education, the science behind teaching and learning in nursing, has been firmly established as a separate discipline. Parallel to the advancement in nursing science, nursing education has seen tremendous progress as a discipline. The beneficial effects of such development are readily evident. Teaching and learning have become more scientific and rigorous curricula are based on good pedagogical principles, and problem-based and other forms of active and self-directed learning are no longer viewed as an anomaly but are now considered to be mainstream. There is a strong emphasis on evidence-based education.

This is a time of great excitement and opportunity for anyone who is interested in teaching and learning in nursing. Parallel to its spectacular growth, nursing education has become more specialized as a discipline. In recent years, there is extensive publication by international and national authors in nursing education. There are several scholarly journals dedicated to nursing education that are published regularly and enjoy a good readership base. Moreover, most clinical professional journals also publish articles on nursing education. There are also many authentic books on the various aspects of nursing education written by renowned scholars and leaders.

But the rapid development and specialization in nursing education has not come without a price. The more developed the discipline became, the more specialized and fragmented became the books and publications on nursing education. Many books are too intimidating and esoteric to meet the needs of general nursing teachers and learners. In contrast to the prolific publication trend in specialized aspects of nursing education, there is a marked paucity of books written for the general reader in nursing education. More importantly, there are few books that are easy to understand, portable as well as affordable for the individual reader. The issue of nonavailability is evident from our interactions with our colleagues. Frequently, we engage our friends and colleagues in a passionate discussion about nursing education and the benefits that they may get from knowing the science of teaching and learning. When we have managed to instill enough interest, our colleagues' response is typical—'It seems nursing education is interesting. Can you name a book where I can read more about it?' Our defeat comes now. It is hard to recommend a book about communication and educational technology that meets all four criteria of syllabus requirement, understandability, portability and affordability.

Therefore, in this simple nonintimidating book, we promise to tell the undergraduate-level nursing students and teachers what they need to know about communication and educational technology. We strive towards making the book a readable, jargon-free, precise yet complete guide to communication and educational technology in nursing, which is written exactly as per the syllabus prescribed by the Indian Nursing Council.

—Authors

Contents

CHAPTER 1

Education and educational technology

LEARNING OBJECTIVES

This chapter is designed to enable the reader to:

- Define and discuss the meaning, aims, approaches and scope of education and educational technology.
- Explain the role of hardware and software technology in educational practices.
- Discuss the aims, characteristics, principles and outcomes of transformative education.
- Define and discuss the aims, elements, importance and challenges of relationship-based education.
- Discuss the meaning, elements and principles of competency-based education.

KEY TERMS

INTRODUCTION

In India, nursing education has evolved from hospital-based training to university-based undergraduate, postgraduate and doctoral level education. Today, nurses are progressively more involved in education of patients, family, colleagues and student nurses. There are wide varieties of nursing courses offered in India, like 1½ year Auxiliary Nurse Midwifery programme, 3-years General Nursing and Midwifery diploma programme, undergraduate, postgraduate, nurse practitioners and doctoral nursing programmes, where Indian Nursing Council plays a significant role in establishing uniformity of these programmes across the country. Recently, technology has crucially impacted every sphere of the human life including education and nursing education. It has remarkably influenced the curriculum, teaching-learning pedagogy, infrastructure requirements and assessment practices in nursing education. Evidence generation related to nursing education happening globally, which helping in continued quality improvement in nursing education. There are growing challenges in preparing future nurses, who are clinical-practice ready to immediately take up the registered nurses' role in the healthcare system. Frances Payne School of Nursing, Case Western Reserve University, Cleveland, Ohio, United States, brought a Quality and Safety Education for Nurses (QSEN) project with a purpose to meet challenges of preparing future nurses, who have knowledge, skills and attitude essential to continuously improve quality and safety of the healthcare systems within which they work. The QSEN competencies are listed under six domains: patient-centred care, teamwork and collaboration, evidence-based practice, quality improvement, safety and informatics.

EDUCATION

The term education has its origin in the Latin words *educo*, *educare* and *educatum*. Etymologically, the word education is derived from the Latin words *educo* where *e* means 'out of' and *duco* means 'I lead'. According to this view, *education* means 'I lead out of darkness into brightness'.

In another perspective, the word education is derived from the Latin word *educare* which refers to breed, to bring up and to rear. Also *educatum* denotes education that means 'an act of teaching or training'. Therefore, education means to lead, to lead forth or to unfold the hidden talents of man. It is very much the art of developing and cultivating the various powers of mind, physical, mental and moral. Education is a social process and the main concern is the modification of behaviour.

DEFINITION OF EDUCATION

Indian philosophers have beautifully defined education; some definitions are given below:

> *Education means the training for the country and love for the nation.*
>
> **—Chanakya**

> *Education is realization of self.*
>
> **—Shankaracharya**

> *Education is self-realization and service of the people.*
>
> **—Guru Nanak Dev**

> *Education is the manifestation of divine perfection already existing in man.*
>
> **—Swami Vivekananda**

> *Educations means enabling the mind to find out that ultimate truth which emancipates us from the bondage of dust and gives us the wealth not of things but of inner light, not of power but of love, making the truth its own and giving expression to it.*
>
> **—Rabindranath Tagore**

> *Education is an all-round drawing out of the best in child and man-body, mind and spirit.*
>
> **—Mahatma Gandhi**

Several international educationists and philosophers have also given outstanding definitions of education, some of which are presented below:

> *Education is the capacity to feel pleasure and pain at right moment. It develops in the body and in the soul of the pupil all beauty and all perfection which he is capable of.*
>
> **—Plato**

> *Education is the process of living through a continuous reconstruction of experiences. It is the development of all those capacities in the individual which will enable him to control his environment and fulfil his possibilities.*
>
> **—John Dewey**

> *Education is the natural, harmonious and progressive development of man's innate power.*
>
> **—Pestalozzi**

Education is the creation of a sound mind in a sound body.

—Aristotle

Education is the organization of acquired habits of such action as will fit the individual to his physical and social environment.

—James

AIMS OF EDUCATION

The aim of education guides the child to fulfil the goals of life. The main aims of education are detailed below (Fig. 1.1):

1. **Social aim:** Society is considered to be the result of interactions between individuals in small or large groups and education ensures the peaceful existence of the society. Through education, students realize the importance of social values like justice, fair play, healthy competition and harmony. Education makes the individual accountable to the community, society and the nation. Education along with social objectives gives direction to the society for its positive and inclusive development.
2. **Vocational aim:** The process of education enables the individual for his livelihood so that he can lead a useful and productive life in society. Vocational aim of education enable person to respect dignity of labour and make him self-sufficient. Furthermore, vocational education facilitates the individual to easily get into a vocation, and it is essential to reduce unemployment rate in a country.
3. **Cultural aim:** Mankind has a rich heritage in the form of traditions and customs called culture. It has to be preserved and disseminated through the agency of education to increase generalization, which is both a conservative and a dynamic force. The education aim of culture involves a better

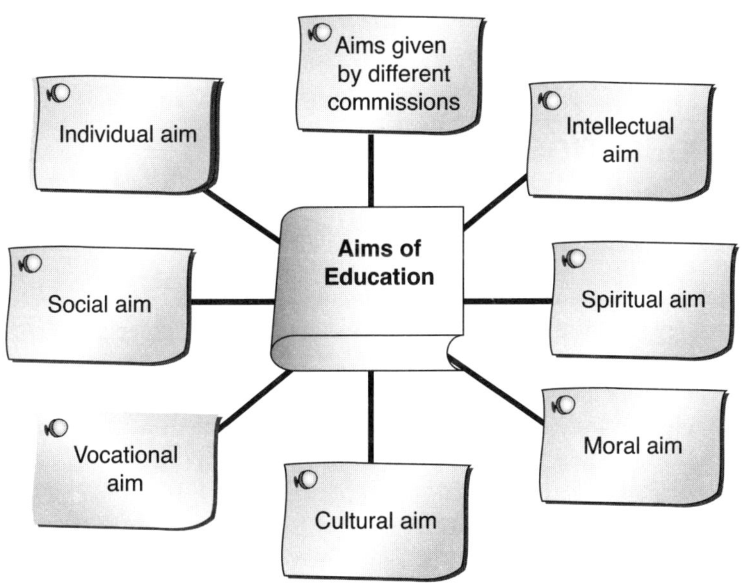

Figure 1.1

Aims of education.

understanding about the existing beliefs, arts, morals, laws and so on of the society. An educated person develops an aesthetic sense and respects the cultures of others, which promote mutual respect and cooperation.
4. **Moral aim:** Incorporating education into the soul or imparting moral education is the main task of education. Education helps in building the character of a person. Most of the values like honesty, truthfulness, justice, goodness, purity, courage, punctuality and dutifulness are nurtured through education.
5. **Spiritual aim:** Education is necessary to promote spirituality among individuals through which they elevate themselves above selfishness and work for the welfare of others and society, which is called a state of self-realization. According to an idealist, the sole aim of education is to develop the spiritual-self of the individual.
6. **Intellectual aim:** Education provides an opportunity for a person to develop innate power or intellectual capabilities, so that one can think logically and lead a meaningful life independently with fullest possible confidence.

EDUCATIONAL TECHNOLOGY

According to Leith, 'Educational technology as the systematic application of scientific knowledge about teaching-learning and conditions of learning to improve the efficiency of teaching and training'.

An Indian educationist Sh. S.S. Kulkarni mentions that 'Educational Technology can be defined as the application of the laws as well as recent discoveries of science and technology to the process of education'.

The use of technology, processes and procedures to improve learning experiences is called educational technology. Educational technology has significantly impacted the nursing education, and it is widely used in variety of settings such as workplace learning, formal learning, informal education, just-in-time learning and lifelong learning in nursing. Educational technology has rapidly expanded and now includes more advanced approaches and devices, such as virtual and augmented reality, simulations and immersive environments, mobile technology as well as collaborative learning, social networking and cloud computing.

NATURE OF EDUCATIONAL TECHNOLOGY

The nature of educational technology is not limited to the use of technology in the field of education but it encompasses a wide range of scientific activities and applications in teaching and learning as detailed below:
- The science is the foundation of educational technology.
- Education technology studies the impact of science and technology on education.
- Educational technology is an ever-changing, progressive and effective method of educating students.
- Educational technology is the key to new conceptions, such as micro-teaching and simulated teaching, programmed learning, simulation, interaction analysis, programming and tape recorder.
- Educational technology considers educational institute as a system. This system includes building, furniture and teacher as **input**. Various methods, techniques, strategies and the teaching and exam with the aid of audio-visual aids function as a **process**. **The output** comes in the form of the abilities and capabilities of the students.

- Engineering technology is a component of educational technology; technologies such as television, radio, tape recorder and videotape, which are also known as audio-visual aids, are one component of educational technology only.
- Technology-driven audio-visual aids are only the input components of educational technology, while educational technology encompasses as input, process and output.
- Programmed instruction not educational technology, but it is only an activity within it, where student learns the instructions by himself following programmed pathway of learning with the help of computer. It can only be used for specific objectives and subject matter. Programmable instruction is therefore only a part of educational technology.
- Educational technology is not the solution of all the problems in education, but it can be used to enhance teaching and learning processes.
- There are three components of educational technology: (1) Input; (2) Process; and (3) Output. Within this, the teacher is still the most important aspect of education as input and cannot be replaced by any type of educational technology.

AIMS OF EDUCATIONAL TECHNOLOGY

The educational technology encompasses a wide range of activities ranging from the analytic methods of psychology of learning to teaching the audio-visual communication and mass media technology. Thus educational technology has the following main aims:

1. Educational technology is concerned with the systematic application of science and technology in the field of education, and thus may be defined as the application of technology to education in order to further the case of the latter.
2. Just as science and technology help in carrying out the practical task in general, educational technology helps in providing efficiency to the task of teaching and learning.
3. Educational technology provides technical guidance and solution to the problems of education.
4. Teaching is communicating and education technology can play an effective role in the communication between teacher and student.
5. Education technology encompasses a wide range of teaching and learning activities and processes involving elements such as:
    - Help in specification of goals and behavioural objectives.
    - Analysis of the ability and characteristics of the learner.
    - Selection and organization of the content or subject matter to be learned.
    - Methods and strategies of the presentation of the content.
    - Use of aid-materials, software and hardware, mass media and communication techniques.
    - Effective arrangement of learning situations, learning environment and learning experiences.
    - Effective classroom control and management.
    - Continuous feedback and evaluation of the educational outcomes.
6. Educational technology is not limited to the use of audio-visual aids and does not symbolize merely educational hardware, such as sophisticated gadgets and mechanical devices used in education. For the effective management of the total teaching-learning process, it tends to utilize the results of all goods, experiments and researches in the field of human learning and the art of communication and employs a combination of all possible human and nonhuman resources to achieve the desired educational objectives.

In a nutshell, the aim of educational technology is:

1. To develop the teaching methods and learning approaches after systematizing them in order to make them more effective for the new era.

2. To change the behaviour of educators and students through improving teaching, learning and evaluation conditions.
3. To make classroom teaching simple, clear, engaging, effective, understandable and scientific.

In brief, the main aim of educational technology is wise application of the available human and non-human resources for providing appropriate solution to the educational problems and to improve the process and products of education.

APPROACHES OF EDUCATIONAL TECHNOLOGY

Lumsdaine (1964) described three different approaches of educational technology: Hardware, Software and System approach.

I. **Hardware approach of educational technology:**
   - It involves technology developed from engineering and physical sciences such as microphones, speakers, liquid crystal display projectors, computers, cameras, slide projectors, and overhead projectors. These technological hardware of multimedia, multisensory audio-visual aids has revolutionized teaching-learning in nursing education.
   - This hardware approach of educational technology has been developed through engineering and physical sciences, which has significantly revolutionized education. For instance, if a teacher is teaching in a large hall and uses a microphone to hear his voice, it could be said that he approaches such technology for his teaching effectiveness. These types of teaching technology have markedly impacted the teaching-learning processes and outcomes. In another example, use of hardware in teaching and learning is: During COVID-19 pandemic, educationists have used personal computers or laptops, smart phones or other similar devices, internet and remote teaching platforms for teaching-learning purposes. Most of the equipment and materials used as hardware are from areas other than education and used for educational purposes.

II. **The software approach of the educational technology:**
   - It is also known as instructional technology, which includes teaching-learning strategies, processes and instructional methods based on psychological principles of learning to achieve best possible results of these processes, methods and techniques.

     Psychology of learning was a solid technology that enabled students to make desirable behavioural changes. This serves education by establishing a clear instructional process, teaching behaviour and behavioural modification devices. Sometimes, the second type is called instructional technology.
   - This technology adopts a process-oriented approach and seeks to produce the most effective teaching-learning material and teaching-learning strategies. It also aims at evaluating teaching-learning techniques in order to achieve the best possible results in the teaching and learning processes. Educational technology basically stands for the technique of developing and utilizing software and, that is why, it is referred to as the software approach. The materials, such as programmed material and teaching-learning strategies based on the psychology of learning are usually known as software, and the equipment and gadgets are called hardware.

III. **The system approach of educational technology:**
   - It is also known as management technology of education, which consists 'a set of inputs', 'processes' and 'designed to produce intended outcome' of education to achieve desired objectives of particular discipline of education.
   - System analysis as educational management technology developed after World War II. It provided a scientific basis for the decision-making regarding the problems associated with

administration, management, commerce, industry and the army. It helps to study the problems of educational administration and management in a scientific and conclusive way.

- This type of educational technology is related to the concept of system engineering which owes its origin to computer science. It represents the latest concept in educational technology of education.
- This system approach views education as a system with a set of inputs that are subject to a process and designed to produce certain outcomes which meet the defined objectives of the system.
- System approach of educational technology is the dynemic role played by machines, man, and media in a system for education, which is supported by development of an instructional design and strategies according to related objectives.

ROLE OF HARDWARE AND SOFTWARE TECHNOLOGIES IN EDUCATIONAL PRACTICES

- It helps in organizing and arranging individualized instructions.
- Use the multimedia and multisensory approach to teaching-learning
- Management of the affairs of educational practices in an efficient and productive way.
- Providing proper input and process for the best possible outcomes (products).
- Fulfilling the expectation of distances and correspondence education.
- Making the task of teaching-learning interesting, purposeful and productive.

The hardware, software and system approach of the technology has significantly impacted the education system but it has several issues, which have been illustrated in Fig. 1.2.

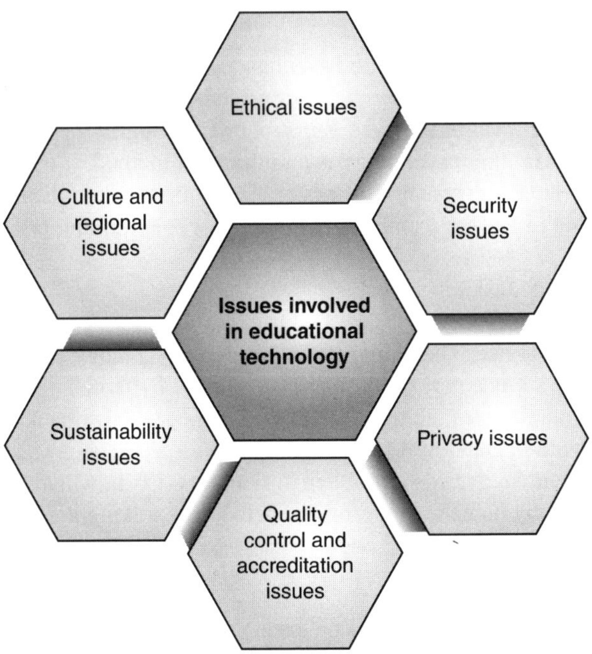

Figure 1.2

Issues involved in educational technologies.

SCOPE OF EDUCATIONAL TECHNOLOGY

The scope of educational technology is quite large as it involves the application and practice of using technologies (in the form of tools, techniques, resources, processes, etc.) to support, facilitate and enhance learning, performance and instruction. While educational technology has emerged as a recognized discipline and profession in the last 50 years, it is a dynamic, complex and interdisciplinary enterprise. It is dynamic in part due to the rapid changes occurring in technology. It is complex due to the many interacting factors, components and people involved in an education system or learning environment; moreover, many of the relationships among those factors, components and people are nonlinear and change over time. Educational technology is inherently an interdisciplinary enterprise involving, among others, content experts, technical specialists, teachers and administrators, who have different backgrounds and formal training.

Educational technology is as wide as education itself. Educational technology implies the use of all educational resources – Men, Materials, Methods and Techniques, Means and Media in an integrated and systematic manner for optimized learning. The main scope of educational technology are detailed as below:

- **Behavioural Technology:** It is one of important components of educational technology, which puts emphasis on the use of psychological principles in learning and teaching, so that the behaviour of the teacher and pupils may be modified in accordance of the teaching objectives.
- **Instructional Technology:** Instructional technology means a network of techniques or devices employed to accomplish certain defined set of learning objectives. Instructional technology implies the application of psychological, sociological and scientific principles and knowledge to instruction for achieving the specific objectives of learning.
- **Teaching Technology:** Teaching is the social and professional activity. It is a process to develop teaching as system of actions which induce learning through interpersonal relationship. Teaching technology is the application of philosophical, sociological and scientific knowledge to teaching.
- **Instructional Design:** In order to bring desired changes in the pupils' behaviour, the teaching situations, working tools and new approaches were considered important in addition to the learning principles. The composite form of all these is instructional design.
- **Training Psychology:** Training psychology is an important method of teaching and learning. Its development resulted out of the research work carried out on the complicated training problems and situations. Training psychology emphasizes that the whole training task should be divided into three parts. These are:
    - Preparing outline of the task.
    - Task analysis.
    - Putting the task in sequence. The main role of training psychology is in Teacher Education.
- **Cybernetic Psychology:** It is a part of training psychology. Cybernetic psychology accepts human beings as machine. It emphasizes the fact that all the methods of feedback bring the desired changes by controlling the behaviour of the pupil.
- **System Analysis:** System analysis is a problem-solving process in which the needs of the management are diagnosed, and by using an appropriate method for solving the problem, evaluation is carried out.

LATEST APPROACHES TO EDUCATION

Contemporary development constantly imposes new trends in education in order to gain future workforce that will be able to solve complex tasks which modern society imposes. Technology development accelerates teaching, which implies a faster way of transferring knowledge, skills and competences. The system of education and training should prepare and train individuals for the world of work. Professional development and education of individuals as educated, responsible, entrepreneurial and efficient people and the development of their careers in the service of progress and contribution to the community, economy and society should start early in the process of learning. Individuals need to be trained so they can solve problems, independently conclude and make decisions in life and social environment.

These new approaches to education are also termed as latest or modern approaches to education. Today educational systems and educational institution programmes that have traditional methods of learning and teaching do not go hand in hand with modern society. New forms of acquiring knowledge, skills and competences are increasingly being imposed as the needs of today's generation are continuously changing.

However, with time being changed to an extent, learners demand new techniques and methods to gain knowledge, which specializes them not only in theoretical study but also ensures them to provide practical knowledge, sharpen their skills and make them educated to face any kind of challenges. Modern teaching methods are the only way to meet the requirements of modern times. This needs an introduction of new approaches to education which focus more on questioning, demonstration, explaining, practical, collaboration methods and are more activity-based. The key characteristics of latest approaches of education are (1) Learner-centred; (2) Task-based or activity-based; (3) Resource-based; (4) Interactive in nature; (5) Integrative nature; and (6) Peer collaboration.

Like other fields, education has also revolutionized drastically over the period. Earlier, teachers were the only means to create a bridge between education and learners. They were using conventional pedagogical methods to explain the topic or to provide content. However, modern education approach has changed significantly, which is learner-centric and activity-oriented and encourages learners to holistically develop in all dimensions of life. Recently, different modern teaching approaches and methods have emerged, and the introduction of technology along with innovative ways to teach has brought a rapid revolution in the field of education.

The three main latest educational approaches are Transformational Education, Relationship-Based Education and Competency-Based Education, which have been discussed in this chapter.

TRANSFORMATIVE EDUCATION

Transformative education is defined as 'the process of encouraging students to change from being recipients of the knowledge to be more meaningful learner through considering different viewpoints and questioning their own beliefs, values and assumptions'.

Transformational education or transformative education views education as a means of helping people understand and acknowledge the interconnectedness between their inner and outer world. This is a new learning process that involves expanding consciousness and working towards a life of meaning and integration, as demonstrated in authentic relationships with others.

Transformative education is a process of recognizing the structures of injustice and recognizing one's own ability to redress those roots of injustice. Further, such transformation is not a one-off event but an ongoing process of continuous reflection and action, described by transformative educators as praxis.

AIM OF TRANSFORMATIVE EDUCATION

Transformative education is a holistic approach, which aims for education of the whole person – mind, body and animating spirit, including their emotional, social and physical development as well as values, multiple divergent and creative/artistic intelligence important to problem-solving in a complex world. Some of the main aims of the transformative education approaches are:

- Transformational education approach is used to facilitate and empower learner to view social world distinctly considering basic ethical principles, so that they can understand, challenge self and satiation to become a change agent for positive social changes.
- Transformational education approach helps teachers to identify and connect with learner's personal and emotional experiences.
- This approach also helps teachers in engaging with learners through dialogues, social interactions, considering importance of emotions, feelings and experiences of learners.
- The ultimate aim of transformative education approach is to encourage learner to achieve personal transformations in the light of emotions, feelings and experiences.

CHARACTERISTICS OF TRANSFORMATIVE EDUCATION

The transformative education has the following key characteristics:

1. Learning by means of discovery
2. Reciprocal learning
3. Collaborative learning
4. Learner-centred approach
5. Focus on self-regulation and a real issues orientation
6. Student self-evaluation, self-government
7. Cognitive (inquiring), as well as emotional, knowledge-oriented targets
8. Discussion, development of the diversity of viewpoints
9. Practice oriented learning that combines theory with practice
10. Emphasis on self-regulatory learning and realization of the real gains
11. Cognitive, affective and skill-related objective
12. Learning with and from outside

PRINCIPLES OF TRANSFORMATIVE EDUCATION

There are 12 principles of transformative education, which are intended to transform older, obsolete models of human learning to create a sustainable, diverse, conscientious global citizen with the ability to problem-solve complex issues for a better, more equitable and viable world. The first five principles listed are core principles of transformative education, and the rest subsequent seven principles are more specific elements that are essential to the concepts of transformative education as it is practised pedagogically.

1. **Principle of Human Rights:** Transformative education shall promote and support the Universal Declaration of Human Rights to reinforce the full development of the human personality and the strengthening of respect for human rights and fundamental freedoms. Transformative education acknowledges the right of all people, from all nations, all races, all ages and economic standing – in particular for girls and women in all nations, to access a transformative education equal to that of men.
2. **Principle of Sustainability:** Transformative education shall promote and support the practice of sustainable development, meshing economic growth, respect and protection for the environment

with social equity and well-being. Humans are entitled to a healthy and productive life in harmony with nature.

3. **Principle of the Importance of Value Systems (i.e. Morality, Ethics and Spirit):** Transformative education shall embrace thc values, ethics, morality and spirit that have stood the test of time worldwide because these values recognize and honour the interconnectedness of all life. Transformative education shall lead to a more conscientious global citizen with an emphasis on empathy and compassion and with the understanding that science, technology, engineering and mathematics, without the underlying values of planet and human sustainability, are devoid of meaning.
4. **Principle of Diversity:** Transformative education shall promote values of diversity, welcome cultural differences, and recognize heterogeneity as a gift of strength and adaptability and the critical concept in developing any viable solutions for sustainability in a diverse and complex world.
5. **Principle of Economic and Social Justice/Equity:** Transformative education shall inform, promote and support the special situations and needs of developing countries, particularly the least developed and those most environmentally vulnerable, as a special priority. Transformative education should also address the interests and needs of all countries, including developed countries where poverty and racial and economic inequities still exist, and thereby contribute to the prevention and reduction of economic global inequality.
6. **Principle of Peace Education and Conflict Resolution:** Transformative education shall promote and teach the tools of peaceful conflict resolution, including alternative dispute resolution, which is defined as any process or collection of processes established to resolve disputes without trial or violence.
7. **Principle of Holistic Education:** Transformative education shall be holistic and aim at education of the whole person – mind, body and animating spirit, including their emotional, social and physical development as well as values, multiple divergent and creative/artistic intelligences important to problem-solving in a complex world.
8. **Principle of Community-Based Learning and Indigenous Wisdom:** Transformative education shall be community-based and take local needs into account as well as value indigenous wisdom and their contexts while promoting service learning, including an ability to identify community needs and the skills to address them.
9. **Principle of Simulation/Experiential Learning:** Transformative education shall encourage and promote the use of simulation and experiential learning programmes such as Model United Nations, Model Governments and Model Corporations to build dynamism, active complex problem-solving, emotional, social and cultural intelligences and other core elements of human capacity.
10. **Principle of Incorporating New Brain Neuroscience and Skills of Critical Thinking:** Transformative education shall support the inclusion, application and integration of recent educational neuroscience findings, including integrative neurophysiology and pedagogical learning theory on how the integrated brain actually learns best. Transformative education shall promote and incorporate transformative, pedagogical practices that develop the whole brain, critical thinking/feeling abilities and capacities.
11. **Principle of Use of Technology for Greater Connection:** Transformative education shall utilize technology in a manner that does not impede but enhances the education of children and enables transformative education, which cannot be delivered in any other manner.
12. **Principle of Sanctity of Human Learning and Life:** The learning environment shall be sacred, trust in the wisdom of imagination, teach the wonder and potential of every human child, the interrelationship of life and that we can no longer afford to live with privileged disregard of this planet, all its diverse and valuable species and each other.

OUTCOMES OF TRANSFORMATIVE EDUCATION

Transformative education offers students a range of outcomes from their education:

1. Cognitive development
2. Emotional and social development
3. New knowledge and skills
4. Develop attitudes and values that reflect human rights
5. Ability to participate fully in classroom and school
6. Connection between school, home and community
7. Ability to think critically, to question and to act.
8. Helping students develop the core attributes of active citizenship that empower them to take action to improve the world they see around them through democratic processes.
9. Encourages wider social change by imbuing students with an inherent knowledge of their right to participate and have a voice in society.

RELATIONSHIP-BASED EDUCATION

Students today have all the information at their fingertips through a flurry of devices, applications and social media platforms. The teacher no longer disseminates information; instead, he or she tells students how to use information. Relationship-based education recognizes that all learning is rooted in relationships, and that environment affects learning.

Relationship-based education is a student-centred approach to classroom management that depends on teacher-student collaboration to maintain a safe, positive learning environment. Relationship-based education, as its name suggests, relies on strong, mutually respectful, personal relationships to engage cooperation in the classroom. Teachers help students meet academic and behavioural expectations by emphasizing teacher-taught empathy, unconditional positive regard, genuineness, encouragement and trust. In such an environment, students behave not because they are afraid of punishment or because they seek a reward, but because they know they are valued members of the classroom community.

In this model, teachers are often more concerned with a student's respect, honesty, care, appreciation, ambition and joy in learning than they are with any specific academic lesson.

AIMS OF RELATIONSHIP-BASED EDUCATION

1. This approach of education provides opportunity to know students' strengths, challenges, passions, etc.
2. Identify students' abilities and needs such as empathy, movement, and time.
3. This approach enables teachers to work with students closely for holistic development of students.

ELEMENTS OF BUILDING RELATIONSHIP

Elements of building relationship are true equity, consistent communication, expanded possibilities, mutual respect, trust, hope, forgiveness, integrity, compassion, expressed care, etc. (Fig. 1.3).

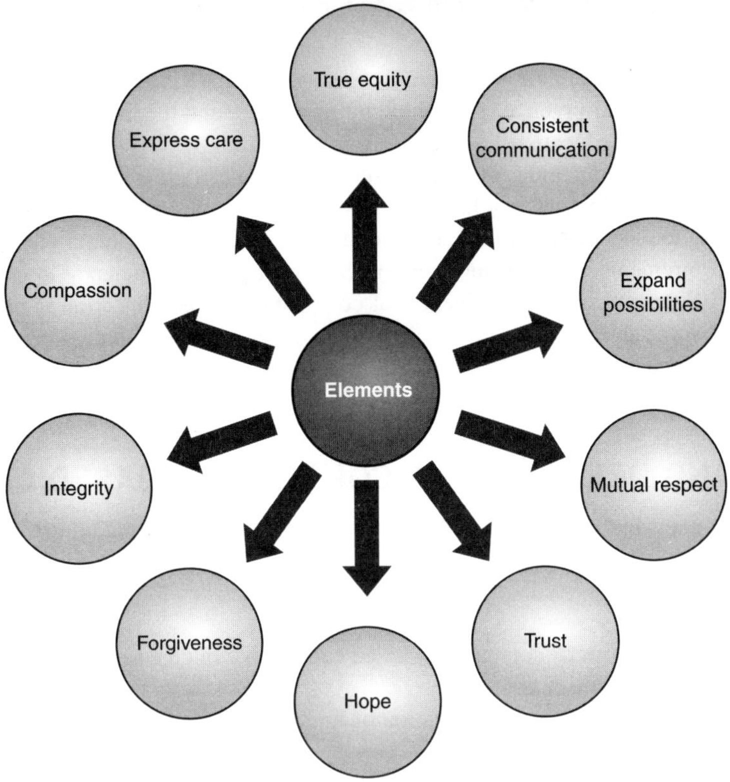

Figure 1.3

Elements of building relationship.

IMPORTANCE OF RELATIONSHIP-BASED EDUCATION

1. It provides a foundation for student engagement, belonging and, ultimately, learning and academic performance.
2. It helps to relive stress, calm anxiety and let students know how much they matter.
3. Classrooms can be safe havens for students who struggle and can enable them to trust others, believe in themselves and flourish.
4. It helps to increased self-control and enhance emotional well-being.
5. It prevents school dropout.
6. It increases pursuit of social goals and development of social skills.
7. It enhances internalization of adult values and goals.

CHALLENGES OF RELATIONSHIP-BASED EDUCATION

The relationship-based educational approach has several challenges. Some of the challenges are listed below:

1. It is complex and confusing to maintain continued relationship.
2. Thinking relationally and focusing on what students need is difficult.

COMPETENCY-BASED EDUCATION

There is a significant gap in theory and practice in nursing, and there is an emerging echo that currently trained nurses are not clinical-practice ready though they have sound theoretical knowledge. Therefore, need of competency-based education has been felt globally. Competency-based education is different from traditional models of education, as it tends to be divorced from the traditional credit hour model, also known as 'seat time'. Competency-based education programmes are also typically self-paced and utilize prior learning to meet competencies. Instead of students completing required assignments, meeting credit hour requirements and then moving on, they must prove proficiency in competency before advancing in the programme. A key distinction of competency-based education is that the learning is flexible and time is variable. Moradi et al. (2019) has given six core clinical competencies for the graduate nursing students (Fig. 1.4).

MEANING AND DEFINITION OF COMPETENCY-BASED EDUCATION

In basic terms, competency-based education means that, instead of focusing on grades and yearly curriculum schedules, the main focus is placed on how competent each student nurse is in the subject or specialty area. This means that students can only move forward when they can demonstrate mastery in initial found subjects.

There are several definitions of competency-based education, which can also be explained in various educational programmes and disciplines.

- Competency-based education is a combination of knowledge, attitude and skills necessary to meet a certain standards of practice.

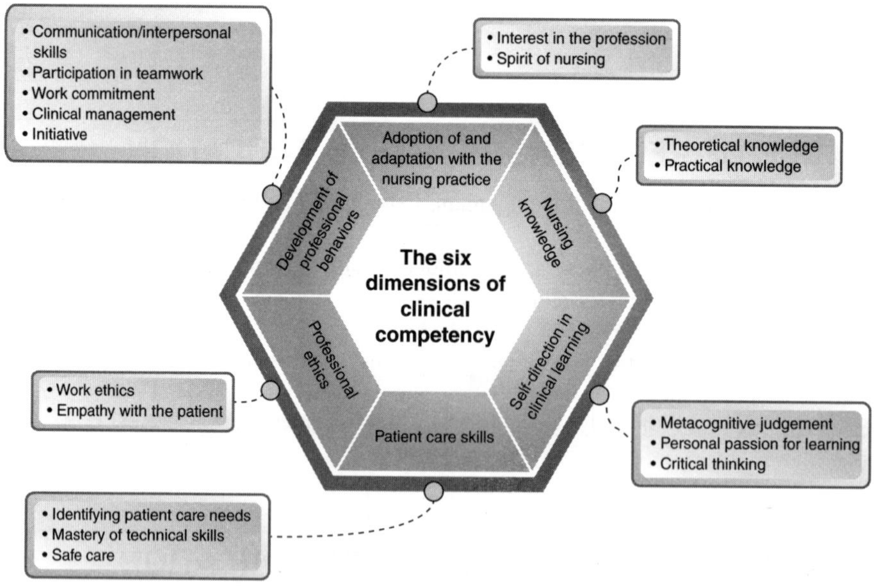

Figure 1.4

Core clinical competencies for a graduate nursing student.

Source: From Moradi, Y., Ahmadi, F., Sadeghi, A., & Oshvandi, K. (2019). Conceptualizing and determining core clinical competencies in nursing students: A qualitative study. International Nursing Review, 66(4), 530–540.

- Competency-based education is defined as an 'outcome-based approach to education that incorporates modes of instructional delivery and assessment efforts designed to evaluate mastery of learning by students through their demonstration of the knowledge, attitudes, values, skills, and behaviors required for the degree sought'.
- 'The competency-based education is an approach allows students to advance based on their ability to master a skill or competency at their own pace regardless of environment'.

A competency-based education working definition that includes five elements:

1. *Students advance upon demonstrated mastery:* Students can work harder in areas they are not proficient in and move towards mastery. Some domains may allow them to go above grade level while others require more effort. The teacher can help students focus their attention on the areas they need most assistance while also making sure that they are learning the necessary skills to move up the ladder.
2. *Competencies can be defined as specific, measurable and transferable learning goals that empower learners:* Students will feel more in control of their education if they have clearer learning objectives. They also have more choice over how and when they learn. This allows teachers to collaborate with students more effectively as they become more intentional about what they want students know and can do.
3. *Assessment is valuable and provides a decisive learning experience for learners:* Formative assessments are stressed so that teachers can better understand students' misconceptions and students get the feedback they need.
4. *Students get personalized and timely support based on their learning needs:* Students have the option to take advantage of flexible time during the day for additional instruction and clarifications. Instead of retaking a course they do not want to complete, students focus on developing the skills they need.
5. *Students acquire and use a variety of skills and dispositions:* Students learn and actively apply critical-thinking, problem-solving and communication skills to be able to work in ever-changing and diverse workplaces.

ELEMENTS OF COMPETENCY-BASED EDUCATION

There are three main elements at the core of competency-based education (Fig. 1.5):

1. **Mastery**: Students advance to the next level, course or grade based on demonstration of skills and content knowledge.

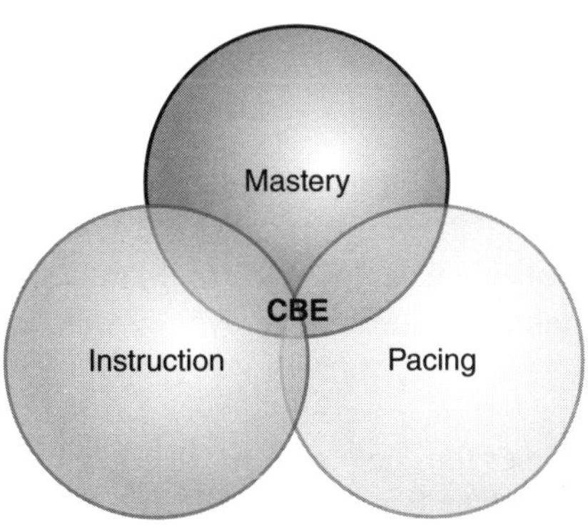

Figure 1.5

Elements of competency-based education.

2. **Pacing:** Students progress at different rates in different areas, rather than on a teacher-driven, class-wide schedule.
3. **Instruction:** Students receive customized supports to match their individual learning needs to keep them learning increasingly challenging material in a developmentally appropriate and motivating manner.

PRINCIPLES OF COMPETENCY-BASED EDUCATION

There are six main principles of competency-based education, which are detailed below:

1. **Principle of equity:**
    - Equity does not mean giving each student the same learning experiences. Instead, it means giving each student what they need to reach the same end goal.
    - This is the main principle of competency-based education because students are taught and supported based on their personal strengths and weaknesses, giving each individual the same chances for success.
    - Thus, the predictability of achievement based on culture, social class, household income or language is completely removed. Further, competency-based education also helps create an inclusive culture where all students feel safe and respected.
2. **Principle of predetermined measurable competencies:**
    - Competencies must be defined in advance and set as learning objectives for each student.
    - Rather than just testing for knowledge, competencies focus on the practical understanding that a student has of the subject. These competencies can be based on:
        - Understanding of key concepts
        - Ability to apply knowledge to meaningful problems
        - Mastery of relevant skills
    - In order for the results to be measured, competencies must be defined in advance by educational institute administration with help and input from teaching staff to develop ideas on what knowledge and skills are necessary to determine mastery.
3. **Principle of transparency and ownership:**
    - What is the end goal for each student in a particular group? The answer to this question should not only be available to teachers.
    - The learning objectives that are set for the group (and the educational institute as a whole) should be clear to both students and parents. In a competency-based education system, students understand these three things when starting the educational programme:
        - What they need to learn
        - How mastery is defined
        - How they will be assessed
    - When each student has the end goal clear in mind, they will take more responsibility for their own education.
    - If the student clearly understands what he needs to do in order to be proficient and move forward in the class, he will take more ownership over his education. Then, when he hits a snag in the project or lacks the knowledge to finish it properly, he will realize on his own that he needs help.
    - Transparent goals and outcomes thus help students take responsibility for their learning path. This ownership, in turn, helps them become better learners now and into adulthood.

4. **Principle of individuality:**
   - This is where teacher availability comes into the picture. In a competency-based education environment, students should have a framework to understand how long they should work on a problem before asking for help, and when in the class time they can approach the teacher.
   - Competency-based education works through bias and produces equity, as discussed above. So, as teachers work with students through their different weaknesses and help them draw on their strengths, each student is moved forward towards mastery on a unique (but equally effective) path. This personalized learning experience gives each student an equal opportunity for success.
   - For this process to work smoothly, though, teachers must be available to help students. Also, they cannot just rely on students asking for help: teachers need to be fully aware of each student's progress.
5. **Principle of continued feedback and assessment:**
   - Assessments come in many shapes and sizes. Here are three types of assessments that are especially useful for competency-based education:
     - *Formative assessments*: These assessments help teachers to determine where each student is in the learning process and adjust their teaching as necessary. Formative assessments give teachers the ability to adjust in real time by clearly identifying the key areas where students need to improve.
     - *Authentic assessments*: Getting students to take their knowledge and apply it to real world situations is another great way to demonstrate mastery. Plus, students get to develop skills that they will need in the future. Authentic assessments might include using English knowledge to write a cover letter for a job application, or using an understanding of physics to design and build a stable tower out of toothpicks and marshmallows.
     - *Digital content assessment*: When using tech in the classroom, assessment becomes a lot easier. Much classroom software includes assessment and progress reporting, which helps teachers see exactly where each student is in the learning process.
   - Teachers can create spiral assessments by selecting certain topics to be covered, which are updated in-game for students. Then, they can check the Topic Coverage Report to see how much of each domain students have already covered and where they are struggling.
6. **Principle of continued growth and mastery:**
   - By including regular assessments and data-based progress reporting, teachers understand where each individual student is in the learning process.
   - When students demonstrate a clear understanding of the topic, prove their ability to apply that understanding, and show how they have developed important skills; it is time for them to move forward.

REVIEW QUESTIONS

LONG-ANSWER QUESTIONS

1. Define and discuss the aims of education and educational technology.
2. Explain the different approaches to educational technology.
3. Discuss the nature and scope of educational technology.
4. Elaborate the latest approach of education.

SHORT-ANSWER QUESTIONS

1. Write a short note on transformative education.
2. Write a short note on relations-based education.
3. Discuss competency-based education in brief.
4. Explain the role of software technologies in educational practices.

MULTIPLE-CHOICE QUESTIONS (MCQs)

1. What is the primary aim of nursing education?
   (a) To provide job opportunities for nurses
   (b) To develop clinical skills in nursing students
   (c) To foster professional growth and competence
   (d) To enhance social interactions among nurses
2. Which of the following best describes the aim of nursing education?
   (a) To prepare students for licensure and professional practice
   (b) To equip students with theoretical knowledge only
   (c) To provide hands-on training in healthcare facilities
   (d) To focus solely on technical skills development
3. What is the overarching aim of nursing education programs?
   (a) To produce nurses with high leadership qualities
   (b) To train nurses in basic patient care skills
   (c) To ensure patient safety and quality care delivery
   (d) To enhance nurses' administrative and managerial skills
4. The primary aim of nursing education is to:
   (a) Prepare students for medical school
   (b) Promote evidence-based practice in nursing care
   (c) Develop specialized nursing roles within the profession
   (d) Focus on administrative tasks and healthcare management
5. The aim of nursing education is to:
   (a) Promote a standardized approach to patient care
   (b) Encourage nurses to focus solely on technical skills
   (c) Establish nurses as the primary decision-makers in healthcare settings
   (d) Develop critical thinking and clinical reasoning abilities
6. What is the primary aim of integrating educational technology in nursing?
   (a) To replace traditional teaching methods entirely
   (b) To reduce the workload of nursing faculty
   (c) To facilitate effective and efficient learning experiences
   (d) To decrease the need for clinical practice
7. How does educational technology contribute to nursing education?
   (a) By providing access to online nursing courses
   (b) By improving communication between nurses and patients
   (c) By enhancing critical thinking and problem-solving skills
   (d) By automating nursing tasks and procedures

8. Which statement best describes the relationship between education and nursing technology?
   (a) Education is essential to the effective use of nursing technology
   (b) Nursing technology can replace the need for nursing education
   (c) Education and nursing technology have no relationship
   (d) Nursing technology can hinder the educational process
9. How does educational technology promote collaborative learning in nursing?
   (a) By allowing students to interact with their peers in online forums
   (b) By providing access to virtual simulations and case studies
   (c) By automating group assignments and assessments
   (d) By reducing the need for classroom discussions and debates
10. What role does educational technology play in nursing practice?
    (a) It replaces the need for human interaction in patient care
    (b) It enables nurses to access patient records more quickly
    (c) It facilitates lifelong learning and professional development
    (d) It reduces the need for continuous training and education
11. What is the significance of educational technology in nursing research?
    (a) It eliminates the need for data analysis and interpretation
    (b) It enables nurses to conduct experiments more efficiently
    (c) It provides access to online databases and research resources
    (d) It hinders the dissemination of research findings
12. Which of the following is NOT a potential benefit of educational technology in nursing?
    (a) Increased access to educational resources
    (b) Improved patient outcomes and quality of care
    (c) Enhanced critical thinking and clinical reasoning skills
    (d) Reduction in the need for evidence-based practice
13. How does educational technology contribute to the development of nursing skills?
    (a) By replacing the need for clinical practice and hands-on experience
    (b) By providing virtual simulations and scenarios for practice
    (c) By reducing the need for critical thinking and decision-making
    (d) By limiting the scope of nursing practice to technical skills
14. What is the primary approach of educational technology in nursing?
    (a) Enhancing patient care through advanced technology
    (b) Automating administrative tasks for nurses
    (c) Supporting effective teaching and learning methods
    (d) Minimizing the need for clinical practice
15. How does educational technology support personalized learning in nursing?
    (a) By providing individualized study materials for each student
    (b) By automating the grading process for assessments
    (c) By reducing the need for interaction with nursing faculty
    (d) By eliminating the need for group discussions and collaboration

ANSWERS OF THE MULTIPLE-CHOICE QUESTIONS

1 (c), 2 (a), 3 (c), 4 (b), 5 (d), 6 (c), 7 (c), 8 (a), 9 (a), 10 (c), 11 (c), 12 (d), 13 (b), 14 (c), 15 (a)

FURTHER READING

AACN's definition of competency-based education [Internet]. American Association of Colleges of Nursing: The Voice of Academic Nursing. [cited June 1, 2022]. https://www.aacnnursing.org/Essentials/Definition-of-Competency-Based-Education

Agarwal, J. C. (2003). *Educational technology and management*. Agra: Vinod Pustak Mandir.

Arbeiter, J., & Bucar, M. (2020). *Transformative education: Bridging education for change*. https://www.researchgate.net/publication/354209422_Transformative_Education_Bridging_Education_for_Change?channel=doi&linkId=612ca13d0360302a0068b66b&showFulltext=true. Accessed March 16, 2022.

Archibaalt, R. (2009). *Philosophical analysis and education*. New Delhi: Oxford University Press.

Balsiger, J., Förster, R., Mader, C., Nagel, U., Sironi, H., Wilhelm, S., & Zimmermann, A. B. (2017). Transformative learning and education for sustainable development. *GAIA*, *26*(4), 357–359.

Bastable, S. B. (2021). *Nurse as educator: Principles of teaching-learning for nursing practices* (6th ed.). Sudbury: Jones & Bartlett Publisher.

Brubacher, J. S. (1971). *Modern philosophies of education*. New Delhi: Tata McGraw Hill, Pvt. Ltd.

Cronenwett, L., Sherwood, G., Barnsteiner J., Disch, J., Johnson, J., Mitchell, P., ... Warren, J. (2007). Quality and safety education for nurses. *Nursing Outlook*, *55*(3), 122–131.

Gravina, E. W. (2017). Competency-based education and its effect on nursing education: A literature review. *Teaching and Learning in Nursing*, *12*(2), 117–121.

Lee, B., Del Rosario, K., & Byron-Iyamah, C. (2017). Incorporating relationship-based care into a nurse education program for managing disruptive patient behaviors. *Clinical Nurse Specialist CNS*, *31*(4), 201–209.

Lumsdaine, A. A. (1964). Educational technology, programmed learning and instructional science. *Teachers College Record: The voice of Scholarship in Education*, *65*(9). https://doi.org/10.1177/016146816406500914

Mani, R. S. (1996). *Educational ideas and ideals of Gandhi and Tagore (a comparative study)*. New Delhi: New Book Society of India.

Moradi, Y., Ahmadi, F., Sadeghi, A., & Oshvandi, K. (2019). Conceptualizing and determining core clinical competencies in nursing students: A qualitative study. *International Nursing Review*, *66*(4), 530–540.

National Council of Educational Research and Training. (2005). *National curriculum framework*. New Delhi: NCERT.

Parankimalil, J. (2015). *Approaches to educational technology* [Internet]. [cited May 16, 2022]. https://johnparankimalil.wordpress.com/2015/01/22/approaches-to-educational-technology/

Teaching for Transformation. (2022). *Transformative education* [Internet]. [cited December 16, 2022]. https://www.teachingfortransformation.com/transformative-education/

CHAPTER

Principles and philosophies of education

2

LEARNING OBJECTIVES

This chapter is designed to enable the reader to:

- Understand the Indian and international concept of education
- Identify the aims and functions of education and nursing education
- Define philosophies of education
- Explain the interdependence of philosophy and education
- Classify the traditional and modern philosophies of education
- Describe the traditional and modern philosophies of education

KEY TERMS

INTRODUCTION

According to Albert Einstein, education is what remains after one has forgotten what one learned in school. Education may be looked upon as the process of providing desirable knowledge and experience to a child to develop his inner powers to the maximum possible extent, which helps the child lead a full and worthy life. It is a process of training the individual through various experiences of life, so as to draw out the best in him.

MEANING OF EDUCATION

The term *education* has its origin in the Latin words *educo*, *educare* and *educatum.* Etymologically, the word *education* is derived from the Latin words *educo*, where *e* means 'out of' and *duco* means 'I lead'. According to this view, *education* means 'I lead out of darkness into brightness'.

In another perspective, the word education is derived from the Latin word *educare*, which refers to breed, to bring up and to rear.

Also, *educatum* denotes education that means 'an act of teaching or training'.

Therefore, education means to lead, to lead forth or to unfold the hidden talents of man. It is very much the art of developing and cultivating the various powers of mind, physical, mental and moral.

I. INDIAN CONCEPT OF EDUCATION

In India, disciplining the mind and imparting knowledge have always been the foremost priorities. There are various synonyms prevailing in the Indian society for the word *education*.

- One of them is *shiksha*, which is derived from the Sanskrit root *shas* referring to 'discipline', 'control', instruct' or 'teach'.
- Another synonym of the word *education* is *vidya*, which is derived from the Sanskrit root *vid*, which means 'to know'. Vidya is thus the subject matter of knowledge.
- It is mentioned in the Upanishads that the end product of education is salvation. Also, it is stated in the *Bhagwad Gita* that nothing is more purifying on the earth than knowledge.

II. DEFINITIONS OF EDUCATION BY INDIAN PHILOSOPHERS

Famous Indian philosophers or educationists have given the following concepts of education with their own meanings:

> *Education means the training for the country and love for the nation.*
>
> **—Chanakya**

> *Education is realization of self.*
>
> **—Shankaracharya**

> *Education is self-realization and service of the people.*
>
> **—Guru Nanak Dev**

> *Education is the manifestation of divine perfection already existing in man; education means the exposition of man's complete individuality.*
>
> **—Swami Vivekananda**

> *Education means enabling the mind to find out that ultimate truth which emancipates us from the bondage of dust and gives us the wealth not of things but of inner light, not of power but of love, making the truth its own and giving expression to it.*
>
> **—Rabindranath Tagore**

> *Education is an all-round drawing out of the best in child and man—body, mind and spirit.*
>
> **—Mahatma Gandhi**

III. DEFINITIONS OF EDUCATION BY INTERNATIONAL PHILOSOPHERS

Education has been viewed in various ways by philosophers or educationists internationally as given below:

> *Education is the capacity to feel pleasure and pain at right moment. It develops in the body and in the soul of the pupil all beauty and all perfection which he is capable of.*
>
> **—Plato**

Education is the process of living through a continuous reconstruction of experiences. It is the development of all those capacities in the individual which will enable him to control his environment and fulfil his possibilities.

—John Dewey

Education is the natural, harmonious and progressive development of man's innate power.

—Pestalozzi

Education is the deliberate and systematic influence, exerted by the mature person upon the immature through instruction, discipline and harmonious development of physical, intellectual, aesthetic, social and spiritual powers of the human being according to their essential hierarchy, by and for the individual and social uses and directed towards the union of educand with his creator as the final end.

—Redden and Ryan

AIMS OF EDUCATION

Education is a purposeful and planned activity undertaken by the educator and the learner for achieving clearly defined objectives or ends in view. Without an end or objective, no purposeful activity will have the real force which directs it and makes it meaningful. An aim is a predetermined goal which determines the individual to attain it through appropriate activities. Some suggested aims of education are discussed below:

- **Individual aim:** Education should aim at the training and development of an individual. Only a well-trained individual can understand his rights and obligations towards the society. Biologists recognize every individual as different from another. Naturalists make nature supreme which would make an individual what he ought to be. Psychologists favour flexible curriculum development based on individual mental capacity and emotional disposition. Though qualities of individual aim, criticism says that it makes education selfish and self-centred and ignores society and culture. Some important individual aims of education are as follows:
  - Development as an individual of a human being
  - Moral and spiritual development
  - Cultural development
  - Harmonious development
  - Promote positive physical development
  - Provide a sense of complete living
  - Development of a right personality
  - Development of good citizenship
  - Development of good leadership
  - Vocational development of an individual
  - Emotional and mental development
  - Create national consciousness
  - Promote good social development
  - Character building
  - **Social aim:** An individual is born with certain potential and natural endowments. It is the task of education to develop this into distinct individual personality. Personality development does not take place in a vacuum. It takes place in association with others, in cooperative living and in working together for the welfare of group or society. As per historical evidences, in ancient Sparta, it

was believed that each individual was born not for himself but for his country. A socially efficient individual conforms to certain standards of conduct known as *moral conduct*. John Dewey once said that in the democratic and technological environment, the aim of education should be to enable the individual to control his environment and fulfil his responsibilities. He further added that all education proceeds by the participation of an individual in the social consciousness of race. This process begins almost at birth and is continually shaping individual powers.

The critics consider the social aim makes an individual only a tool of the government. The extreme notion of an all-powerful state or society ignores the legitimate needs, desires and interests of the individual and suppresses his creative power.

- **Vocational aim:** Education should have a utilitarian aim. This means that education should help an individual earn his livelihood himself, which is an essential function of life that cannot be ignored. This aim makes an individual economically self-sufficient, gives purpose to the educational activity and bridges the gap between pure literary education and vocation.

  The major limitation of the vocational aim is that it is not a complete aim on its own as life and education are much more than bread and butter only.
- **Cultural aim:** Culture is a complete whole and includes knowledge, belief, art, morals, law, custom and other capabilities and habits acquired by man as a member of society. True education is not satisfied if members of a society take up and preserve only the existing manners and customs. On the other hand, it is satisfied when men and women try to form better and still better habits of thought and action and thereby help in the establishment of a future society which is an improvement over the existing one.

  The major drawback of the cultural aim is that it may create controversies as there is high diversity in culture and the so-called cultured persons usually belong to the high strata of society.
- **Moral aim:** A strong character includes physical fitness, resolution and will power. Moral virtues like honesty, loyalty, tolerance, justice, self-control and sincerity promote the social efficiency of an individual.
- **Spiritual aim:** Ancient Indian educators defined education as a means for salvation. Dr Radhakrishnan said that the aim of education is neither national efficiency nor world solidarity but making individual feel that he has within himself something deeper than intellect, call it spirit, if you like. But spiritual aim does not find any place in the western education system.

  The criticism follows the spiritual aim by mentioning that it might lead us to an attitude of escapism, renunciation of the world and complete inaction. Only the realization and preaching of this philosophy is not enough, but practising it in daily life is also mandatory.
- **Intellectual aim:** Education in ancient times did not have much vocational aim but emphasized mostly on the development of intellectual powers and imbibing culture. Knowledge aim is the exact antithesis of vocational aim. The former glorifies material possessions while the latter emphasizes intellectual possessions.
- **Aims of education as stated by Secondary Education Commission, 1952–1953:** The Secondary Education Commission formulated the following aims of education:
  - ***Development of democratic citizenship:*** It includes developing clear thinking, clear speech and writing, receptivity to new ideas, social justice, tolerance, patriotism and internationalism.
  - ***Improvement of vocational efficiency:*** It refers to the appreciation of dignity of work and promotion of technical skills.
  - Development of personality by inculcating creative energy, interest and the development of hobbies.
  - Development of qualities of leadership.

- **Aims of education as stated by Kothari Commission Report, 1966:** This report gave a fourfold aim of our national education system which are as follows:
  - Increasing productivity
  - Achieving social and national integration
  - Accelerating the process of modernization
  - Cultivating social, moral and spiritual values
- **Aims of education as stated by Education Commission, 1964–1966:** It mentioned a fivefold programme on educational aims which are stated below:
  - Relating education to productivity
  - Strengthening social and national integration
  - Consolidation of democracy through education
  - Development of social, moral and spiritual values
  - Modernization of society through the awakening of society through curiosity, development of attitudes and values and building up certain essential skills.

I. AIMS OF NURSING EDUCATION

Nursing education has its aims in common with the aims of education in general as well as specific. The nursing education aims are determined by the health needs of the society, needs of students, philosophy of nursing, current trends in education and nursing and advancement in science and technology. The many nursing aims are listed below:

- ***Intellectual aim:*** Theoretical and practical knowledge is essential for rendering intelligent and efficient nursing services. Professional nursing practice is based on scientific principles and evidence-based practice.
- ***Leadership aim:*** Nurses plan, organize and manage health care activities and programmes. They have to evaluate the quality and structure of health care services. They have to coordinate and collaborate on the health care services. Thus, education aims at identifying potential nursing leaders.
- ***Professional development aim:*** Each individual nurse should be educated in a manner to enable her to develop the appropriate skills and attitude essential for professional practice.
- ***Personality development aim:*** Nursing education should aim at an all-round development of the individual in all aspects. The nurse should grow and develop as a person of self-awareness, self-direction and self-motivation.
- ***Generating and utilizing research evidences:*** Evidence-based practice and ongoing research is vital for the growth of the nursing profession. Therefore, nursing education must pay emphasis on the utilization and development of resource evidence.
- ***Ensuring a safe, quality and cost-effective case:*** It is the prime responsibility of the nursing education that it equip its professionals to provide safe, quality and cost-effective care to the common man.

II. FACTORS AFFECTING AIMS OF EDUCATION

Educational aims are affected by certain factors such as philosophy of life, elements of human nature, religious reasons, political ideology, socioeconomic reasons, cultural reasons and the intention of exploring new knowledge, which are described as follows (Fig. 2.1):

- ***Philosophy of life:*** Both educational aims and philosophy of life are very closely related just like two facets of the same coin. Education is the best means of propagation of the philosophy of life and philosophy gives the basis for aims of education.

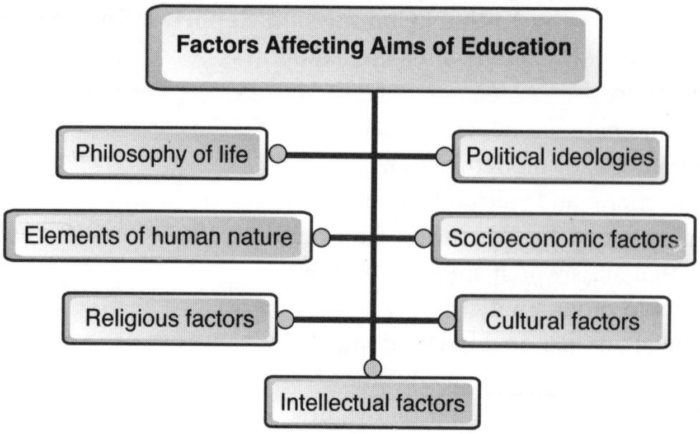

Figure 2.1

Factors affecting aims of education.

- ***Elements of human nature:*** Human nature is always considered for determining educational aims. Idealism infolding divinity in man is considered as the main aim of education.
- ***Religious factors:*** Religion is an inseparable determinant of educational aims. In India, Buddhism focuses on adoption of *ahimsa* and truth in the education system and Sikhism focuses on patriotism as the aim of education.
- ***Political ideologies:*** Political ideologies certainly have a say in determining educational aims. The educational aims of a democratic political system can be quite different from that of an autocratic political set-up.
- ***Socioeconomic factors:*** These factors play an important role affecting the aims of education. The social system, social ideology and economy of a country are important factors to affect the aims of education.
- ***Cultural factors:*** Education plays an important role in transmitting cultural heritage and traditions from one generation to another. Culture also develops educational aims by itself.
- ***Intellectual factors:*** As education is fully scientific today, it has to aim at exploring new information and knowledge.

FUNCTIONS OF EDUCATION

Education is the process of living through a continuous reconstruction of experiences. It is the development of all those capacities in an individual which will enable him to control his environment and fulfil his possibilities. A child is born with certain endowments which are developed in accordance with the demands of the society through education. Education enables the child to manipulate his environment. Thus, education provides important functions towards the individual as well as the society. Functions of education can solely be for an individual or towards the society and nation at large. Some essential functions of education are discussed below (Fig. 2.2):

I. FUNCTION OF EDUCATION TOWARDS AN INDIVIDUAL

Education participates in the growth and direction of an individual as described below:

- ***Growth and development of individual:*** Johann Heinrich Pestalozzi said when we leave the earth carelessly to nature, it bears weeds and thistles. The same way when we leave child's education to

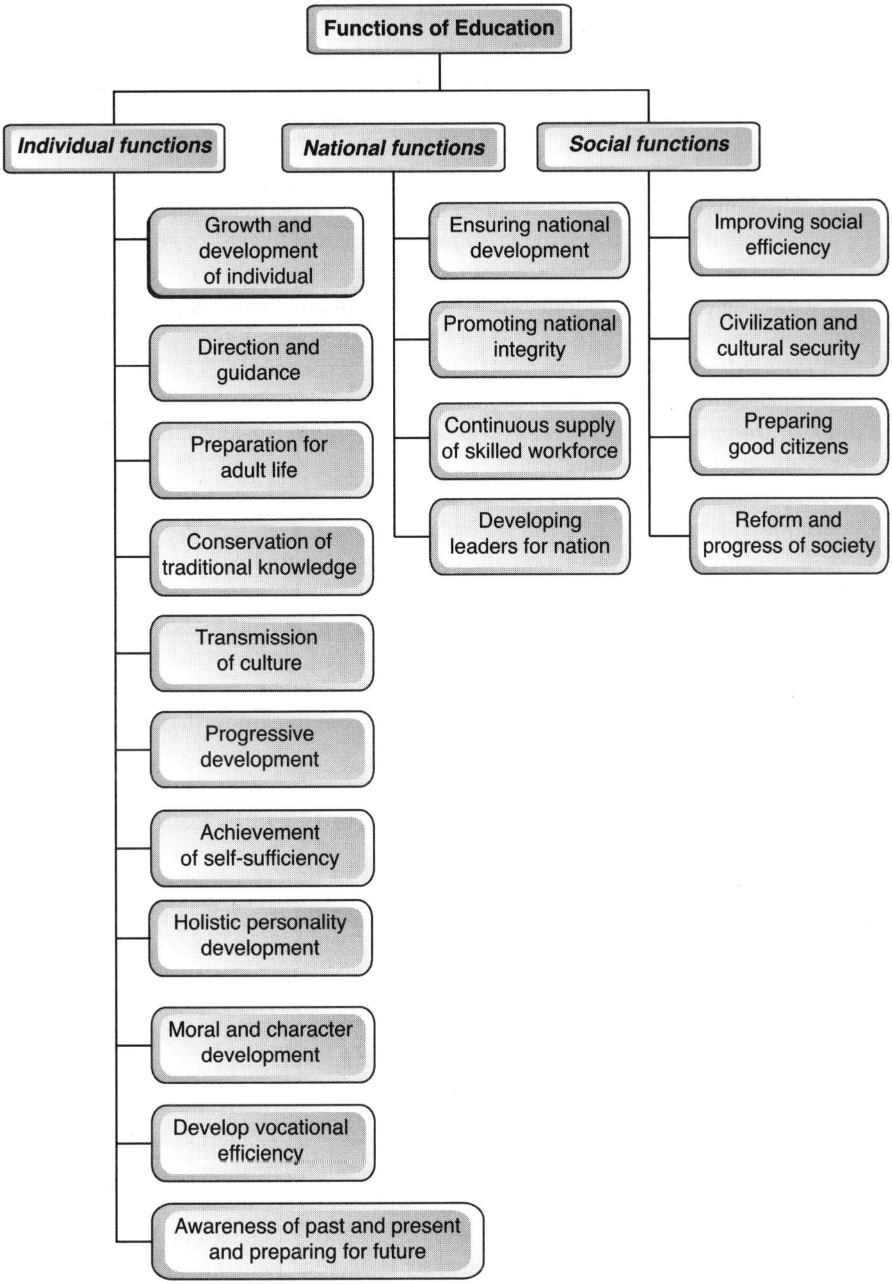

Figure 2.2

Functions of education.

nature alone, he develops only confused impressions in his mind. Thus, only environmental and natural growth is not sufficient for the complete growth and development of an individual. To this must be added a systematic course of formal training. Moreover, only one-sided growth will not serve the purpose. The whole personality of the child should develop physically, intellectually, morally, socially and spiritually.

- ***Direction and guidance:*** Direction refers to minimizing unnecessary and confusing movements. When an immature child responds to stimulus, much of the superfluous energy is wasted. This wastage can be saved if the child's activity is properly directed towards a goal. One can be directed by his internal tendencies or by external stimulus. The teacher, therefore, in the direction programme should take into account the external factors of an environment as well as the child's inborn tendency.
- ***Preparation for adult life:*** Preparation of a child for the responsibilities or privileges of adult life have been considered to be the chief function of education from ancient times.
- ***Conservation of traditional knowledge:*** Preserving old traditions, values, ideals, customs and way of thinking is also a function of education.
- ***Transmission of culture:*** Transmitting the cultural heritage to the younger generation is achieved through education.
- ***Progressive development:*** Reconstructing new experiences, unfolding new dimensions of knowledge and furthering civilization and culture.
- ***Develop vocational efficiency:*** Education enables the person to acquire the knowledge and skills to efficiently perform the tasks related to a particular vocation or professional field.
- ***Achievement of self-sufficiency:*** Self-sufficiency can be gained by the individual through education because after obtaining the required education person is able to earn for her own livelihood as well as become cognitively and economically independent.
- ***Holistic personality development:*** Education must be aimed at developing an individual's holistic personality.
- ***Moral and character development:*** An ideal education must be helpful for an individual to develop good moral values and character.
- ***Creating awareness of past and present and preparing for future:*** Education must make an individual become knowledgeable about the past and present scenarios of social and professional pursuit as well as prepare him to manage future expectations and needs.

II. FUNCTION OF EDUCATION TOWARDS THE NATION

National progress depends on an individual's hard work, energy, selflessness and devotion. Education plays important role to inculcate these qualities in individuals. The Kothari Commission Report rightly said that the destiny of India was being reshaped in its classroom. The important functions of education for a nation are given below:

- ***Ensuring national development:*** National development largely depends on the education of a country. It is directly proportional to the literacy rate as well as availability of human resources.
- ***Promoting national integrity:*** India is a country of diversity having a strong sense of casteism, communalism, provincialism, regionism and linguistic antagonism that could serve as barriers to national integration. Education can be helpful in breaking these barriers and can promote national integration.
- ***Continuous supply of skilled workforce to the nation:*** Every country requires a skilled workforce for the smooth functioning of its service sector. It is the main national function of education to ensure the continuous supply of skilled workforce to the country.

- ***Developing leaders for the nation:*** Leaders are the main role players in the overall development of a country. Leaders are essentially required in social, economic, political and cultural sectors and education can realize this requirement by preparing leaders to meet a country's present and future needs.

III. FUNCTION OF EDUCATION TOWARDS THE SOCIETY

As biological life maintains and transmits by nutrition and reproduction, the same way social life is maintained by education. Education is necessary and an inevitable result of the society's needs to guide the growth and development of its younger members to produce an improved generation. History bears evidence that as education advances, civilization also advances. Some selected social functions of education are as follows:

- ***Improving social efficiency:*** Education ensures the overall holistic development of individuals, who could be good individuals in a society. It ultimately promotes social efficiency and the society flourishes in the right direction.
- ***Civilization and cultural security:*** Education teaches individual gain civic sense so that a positive civilization can be expected for its members. In addition, education must ensure cultural security so that important traditional culture can be preserved and utilized by the future generations.
- ***Preparing good citizens:*** The main function of education is to prepare good citizens in a country so that a civilized society can be expected and each individual has the privilege of enjoying full social freedom, human honour and rights.
- ***Reform and progress of society:*** The progress of a society primarily depends on education. Mahatma Gandhi once said that education acts as fertilizer for social growth and progress. Growth is the law of nature and human existence requires reforms to meet new demands and needs. Therefore, social reform and progress of a society is also one of the important functions of education.

PHILOSOPHIES OF EDUCATION

The term *philosophy* has a Greek origin, that is *philosophia*, which is made up of two words, viz. *phileo* and *sophia. Phileo* means 'love' and *sophia* means 'wisdom'. The literal meaning of *philosophy* is 'love of wisdom' or 'passion of learning'.

I. DEFINITIONS OF PHILOSOPHY

It is said that education without philosophy is blind and philosophy without education is invalid (Thomas, 1968). Philosophy is the earliest and the most original intellectual discipline. It is one of the oldest and most respected disciplines of knowledge. It is rather difficult to define philosophy in a way that is universally acceptable. Some of the most accepted and prevailing definitions of philosophy are given below.

> *Philosophy is the science of knowledge.*
>
> **—Fitch**

> *Philosophy is the science of sciences.*
>
> **—Coleridge**

> *Philosophy is a search for comprehensive view of nature, an attempt at a universal explanation of the nature of things.*
>
> **—Alfred Weber**

Philosophy is critical reviewing of just those familiar things.

—John Dewey

Philosophy is the critical science of universal values.

—Windlband

Philosophy is concerned with everything as a universal science.

—Herbert Spencer

Philosophy is a persistent effort of both ordinary and pertinent people to make life as intelligible and meaningful as possible.

—Bramold

Philosophy, like science, consistent of theories of insight arrived at as a result of systemic reflection.

—Joseph A. Leighton

II. PHILOSOPHY, EDUCATION AND THEIR INTERDEPENDENCE

Philosophy and education are interdependent in nature and that can be clearly understood from the following facts (Fig. 2.3):

- The philosophy of great philosophers reflects from their educational systems and they are great educators of their times.
- Education and philosophy have a common end, that is wisdom and common means directed towards the end, that is inquiry. Separation of philosophy and education would frustrate wisdom. Philosophy can provide the direction and guidance to behave intelligently in the educational process.
- For the educator, philosophy aims at improving the quality of life because it helps us gain a wider perspective on human existence and the world around us.
- The chief task of philosophy is to state the aspects of a good life, whereas for education, the chief task is how to make life worth living. So, philosophy and education are mutually reconstructive, that is they function with a mutual give and take.
- Philosophy handles goals while education provides the means to achieve those goals. In this sense, philosophy of education is a distinct but not a separate discipline. The process of philosophizing about education requires an understanding of education and its problems.

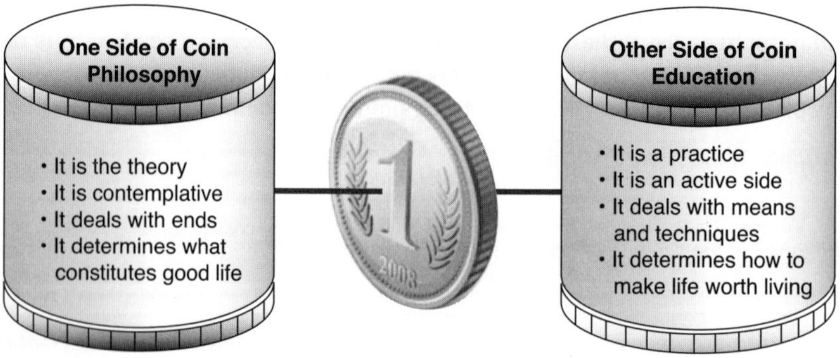

Figure 2.3

Interdependence of philosophy and education as two faces of a coin.

Ross stated that philosophy is the contemplative side while education is the active side. It can be concluded that philosophy is the theory while education is the practice. Practice unguided by theory is aimless and inconsistent just as theory which cannot be translated into practice is useless and confusing.

III. CLASSIFICATION OF EDUCATIONAL PHILOSOPHIES

There are various schools of educational philosophies. Some of the main traditional and modern contemporary educational philosophies are discussed below (Fig. 2.4):

A. Traditional Educational Philosophies

- Naturalism
- Idealism
- Pragmatism
- Realism

B. Modern Contemporary Educational Philosophies

- Perennialism
- Essentialism
- Existentialism
- Reconstructionism
- Progressivism

TRADITIONAL EDUCATIONAL PHILOSOPHIES

In this chapter, the main traditional educational philosophies are discussed. These are naturalism, idealism, pragmatism and realism (a brief review may be seen in Table 2.1).

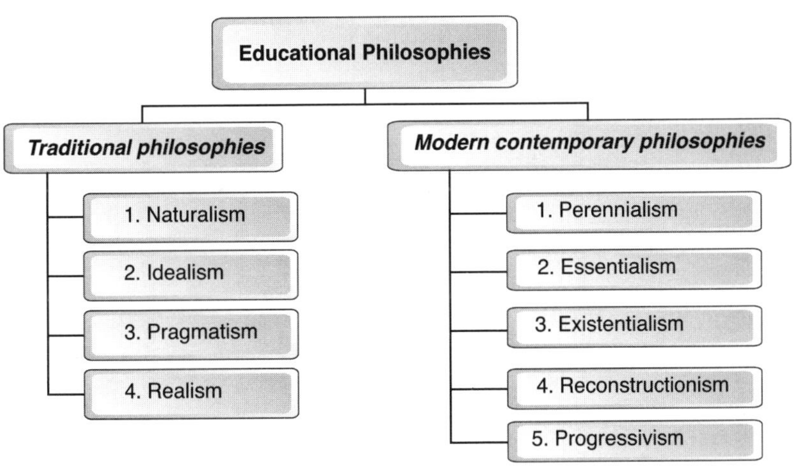

Figure 2.4

Classification of educational philosophies.

Table 2.1 Brief Description About Traditional Philosophies of Education

Concept of Philosophy	Organization and Aims of Education	Curriculum	Methods of Education	Role of Teacher	Discipline
1. Naturalism: Chief proponents were Rabindranath Tagore, Jean Jacques Rousseau, Johann Heinrich, Pestalozzi and Herbert Spencer					
Educating the human generations about and in the nature rather than artificial environment by keeping in mind the individuality of each child.	Nature is considered the classroom. Emphasis on open air schools to teach through direct experience with nature.	Basis of curriculum development was child's nature, interest and needs. Stressed on subjects dealing with nature, such as physics, chemistry, biology, language and mathematics. Tagore also stressed on teaching spiritual values of nature.	As natural as possible considering individual differences. Noble efforts for planned living with nature. Direct experience of nature through observation, excursion, experimentation, play-way and Dalton plan methods.	Teacher is an observer and facilitator of the child to develop in nature; teacher facilitates best possible natural environment for prompt learning.	No emphasis on external rigid discipline; recommended free discipline to child in nature for optimum desired learning.
2. Idealism: Chief proponents were Dr Radhakrishnan, Sir Aurobindo, Plato, Ross and Socrates					
It believes that the act of knowing takes place within the mind for three values, i.e. intellectual, aesthetic and moral values and the purpose of education is the development of the student's mind and self.	Well-planned formal classrooms or formal place of teaching–learning activity is recommended.	The basis of curriculum is inculcating intellectual, aesthetic and moral values or discipline. The intellectual value is represented by subjects such as language, literature, science, mathematics, history and geography; aesthetic through arts and poetry and moral through religion, ethics and metaphysics. Dr Radhakrishnan also advocated for physical education.	Idealism recommended formal classroom teaching methods such as lecture, discussion, presentation and group interaction. Knowledge is transferred from the more mature person (teacher) to the less mature person (pupil) through formal and well-planned teaching–learning methods.	Teacher is considered as centre of education where pupil catches fire from teacher who is himself a flame. Teacher must be ideal and a role model for the child both intellectually and morally. The teacher should exercise great creative skills in providing opportunity for the pupil's mind to discover, analyse, unify, synthesize and creative application of knowledge to life.	Idealism believes in interconnection of discipline and interest. Advocates discipline for self-realization of individual. It does not favour rigid discipline but advocates spontaneous and self-discipline.

3. Pragmatism: Chief proponents were Williams James, John Dewey, Charles Sanders Pierce, S. Kil Patrick and Margaret H.					
It considers self-activity as the basis of all teaching–learning processes in context of cooperative activity; to create optimistic men, who are the architects of their own fate by the process of their efforts. Education should be according to the child's aptitudes and abilities, where he is respected and education is planned to cater to his inclinations and capacities; however, he develops in social context.	Aim of education is to teach one how to think so that one can adjust to an ever-changing society. In order to produce creative, resourceful and adaptable children, we should have conditions in the school which are conducive to the creation of these qualities of mind. Recommends formal schools to have activity-oriented learning based on the needs, interest, aptitude and capabilities of the individual student.	Pragmatists believe in a broad and diversified curriculum, which is composed of both content and process and subjects ranging from humanities to geography and sciences.	Teaching–learning process is a social process where the sharing of experiences between the teacher and the student takes place. Preferred methods are project method and activity-oriented learning.	Role of a teacher is not that of a dictator or a task master but as a leader of group activities. Teacher acts as catalyst where he suggests a problem to students and stimulates them to find a solution. Teacher is a mentor with resources to guide the students.	Pragmatism does not believe in traditional firm discipline; however, it advocates for freedom of self-discipline in a free and conducive teaching–learning environment.
4. Realism: Chief proponents were Aristotle, Johann Friedrich Herbart, Herbert Spencer, John Locke and Franklin Bobbitt					
Realism makes the human being understand and enjoy society in the true sense by getting the multidimensional real joy of life in reality. It also aims for education to make the life of a man useful, where a man can enjoy his activities and comfort in reality. Education should equip individuals to a best possible meaningful life through vocational skills.	Realism emphasizes on scientific attitude based on realistic principles where the child can extend his knowledge, which he learns through books. It has given due emphasis on formal schools, which provides adequate opportunities for learners to learn the vocational skills through observation, experimentation and examination.	Selection of the curriculum for the students must be based on their abilities, interest and capabilities so that education helps the student to adjust to changing circumstances of the society. It also emphasizes on subject matters of real-life use such as science, mathematics, hygiene and vocational subjects. Vocational content has given prominent stress on the curriculum.	Realism believes in objectivity, knowledge of scientific evidences and reality. Methods of teaching should be according to needs, interest and capabilities of students. Vocational education should equip the individual with capacities to earn livelihood such as experimentation, examination and observation.	Teachers must focus on the development of vocational skills in the learners, so that they can be equipped with qualities of race preservation and vocational behaviour activities. Teacher acts as a mentor and must be a role model and skilled to demonstrate vocational skills to the learners.	Realism believes in an optimum level of discipline without imposing undue stress on the learners.

I. NATURALISM

The basic concepts of naturalism are as follows:

- The concept of *naturalism* as a philosophy of education occurred during the 18th century.
- Naturalism is based on the basic assumption that nature as a total system explains all existence including human beings and human nature.
- According to naturalists, the material and the physical world is governed by certain laws, and man, who is the creator of the material world, must submit to it.
- It denies the existence of anything beyond nature, behind nature and other than nature such as supernaturalism.
- In terms of epistemology or theory of knowledge, naturalists highlight the value of scientific knowledge.
- Francis Bacon emphasizes the inductive method for acquiring scientific knowledge through specific observation, accumulation and generalization. He also lays emphasis on empirical and experimental knowledge.
- Naturalists also lay stress on sensory training as senses are the gateways to learning.
- Values are developed from human beings' interaction with the environment.
- Instincts and impulses are expressed rather than repressed. According to this theory, there is no absolute good or evil in the world. All values of life are creations of human needs.
- Naturalism as a philosophy of education has exercised great influence on the theory and practice of education. It describes all external restraint and condemns all necessary formalities.
- There is no place for classrooms, textbooks, time tables, curriculum, formal lessons or examinations in the naturalistic system of education. The teacher has to play the role of acquainting children with their natural environment.
- External discipline is altogether out of place. The only discipline is the discipline of natural consequences. Naturalism believes that formal education is the invention of society and so is artificial.
- Good education can be possible only through a direct contact with nature. Naturalism in education has the following common themes:
  - Look to nature and human nature as part of the natural order for the purposes of education.
  - The key to understanding nature is through the senses. Sensation is the basis of our knowledge of reality.
  - Because nature's processes are slow, gradual and evolutionary, our education should be steady too.

A. Chief Proponents of Naturalism

There are many great names associated with naturalism but the eminent ones are as follows:

- Jean Jacques Rousseau
- Johann Heinrich Pestalozzi
- Herbert Spencer
- Rabindranath Tagore

B. Naturalism and Aims of Education

The main aims of education according to naturalism are given below:

- Development of self-realization, self-expression and self-preservation in children.
- Cultivating self-restrain and a sense of moral values.
- Making a child adjust himself both physically and psychologically to his immediate environment and to the challenging surroundings in his life.

- Equipping the child to struggle for existence and ensuring his survival by making him the fittest.
- Promoting better humanity through the transmission of not only physical characteristics but also moral values.
- Promoting the perfect development of individuality in a child through the development of natural endowments, into a joyous, rational, balanced, useful and natural person.
- Customizing the teaching–learning process according to the child's nature, tenderness, capacities, likes and dislikes.

C. Naturalism and Organization of Education

- According to naturalists, the existence of school is a natural necessity. All of us know that man is the most dependent creature of God as compared to other animals because of the long period of infancy and a child's consequent dependence on adults. The offsprings of other animals have negligible periods of infancy, whereas the human offspring requires at least a few years to perform simple functions of day-to-day living. Because of this important dimension of the dependent nature of man, education becomes an urgent necessity and so do educational institutions like schools.
- Naturalism attaches less importance to the existence of a formal school and textbooks because it hinders the natural development of children. For Rousseau 'everything is good as it comes from the hands of author of nature, but everything degenerates in the hands of man'. According to him, nature is the only pure, clean and ennobling influence. Human society is thoroughly corrupt. Therefore, a man should be freed from the bondage of society, and he should be prepared to live in the state of nature. Human nature is essentially good, and it must be given full opportunities for free development in a free atmosphere.
- Gandhi's philosophy of education is also naturalistic in setting as he believes in the essential goodness of a child's nature. According to him, children should be educated in an atmosphere of freedom, freedom from superimposed restriction and interferences. His main emphasis is on activity or learning by doing and he shows an aversion to artificiality and pedantry. Being a naturalist, he attempts to liberate education from the four walls of the classroom and wishes it be given in a wider sphere of the natural surroundings of a child.

D. Naturalism and Methods of Education

- The school to the naturalist is in no way different from the home; Frobel called the school as *kindergarten* or *garden for children*, whereas Montessori calls it *Case-de-Bambini* or *home for* the children.
- According to Pestalozzi, there should be no difference between school and home. Tagore also believes that education given in natural surroundings develops intimacy with the world. He puts more faith on the individual rather than institutions. Nature, to him, is the focus where the interests and aspirations of human beings meet. It is therefore essential not only to know nature, but to live in nature. *School*, according to him, is like a large home where the children and teachers live together with their families sharing a common life of high aspirations, planned living and noble efforts in contact with nature on one hand, and with the spirit of joy on the other.
- Naturalism also believes in the principle of individual differences, which means that every child has a unique capacity to acquire knowledge. The pace of learning is also unique. The school should have respect for personal diversity and it should cater to the varied and different interests of the child.
- Naturalists advocate the methods of teaching that offer the child an opportunity for self-education, self-expression, creative activity and integrated growth in an atmosphere of unrestrained freedom.

E. Naturalism and Curriculum

- Naturalists emphasize the study of sciences dealing with nature such as physics, chemistry, biology, zoology and botany.
- They also give importance to the study of language and mathematics.
- Naturalism gives a very insignificant place to spiritualism in the curriculum. However, naturalists like Rabindranath Tagore do emphasize spiritual values together with the study of literature and sciences, to facilitate the harmonious development of a child.
- At the same time, teaching of religion according to Tagore can never be imparted in the form of lessons but should be imparted by actual practice. By religion, he does not mean the religion of man or any narrow sectarianism. According to him, truth is the basis of all religions.
- Spencer, an extreme naturalist, thinks that human nature is strictly individualistic and self-preservation is the first law of life. He wants all activities to be classified in order of their importance and priority should be given to activities that minister self-preservation. Thus, he assigns a special place to *laws of life and principles of physiology* in the curriculum. He gives a very high place to science, which he considers best both for intellectual and moral discipline. According to him, all studies should be correlated with science.
- T.H. Huxley does not agree with Spencer for giving undue importance to science. He wants aesthetic culture to be imparted to children as a subject of priority.
- Rousseau promotes negative education, a typical feature of the naturalistic philosophy: the subordination of the child to natural order and his freedom from the social order. He defines negative education as one which perfects the senses that are the instruments of knowledge before giving them this knowledge directly.
- For naturalists, genuine education is based on the laws of readiness and needs of human beings. According to them, child's nature, interests and needs provide the basis of curriculum.

F. Naturalism and Teacher

- According to naturalists, the teacher is not only the provider of information, ideas, ideals and will power or a moulder of character but is the observer and facilitator of the child's development. Ross stated that teacher in a naturalistic set-up is only a setter of the stage, a supplier of materials and opportunities, a provider of an ideal environment, a creator of conditions under which natural development takes place. Teacher is only a noninterfering observer.
- Like Rousseau, Tagore is also an individualist and a naturalist. He says that everyone is unique and every individual is different from another. He believes that the natural teachers, that is the trees, dawn, evening, moonlight, etc., nourish the child's nature spontaneously. Nature inspires human beings differently at different stages of human development. He gives an important place to the teacher because according to him, a real teacher humanizes the learning process and activates the mind instead of stuffing it. It is the teacher who kindles independent thinking, imagination and judgement.
- Rousseau said that the teacher should not be in a hurry to make the child learn but should be patient, permissive and nonintrusive. Demonstrating great patience, the teacher cannot tell the student what the truth is but rather must stand back and encourage a student's self-discovery. Naturalists view that the teacher is not one who stresses on books, recitations and massing information in literary forms, rather he should give emphasis on learning by doing.

G. Naturalism and Discipline

- Naturalism has given no emphasis on external rigid discipline. However, he recommended free discipline to child for optimum desired learning to take place in nature.

- Naturalists believed that external discipline should be altogether out of place in education. The only discipline is the discipline of natural consequences. Naturalism also believes that formal education is the invention of society which is artificial. Therefore, rigid man-made discipline must be avoided in the teaching–learning process.

II. IDEALISM

The basic concepts of idealism are as follows:

- Idealism is the oldest system of philosophy known to man. Its origin goes back to ancient India in the East and to Plato in the West. Generally, idealists believe that ideas are the true reality. According to them, the human spirit is the most important element in life.
- All of reality is reducible to one fundamental substance: spirit. The universe is viewed as essentially nonmaterial in its ultimate nature. Matter is not real; rather it is a notion, an abstraction of the mind. It is only the mind that is real. Therefore, all material things that seem to be real are reducible to mind or spirit.
- For idealists, all knowledge is independent of an experience of sense. The act of knowing takes place within the mind. The mind is active and contains innate capabilities for organizing and synthesizing the data derived through sensations.
- Idealists advocate the use of intuition for knowing the ultimate. Man can immediately apprehend some truth without making use of any of his senses. Man can also know the truth through the acts of reason and examine the logical consistency of his ideas.
- Idealists like Plato believe that the spirit of man is eternal. Whatever he knows is already contained within his spirit.
- In idealist axiology, or value theory, values are more than mere human preferences; they really exist and are inherent intrinsically in the structure of the universe. Value experience is essentially an imitation of the Good, which is present in the absolute universal realm of ideas. According to them values are eternal. They believe in three spiritual values: *the truth*, *the* beauty and *the goodness.* The truth is an intellectual value, the beauty an aesthetic value and the good a moral value.
- The purpose of education is the development of the mind and self of the pupil according to idealism. Idealists like to educate the child for mainly two reasons. First, education is a spiritual necessity and second education is also a social necessity. The school should emphasize on intellectual activities, moral judgement, aesthetic judgement, self-realization, individual freedom, individual responsibility and self-control in order to achieve this development.
- In essence, idealists advocate that:
    - Education is a process of unfolding and developing that which is a potential in the human person. It is unfolding of what is already enfolded.
    - Learning is a process of discovery in which the learner is stimulated to recall the truth present within the mind.
    - The teacher should be a moral and cultural exemplar or model of values that represents the highest and best expression of personal and human development.

A. Chief Proponents of Idealism

There are a number of great names associated with idealism, a few important ones are as follows:

- Plato
- Guru Nanak Dev Ji
- Rabindranath Tagore
- Mahatma Gandhi

- Dayananda Saraswati
- Sri Aurobindo
- Dr Sarvepalli Radhakrishnan
- Socrates
- Ross

B. Idealism and Aims of Education

The main aims of education according to idealism are given below.

- Exaltation of the human personality which leads to perfection in the individual.
- Ensuring self-realization of the individual towards duties of self, cleanliness, satisfaction of all desires, self-control, self-sacrifice, punctuality and regularity, avoidance of obscenity, profanity and immoral language.
- Ensuring the individual realize unity within him and establish harmony between his nature and ultimate universe. Indian idealism advocates for liberation (*mukti* or *nirvana*) as the ultimate aim of life.
- Providing a means for students to acquire achievement in art, literature, mathematics and sciences, so that a man can invent, create and produce new ideas and objects of the community and society.
- Provide an opportunity for the acquisition and enrichment of cultural heritage. Promoting the development of moral sense and moral values, so that he can distinguish between right and wrong.
- Promoting the development of self-culture, which includes polite behaviour, good manners, self-control, respect for others opinion, cooperativeness, reliability, liberality, generosity, sincerity and perseverance.
- Promoting universal education without discrimination in gender, cast, creed, religion, region, culture, country and language.

C. Idealism and Organization of Education

- Idealism recommends well-planned formal classrooms or a formal place for teaching–learning activity where the teacher is considered as a mature person and gets an opportunity to share or transfer his knowledge to students.

D. Idealism and Methods of Education

- Idealism recommends formal classroom teaching methods such as lectures, discussions, presentations and group interaction, self-activity, project methods, questioning and role play.
- Knowledge is transferred from a more mature person (teacher) to a less mature person (pupil) through formal and well-planned teaching–learning methods.

E. Idealism and Curriculum

- Idealism emphasizes the spiritual side of a man. For idealists, curriculum is based upon the idea or assumption of the spiritual nature of man. They are of the view that the curriculum is a body of intellectual or learned disciplines that are basically ideational or conceptual. They arrange their curriculum in the form of a hierarchy in which the general discipline occupies the top most position and gradually comes down to the particular subjects in their relationship to general discipline.
- Plato, a great exponent of idealism, conceives of the curriculum from the point of ideas. He believes that the highest idea of life is the attainment of the highest good or God; hence curriculum ought to impart inherent values to enable the educand (student) to attain his highest good. The spiritual values, according to him are truth, beauty and goodness. These three values determine

three types of activities: intellectual, aesthetic and moral. Each type of activity is represented by different subjects and should form a part of the curriculum. Intellectual activities are represented by subjects such as language, literature, science, mathematics, history and geography; aesthetic activities will be possible through the study of art and poetry, and moral activities are possible through the study of religion, ethics and metaphysics.

- Ross talks of two types of activities, that is physical and spiritual, to be included in an idealistic curriculum. Physical activities include subjects such as health and hygiene that foster physical skills (such as gymnastics and athletics) that lead to good health and fitness and thus make the pursuit of spiritual values possible. Spiritual pursuits imply intellectual, aesthetic, moral and religious studies. Hence, subjects such as history, geography, language, fine arts, morality, ethics, religion, science, mathematics and others should be included in the curriculum.
- Sri Aurobindo in his *Integral Philosophy of Education* gives importance to moral, religious and physical education. By moral education, he means the training of moral faculty, that is the ability to distinguish between right and wrong. Another important thing in moral education is the value of suggestion. A suggestion by the teacher has to be exercised by personal example, daily talks and *svadhyaya* or reading good books. Narration of the deeds of great men in an interesting style always makes a large amount of impression on the young minds. In addition, Aurobindo advocates that religious education should be imparted not only through religious books or religious sermons but by the practice of religious life and spiritual self-training. Theoretical teaching of religion must be complemented with actual practice. Along with moral and religious education, he stresses on the importance of physical education. With regard to physical education he says, 'if our seeking is for a total perfection of the being, the physical part of it cannot be left aside; for the body is the material basis, the body is the instrument which we have to use'.
- Another Indian idealist Dr Radhakrishnan wants to make moral education a compulsory part of education at the primary and secondary level. Without moral education, he states, 'the educational institutions cannot fulfil their objectives of educating the youth of the country'. According to him, the greatness of a country cannot be measured by its physical civilization but by its moral and spiritual advancement. He also supports religious education which for him is not the instruction of a particular religion but a means for developing spiritual intuition because the aim of religion is spiritual and not merely a change in metaphysical ideas. Further he suggested the inclusion of physical education in the curriculum. In his words, 'the body is the means of the expression of the human soul; physical education therefore must be properly given'.

F. Idealism and Teacher

- Idealism believes in the maxim that pupils catch fire from a teacher who is himself a flame. Idealists have high expectations of the teacher. The teacher must be ideal both intellectually and morally to serve as an example for the student. They believe that the teacher is an important ingredient in a child's education. The teacher should not only understand the stages of learning but also maintain constant concern for the ultimate purpose of learning.
- Some idealists emphasize the importance of emulation in learning. They feel the teacher should be the kind of person we want our children to become. Socrates has been used by idealists not only as a prototype of learning but also as a model for emulation.
- In this connection, Dr Radhakrishnan opines, 'the type of education which we may give to our youth depends on the fact that what type of teachers we get'. According to him, teachers have a special place in the formation of the mind and heart of the youth. Besides knowledge and scholarships, the teacher should be devoted to teaching. It is the teacher who has to provide the right environment in the school. He must be himself an ideal person in order to exercise wholesome

influences on the young ones. It is the teacher's forceful personality, his effective methods, his sense of dedication to the work which encourages the child to perceive him as exemplary. The teacher must also exercise great creative skill in providing opportunities for the students' mind to discover, analyse, unify, synthesize and create applications of knowledge to life and behaviour. The teacher should respect the learner and assist the learner to realize the fullness of his or her own personality. To the idealist 'the school is a garden, the educand (student) is a tender plant, and the educator the careful gardener'.

- In the words of Ross, 'the educator constitutes the special environmental factor whose function is to lead the child nearer to reality, to guide him towards his utmost possible perfection'. J. Donald Butler has identified the desired qualities of a good teacher. According to him, the teacher should:
  - Personify culture and reality for the student
  - Be a specialist in the knowledge of the pupils
  - Be the kind of person who commands the student's respect by virtue of what he is himself
  - Be a personal friend of the individual student
  - Awaken students' desires to learn
  - Be a master of art of living
  - Be one who capably communicates on his subject
  - Appreciate the subject he teaches
  - Aid in the cultural rebirth of generations

G. Idealism and Discipline

- Interest and discipline are interconnected devices of education. The concept of interest and discipline can be better understood with the help of another concept called *effort*. By interest, we mean the totally positive attraction of a child for the work at hand without any conscious or voluntary exertion and also a minimum persistence on the part of the teacher.
- Effort is the conscious and voluntary exertion by the student for doing the work without any self-interest. By discipline, we mean some extraneous action by the teacher to stimulate the pupil to complete the task in hand.
- According to Home, interest and effort cannot be distinctly separated as interest evokes effort and effort may give rise to interest. Effort is not a substitute to interest, but it supplements interest. It acts as a faithful friend. He says, 'effort is the will to do one's duty'.
- Idealist educators like Fredrick Froebel, the founder of the kindergarten, emphasize the principle of the learner's own self-activity. The learners self-activity is related to the learner's interests and willingness towards an effort. Students have their own intuitive self-interest, which attracts them to certain acts, events and objects for which they readily put in effort.
- *Gentile* finds discipline that is separated from the constructive teaching process as undesirable. According to him, discipline should be considered as an end product instead of an input and it is a part of the teaching process and should be in the teacher's personality. Teacher should achieve discipline through freedom and not conversely. But today education has bypassed this concept by beginning with discipline and moving towards freedom. Idealists do not favour rigid discipline. In fact, their theory of discipline is based on their concept of freedom. Freedom does not mean waywardness, it implies responsibility. It should be regulated, guided and restrained freedom.
- Mahatma Gandhi also believed that real freedom comes through self-discipline; discipline that arises spontaneously from the inner spring of life rather than that which is imposed from without. His concept of discipline is a synthesis of both freedom and external control. Idealists believe that human behaviour should have internal rather than external control. Discipline begins externally but ends internally through self-control.

III. PRAGMATISM

The basic concepts of pragmatism are as follows:

- Pragmatism is popularly regarded as an indigenous American philosophy. But its roots can be traced to ancient Greek philosophy.
- The term *pragmatism* is derived from the Greek word *pragma* which means 'work'. Heraclitus and Sophist of ancient Greece are considered to be pragmatic in their approach to life.
- There were other contemporaries such as Protagoras and Gorgias. The background of pragmatism is associated with the works of Francies Bacon, John Locke, Jean Jacques Rousseau and Charles Darwin. But the philosophical elements that give pragmatism a consistency and system as a philosophy in its own right are primarily the contributions of Charles Sanders Pierce, William James and John Dewey though they differ considerably in their methods and conclusions. Pierce's view of pragmatism is oriented towards physics and mathematics and Dewey's towards social science and biology. James's philosophy, on the other hand, is personal and psychological and is motivated by religious considerations.
- Pragmatists reject metaphysics as a legitimate area of philosophical inquiry. Reality, they opine, is determined by an individual's sense experience. Man can know nothing beyond his experience. Questions relating to the ultimate nature of man and the universe simply cannot be answered because these problems transcend one's experience. For example, there is no way for any living being to determine whether there is life after death because one cannot experience life after death while living. Any conclusion we make about life after death in merely conjecture or a guess.
- Pragmatists believe that reality is in constant flux. There is nothing in the world which is static, permanent or eternal. According to pragmatism, knowledge based on experience is genuine and worthy of acquisition. Since the phenomena are constantly changing, knowledge and truth must change accordingly.
- Knowledge which is helpful in solving present-day problems is most preferred. Pragmatists emphasize on functional knowledge and understanding.
- Pragmatism does not believe in standard, permanent and eternal values. According to this philosophy, values are derived from the human condition. Because man is a part of the society, the consequences of his actions are either good or bad according to their results. If the consequences are worthwhile, the value of the action is proven to be good. Thus, values in ethics and aesthetics depend on the relative circumstances of situations as they arise. Definitive values cannot exist.
- Pragmatism, being a practical and utilitarian school of philosophy, has influenced education to the maximum extent. It considers activity as the basis of all teaching and prefers self-activity in the context of cooperative activity. It creates optimistic men who are the architects of their own fate by the process of their efforts. Pragmatists want that education should be according to one's aptitudes and abilities.
- Individuals must be respected and education should be planned to cater to their inclinations and capacities. Individual development, however, must take place in a social context.
- According to pragmatism, the aim of education is to teach individuals how to think so they can adjust to an ever-changing society. To produce creative, resourceful and adaptable children, we should have conditions in the school which are conducive to the creation of these qualities of mind.
- Children should not be asked to work according to predetermined goals. They should determine their goals according to their needs and interests and in conformity with the demands of the activities that they have undertaken. For them the teaching–learning process is a social process where the sharing of experiences between the teacher and the student takes place.

A. Chief Proponents of Pragmatism

Many great names are associated with pragmatism but the important ones are as follows:

- Williams James
- John Dewey
- Charles Sanders Pierce
- S. Kil Patrick
- Margaret H.

B. Pragmatism and Aims of Education

- *All-round development of the individual:* Pragmatism believes in the holistic development of physical, psychological, social, moral and aesthetical domains of an individual so that an individual's full potential can be utilized to live a fruitful life.
- *Personal and social adjustment of an individual:* Human beings are social animals; however, they have to fulfil their personal as well social needs to attain ultimate satisfaction in life. Pragmatism believes that education must equip the individual to have a harmonious adjustment in the achievement of personal and social needs.
- *Learning through activity and experience:* Pragmatism believes that education must be based on the activity and experiences of an individual so that it can help the individual in the creation of new values, activities and experiences that are essential for a man to be a social being.
- *Reconstruction of experiences:* Pragmatism emphasizes on the adaptation of an individual on contraction and reconstruction of experiences to develop specific capabilities in an individual to control the new or existing environment.
- *Creation of new moral and aesthetic values:* The main aim of education is to develop the individual's moral and aesthetic values so that these new values can serve as a guiding path to handle and manage the new complex life environment.

C. Pragmatism and Organization of Education

- The aim of education in pragmatism is to teach one how to think so that one can adjust to an ever-changing society. To produce creative, resourceful and adaptable children, we should have conditions that are conducive to the creation of these qualities of mind in schools. They recommend formal schools to have activity-oriented learning based on the needs, interests, aptitude and capabilities of individual students.

D. Pragmatism and Methods of Education

- Pragmatism primarily believes in the principle of learning by doing, where the learner is encouraged to learn in real-life situations by self-activity, self-effort and creative activity like project methods and practice-oriented learning.
- Pragmatism also advocates for programmed learning in either real-life situations or artificial situations such as real-life laboratories or simulated laboratories for practical learning of the individuals.

E. Pragmatism and Curriculum

- According to pragmatists, the focus of education is a good life in the present and future. The standard of social good is dynamic so it should be tested and verified through changing experience. John Dewey, however, is of the view that acquaintance with past experience is very important for handling the present and the future effectively.

- School curriculum should reflect the society. Pragmatism refused the traditional approach to subject matter curriculum, which is associated with formal schooling, where knowledge is fragmented or compartmentalized.
- Dewey viewed that all learning should be contextual to the given time, place and events. For example, history is taught to students without considering its relevance to everyday life.
- Dewey recommended three levels of curricular organization: (1) making and doing, (2) history and geography and (3) organized sciences.
  - The first curricular level, making and doing, engages students in activities and projects based on their experiences. This idea is similar to that of Mahatma Gandhi, who is considered as an idealist, a naturalist as well as a pragmatist. He believes in the principle of learning by doing. There is a lot of similarity between the craft-centred activities advocated by him and the project method of Dewey. Though Rabindranath Tagore is a naturalist, his views regarding curriculum are pragmatic in nature. To him, curriculum is not a number of subjects to be learnt but relevant activities to be undertaken.
  - The second level curriculum, history and geography, helps in enlarging the scope and significance of the child's temporal and spatial experience to the larger community and the world.
  - The third stage of curriculum is that of the organized subjects, the various sciences, that is bodies of tested knowledge. Pragmatists endorse a more general education than narrow specialization.

F. Pragmatism and Teacher

- Pragmatism neither treats the teacher merely as a spectator like naturalism nor regards him as a pragmatist, the teacher is not a dictator or task master but a leader of group activities.
- The chief function of a pragmatic teacher is to suggest problems to his pupils and to stimulate them to find solutions. Teachers should not try and pour information and knowledge into the puppet because what students learn depends on their own personal needs, interests and problems.
- Dewey views the teacher as a resource person who guides rather than directs learning. The teacher's role is to guide learners who need advice or assistance and the direction comes from solving particular problems. Educational aims always belong to the learner majorly rather than the teacher. Since pragmatists are concerned with teaching children how to solve problems, they should select real-life situations that encourage the problem-solving ability in children. For a problem to be solved correctly, the learner needs to establish a correct procedural sequence with the help of teacher guidance to solve a particular problem.
- A pragmatist teacher needs to be patient, friendly, enthusiastic and cooperative. Although coercion might force students to achieve immediate results, it is likely to limit the flexibility needed for future problem solving.
- The teacher's control of the learning situation is ideally indirect rather than direct. Direct control, coercion or external discipline generally fails to enlarge the learner's internal disposition and does not in any way contribute to the learner in becoming a self-corrected person.
- As a resource person, the pragmatic teacher needs to be noninterfering or what Dewey refers to as *permissive* and allow students to make errors and to experience the consequences of their actions. In this way, the teacher helps students become self-directed individuals. For Dewey, permissiveness does not mean that children's whims should dictate the curriculum. Rather, the teacher as a mature person should exercise professional judgement and expertise so that the consequences of action do not become dangerous to the students or their classmates.
- The pragmatic teacher should constantly be aware of the motivation factor. Dewey opined that children are naturally motivated and the teacher should capture and use the motivation that is already present.

- Dewey also pointed out that the teacher should respect the principle of individual differences and treat students accordingly. A pragmatic teacher wants his students to think and act for themselves, to do rather than to know and to originate rather than to repeat. The pragmatic teacher is a pragmatist first and a teacher afterwards.

G. Pragmatism and Discipline

- Pragmatism advocates a discipline that can be maintained through play as work. It is the mental attitude that converts work into play and vice versa. For example, a football game becomes work if it is played due to some external pressure and difficult algebraic sums become a play if solved out of zeal.
- Pragmatism does not believe in external discipline exercised by the authority of the teacher.
- Discipline is based on the principles of child's activities and needs, and the interest of the child should be aroused and satisfied.
- Control is achieved from the cooperative aspect of shared activity, which involves working with the fellow mates.
- There is no place for rewards and punishments. In pragmatism, every activity is to be pursued in a social setting where the teacher should come down to the children's level, mix with them, share their interests and participate in their activities.

IV. REALISM

The basic concepts of realism are as follows:

- Realism is also known as *objectivism* and basically opposes idealism and has the opposite viewpoints of spiritualism. However, realism propagates for the true and real in daily life.
- Scientific development ultimately gave birth to realism, through experimentation, examination and observation, what is found true and evident and considered real and is the basis of realism. Therefore, realism is directly associated with man and society.
- Realism makes human beings understand and enjoy the society in the true sense by getting multidimensional real joy of life in reality.
- Realism aims at education in making the man's life useful, where a man can enjoy his activities and comfort in reality.
- The main types of realism are naïve realism, representationism, neorealism and critical realism.

A. Chief Proponents of Realism

Many great names are associated with realism, the important ones are as follows:

- Aristotle
- Johann Friedrich Herbart
- Herbert Spencer
- John Locke
- Franklin Bobbitt

B. Realism and Aims of Education

Realism propagates for the following aims of education:

- Education can facilitate the individual enjoy a happy, comfortable, integrated and meaningful life.
- Franklin Bobbitt mentioned that the basic aim of education is bringing happiness in life of an individual that can be achieved by fulfilment of human responsibilities and obligations, such as activities concerned with language, hygiene, citizenship activities, ordinary social activities, leisure

activities, activities of mental health, religious activities, activities concerning race preservation, vocational behaviour activities and vocational activities.

- Realism emphasizes on developing a man's capabilities of earning by vocational means.
- It also emphasizes on developing and strengthening the wisdom and power of decision making.
- Education must develop the capacity to patiently fight and struggle against adverse situations arising in everyday life.
- Education must enable individuals to develop the capacities to handle the reality of life and making the child successful in fighting with routine and adverse difficult situations.

C. Realism and Organization of Education

- Realism emphasizes on scientific attitude based on realistic principles, where the child extends the knowledge he learns through books. Spiritual needs are not given due consideration as a real need of education.
- It gives due emphasis on formal schools that provide adequate opportunities for learners to learn vocational skills through observation, experimentation and examination.

D. Realism and Methods of Education

- Proponents of realism believe that objectivity and knowledge of scientific evidences and reality are key in deciding what methods should be used for the teaching–learning process. Teaching methods should be according to the needs, interest and capabilities of student.
- Vocational education equips the individual with capacities to earn livelihood and enjoy leisure time utilization through experimentation, examination and observation.

E. Realism and Curriculum

- Selection of curriculum for students must be based on their abilities, interest and capabilities so that education helps the student to adjust to changing circumstances of the society. The curriculum must have practical utility and must equip the child to adjust to the needs of the day-to-day life.
- Realism emphasizes on subject matters of real life use such as science, mathematics, hygiene and vocational subjects. Vocational content has given prominent stress on curriculum.

F. Realism and Teacher

- Teachers must focus on the development of vocational skills in learners so that they can be equipped with qualities of race preservation and vocational behavioural activities.
- According to realism, teachers are the mentors who must be role models and skilled to demonstrate the vocational skills to their learners.

MODERN CONTEMPORARY EDUCATIONAL PHILOSOPHIES

Modern contemporary educational philosophies are also known as *normative philosophies*. These are actually the theories of education that are based on the results of philosophical thought and of factual inquiries about human beings and the psychology of learning. However, they guide about what education should be, what dispositions it should cultivate in learners, why it ought to cultivate them, how and in whom it should do so and what forms it should take. Some of the major modern contemporary education philosophies are discussed below (a brief review may be seen in Table 2.2).

Table 2.2 Brief Description About Modern Contemporary Educational Philosophies of Education

Concept of Philosophy	Organization and Aims of Education	Curriculum	Methods of Education	Role of Teacher	Discipline
1. Perennialism: Chief proponents were Thomas Aquinas, Robert Hutchins and Mortimer Adler					
Education ensures that students acquire an understanding about the great ideas of civilization. These ideas have the potential for solving problems in any era. The focus is to teach ideas that are everlasting, to seek enduring truths which are constant, as the natural and human worlds at their most essential level.	The aim of education is to develop the rational person, who has intellectual abilities to uncover universal truth. Character training is also important for moral and spiritual development of an individual.	Accepts little flexibility in the curriculum that emphasizes on language, literature, mathematics, arts and sciences. Common curriculum for all the students with minimal opportunities for elective subjects. Teaching–learning process must create liberalism, tolerance and discretion among learners.	Perennialism portages for the educational methods, which promotes constant teacher–taught interaction such as oral exposition, lecture and explication. Emphasis is placed on teacher-guided seminars, where students and teachers engage in mutual inquiry sessions. Students may also learn directly from reading and analysing the great books.	Teacher must be competent and master of his subject so that he can help their students to develop the power to think deeply, analytically, flexibly and imaginatively. Teacher is also authoritative and a guide of the students.	Education should be organized and conducted in a manner that problem of indiscipline does not arise at all.
2. Essentialism: Chief proponents were William Bagley, Arthur Bestor, Admiral Hyman Rickover, James D. Koerner, Paul Copperman and Theodore Sizer					
Essentialists believe that there is a common core of knowledge that needs to be transmitted to students in a systematic, disciplined way. The emphasis placed on intellectual and moral standards that schools should teach and preparing students to become valuable members of society.	Essentialism has recommended for the formal schools or teaching–learning places. The aims of education is to promote intellectual growth and academic competitiveness of the individual to become a model citizen.	This philosophy recommended intellectual content with quality and capacity of the learner. The recommended subjects are English, mathematics, natural science, history and foreign languages.	Essentialism recommended formal and well-planned classroom teaching methods such as lectures, discussions, presentations and group interaction.	Teacher must be a master of subject matter and role model for learners with high level of authority and control over teaching–learning process and learner.	Essentialism believes in rigid discipline and devoted hard work of learners in his studies.

3. Existentialism: Chief proponents were Soren Kierkegaard, Friedrich Nietzsche, Maxine Greene, George Keller and Van Cleve Morris					
This philosophy believes that education must develop the consciousness about the freedom of choices among learners because a man becomes what he chooses for his self. Education must equip the individual for better choices.	The ultimate aim of education is to develop child's knowledge about human conditions and the choices that person has to make for self. Therefore, organization of education must be formal with sufficient opportunities of choices.	Curriculum must be that which provides the free opportunities for children to select from many available learning situations and choosing the subjects that learner wish to learn. Humanities are commonly given tremendous emphasis, which helps the student to unleash their own creativity and self-expression.	Existentialism promotes the methods of education, which emphasizes on self-activity of the learner, such as self-expressive activities, experimentation, methods and media that illustrate emotions, feelings and insight.	Teacher must promote freedom for a learner to make personal choices and individual self-definition.	Existentialism believes in self-discipline but not in the strict discipline. Teacher creates an environment in which students may freely choose their own preferred way.
4. Reconstructionism: Chief proponents were Theodore Brameld, George Counts and Paulo Freire					
This philosophy of education believes on reorganizing and restructuring the process of education to being about social and cultural contrastive changes in community, society and country, where emphasis is placed on cultural pluralism, equality, futurism, national interest-oriented education.	Reconstructionism recommends for formal as well as informal ways of organizing education so that desired aim of education can be achieved to bring the reconstruction of the society.	Curriculum should be conceived with a new socioeconomic and political interest. Therefore, the subject content must be oriented towards aspects of new changes expected social, economic and political discipline such as sociology, economics and science and technology.	This philosophy of education believes that teaching methods must be organized in manner that student become self-reliant, education must be activity oriented to develop necessary activities and abilities.	The role of a teacher is to take the social responsibilities and along with students must become the agent to improve society.	This philosophy of education propagates about optimum level of discipline but not a rigid discipline.
5. Progressivism: Chief proponents were Horace Mann, Henry Barnard and Johan Dewey					
Progressivism believe that learning must be through problem solving and scientific inquiry in a cooperative and self-discipline way, which promote the democratic living and transmits the culture of society while preparing students to adapt in changing world.	Progressivism recommended democratic school procedures, which promote the community and social reforms. The aim of education is to promote the democratic social living.	Progressivism recommended curriculum, which is interdisciplinary in nature, which promotes written textbooks and subject content that are the part and process of learning rather than ultimate source of knowledge. Further, curriculum is based on child's interest, problems and life affairs.	Child is considered as learner rather than subject, who primarily learned through cooperative group activities and experiences.	Teacher must act as guide for problem solving, leader for group activities and partner in planning the learning activities.	Has not recommended any sort of specific formal discipline.

I. PERENNIALISM

The basic concepts of perennialism are as follows:
- It is the oldest and most conservative educational philosophy that has roots in realism and relies in the past views about changes in the nature of universe, human beings, knowledge, truth, virtue, etc.
- The major aim of education is to ensure that students acquire understanding about the great ideas of western civilization that focuses on enduring truths, which are constant, not changing, as the natural and human worlds, at their most essential level, do not change.
- The curriculum focuses on attaining cultural knowledge and stressing on students' growth in enduring disciplines.
- *Perennial* means 'everlasting', like a perennial flower which grows year after year. Some ideas have lasted over a long time and are as relevant today as when they were first conceived. Perennialism urges these ideas should be the focus of education. When students are immersed in the study of those profound and enduring ideas, they will appreciate learning for themselves and become true intellectuals.

A. Chief Proponents of Perennialism

Many great names are associated with perennialism but the important ones are as follows:
- Roots lie in the philosophy of Plato and Aristotle
- Thomas Aquinas
- Robert Hutchins
- Mortimer Adler

B. Perennialism and Organization of Education

- Aims to rigorously develop students' intellectual powers in a classroom-centred environment by the teachers.
- It further aims to develop a rational person who has intellectual abilities to uncover the universal truth.
- Character training is also important for moral and spiritual development of an individual. It further develops the power of an individual to think deeply, analytically, flexibly and imaginatively.
- Perennialists criticize the vast amount of discrete factual information students are required to absorb. Perennialists urge schools to spend more time teaching how these concepts are meaningful to students.

C. Perennialism and Curriculum

- Accepts little flexibility in the curriculum that emphasizes on language, literature, mathematics, arts and sciences.
- This philosophy allows no curricular electives except in the choice of a second language.
- Common curriculum for all students with minimal opportunities for elective subjects. The teaching–learning process must create liberalism, tolerance and discretion in the learners.
- Perennialists oppose vocational curriculum or life-adjustment courses because they believe that this type of curriculum blocks the opportunity to fully develop students' rational powers.

D. Perennialism and Methods of Education

- Greater emphasis is placed on students and teachers engaging in Socratic dialogues or mutual inquiry sessions to develop an enhanced understanding of concepts.
- They recommend that students learn directly from reading and analysing great books.
- Perennialism portages for the educational methods that promote constant teacher–student interaction, such as oral exposition, lecture and explication.

- Students must spend considerable time in classroom for mastering the three 'Rs', *Reading*, *Riling* and *Rithmetic*.

E. Perennialism and Teacher

- The teacher must be competent and a master of his subject so that he can help his students develop the power to think deeply, analytically, flexibly and imaginatively.
- They must also be authoritative and a guide to manage a classroom as well as the teaching–learning activities.

F. Perennialism and Discipline

- Education should be organized and conducted in a manner such that problems of indiscipline do not arise at all. Perennialism believes on laying a significant amount of external discipline on the learner along with a good amount of freedom to think rationally and logically.

II. ESSENTIALISM

The basic concepts of essentialism are as follows:

- This philosophy has its roots in both idealism and realism that has a primary focus on the development of academic standards and improving the mind and workability of a child.
- *Essentialism* means a 'traditional' or 'back to the basics' approach towards education. It strives to instill in students the essentials of academic knowledge and character development.
- The term *essentialism* was popularized in the 1930s by the American educator William Bagley.
- It is a dominant approach to education in America from the beginnings of American history. Early in the 20th century, essentialism was criticized for being too rigid to prepare students adequately for life.
- But with the launching of Sputnik in 1957, interest in essentialism revitalized. Among the modern supporters are members of the President's Commission on Excellence in Education.
- Essentialists believe this conservative perspective is on intellectual and moral standards that schools should teach in a systematic and disciplined way.
- The schooling should be practical which may prepare students to become valuable members of the society. It should also focus on facts, the objective reality and train students to read, write, speak and compute logically.

A. Chief Proponents of Essentialism

Many great names are associated with essentialism but the important ones are as follows:

- William Bagley
- Arthur Bestor
- Admiral Hyman Rickover
- James D. Koerner
- Paul Copperman
- Theodore Sizer

B. Essentialism and Organization of Education

- Essentialism recommends that formal schools or teaching–learning places and classrooms should be oriented around the teacher.
- It emphasizes that American schools should transmit the traditional and moral values and intellectual knowledge that students need to become ideal citizens.

- The aims of education are to promote intellectual growth and academic competitiveness of the individual.

C. Essentialism and Curriculum

- This philosophy recommends intellectual content with quality and capacity of the learner. Essentialists emphasize on instruction in natural science.
- Essentialists urge that the most essential or basic academic skills and knowledge such as mathematics, natural science, history, foreign language and literature form the foundation of curriculum.

D. Essentialism and Methods of Education

- Essentialism recommends formal and well-planned classroom teaching methods such as lecture, discussion, presentation and group interaction.
- It believes that elementary students should receive instructions for writing, reading, measurement and computers.
- Even while learning art and music, the subjects associated with the creativity development, the students are required to master information and basic techniques, moving from less to more complex skills and knowledge.

E. Essentialism and Teacher

- The teacher must be a master of the subject matter and a role model for learners with a high level of authority and control over the teaching–learning process and the learner.
- Teachers decide what students should learn and place little emphasis on student interests, especially when students divert their time and attention away from academic curriculum.
- Teachers focus on achievement test scores as a means of evaluating the student's progress.

F. Essentialism and Discipline

- Essentialism believes in a significant amount of external discipline and complete devoted hard work of learners in their studies.
- Students should be taught hard work, discipline and respect authoritatively. Teachers are to help students keep their nonproductive instincts such as aggression or mindlessness in control.

III. EXISTENTIALISM

The basic concepts of existentialism are as follows:

- Existentialism refers to a set of ideas about human existence beyond the terms used in ancient philosophy and objective science. Jean Paul Sartre mentioned that 'man is nothing else but what he makes of himself', which is the essential principle of existentialism.
- This philosophy believes that education must develop a consciousness of the freedom of choice in learners because a man becomes what he chooses for his self.
- Education must provide the individuals with opportunities so they can make wise choices and live a meaningful and productive life.
- Individuals are responsible for determining for themselves what is 'true' or 'false', 'right' or 'wrong' and 'beautiful' or 'ugly'. There is no existence of any source of objective and authoritative truth about metaphysics, epistemology and ethics.
- Existentialists believe that there exists no universal form of human nature and each of us have the free will to develop as we see fit.

A. Chief Proponents of Existentialism

Many great names are associated with existentialism but the important ones are as follows:

- Soren Kierkegaard
- Friedrich Nietzsche
- Maxine Greene
- George Keller
- Van Cleve Morris

B. Existentialism and Organization of Education

- The subject matter is secondary in helping the students appreciate themselves as unique individuals with responsibility for their thoughts, feelings and actions.
- The ultimate aim of education is to develop a child's knowledge of human conditions and the choices that a person has to make for himself. The organization of education must be formal with sufficient opportunities for choices.

C. Existentialism and Curriculum

- Existentialist advocates education of the whole person and not just the mind. Although many existentialists provide some curriculum, existentialism affords students great freedom in their choice of subject matter. Students are given a wide variety of options to choose from.
- Curriculum must provide free opportunities for children to select from the many available learning situations and choose the subjects that the learner wishes to learn.
- The humanities are explored as a means of providing students with vicarious experiences that will help unleash their own self-expression.

D. Existentialism and Methods of Education

- Existentialist methods focus on the individual. Learning is self-paced, self-directed and includes a great deal of individual contact with the teacher, who relates to each student openly and honestly.
- Existentialism promotes the methods of education which emphasize on self-activity of the learner, such as self-expressive activities, experimentation and methods and media that illustrate emotions, feelings and insight.

E. Existentialism and Teacher

- The teacher must promote the freedom for a learner to make personal choices and individual self-definition.
- The teacher's role is to expose students to various paths they may take in life and create an environment where they can freely select their own way.

F. Existentialism and Discipline

- Existentialism believes in self-discipline but not in a rigid and strict discipline.

IV. RECONSTRUCTIONISM

The basic concepts of reconstructionism are as follows:

- Reconstructionism is a philosophical theory with the belief that societies should continually reform themselves in order to establish more perfect governments or social networks. Thus, social questions will emerge as there are quests to create a better society and worldwide democracy.

- Reconstructionism is an ideology that emphasizes on the importance of changing for the better. In other words, reconstructionism is a philosophy that centres on the idea of constant change.
- This philosophy of education believes on reorganizing and restructuring the process of education to bring about social and cultural contrastive changes in community, society and country, where emphasis is placed on cultural pluralism, equality, futurism and national interest-oriented education.
- Reconstructionists encourage others to make necessary changes that will be beneficial to their future. These are positive changes that will help make life better and solve social problems. These changes are completed through a systematic outlook called the *reconstructionist philosophy*.

A. Chief Proponents of Reconstructionism

Many great names are associated with reconstructionism but the important ones are as follows:

- Theodore Brameld
- George Counts
- Paulo Freire

B. Reconstructionism and Organization of Education

- Reconstructionism recommends for formal as well as informal ways of organizing education so that the desired aim of education can be achieved to bring about reconstruction of the society.

C. Reconstructionism and Curriculum

- Reconstructionism is more concerned with the broad social and cultural fabric in which humans exist. Reconstructionist educators focus on a curriculum that highlights social reform as the aim of education.
- Curriculum should be conceived with the new socioeconomic and political interest. Therefore, the subject content must be oriented towards aspects of new changes and expected social, economic and political disciplines, such as sociology, economics, science and technology.
- Curriculum focuses on student experience and taking social action on real problems (violence, hunger, international terrorism, inflation and inequality). Strategies for dealing with controversial issues, inquiry, dialogue and multiple aspects are also the focus of the curriculum.

D. Reconstructionism and Methods of Education

- This philosophy believes that the educator does not deposit information into students' heads, and teaching and learning is a process of inquiry in which the child must reinvent the world.
- This philosophy of education believes that the teaching methods must be organized in a manner such that the student becomes self-reliant. Education must be activity oriented to develop necessary activities and abilities.
- Community-based learning and bringing the world into the classroom are also considered as effective methods and strategies of education in reconstructionism.

E. Reconstructionism and Teacher

- The role of a teacher is to take social responsibilities and become an agent to improve society along with students.

F. Reconstructionism and Discipline

- This philosophy of education propagates about the optimum level of discipline but does not stress on rigid discipline.

V. PROGRESSIVISM

The basic concepts of progressivism are as follows:

- Progressive philosophy believes that the school must play a leading role in preparing citizens for active civic participation in a democratic society.
- Progressivism believes that learning must be done through problem solving and scientific inquiry in a cooperative and self-discipline way, which promotes democratic living and transmits the culture while preparing students to adapt in changing world.
- Progressivists believe that education should focus on the whole child rather than on content or the teacher.

A. Chief proponents of Progressivism

Many great names are associated with progressivism but the important ones are as follows:

- Horace Mann
- Henry Barnard
- Johan Dewey

B. Progressivism and Organization of Education

- This educational philosophy stresses on active experimentation by students.
- Learning is embedded in the queries of learners that arise through experiencing the world. The learner is a problem solver and thinker who learns through her individual experiences in the physical and cultural context.
- Progressivism recommends democratic school procedures that promote community and social reforms. The ultimate aim of education must be to promote democratic social living.

C. Progressivism and Curriculum

- Curriculum is drawn from student interests and questions. The scientific method is used so that students can study matter and events systematically.
- Progressivism recommends curriculum that is interdisciplinary in nature, which promotes written textbooks and subject content as part and process of learning rather than the ultimate source of knowledge. Further, curriculum is based on child's interests, problems and life affairs.

D. Progressivism and Methods of Education

- A child is considered as a learner rather than a subject who primarily learns through cooperative group activities and experiences.
- Lessons that are planned provoke curiosity to make school interesting and useful.
- Students are active learners. The students interact with one another and develop cooperation and tolerance for different points of view.

E. Progressivism and Teacher

- Effective teachers provide experiences so that students can learn by doing.
- The teacher must act as a guide for problem solving, as a leader in group activities and as a partner in planning learning activities.

F. Progressivism and Discipline

- Progressivists believe that education should be a process of ongoing growth, not just a preparation of becoming an adult. Therefore, they do not recommend any sort of specific formal discipline. However, they believe in an individual's self-discipline and self-governance.

PHILOSOPHY OF NURSING EDUCATION

The nursing educational institutes establish a set of values that guide their curriculum, teaching–learning processes, evaluation and discipline of students in nursing education for different nursing programmes, namely undergraduate, postgraduate, doctoral and other short-term specialty nursing programmes. A nursing school or college can develop its own philosophy or a philosophy for a particular nursing programme to guide and motivate for its most effective implementation.

The term philosophy means 'love of wisdom' or 'love of learning'. The philosophy of nursing education is a mission statement that outlines an educational institute's values, beliefs and professional ethics that act as guiding principles of the educational behaviour of the teaching team, administration and nursing educational institute.

In other words, the philosophy of nursing education is the fundamental nature of knowledge, reality, existence and academic discipline of nursing education. The philosophy of nursing education is a written statement of the values, beliefs, attitudes and ideas that the faculty and administration of an educational institute or the university as a team agreed upon in relation to the particular nursing educational programme.

Philosophy of nursing education is a field of study or academic discipline of nursing education that 'seeks to uncover the nature, root, and meaning of nursing and nursing education, being as a nurse, reality (metaphysics), ethics, and knowledge of nursing (epistemology)'. In a broader sense, philosophy of nursing education has seven dimensions: Metaphysics, Epistemology, Ethics, Aesthetics, Logic, Axiology and Political Philosophy of nursing education (Fig. 2.5).

IMPORTANCE OF PHILOSOPHY OF NURSING EDUCATION

There are various benefits of philosophy of nursing education; some of the key benefits are listed below:

1. Guide development and revision of nursing curriculum, teaching–learning methods, teaching–learning processes and evaluation methods for a particular nursing programme or course.

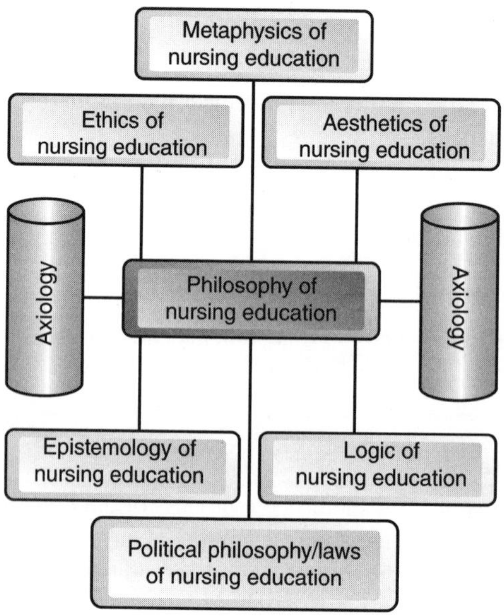

Figure 2.5

Dimensions of philosophy of nursing education.

2. It promotes effective and meaningful teacher-taught interactions and teaching–learning processes.
3. Nursing educational philosophy keeps teachers and students motivated and focused to achieve expected outcomes of nursing education.
4. Philosophy also helps to guide to choose appropriate and effective teaching–learning methods, disciplinary mechanisms and content of the curriculum for a particular nursing programme or course.

PRINCIPLES OF PHILOSOPHY OF NURSING EDUCATION

1. The pursuit of reality and truth that results in ideas and aspirations is referred to as nursing educational philosophy.
2. It is dynamic and evolves over time in accordance with societal, educational, professional and environmental developments.
3. It is affected by the setting in which it is used.
4. It may be unique and reflect the values, beliefs, reasoning, morality and ethics of the nursing institute particularly.
5. It may exist on a global scale, be a part of a nursing organization or institution, etc.
6. It expands the nursing profession's scope of practice.

REVIEW QUESTIONS

LONG-ANSWER QUESTIONS

1. Describe the philosophy of education.
2. Discuss the aims of education.
3. Discuss about social aim of education.
4. Describe the aims of nursing education.
5. Briefly explain the philosophies and aims of education.
6. Discuss the relationship between education and philosophies.
7. Define education and discuss the various aims of education.
8. Explain the various philosophies of education and formulate a philosophy for a B.Sc. Nursing programme.
9. Describe idealism.
10. Define education and discuss the functions of education.
11. Describe pragmatism.
12. Discuss the traditional philosophies of education.
13. Discuss the differences between philosophy and education.
14. Define curriculum and discuss the curriculum development process.

SHORT-ANSWER QUESTIONS

1. Define education, as given by Mahatma Gandhi.
2. List down the methods of teaching under Naturalism.
3. Mention four educational philosophies.

4. Discuss briefly the four aims of education.
5. Mention four aims of nursing education.
6. List down the types of education.
7. Discuss any four principles of pragmatism.
8. Define philosophy.

MULTIPLE-CHOICE QUESTIONS (MCQs)

1. The term *education* is derived from a
   (a) Latin word
   (b) Sanskrit word
   (c) Chinese word
   (d) Greek word
2. The word *education* means
   (a) An act of teaching
   (b) An act of training
   (c) An act of teaching and training
   (d) An act of learning
3. Which aim of education allows the student to develop themselves into distinct individual personality?
   (a) Individual aim
   (b) Social aim
   (c) Vocational aim
   (d) Moral aim
4. The aim of education 'achieving social and national integration' was stated by
   (a) Secondary education commission
   (b) Kothari commission
   (c) Education commission
   (d) Planning commission
5. Which of the following factors play an important role in transmitting the cultural heritage and traditions from one generation to another?
   (a) Religious factors
   (b) Cultural factors
   (c) Intellectual factors
   (d) Philosophy of life
6. Which of the following is not a function of education towards nation?
   (a) Ensuring national development
   (b) Promoting national integrity
   (c) Preparing good citizen
   (d) Developing leader for nation
7. ________________ is the social function of education.
   (a) Civilization and cultural security
   (b) Preparation for adult life
   (c) Transmission of cultural
   (d) Moral and character development

8. Philosophy is defined as
   (a) Science of knowledge
   (b) Science of facts
   (c) Review of universal things
   (d) Critical review of critical science

9. Which of the following is not a traditional philosophy of education?
   (a) Naturalism
   (b) Idealism
   (c) Pragmatism
   (d) Essentialism

10. The concept of philosophy 'educating the human generation about and in the nature rather than artificial environment by keeping in mind the individuality of each child' is based on
   (a) Naturalism
   (b) Idealism
   (c) Pragmatism
   (d) Essentialism

11. Which of the following philosophy recommended well-planned classroom for teaching–learning activity?
   (a) Naturalism
   (b) Pragmatism
   (c) Idealism
   (d) Realism

12. Naturalism philosophy emphasizes
   (a) Rigid discipline to child
   (b) Free discipline to child in nature
   (c) Spontaneous and self-discipline to child in nature
   (d) No discipline to child in nature

13. Existentialist method focuses on
   (a) Individual
   (b) Group
   (c) Society
   (d) Nation

14. Reconstructionist educators should emphasize on curriculum that highlights
   (a) Social reforms
   (b) Traditional facts
   (c) Scientific knowledge
   (d) Logical studies

15. __________ believe that education should focus on whole child rather than content or teacher:
   (a) Reconstructionists
   (b) Existentialists
   (c) Progressivists
   (d) Naturalists

ANSWERS OF THE MULTIPLE-CHOICE QUESTIONS

1. (a), 2. (c), 3. (a), 4. (b), 5. (b), 6. (c), 7. (a), 8. (a), 9. (d), 10. (a), 11. (c), 12. (b), 13. (a), 14. (a), 15. (c)

FURTHER READING

Acemoglu, D., Johnson, S., & Robinson, J. A. (2001). The colonial origins of comparative development: An empirical investigation. *American Economic Review*, *91*(5), 1369–1401.

Armstrong, J. S. (1979). *The natural learning project* (pp. 5–12). North-Holland: Elsevier.

Armstrong, J. S. (1983). *"Learner responsibility in management education, or ventures into forbidden research (with comments)". How the world's best-performing school systems come out on top*. Mckinsey.com. September 2007.

Asimov, M. S., & Bosworth, C. E. (1999). *The age of achievement* (Vol. 4, pp. 33–35). Motilal Banarsidass.

Barbe, W. B., Swassing, R. H., & Milone M. N. (1979). *Teaching through modality strengths: Concepts and practices*. Columbus, OH: Zaner-Bloser.

Blurton, C. (1999). *New directions of ICT-use in education (PDF)*. Retrieved February 6, 2007. https://unesdoc.unesco.org/ark:/48223/pf0000119077

Bowles, S., & Herbert, G. (2011). *Schooling in capitalist America: Educational reform and the contradictions of economic life*. Chicago, IL: Haymarket Books. Retrieved October 21, 2011.

Cahn, S. M. (1997). *Classic and contemporary readings in the philosophy of education* (p. 197). New York: McGraw Hill.

Card, D. (1999). Causal effect of education on earnings. In O. Ashenfelter & D. Card (Eds.). *Handbook of labor economics* (pp. 1801–1863). Amsterdam: North-Holland.

De Grauwe, A. (2009). *Without capacity, there is no development*. Paris: UNESCO-IIPE.

Dewey, J. (1916/1944). *Democracy and education* (pp. 1–4). New York: The Free Press.

Dubois, H. F. W., Padovano, G., & Stew, G. (2006). Improving international nurse training: An American–Italian case study. *International Nursing Review*, *53*(2), 110–116.

Finn, J. D., Gerber, S. B., & Boyd-Zaharias, J. (2005). Small classes in the early grades, academic achievement, and graduating from high school. *Journal of Educational Psychology*, *97*(2), 214–233.

Frankena, W. K., Raybeck, N., & Burbules, N. (2002). Philosophy of education. In J. W. Guthrie (Ed.). *Encyclopedia of education* (2nd ed.). New York: Macmillan.

Gutek, G. L. (2009). *New perspectives on philosophy and education* (p. 346). New Jersey: Pearson Education, Inc.

Hanushek, E. A. (2005). *Economic outcomes and school quality*. International Institute for Educational Planning. Retrieved October 21, 2011.

Hanushek, E. A., & Woessmann, L. (2008). The role of cognitive skills in economic development. *Journal of Economic Literature*, *46*(3), 607–608.

Harriman, P. (1935). Antecedents of the Liberal Arts College. *The Journal of Higher Education*, *6*(2), 63–71.

Heckman, J. J., Lochner, L. J., & Todd, P. E. (2006). Earnings functions, rates of return and treatment effects: The Mincer equation and beyond. In E. A. Hanushek, & F. Welch (Eds.). *Handbook of the economics of education* (pp. 307–458). Amsterdam: North Holland.

Kneller, G. (1964). *Introduction to the philosophy of education* (p. 93). New York: John Wiley & Sons.

Locke, J. (1996). *Some thoughts concerning education and of the conduct of the understanding* (p. 10). In R. W. Grant & N. Tarcov (Eds.). Indianapolis: Hackett Publishing Co., Inc.

May, S., & Aikman, S. (2003). Indigenous education: Addressing current issues and developments. *Comparative Education*, *39*(2), 139–145.

Mincer, J. (1970). The distribution of labor incomes: A survey with special reference to the human capital approach. *Journal of Economic Literature*, *8*(1), 1–26.

Munari, A. (1994). Jean Piaget (1896–1980). *Prospects: The Quarterly Review of Comparative Education*, *XXIV*(1/2), 311–327.

Noddings, N. (1995). *Philosophy of education* (p. 1). Boulder, CO: Westview Press.

Pashler, H., McDonald, M., Rohrer, D., & Bjork, R. (2009). Learning styles: Concepts and evidence. *Psychological Science in the Public Interest*, *9*(3), 105–119.

Phenix, P. H. (1963). Educational theory and inspiration. *Educational Theory*, *13*(1), 1–64.

Potashnik, M., & Capper, J. (2005). *Distance education: Growth and diversity (PDF)*. Retrieved February 6, 2007. chrome-extension://efaidnbmnnnibpcajpcglclefindmkaj/https://www.imf.org/external/pubs/ft/fandd/1998/03/pdf/potashni.pdf.

Rizvi, S. H. (2006). *Avicenna/Ibn Sina (c. 980–1037)*. Internet Encyclopedia of Philosophy.

Robinson, K. (2006). *Schools kill creativity*. Monterrey, CA: TED Talks.

Russell, G. A. (1994). *The 'Arabick' interest of the natural philosophers in seventeenth-century England* (pp. 224–262). Leiden: The Netherlands Brill Publishers.

Schofield, K. (1999). *The purposes of education*. Brisbane, Australia: Queensland State Education board.

Steer, L., & Baudienville, G. (2010). *What drives donor financing of basic education?* London: Overseas Development Institute. news room/latest news/press_releases/2010/2010_02_23_AEW_launch_en. Transparency.org (2010-02-23). Retrieved October 21, 2011.

Swassing, R. H., Barbe, W. B., & Milone, M. N. (1979). *The Swassing-Barbe modality index: Zaner-Bloser modality kit*. Columbus, OH: Zaner-Bloser.

Thomas, G. W. P. (1968). *Introduction to philosophy*. London: Novello and Company.

Thomson, I. (2002). Heidegger on ontological education. In M. A. Peters (Ed.). *Heidegger, education, and modernity* (pp. 141–142). New York: Rowman and Littlefield.

Tremblay, E. (2010). Educating the mobile generation: Using personal cell phones as audience response systems in post-secondary science teaching. *Journal of Computers in Mathematics and Science Teaching*, *29*(2), 217–227.

UNESCO. (2008). *Education for all monitoring report 2008, Net enrollment rate in primary education*. https://learningportal.iiep.unesco.org/en/glossary/net-enrolment-rate-ner.

Webb, D. L, Metha, A., & Jordan, K. F. (2010). *Foundations of American education* (6th ed., pp. 55–91, 77–80, 192–193). Upper Saddle River, NJ: Merill.

Whyte, C. B. (1989). Student affairs: The future. *Journal of College Student Development*, *30*(1), 86–89.

CHAPTER

Teaching–learning process

3

LEARNING OBJECTIVES

This chapter is designed to enable the reader to:

- Understand the concept and nature of teaching and learning
- Describe the characteristics, principles and domains of learning
- Recognize the factors influencing learning
- Discuss the characteristics, principles and maxims of teaching
- Identify the meaning, characteristics, importance, domains and types of educational objectives
- Demonstrate skills in framing the educational objectives
- Explain meaning, functions, importance, characteristics, prerequisites, types and format of lesson planning
- Design the format of lesson plan to use for teaching the assigned group
- Explain the meaning, dimensions, principles, problems and strategies of classroom management and role of teacher in it

KEY TERMS

INTRODUCTION

Teaching and learning activities are twin activities involved in the total educational process. Teaching and learning are closely related and they are reciprocal to each other. Teaching cannot be thought without an idea of learning, and learning is not possible without teaching activities. The main focus of teaching is to facilitate learning, where the teaching–learning process occurs smoothly and continuously. The teaching–learning process has four pillars: teacher, student, learning process and learning activities. Interaction between the teacher and learners is the core of the teaching–learning process.

MEANING OF LEARNING

Learning is said to be equivalent to change, modification, development, improvement and adjustment. It is a comprehensive term which leaves permanent impressions on individuals. Learning is central to our behaviour as we learn to speak, write, think and perceive. Our attitudes and emotional expressions are also learned behaviours.

Meaning of efficient learning: Efficiency in learning can be measured by three factors, namely accuracy, speed and retention. The meanings of accuracy, speed and retention are given below:

- *Accuracy:* How accurately do learners remember?
- *Speed:* How soon do learners remember?
- *Retention:* How long do learners remember?

DEFINITIONS OF LEARNING

Learning is acquisition of habits, knowledge and attitudes. It involves new ways of doing things and it operates in an individual's attempt to overcome obstacles or to readjust to new situations. It represents progressive change in behavior. It enables him to satisfy interests to attain goals.

—Crow and Crow

Any activity can be called learning so far as it develops the individual and makes his/her behavior and experiences different from what that would otherwise have been.

—Woodworth R.S.

Learning is a process that results in the modification of behavior.

—J.F. Travers

Learning may be considered as a change in insights, behavior, perception, motivation or a combination of these.

—M.L. Bigge

Learning is the process by which behavior is originated or changes through practice and training.

—Kingsley H.L. and Garry R.

Learning is the process by which an activity originates or is changed through reacting to an encountered situation, provided that the characteristics of the change in activity cannot be explained on the basis of native responses tendencies maturation or temporary states of the organism.

—B.L. Hilgard

Learning is the acquisition of new behavior or strengthening or weakening of old behavior as the result of experience.

—H.P. Smith

Learning is the process by which an organism is satisfying its motivation, adopts and adjusts its behavior in order to overcome obstacles or barriers.

—Hunter and Hilgard

Learning is an episode in which a motivated individual attempts to adapt his behavior to succeed in a situation, which he perceives as requiring action to attain a goal.

—Pressey, Robinson and Horrocks

Learning can be defined as changing one's potential for seeing, feeling and doing through experiences partly perceptual, partly intellectual, partly emotional and partly motor.

—W.C. Morse and G.M. Wingo

There are three important factors in the definition of learning:

- Learning brings change in behaviour (usually for betterment).
- Change takes place through practice or experience and not due to maturation.
- The change in behaviour should be relatively permanent lasting for years, months or weeks.

CONCEPT OF LEARNING

People learn, but they also forget. Learning may or may not be useful in few situations. According to Crow and Crow, learning is the acquisition of knowledge, habits and attitude in an individual for the betterment of self and society.

According to Woodworth, the process of acquiring new knowledge and new responses is the process of learning. Learning is not only getting knowledge of the subject matter or skills in art by study, by experience or by being taught, it is also an acquisition of habits, attitudes, perceptions, preferences, interests, social adjustments, values and ideals. Learning is a modification of observation, overt activity, thinking and associated motivational and emotional reactions.

A change in behaviour may occur through maturation which implies progressive advancement towards maturity. Learning is a change in performance through conditions of activity, practice and experience. In classroom situations, the activity or experience which leads to change in performance may be listening or judging, reading or reciting or observing a demonstration of a procedure. Through these activities or experiences, an effective teacher can bring out changes in behaviour. Desirable changes are those changes that serve educational purposes, aims, objectives and goals.

A learning pyramid is depicted in Fig. 3.1, which illustrates the average retention rate among students through the different learning methods.

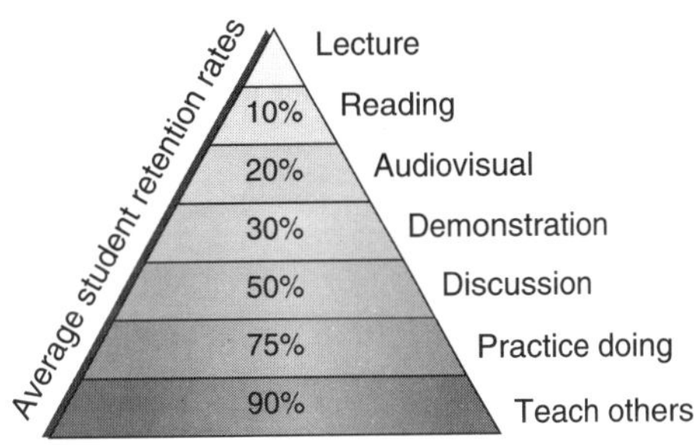

Figure 3.1

Learning pyramid.

TEACHING–LEARNING PROCESS

Teaching–learning is a process of interaction between the teacher and students. This process endeavours to harmonize various activities, including learners, their individual differences, the method of teaching, the material to be taught, classroom management, teaching aids and teaching methods. The teacher uses all the techniques and teaching strategies to fulfil the desired objective of teaching. The concept of teaching–learning process can be understood from the following points:

- It is an interaction between teachers and students, where teachers try to transmit knowledge and content to students according to their age, capabilities, skills and living conditions.
- It is a combined process, where an educator assesses learning needs, establishes specific learning objectives, develops teaching and learning strategies, implements a plan of work and evaluates the outcomes of the instruction.
- It is a process to transfer knowledge from a teacher to a student. It is a combination of various elements within the process where an educator identifies and establishes the learning objectives and develops teaching resources and implements the teaching and learning strategy.
- Teaching–learning is a process through which the teacher, the learner, the curriculum and other variables are organized in a systematic way in order to achieve predefined goals.

Teaching–learning process includes four main components: (1) content and curriculum; (2) course design and learning environment; (3) student and learning; and (4) teacher and teaching (Fig. 3.2).

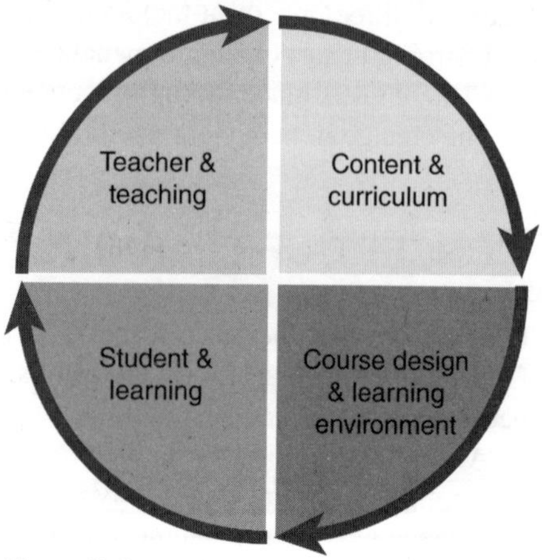

Figure 3.2

Components of teaching–learning process.

STEPS OF TEACHING–LEARNING PROCESS

Teaching–learning is an ongoing process that involves many steps. It is hard to distinguish between steps. Wilson and Gallup outlined the steps of the teaching–learning process in AIDCAS (Attention, Interest, Desire, Conviction, Action, and Satisfaction – Fig. 3.3).

1. **Attention:** Educators' first task is to draw the attention of the learner for better ideas and new ways of working. It is also important to inform learners about their improvements through regular feedback.
2. **Interest:** Once attention has been caught, it is possible for the teacher or trainer to appeal to the basic needs and urges of the student and to arouse their interest in the idea or subject matter.
3. **Desire:** The desire refers to the learner's continued interest in the idea, better practice or alternative until it becomes a desire or motivating factor.
4. **Conviction:** Action is the result of desire, conviction and satisfaction. This step teaches the learner what actions are necessary and how to do them. He ensures that the learner is able to visualize the action within his particular situation and has gained confidence in his abilities to complete the task.
5. **Action:** Without conviction being converted into action, all efforts will be in vain. Teachers have the responsibility of making it easier for learners to take action. If you do not act quickly to fulfil your desire, the idea will soon fade away. This is why it should never be overlooked.
6. **Satisfaction:** This is the final result of the entire process. Teachers will continue to follow up with learners in order to help them evaluate their strengths and progress. Satisfaction allows the learner to carry on his work with greater satisfaction. Satisfaction drives us to learn more.

These six steps can be mixed together and at times can be utilized without a particular sequence.

NATURE OF LEARNING

Following are some of the significant views about the nature of learning:

- **Behaviourist view:** Learning is a change in behaviour as a result of experience. Men and other living beings react to the environment.

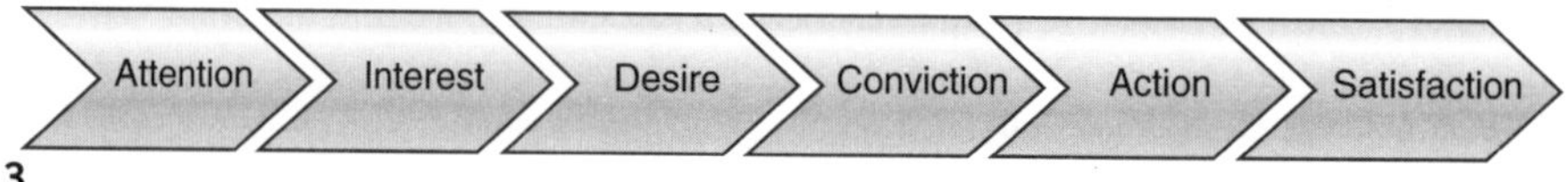

Figure 3.3

Steps of teaching–learning process.

- **Gestalt view:** According to this view, learning depends on gestalt or configuration (wholeness of the situation). Learning is a total reaction to the total situation.
- **Hormic view:** This view was developed by McDougall. It stresses on the purposeful nature of learning, that is, learning is a goal-directed activity.
- **Trial and error view:** This view was put forward by Thorndike. He conducted many experiments on dogs, cats and fish and concluded that most learning takes place by trial and error.
- **Learning is a process which involves a series of steps** (Fig. 3.4)**:**
  - ***Motive of the learner:*** Motive or need arises first. Motive is the force that impinges or compels the individual to behave or react or do a particular task.
  - ***Establishing goals:*** If a motive or need is present, the goal is set up by the teacher and learner.
  - ***Teacher–student adjustment:*** Adjustment on the part of the students and teacher to each other and the environment.
  - ***Change in the student's behaviour:*** During this phase, inappropriate behaviours are dropped and new behaviours are acquired by the student. Changes in behaviour in an individual take place after due interaction of the student with the educational environment and/or teacher.
  - ***Fixation or stabilization of behaviour:*** Later the changes in the behaviour of the learner acquainted are expected to be fixed and stabilized for permanence.
- **Learning is a cooperative process:** Learning is cooperative, which involves five essential elements (Fig. 3.5):
  - Group processing
  - Individual and group accountability
  - Promote face-to-face interaction
  - Positive interdependence
  - Learning social skills

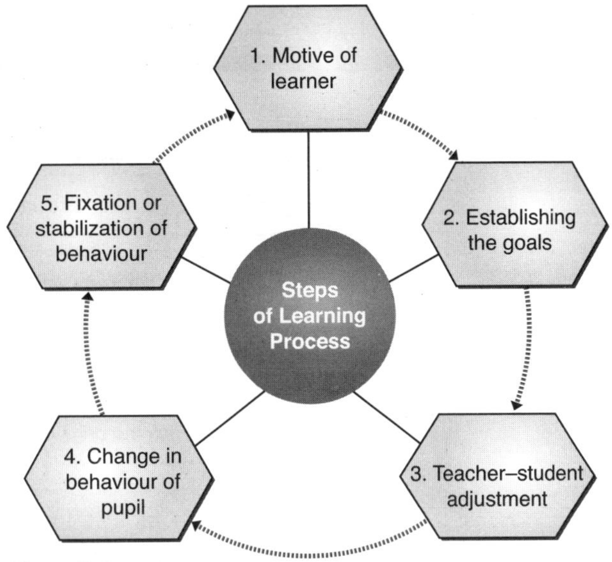

Figure 3.4

Learning process.

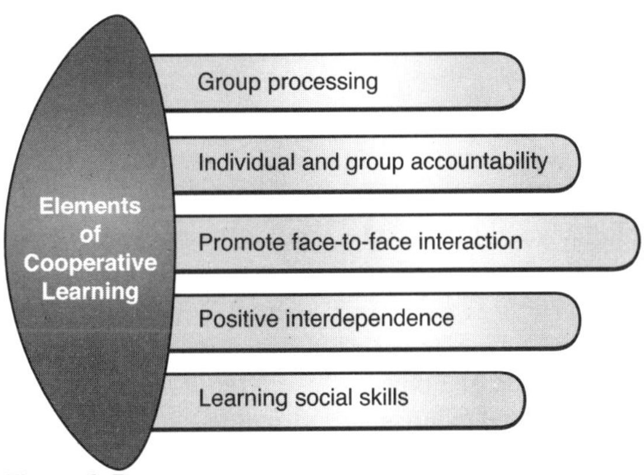

Figure 3.5

Elements of cooperative learning.

CHARACTERISTICS OF LEARNING

Learning is the acquisition of knowledge and/or skill through education and experience. Our ability to learn and our intellectual capacity are intangibles. These intangibles are our greatest assets because

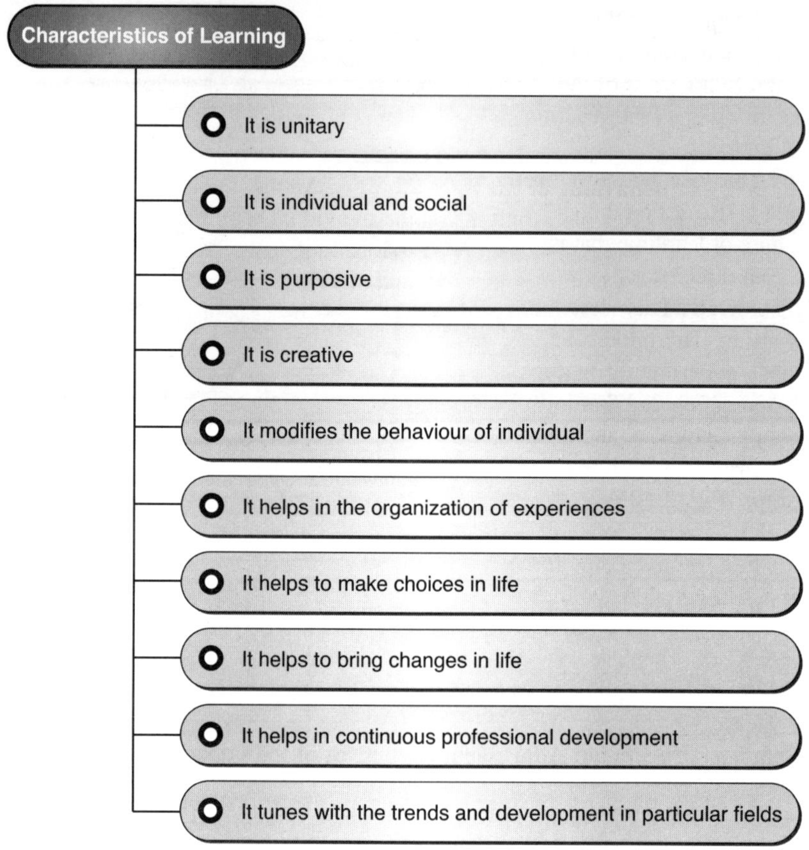

Figure 3.6

Characteristics of learning.

everything we do to reinvent and update our knowledge allows us to grow from where we are today to where we want to go. Learning is a prerequisite to growth, some may think that learning is a luxury for a few individuals or learning should be concerned with our early years. It should be looked at as something beyond formal schooling. Detailed discussion about the characteristics of learning is given below (Fig. 3.6):

- **Learning is unitary:** The process of learning helps the learner respond as a whole person in a unified way to the whole situation or total pattern. He responds intellectually, emotionally, spiritually and physically and these occur simultaneously. He reacts to the whole learning situation rather than to any single stimulus.
- **Learning is individual and social:** Learning is in a sense an entirely individual matter. Each individual must learn his or her own activity. In a larger sense, all learning is social, as it takes place in response to the environment in which there are other individuals as well as physical things. Learning is social because it takes place as a type of response to an individual's social environment. It is important that each person do his or her own learning irrespective of their individual differences, their capacities and level of intelligence.
- **Learning is purposive:** Learning is not only active but active in a specific direction. It helps the individuals achieve goals or purposes in their life. Learning cannot be meaningful and efficacious

without persistent selective and purposeful effort. Learning not only contributes to an individual's purposes at times but enables him/her to make more intelligent adjustments in future.

- **Learning is creative:** Human learning is both selective and creative. Man is the only creature on earth who is not merely a creature but a creator as well. Learning helps a man to be more creative in life. It is the process of personal choice making. Learning helps him be creative for the betterment of the society.
- **Learning modifies the behaviour of the individual:** Learning affects the conduct of the individual. True learning takes place only when the individual acquires a type of knowledge or a skill that changes his or her attitudes and appreciations in response to a real need and modifies his or her conduct in accordance with new learning and therefore is changed.
- **Learning helps in the organization of experiences:** The process of learning is not mere acquisition of facts and skills through drill and repetition. It involves organization and evaluation of learning materials. The learner reorganizes his or her experience and behaviour.
- **Learning helps make choices in life:** Change is a law of nature and things are changing around us in the universe at every movement. Therefore, learning is as essential as food and physical exercise so that one can make wise decisions and adaptations with the changes one witnesses in his surroundings. Thus, it will not be wrong to state that changes as well as learning are lifelong processes because as changes in life take place every day, learning is also needed every moment to make best choices and decisions in life.
- **Learning helps bring changes in life:** Everyone of us needs change and progress in life; however, questions arise on how one can achieve fast and prompt changes and progress in life. The answer is learning because when one acquires new knowledge, he/she tries to apply it on the ground that ultimately brings about change and progress in life. All rapid changes and human progress in the world is the result of new learning.
- **Learning helps in continuous professional development:** Learning does not end at the completion of a particular course or educational programme but is needed throughout life for continuous professional development of the individual. For example, health care professionals including nurses regularly engage in professional education such as seminars, symposiums, workshops and conferences essential for their continuous professional development.
- **Learning helps keep in tune with trends and development in particular fields:** Learning provides an individual a new way of thinking, and professionals must acquire new knowledge to meet the pace with emerging new demands of their consumers. For example, India is catching up with medical tourism; nurses and health care professionals have to equip themselves with the emerging health care demands of these new health care consumers. Learning helps such individuals be in tune with new trends and development of their profession.

PRINCIPLES OF LEARNING

The main principles of learning (also listed in Box 3.1) are discussed below.

- **Brings progressive change in behaviour:** Learning brings progressive change in behaviour as the individual reacts to situations, and this is how learning leads to improvement in an individual.
- **Learning is motivated by adjustment:** The individual has to adjust to the new environment.
- **Learning is universal in nature:** Man is a rational animal and learns more than other animals from nature; however, learning does occur in other animals, since it is an omnipresent phenomenon.
- **Learning is never-ending growth:** Every individual has an inspiration to learn more. One achievement leads to further incentive, pursuit and effort. Therefore, learning is the never-ending growing phenomenon of an individual.

BOX 3.1 PRINCIPLES OF LEARNING

I. *Basic fundamental principles of learning*
Learning is
- motivated by adjustment with new things
- universal in nature
- never-ending growth
- a continuous process
- goal directed or purposive
- active and creative
- aroused by individual and social needs
- response of the whole individual to the total situation
- transferable
- possible on cognitive, affective and conative side
- a process not a product
- learning brings progressive change in behaviour of learner

II. *Ten principles of learning given by JTFSL**
Learning is
- a constant interaction between learner and environment
- an outcome of stimulation and motivation of learner
- an active process
- ongoing, developmental and cumulative process
- an outcome of cooperation and support
- an essential influence of environment
- through practice, feedback and evaluation
- a formal as well as an informal act
- an individual phenomenon
- an act of self-awareness

*The Joint Task Force on Student Learning.

- **Learning is a continuous process:** Learning is continuous and not restricted to the childhood but grows with life. Death is the end of learning.
- **Learning is goal directed or purposive:** When the purpose or goal of learning is clear, vivid and explicit, learning becomes meaningful and effective to the learner.
- **Learning is active and creative:** Learning largely depends on the activities of a learner. It is said no learning can take place where there is no self-activity. Learning results from the activity and experience.
- **Learning is aroused by individual and social needs:** Learning depends on individuals: their needs, problems, interests, attitudes, ambitions and needs of the society. Learning may be quick and fast for some individuals and in others it may be slow or steady. No learning can take place in the absence of social environment.
- **Learning is the response of the whole individual to the total situation:** Learning does not take place in one dimension at a single time; it usually happens in a holistic manner and takes place in several dimensions together (such as cognitive, affective and psychomotor). Generally, individuals respond to the total situation in a wholesome manner rather than in an impendent and isolated manner.
- **Learning is transferable:** Learning is a transferable phenomenon, which may transfer from one learning generation to the next generation learners. A transfer of learning content may take place but the amount of transfer may vary from situation to situation and from individual to individual. Transfer occurs when there is similarity of content, techniques, ideals, procedures, interest and attitudes.
- **Learning is possible on cognitive, affective and conative side:** Acquisition of knowledge is cognitive, modification of emotions is affective and acquisition of skills and habits is conative learning. Generally, learning takes place in these three dimensions.

- **Learning is a process not a product:** Learning is an ongoing process as it goes on and on and is a never-ending process; death of an individual is considered as the end point of learning. Therefore, it is considered a lifelong process rather than an end product of a particular point of life.

I. JTFSL'S PRINCIPLES OF LEARNING

The Joint Task Force on Student Learning (JTFSL) created by the American Association of Higher Education gave 10 principles of learning, as discussed below:

1. ***Learning is a constant interaction between the learner and environment:*** Learning is fundamentally about making and maintaining connections; biologically through the neural network; mentally between concepts, ideas and meanings; and experimentally through interaction between the mind and the environment, self and others, generality and context, deliberation and action.
2. ***Learning is an outcome of stimulation and motivation of the learner:*** Learning is enhanced when taking place in the context of a compelling situation that balances challenges and opportunities, stimulates and uses the brain's ability to conceptualize quickly and its capacity and need for contemplation and reflection upon experiences.
3. ***Learning is an active process:*** Learning is considered as an active process rather than passive. It is commonly said that one can take a horse to the water but cannot make it drink water until and unless the horse itself does it. The same way, learning is also an active process and cannot be achieved passively.
4. ***Learning is a continuous ongoing, developmental and cumulative process:*** Learning is considered as a continuous ongoing, developmental and cumulative process. It is a regular process of the storing of new knowledge over the past knowledge that leads to ultimate development of an individual.
5. ***Learning is an outcome of cooperation and support:*** Learning cannot be imagined without the help, cooperation and support of other individuals in the society. For example, learning occurs with the help of a teacher who teaches; a headmaster who coordinates in the educational activity and a writer who writes the textbook and so on.
6. ***Learning has an essential influence of environment:*** It is generally believed as well as empirically provided that learning is largely influenced by the environment and even some educationists believe that environment is the most important and crucial factor leading to learning. They believe that a man cannot force other men but it is the conducive educational environment created by one mature man that ultimately leads to learning in other individuals.
7. ***Learning takes place through practice, feedback and evaluation:*** Learning requires consistent practice as practice makes a man perfect. In addition, frequent evaluation and feedback to the learners also helps them in improvement during the ongoing learning process.
8. ***Learning is a formal as well as an informal act:*** Learning takes place formally as well as informally. Formal learning occurs during a planned teacher–taught interaction such as classroom teaching, interaction during a formal couching session and so on. Informal learning takes place during informal interaction of learning in the educational environment, such as campus social interactions, active community activity participations and so on.
9. ***Learning is an individual phenomenon:*** Every individual is a unique creature of nature; therefore, he/she also learns in a unique pattern.
10. ***Learning is an act of self-awareness:*** In the true sense, learning is more of knowing about the self and then learning about others. Learning leads to great strength of introspection and ultimately improved self-awareness.

DOMAINS OF LEARNING

Learning does not take place in an aspect. It is identified that learning mainly occurs in three areas: intellectual, emotional and motor aspects, also called cognitive, affective and psychomotor domains of learning (Fig. 3.7). These domains are discussed below.

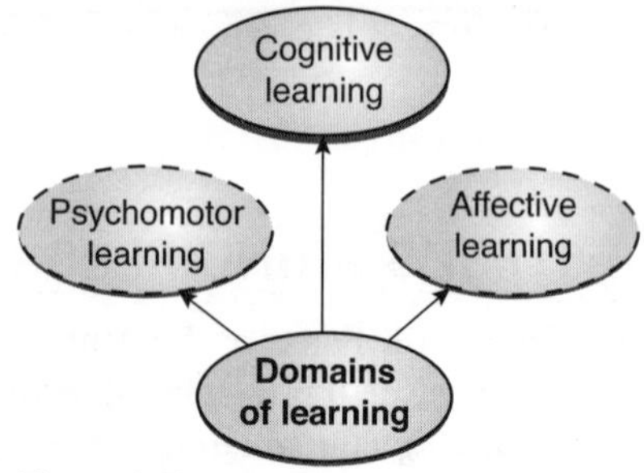

Figure 3.7
Domains of learning.

- **Cognitive domain:** This domain includes intellectual skills such as thinking, knowing and understanding. Cognitive learning is generally provided starting from a simple to a complex manner, which requires various teaching–learning and evaluation methods. The teaching–learning methods or strategies used to achieve this domain of learning are lectures, discussions, lectures enforced with discussion, seminars, panel discussions, conferences, etc. This domain of learning has further sublevels that are expected to be achieved by a learner, that is knowledge, comprehension, application, analysis, synthesis and evaluation. This domain of learning is generally evaluated by formal written examinations such as essay-type or objective written examinations.
- **Affective domain:** This domain includes feelings, emotions, interests, attitudes and appreciations. This domain of learning has further sublevels that are expected to be achieved by a learner, that is receiving, responding, valuing, conceptualizing, organizing and characterizing. The teaching strategies needed for the successful achievement of this domain of learning are simulations, role-plays, discussions, etc.
- **Psychomotor domain:** This domain of learning is also known as the *conative* or *skill learning domain*. This domain involves learning motor skills that require the acquisition of combined psychological and masculine ability to perform a task. Examples are taking blood pressure, performing head-to-toe assessment. This domain of learning has further sublevels that are expected to be achieved by a learner, that is impulsion, imitation, manipulation, coordination and habit formation. Teaching–learning strategies involve demonstrations, laboratory practice, skill practice on simulators, clinical practice, case studies, clinical conferences, etc.

FACTORS INFLUENCING LEARNING

Factors influencing learning are classified under two main headings: intrinsic and extrinsic factors (Fig. 3.8). Details of the intrinsic and extrinsic factors influencing learning are given below.

I. INTRINSIC FACTORS

Intrinsic factors are from within the individual learner such as age, intelligence, attention, interest, holistic health, maturation, fatigue, insight, ability, capacity and motivation.

- ***Age:*** Age can impact the capability to learn. A child can learn faster and an aged person will have difficulty learning the modern ways of knowledge.
- ***Intelligence:*** Mental ability of an individual can affect learning. Individuals with subaverage intelligence will learn later than individuals with normal intelligence level.
- ***Attention:*** Attention plays an important role in the education and training process. Attention is not static. It fluctuates from one object to another. Inattention by trainees is responsible for poor learning.

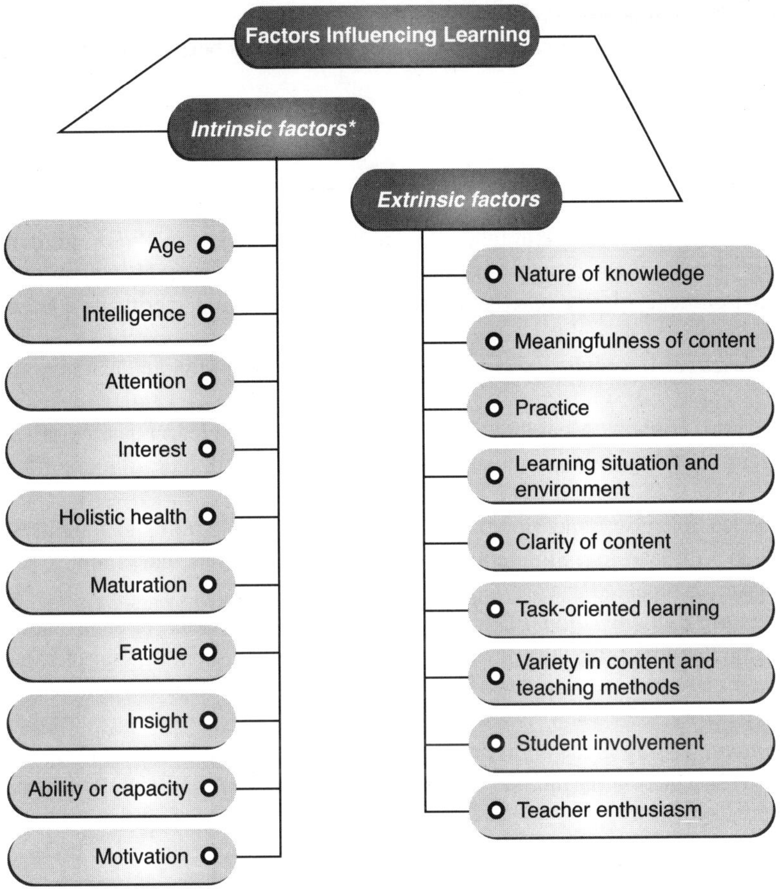

Figure 3.8

Factors influencing learning. **Indicates that the factors belong to the learner.*

- ***Interest:*** Interest is an inner disposition or a tendency of readiness to perceive. Effective learning requires assimilation and interest. Interest should be aroused before learning begins, and for satisfactory results, it should be maintained throughout the learning period.
- ***Holistic health:*** Physical and intellectual health promotes effective learning. Without sound intellectual or physical health, an individual is unable to fulfil the demands of the learning process.
- ***Maturation:*** Learning depends on intellectual age. Maturation means intellectual, social maturity and psychological readiness. The changes associated with normal growth are called *maturation*.
- ***Fatigue:*** Every physical activity involves the consumption of energy. Human efficiency is the ratio between achievement and energy spent. Mental fatigue is caused by a loss of interest and the monotonous nature of work. When an individual is tired, he/she cannot pay attention or concentrate towards learning activities.
- ***Insight:*** Insight also plays an important part in learning. Without clear insight, it is impossible to achieve predetermined goals of learning. Insight is based on the ability of synthesizing the perceived facts and factors. It involves creative and imaginative thinking.
- ***Ability or capacity:*** Different species of animals have a different capacity to learn. Man is known to have a greater capacity to learn than other living beings. Even men vary in their ability to learn.

- ***Motivation:*** Motivation is a general term that encompasses the states of the individual under which he attends to certain aspects of his environment. As a result, his behaviour is both initiated and directed.

II. EXTRINSIC FACTORS

Extrinsic factors are from outside the individual learner and interfere directly or indirectly with an individual's learning process, such as nature of knowledge, meaningfulness of content, practice, learning situation and environment, clarity of content, task-oriented learning, verity in content and teaching methods, student involvement and teacher enthusiasm.

- ***Nature of knowledge:*** If knowledge is interesting in nature, an individual can learn it more efficiently.
- ***Meaningfulness of content:*** Meaningless material can neither be learnt easily nor kept in memory for the long term. If the material is meaningful, the individual will learn it more effectively and easily.
- ***Practice:*** Practice, exercise, repetition or drill are interchangeable terms that are presumed to have something to do with learning. Simple acts are learnt in single trials, but complex acts are learnt through exercises or repeated trials.
- ***Learning situation and environment:*** A learner should have a conducive environment to learn that will promote the learning process. For example, adequate ventilation, lighting, temperature, odour-free environment, absence of nose disturbance, rodent- and insect-free environment and availability of good library resources.
- ***Clarity of content:*** Clarity is the ability of the learner to clearly see, hear and understand what is being said. Threats to clarity include small fonts, slurred speech, obstructions to sight and ambiguous language.
- ***Task-oriented learning:*** People tend to learn better when they are engaged in tasks.
- ***Variety in content and teaching methods:*** A variety of ways used by the teacher can enhance the students' learning. Some people learn by listening, some by seeing and some by doing.
- ***Student involvement:*** Student involvement in the whole teaching–learning process is very crucial for his or her learning. Active involvement of students not only motivates them but also arouses interest in particular activities.
- ***Teacher enthusiasm:*** Enthusiasm of the teachers or presenters is contagious. If the teacher shows interest in a topic, the learners are more likely to be interested.

BARRIERS OF TEACHING AND LEARNING

The barriers of teaching and learning are the factors that stands in the way of a teacher to teach and learner to leaner effectively. It is observed that teachers and learners experience one or more barriers to learning throughout their teaching–learning process. The barriers could be within the individual, within the education system, within the centre of learning, and within the broader social, economic and political context. The teaching–learning barriers could be extrinsic or intrinsic. The extrinsic barriers of teaching–learning process could be organizational/systemic barriers, socio-economic barriers, educational environmental barriers, cultural barriers and situational barriers. Further, intrinsic factors of teaching–learning process could be individual physical and physiological barriers, emotional barriers, motivational barriers and cultural barriers (Fig. 3.9; details may referred from Table 3.1).

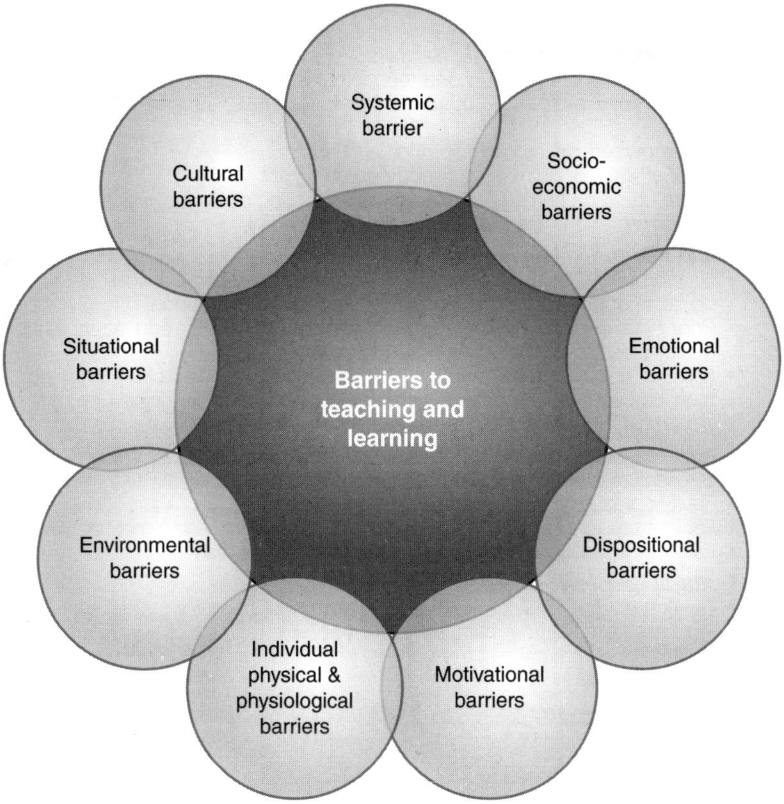

Figure 3.9

Barrier to teaching and learning.

THEORIES OF LEARNING

Learning theories help shape one's perceptions, and nurses can apply these theories at individual, group and community levels not only to understand and teach new material and tasks but also to solve problems and build constructive connections. They can also learn to manage emotions and develop effective behaviour. There are some theories which gave new concepts and ideas to link theories with practice. Some of the theories are as under (Fig. 3.10):

I. **Behaviourist Theory:**
   - Every teacher knows that they will usually have one student in the classroom who is difficult to manage and work with. Their behaviour is usually difficult to control and they may have to work extra hard to get attention and stop distractions. Additionally, it is extremely valuable to learn about the theories of learning and to recognize different ways and ideas about how people learn.
   - This theory focuses on how students learn and states that behaviours are learned from the environment and that innate or inherited factors have little effect on behaviour. Here, positive reinforcement plays an important role, for example if students should get badges every time they get an 'A' grade on a test and on the other hand if teachers do not reward them, there is a possibility that fewer students may get an 'A' grade on their tests because the behaviour here is not associated

Tables 3.1 Barriers of Teaching and Learning

Extrinsic barriers	**I. *Organizational or systemic barriers:*** • Lack of adequate physical and technological infrastructure in the institution. • Lack of required learning materials (books, journals, etc.), technological devices and learning assistance. • Overcrowded classrooms, libraries and hostels. • Lack of trained, qualified and competent faculty. • There could be curriculum-related barriers, such as rigid curriculum, content loaded curriculum and unclear educational objectives. **II. *Socio-economic barriers:*** • *Unaffordability:* Lack of access to the quality education because of unaffordability, because of people from poor socio-economic status cannot afford it. • *Poor funding:* These is limited funding of government for education, which leads to poor quality of education for marginalized social groups. • *Lack of financial support:* People from poor socioeconomic strata cannot afford to send their kids schools or colleges without scholarships or financial support. **III. *Educational environmental barriers:*** • Poor teaching–learning methods, procedures and process. • Stressful classroom environment because of overstrictness. • Faulty curriculum and assessment methods. • Lack of student support system and academic counselling mechanisms. • Lack of appropriate discipline for the motivation of learning. **IV. *Cultural barriers:*** • Cultural diversity may become a hindrance in learning for students because students and teachers from different culture may not be able to interact openly and freely. • Cultural beliefs, customs, stereotype, prejudice, language and behaviour could act as barriers in learning. **V. *Situational barriers:*** • Some of the situations are lack of transportation, harsh weather (extreme cold or heat or humidity), shortage of time, rigid time-table schedules, lack of freedom and nonavailability of crèche for women teachers and students, etc.
Intrinsic barriers	**I. *Individual physical or physiological barriers:*** • Individual physical or physiological barriers could be acute or chronic illness, pain, sensory deficits, poor memory, physical or cognitive disability and mental illnesses like attention deficit hyperactivity disorder (ADHD) and autism. **II. *Emotional barriers:*** • The common emotional barriers which can hinder learning are fear of failure, criticism, judgement and rejection. Further, emotionally oversensitive, adjustment problems, emotional instability, etc. **III. *Dispositional barriers:*** • Lack of self-esteem, confidence, interest, weak peer-support, previous bad experience, negative attitude could be some of the common dispositional barriers in teaching and learning process. **IV. *Motivational barriers:*** • Too much or too less to learn, lack of defined learning goals and targets, unorganized study schedules, procrastination, resistance to unlearn and poor parental involvement could contribute towards poor motivation among learners, which deter them from learning.

with a reward for them. Motivation is also a factor responsible for promoting behavioural learning, for example praising a student for a good score in the test is more likely to learn things effectively and do better as compared to the student who did not receive any praise for a good score in the test. The one who receives no praise experiences negative reinforcement and it becomes unimportant for them to do better next time because there is no motivation.

- Learning is a process that takes place through observation that is based on objectively qualified phenomena rather than on introspective psychology. Pavlov's theory of conditioning is a great example to illustrate that concept where he found that he could activate salivation in dogs by associating the bell with food. This phenomenon was also known as 'learning by association'. B.F. Skinner, an American psychologist, then put forward a theory of operant conditioning that supported the view that learners can be influenced by positive or negative reinforcement.

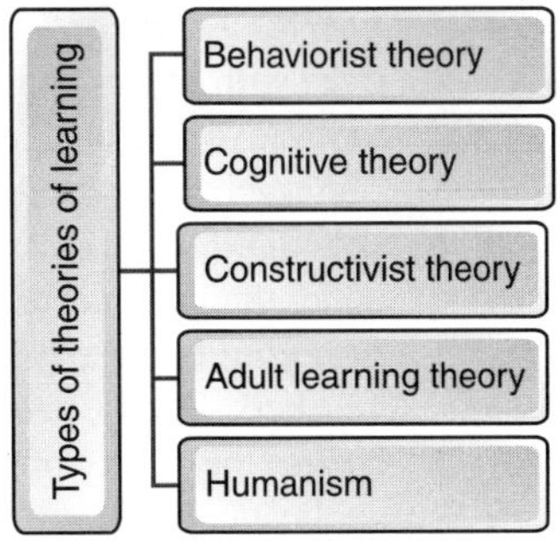

Figure 3.10

Theories of learning.

II. Cognitive Theory:

- This theory of learning puts emphasis on the acquisition of knowledge as well as growth of the mental structure. Cognitive, the word comes from cognition meaning 'thinking' or 'ability to think'. Thinking in all ages is different as individual thinks differently in all his or her life stages. A child will not think like an adult and an adult will not think like an aged individual. It focuses on how the information is received, processed and organized in the existing schema by the student or learner. According to this theory, learning is a process that depends on learner's existing information or what he already knows.
- Cognitive theory also includes stages of development, understanding the multiple forms of intelligence, problem solving, critical thinking and creativity; for example development of children based on nature and nurture, which means what they have inherit and what they are exposed to in their environment. Developmental stages are important to understand whether the child is ready to learn. It helps the teachers to understand if the student is capable of handling certain amount of information.
- For example, a teacher would not teach literature on 'Shakespeare' to the students of class-II standard and similarly would not teach counting in class IV, as it is not at the developmentally appropriate level for the learners or students, and here both the situations will prevent students from learning. A teacher should understand that the work must happen at appropriate levels of development and understanding for their students. We should ensure that content of teaching must be developmentally apprprotiate for the individual learner.

III. Constructivist Theory:

Constructivism is based on the idea that individuals or students actively construct and teachers create a collaborative environment, where the students are actively involved in their own learning or knowledge. Here, the teacher acts as a facilitator of learning than the actual instructor. It makes students understand their previous knowledge and help them to bring their own unique experiences every day. There are some principles on which this theory is based which are as follows:

- ***Knowledge is created rather than innate, or passively absorbed:*** It states that a learner builds new knowledge on the basis of previous learning and forms new ideas. What they see and learn helps them to construct their own unique way and build something different from what another learner will build. So, the previous knowledge of a student plays a role in influencing his ideas to construct new learning experiences.
- ***People learn to learn, as they learn:*** Since learning is constructive, it helps the learner to understand other things better in future. The learning here works with some of the other concepts as well. For example, if a student is learning about the chronology of dates for a series of historical events, he or she also learns or understands the meaning of chronology. Learning one thing like this can always add new learning.

- ***Learning is an active process:*** Active learning means that a learner participates, collaborates with others and applies concepts to the real world as well. It is learner-centred, has an innovative approach and explores how one can have a more effective learning experiences. The teacher can facilitate learning through questioning, discussions and other forms of structured learning experiences that helps learners to listen, reflect, write, solve problem under the guidance of the teacher.
- ***Learning is socially constructed:*** People also learn through interactions with other people. Teachers, family, peers and acquaintances influence our learning. Social constructivism creates the reality of society where social interaction is the key to learning where group applications help students retain their knowledge.
- ***Learning is circumstantial:*** Students learn in ways involving things we already know, what they believe and more. The things one learn and the points we tend to remember are related to other things around us.
- ***Learning exists in the mind:*** Learning is more fruitful if one engages his or her mind in activities, such as hand on experiences is the key to successful learning.
- ***Knowledge is personal:*** Everyone has their own experiences and beliefs that makes knowledge personal. Therefore, each individual has their own way of learning and gaining from education.

IV. Adult Learning Theory:

- There are various theories that explains about the concepts of adult learning that has defined adult learning differently but what these theories have in common is the goal of creating an effective learning experiences for the adult learner. There are three common theories that illustrate the concept of adult learning. These are andragogy, transformational learning and experiential learning (Fig. 3.11).
- **Andragogy:** It was given by *Malcolm Knowles*, who proposed the methods and principles of adult learning. According to him, adult learners differ from children as adults are driven by internal motives and they are willing to learn when the learning is considered to be relevant to the environment. Adults use their past experiences to link learning and are independent learners. They are more task oriented and believe in learning as problem solving.
- **Transformational learning:** This theory was developed by *Jack Mezirow*, who hypothesized that adults learn when new meaning is related to a previous experience. It occurs in three stages where first is identifying a dilemma or crisis and to realize that what we know may not be right or that we do not know what we need to know. Second, establishing personal relevance to determine what is store for oneself, and the third step is about providing opportunities for critical thinking.
- **Experiential learning:** Given by *David A. Kolb* who explained that successfulness of learning is creating meaning from experiences. He conceptualized that learning occurs through concrete experience, reflective observation, abstract concepts and active experimentation. The focus is more on the learning process rather than outcomes.

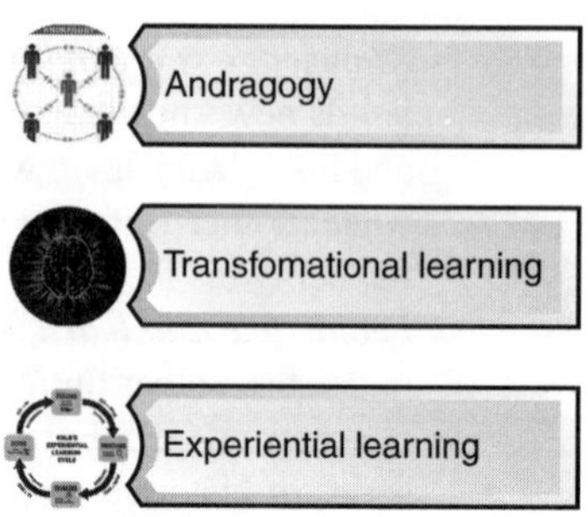

Figure 3.11

Theories of adult learning.

V. Theory of Humanism:

- This theory focuses on the personal worth of the individual, human values, dignity, creative and active nature of the human beings. This theory emphasizes human factors rather than religious, divine or spiritual matters. Humanistic approach looks at the whole person and favours concepts such as free will, self-efficacy and self-actualization.

- It transfers the power from the teacher to the students or it can be said that it encourages independent learning. This theory is about self-directed learning where students take responsibility for their own learning by creating their own realistic goals and figuring out best way to achieve them. It promotes cooperative learning and small group learning rather than competitive and large group learning. Teacher discusses and guides which tools they can use to facilitate learning. This can be achieved by organizing open seminars, individual lesson plans or presentations where the student can participate voluntarily and at an individual pace.
- The teacher can also initiate discovery education in which a teacher gives a concept to student and gives him or her the freedom to discover own way to learn more about the concept. It encourages multiple intelligences and the student explores more options for obtaining answers to gain more knowledge of the concept.

LATEST APPROACHES TO LEARNING

There are several new approaches of learning, of which few of them, such as experiential learning, reflective learning, scenario-based learning, simulation-based learning and blended learning, are discussed below.

EXPERIENTIAL LEARNING

There are several humanistic and constructive approaches to education, which postulate that learning occurs naturally through experiences. One such key experiential leaning theory is given by '*David Kolb*' popularly known as 'Kolb cycle'. He believed that experiences are critical in the development of knowledge construction, as learning occurs through discovery and active participation.

> *Kolb defined learning as 'the process whereby knowledge is created through the transformation of experience'.*
>
> **(Kolb, 1984)**

There are two parts to Kolb's Experiential Learning Theory. The first is that learning follows a four-stage cycle, as outlined in this chapter. Kolb believed that, ideally, learners progressed through the stages to complete a cycle, and, as a result, transformed their experiences into knowledge. The second part of Kolb's theory focused on learning styles, or the cognitive processes that occurred in order to acquire knowledge. Essentially, Kolb believed that individuals could demonstrate their knowledge, or the learning that occurred, when they were able to apply abstract concepts to new situations. Refer Fig. 3.12 for integrated understanding of Kolb's experiential learning cycle and learning styles.

Completion of all stages of the cycle allows the transformation of experience to knowledge to occur. Kolb's entire theory is based on this idea of converting experience into knowledge. With each new experience, the learner is able to integrate new observations with their current understanding. Ideally, learners should have the opportunity to pass through each stage.

KOLB'S FOUR STAGES OF LEARNING

Kolb's learning cycle is based on Jean Piaget's focus on the fact that learners create knowledge through interactions with the environment.

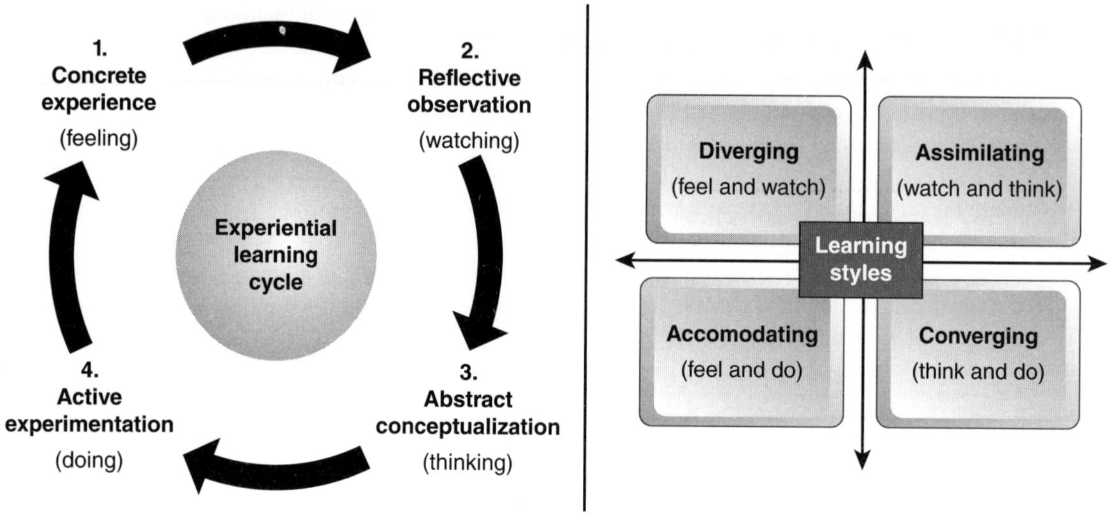

Figure 3.12

Experiential learning cycle and learning styles, based on Kolb's concepts.

1. CONCRETE EXPERIENCE (FEELING)

Kolb's learning process cycle begins with a concrete experience. This can either be a completely new experience or a reimagined experience that already happened. In a concrete experience, each learner engages in an activity or task. Kolb believed that the key to learning is involvement. It is not enough for learners to just read about it or watch it in action. In order to acquire new knowledge, learners must actively engage in the task.

2. REFLECTIVE OBSERVATION (WATCHING)

After engaging in the concrete experience, the learner steps back to reflect on the task. This stage in the learning cycle allows the learner to ask questions and discuss the experience with others. Communication at this stage is vital, as it allows the learner to identify any discrepancies between their understanding and the experience itself. Good vocabulary also allows a solid review of the events that occurred.

3. ABSTRACT CONCEPTUALIZATION (THINKING)

The next step in the learning cycle is to make sense of these events. The learner attempts to draw conclusions of the experience by reflecting on their prior knowledge, using ideas with which they are familiar or discussing possible theories with peers. The learner moves from reflective observation to abstract conceptualization when they begin to classify concepts and form conclusions on the events that occurred. This involves interpreting the experience and making comparisons to their current understanding on the concept. Concepts need not be 'new'; learners can analyse new information and modify their conclusions on already existing ideas.

4. ACTIVE EXPERIMENTATION (DOING)

This stage in the cycle is the testing stage. Learners return to participating in a task, this time with the goal of applying their conclusions to new experiences. They are able to make predictions, analyse tasks and make plans for the acquired knowledge in the future. By allowing learners to put their knowledge into practice and showing how it is relevant to their lives, you are ensuring that the information is retained in the future.

As Kolb's learning theory is cyclical, one can enter the process at any stage in the cycle. However, the cycle should then be completed in entirety to ensure that effective learning has taken place. Each stage is dependent on the others and all must be completed to develop new knowledge.

Although the stages work together to create a learning process, some individuals may prefer some components over others. While one may depend heavily on concrete and reflective experiences, they may choose to spend less time on the abstract and active stages. Because of this, Roger Fry worked with Kolb to identify four unique learning styles.

KOLB'S LEARNING STYLES

1. **Diverging (Feel and Watch):** These people can look at things differently. They are sensitive. They are sensitive and prefer to watch more than they do. They excel at seeing concrete situations from multiple perspectives. This style Kolb called Diverging because they are better at generating ideas, such as brainstorming. People who have a Diverging learning style are open to new ideas and have broad cultural interests. Diverging learners are curious about people and have strong artistic and creative skills. The Diverging style is more comfortable working in groups and listening to others. They also prefer to get personal feedback.
2. **Assimilating (Think and Watch):** The Assimilating learning preference promotes a clear and logical approach. Ideas and concepts are more valuable than people. These people want a clear explanation and not just a practical opportunity. These people excel at understanding large amounts of information and organizing it in a clear and logical manner. People who have an Assimilating learning style are less interested in people and more interested in ideas and abstract concepts. This learning style attracts people who are more interested in logically sound theories and not approaches that have practical value. These types of people are important for information and science careers. These people prefer to read, listen, analyse and think through things informal learning settings.
3. **Converging (Think and Do):** People who use a Converging learning approach can solve problems, and they will apply what they have learned to solve real-world problems. They are more concerned about technical tasks than people and interpersonal aspects. People with a Converging learning approach are better at finding practical ways to apply ideas and theories. They can solve problems, make decisions and find solutions by combining knowledge and experience. People with a Converging learning approach are more inclined to solve technical problems and social issues than those who have an interpersonal or social learning style. Converging learning styles allow for technology and specialist skills. People with a Converging learning style love to experiment with new ideas and to create simulations. They also enjoy working with practical applications.
4. **Accommodating (Feel and Do):** Accommodating learning style is hands-on and relies on intuition more than logic. These people do not trust the opinions of others, prefer practical and experiential approaches and tend to use analysis from other people. These people are drawn to new challenges and opportunities, and they enjoy executing plans. They are more inclined to act on their intuition

than on logic. People with an Accommodating learning approach will rely more on others for information than they do on their own analysis. This learning style can be useful for those who need to take initiative and act. Accommodating learners are more comfortable working in teams to accomplish their tasks.

BENEFITS OF EXPERIENTIAL LEARNING

- It creates real-world relevance.
- It provides opportunity for creativity.
- It provides opportunity for reflection.
- It teaches the value of mistakes.
- It accelerates learning.
- It guides students towards the future.
- It prepares students for adult life.
- It enhances teamwork.
- It improves communication skills.

REFLECTIVE LEARNING

The process of reflection occurs in many aspects of our lives; whether it is personal or professional, the events of the weekend or a recent problem we encountered and how we might have handled the situation differently.

In a professional context, 'reflection' often means critically assessing the ways in which we can improve upon a certain task or performance, how we cope with certain situations, or even how we interact with people we meet. Some of the **meaning, definitions and description of reflective learning** have been given below:

- *Reflective learning* is a kind of learning practice encompassing stepping back from one's learning experience in order to develop critical thinking skills and progress on future performance via analysing past experience.
- *Reflective learning* is a form of education in which students reflect upon their learning experiences and think about how they can further improve in future.
- According to researchers from Kent University, *reflective learning* derives from students' experiences and could be constantly updated.
- *Reflective learning* involves students thinking about what they have read, done or learned, relating the lesson at hand to their own lives and making meaning out of the material. It is more than just memorizing some facts, formulas or dates.

REFLECTIVE LEARNING THEORIES

There are many notable individuals who have proposed their own theories of reflective learning. We will, however, focus on three individuals who are probably the most popular among reflective practitioners.

- ***John Dewey*** is a renowned name in education. Dewey believed that reflection was essential before action. Dewey also advocated that students think about and reflect upon what they read or encounter so that they can better apply the knowledge.

- ***Donald Schon*** had a close look at Dewey and his theories. He believed that there were two types of reflection:
  - *Reflection-on-action:* It is an unconscious event that deals with the knowledge we use to solve problems and carry out actions.
  - *Reflection-in-action:* It occurs as the action is happening. Also, reflection-in-action is when you look back at what you are doing as you do it.
- ***David Kolb*** also talked about reflective observation in his theory of experiential learning. Where he has highlighted two key learning styles, i.e. diverging (feel and watch) and assimilation (thin and watch) and mentioned that the watching is a component of reflection. Thus, Kolb's cycle of learning also includes principle component of reflection.
- ***Graham Gibbs*** gave the most famous model of reflective learning, which includes six cyclic sequential steps of reflecting on an experience, that is description, feeling, evaluation, analysis, conclusion and action plan. This model is popularly known as Gibbs' reflective cycle. As it is the most famous and commonly used theory for reflective learning, it is described in detail in this chapter.

GIBBS' REFLECTIVE CYCLE

Gibbs' reflective cycle is a self-reflection and management tool that helps people to think clearly and systematically about the different experiences they have gone through during specific activity or similar situation and draw conclusions.

Graham Gibbs' plan was to use different stages to describe the situation and make sense of the cycle. He believed that people learned from their experiences and if they did not think about how to do better next time then they were not learning anything from the experience. Gibbs' reflective cycle is one of the important teaching and learning methods that describe the situation and help people to make sense, understand and reflect on how to do better next time.

Reflective learning emphasizes that learning derives from our experiences and can be constantly updated through the process of recording and thinking about the experiences we have. A very important aspect of reflective learning is that it is a process in which we can learn about ourselves. Gibbs' reflective cycle identifies six stages of reflection which help students to make sense of their learning experiences. The six stages of Gibbs' reflective cycle are description, feelings, evaluation, analysis, conclusion and action plan that are described below (Fig. 3.13):

I. ***Step-1: Description:*** In this reflective practice, people describe the situation or their experience. This is not the stage to draw conclusions but to know what has happened. The focus is on the relevant information that will provide a factual description of the situation. This stage helps to create a suitable background for understanding the incident.

   Take the help of the following questions to know about the situations in the description part of the Gibbs' reflective cycle:
   - What happened?
   - Where and when did it happen?
   - Why were you there?
   - What did you do?
   - What did other people do?
   - Who was present?
   - What was the outcome of the situation?
   - What did you want to happen?

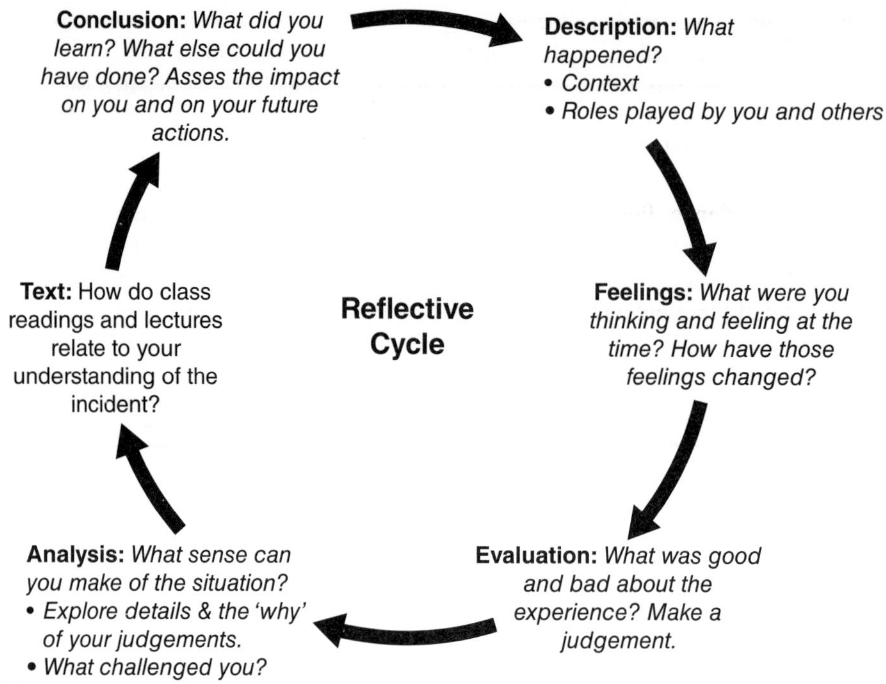

Figure 3.13

Gibbs' reflective cycle. *Source: Oviawe, J. Application of Graham Gibbs Model of Reflection to Improve Teaching Understanding among Technical Education Students in Ambrose Alli University Ekpoma Edo State. 2020. 3. 2617-1201.*

II. ***Step-2: Feelings:*** The second step of Gibbs' reflective cycle is feelings and here people describe their thoughts and description feelings and how it has shown an impact on their experiences. This step is meant to explore your thoughts about the situations and by asking yourself some important questions:

- What were your feelings before this situation?
- What were your feelings during this situation?
- What do you think other people felt during this situation?
- What did you feel after this situation?
- What do you think about the situation now?
- What do you think other people will feel about this situation now?

III. ***Step-3: Evaluation:*** In the third step of Gibbs' reflective cycle, people evaluate their experience positively or negatively both good and bad about the situation. This is the step where you have to be objective and understand what worked in your favour and what did not.

Take the help of the following questions to know about the situations in the evaluation part of Gibbs' reflective cycle:

- What was positive about this situation?
- What was negative about this situation?
- What went well in this situation?

- What did not do so well in this situation?
- What did you do to contribute to this situation? (positively or negatively)
- What did other people do to contribute to this situation? (positively or negatively)

IV. ***Step-4: Analysis:*** The fourth step of Gibbs' reflective cycle is analysis, and here people think, feel and try to make sense of the situation and understand what happened. Earlier a person was focused on details but now is the chance to think and extract meaning from the situation and experience. People who want to include academic literature can do so at this stage. This is the stage to learn what went well and helped the situation or what the cause of the misstep was.

Take the help of the following questions to know about the situations in the analysis part of Gibbs' reflective cycle:

- Why did things go well in this situation?
- Why did not things go well in this situation?
- What sense can you make of this situation?
- What knowledge can help to understand this situation?
- What knowledge of other people can help to understand this situation?

V. ***Step-5: Conclusion:*** The fifth step of Gibbs' reflective cycle is conclusions, and here people think about what they have learned and what could have been done differently. This is the section to come to conclusions by understanding and concluding what are the actions that could have improved the result in the future.

Take the help of the following questions to know about the situations in the conclusion stage:

- What did I learn from this situation?
- How could it have been a more positive situation for everyone?
- What skills do I need to develop to handle this type of situation in a better way in future?
- What else could I have done to better this experience?

VI. ***Step-6: Action Plan:*** The sixth and last step of Gibbs' reflective cycle is action plan, and here people describe how they will deal with similar situations in future and how to do better next time. This is the stage to make changes and come up with a plan to do things differently in future.

Take the help of the following questions to know about the situations in the action plan stage:

- If I had to do the same thing what will my action plan be and what will I do differently?
- How will I develop the required skills that I will need to handle similar situations?
- How can I make sure that I will act differently the next time in similar situations?

BENEFITS OF REFLECTIVE LEARNING

The common benefits of reflective learning approach are:

- Record your development
- Know your strengths and weaknesses
- Understand how you learn
- Develop self-awareness
- Plan your own development
- Learn about yourself
- Articulate your skills/learning to others
- Learn from your mistakes

SCENARIO-BASED LEARNING

Scenario-based learning (SBL) uses interactive scenarios to support active learning strategies such as problem-based or case-based learning. It normally involves students working their way through a storyline, usually based around an ill-structured or complex problem, which they are required to solve. In the process, students must apply their subject knowledge, critical thinking and problem-solving skills in a safe, real-world context. SBL is often nonlinear and can provide numerous feedback opportunities to students based on the decisions they make at each stage in the process.

SBL usually works best when applied to tasks requiring decision-making and critical thinking in complex situations. Tasks that are routine to the students will require little critical thinking or decision-making and may be better assessed using other methods. The **meaning, definitions and description of SBL** are as given below:

- *SBL* is an immersive learning environment where learners meet realistic work challenges and get realistic feedback as they progress, since everything that happens reflects the learner's choices.
- *SBL* is a teaching strategy that involves real-world scenarios to create an immersive, relatable learning experience for learners.
- *SBL* is based on the principle that knowledge is best retained when it is used in context. By working through scenarios, learners can apply critical thinking to decision-making in complex situations – improving understanding, retention and recall.

TYPES OF SCENARIOS

There are several types of scenarios and teachers need to choose the best-fit scenario for the particular teaching–learning situation to ensure seamless, smooth, effortless learning and skill development for the learners. Some of the important scenarios are detailed below:

- ***Skill-based scenario:*** In this scenario, the learner is expected to demonstrate skills and knowledge he has already acquired.
- ***Problem-based scenario:*** This type of scenario is ideal for situations where learners have to integrate their theoretical and practical knowledge to investigate a problem. Decision-making, logical reasoning and critical analyses are integral components of these scenarios.
- ***Issue-based scenario:*** In this type of a scenario, learners get to take a stand on issues, usually with humanitarian perspectives, and explore these issues to an extent that they can understand their effect on decision-making in professional spheres.
- ***Speculative scenario:*** In this scenario, learners have to predict the outcome of an event in the future based on their knowledge and understanding.
- ***Gaming scenario:*** These scenarios involve the use of games as learning tools.
- ***Mini or basic SBL:*** This is used to validate the learner's recall and basic comprehension (essentially for basic problem solving).
- ***Complex or branching SBL:*** This is used to validate the learner's proficiency to apply the learning and practice for proficiency gain.

STEPS TO BUILD AN EFFECTIVE AND ENGAGING SCENARIO

SBL does require planning and time to develop an effective and engaging scenario. *SBL* development is different from the traditional approach and the steps in developing SBL are as follows:

1. ***Know your learners:*** You need to get to know your audience, the students who will be learning. Asking whether they are just starting at their course or are seniors who have been around for a

while will determine the prior knowledge they have. Furthermore, it is important to find what they expect from the learning intervention, if it is to acquire a new skill or simply improve on something they know. Furthermore, it is important to know aspirations of the learners. Generally, students learn because they want to be better version of self tomorrow and reach to their new goals.

2. **Identify the learning outcomes:** Learning outcomes are the goals of the course. These are the objectives (one or more) that particular course sets out to achieve. Of course, the choice depends on the needs of the learners. If as teacher you know your target audience/learner well, you can determine their needs accurately and formulate the outcomes accordingly. Consider the following questions when identifying learning outcomes:
   - What do you expect your learners to experience after they complete the course?
   - What job needs will the course fulfil?
   - What are the situations where the learners will be expected to apply their knowledge?

     This is also the step in which you need to take a look at what the challenging situations are, how frequently they happen and how important they are. Since SBL focuses on real-life issues, these are the best sources for inspiration.
3. ***Decide on your format:*** Is your scenario going to be delivered in the face-to-face or online environments? What media (photographs, audio, video) and other resources will you need? If you are using an online scenario, will you provide other supporting activities, such as wikis and discussion forums?
4. ***Choose a situation for the scenario:*** There may be ample critical situations at the workplace where your learners will be expected to apply their knowledge. But you cannot or should not turn every situation into a scenario. Neither will every situation lend itself to this instructional treatment. So how should you choose a situation to turn it into a scenario?
   - Prioritize critical or challenging situations.
   - Choose nonroutine tasks that do not crop up at the workplace frequently, so learners do not have the chance to exercise their knowledge.
   - Determine how involved the learner needs to be in a situation before creating a scenario from it. In a real-life critical situation at the workplace, the learner may not have to make some high-level decisions. So it is futile to create decision points for these within your scenario. In fact, you may not even want to have a scenario for this topic. Too much interaction can be an overkill!
   - Determine if a scenario can provide the requisite level of interaction that a situation demands. A scenario is akin to a practice activity; it recreates reality within a virtual environment where learners can learn and hone their skills. These practice sessions should compel learners to think and act in a way they would do if they face these situations in real life.
   - Determine if there is an inherent conflict in the situation. The primary goal of a scenario is to teach learners how to resolve a problem. If everything is hunky-dory at their workplaces, why would the learners take your course?
5. ***Write the scenario:*** *SBL* relies heavily on narrative. Each scenario tells a unique story with characters, setting, plot, challenge and resolution. For many designers, crafting the story at the heart of a scenario poses a challenge. The best scenario stories feel authentic, relatable and realistic to the learners. We try to put them in situations they will face on the job. When selecting timing for the scenario components, connect them to specific outcomes for the entire blend. *Here is what to keep in mind:*
   - *Identify a realistic trigger event:* The trigger event sets the scene for the scenario to unfold and a problem or conflict to come to the fore. Of course, the trigger event has to mirror the reality of the learners. Some likely trigger events are activating code blue in the hospital or activating a disaster mock drill alert.

- *Create a believable and relatable protagonist:* The protagonist in your scenario is supposed to inspire the learners to modify or change their behaviour. So he should walk, talk, act and dress in a way that learners can relate to.
- *Give learners space to reflect:* The value of scenarios lies not only in the process of completing the activity but also the opportunity to reflect on the results and learn from mistakes. Learners need to have the opportunity to debrief on their experience. What steps did they take in the scenario? What did they learn from that particular pathway? What did missteps teach them? The instructional design team needs to ensure that learners meet the defined objective. If learners cannot reach the desired end goal, go back to the drawing board and tweak the scenario as needed.

6. ***Discover all possible scenario solutions:*** Learners will navigate a scenario in more than one way. Designers need to contemplate out all the pathways learners may take through the process, account for them and map them out. When planning a scenario, we wonder about things like: 'Is there only one answer? How do I get them to that answer if we designed a choose-your-own adventure? Do we care how learners reach the right answer? How much guidance do we give to get them there? How realistic is this to the job learners do?'
7. ***Peer review your scenario:*** Ask colleagues to work through the scenario to ensure that it flows in the way you expect and achieves the outcomes you intended.

BENEFITS OF SCENARIO-BASED LEARNING

For Learners:

- Creates an authentic experience
- Gets to learn in a safe learning environment
- Increases learner engagement
- Increases knowledge retention
- Speeds up time to competency
- Improves knowledge application
- Allows learners to fail and learn by their own mistakes
- Builds learners' confidence

For Teachers:

- Validate the learning process effectively
- Offer support and guidance to learners as they progress
- Continually refine and improve the learning environment
- Use real-time feedback to gain an insight into learners' behaviour and decision-making
- Receive instant, detailed and accurate results

For Institute:

- *SBL* is cost-effective, efficient and proven to work
- Scenarios can be used multiple times and adapted and refined
- Learners do not require any special equipment or costly software, just a suitable device
- Training results and learner outcomes are improved

SIMULATION-BASED LEARNING

Simulations are increasingly often used in higher education settings. In health sciences and nursing education, it is used to facilitate a deeper understanding of concepts and relationships between them, advance inquiry, problem solving, decision-making and thereby competency development.

Simulation-based learning is a constructivist learning model that provides learners with an experience of working on a usually simplified simulated world or system. Simulation allows learners to experience the real world through interactive simulations and learning is most commonly done in a simulation laboratory setting. Students come for a specific period of time to engage in activities that are specifically tailored around learning objectives. These activities are then turned into simulation scenarios. The **meaning, definitions and description of simulation-based learning** are as give below:

- *Simulation-based learning* is learning or training method that is used to 'replace or amplify real experience with guided experiences'. It is not defined by a technology but rather a learning approach grounded in learning theories.
- *Simulation-based learning* is defined as any educational activity that utilizes simulation aides to replicate scenarios.
- *Simulation learning* is a strategy, which educators can use to not only teach course concepts but to also provide students with opportunities to apply new skills, knowledge and ideas in a practice setting that mirrors the real world.
- *Simulation-based learning* is the pedagogical approach of providing students with the opportunity to practice learned skills in real-life situations.

Simulation-based learning has been shown to offer the best learning outcomes in various educational and workplace settings. Providing learners with a realistic and immersive experience, the technique allows them to obtain practical insights related to a subject or job-related concept.

CHARACTERISTICS OF SIMULATIONS

Typically, simulations incorporate some or all of the following characteristics:

- **Environment:** Simulations replicate in some way an authentic situation or location, such as a pilot's cockpit, hospital room or chemistry lab. These imitation environments can be built in physical or digital spaces.
- **Scenarios:** Simulations present a problem to solve or a situation to react to in a specific context, which could include a certain time frame and/or a set of tools or resources.
- **Open-ended**: Simulations often require you to make a series of decisions. Each decision impacts the progress you make in that scenario and determines what decisions you will make next. There may be multiple potential solutions, with no one right path forward.
- **Role-playing**: Simulations often place you in a specific role within the scenario. Some require you to collaborate with learners in other roles who are working through the same problem but from different perspectives.
- **Guided participation**: Simulations are usually facilitated by an instructor who sets up the scenario and works with you or your team as you proceed. Most simulations can be paused when needed to review students' progress.
- **Reflection**: Simulations rely on structured reflection – through discussion, journaling and other assignments – to evaluate the decisions that were made, connect them to the outcomes they led to and reinforce what you learned from the experience.

Simulation is a generic term that refers to an artificial representation of a real world process to achieve educational goals through experiential learning. A simulation can be defined as a model of reality reflecting some or all of its properties. Robert Gagne identified the following properties of a simulation:

- A simulation represents a real situation in which operations are carried out.
- A simulation provides the user with certain controls over the problem or situation.
- A simulation omits certain distracting variables irrelevant or unimportant for the particular instructional goals.

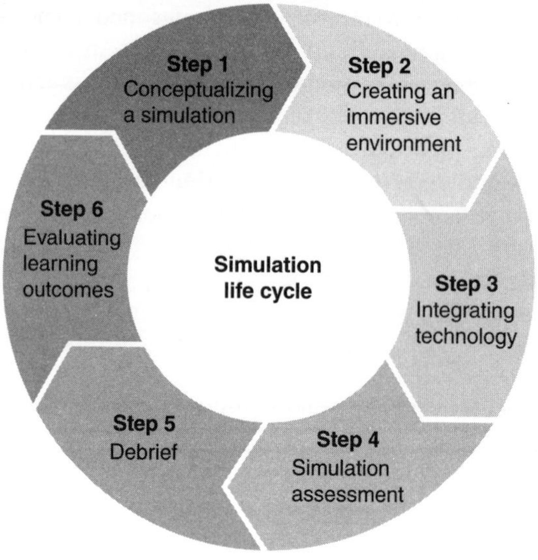

Figure 3.14

Simulation cycle.

The simulation involves conceptualization of a learning experience, formulation of simulation scenario, running simulation scenario, debriefing and evaluation. Dalhousie University has given a practical simulation cycle, which involves six different steps as illustrated in Fig. 3.14.

TYPES OF SIMULATION

The simulation or simulators in medical and nursing education can be classified in different ways. The most simplified classification is presented below and also illustrated in Fig. 3.15.

A. ***On the basis of operating system:*** There are three common types of simulations that are used:

1. ***Live:*** Simulation involving real people operating real systems.
   - Involve individuals or groups
   - May use actual equipment
   - Should provide a similar area of operations
   - Should be close to replicating the actual activity
2. ***Virtual:*** Simulation that involves real people using simulated systems. By exercising, virtual simulations insert Human-In-The-Loop into a central role:
   - Motor control skills
   - Decision skills
   - Communication skills
3. ***Constructive:*** Simulation that involves simulated people using simulated systems. While real people can stimulate (make inputs), they are not involved in the final outcome. The ability to construct simulations allows you to:
   - Analyse concepts
   - Predict possible outcomes
   - Stress large organizations
   - Make measurements

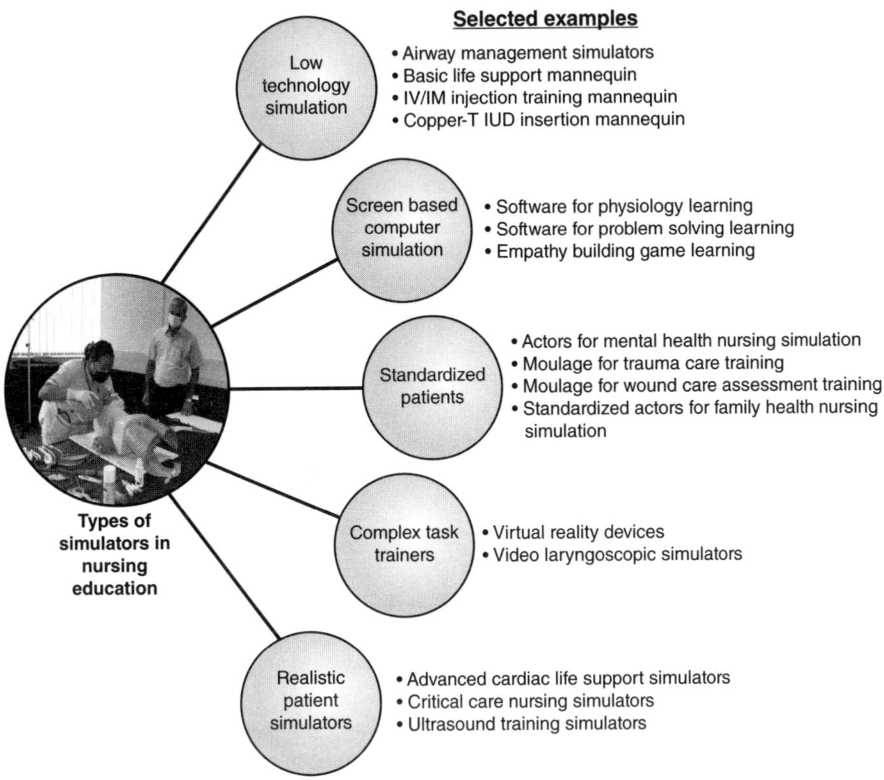

Figure 3.15

Types of simulation in nursing education.

- Generate statistics
- Carry out analysis

B. ***On the basis of simulator's use:***

- ***Physical procedures simulator:*** A simulated object, piece of equipment or machine. It works and functions like the actual physical device. It is used to teach operation of equipment or machinery.
- ***Operational simulator:*** Simulates common procedures used within an organization those are to software or object based or that contains some elements of both. It is used to teach proper steps for completing a desired task.
- ***Principle-based simulator (social simulator):*** Situation in which the learner is placed into an environment in which he or she must interact. Environment changes based on learner's actions. It is used to teach principles, soft skills, skills used when interacting with people.
- ***Problem-solving simulator:*** Learner is presented with a new problem he or she must solve. There is not a single method or process for solving the problem confronting the learner; multiple avenues are available for solving the problem. It is used to teach the learner to confront and solve a new problem amicably.

C. ***On the basis of fidelity:***

Fidelity in simulation has traditionally been defined as 'the degree to which the simulator replicates reality'. Fidelity in simulation is a multidimensional concept corresponding to the degree of realism created through the selection of simulation equipment, setting and scenario. Using this definition, simulators are labelled as 'high' 'medium' and 'low' fidelity depending on how closely they represent 'real life'.

- ***High-fidelity simulators:*** These simulations allow for maximum interaction and realistic learning in an environment that is very similar to reality. These full-body computerized manikins replicate the anatomy, physiology and behaviour of real patients. These manikins can speak, which is a great way for students to learn communication skills and problem-solving. Manikins with high fidelity can also run preprogrammed scenarios.
- ***Medium-fidelity simulators:*** These simulations offer more learning opportunities and make them more realistic. You can use full-body manikins to mimic patients with their breath sounds, bowel sounds, heart sounds and heart sounds. They allow students the opportunity to perform procedures such as intravenous cannula insertions and injections.
- ***Low-fidelity simulators:*** These simulations will feel the least real or most artificial to the learner. These simulations can be either static models or two-dimensional displays. Task trainers are categorized under low-fidelity simulators, which are used to train for specific tasks or procedures, such as intravenous insertion arms, intramuscular injection, and endotracheal tube insertion trainer.

TYPES OF FIDELITY IN SIMULATION

- ***Conceptual fidelity:*** Conceptual fidelity ensures that the scenario makes sense as close as reality, where subject matter expert review scenario to an extent to ensure highest possible conceptual fidelity. For example, signs and symptoms, lab reports, medicines and other physiological parameters are highest possible realistic to the actual situation.
- ***Physical fidelity:*** The degree to which the simulator duplicates the appearance and feel of the real system. Like appearance, anatomical landmarks and quality of skin to feel are as close as real human being.
- ***Emotional or psychological fidelity*** is the extent to which a simulation can duplicate or capture the real task by using a simulated task and make the student feel as if it is real.

BENEFITS OF SIMULATION-BASED LEARNING

- It enhances real-life experiences.
- It helps in better knowledge retention.
- It provides opportunity to get quick and prompt feedback.
- It helps improve the cooperation and teamwork abilities.
- It helps to train many learners at a time.
- It is a faster and most convenient way to improve the leaner's skills and competences.
- It provides personalized and diverse learning.
- Allows students to apply abstract concepts to active hands-on practice.
- It increases helps to ensure patient safety.
- It also helps for swift acclimatization of newly inducted nursing students to the clinical area and reducing chances of clinical placement anxiety among them.

BLENDED LEARNING

Blended learning refers to the use of both online and in-person learning opportunities when teaching students. For example, a blended-learning course might have students take a class in a traditional classroom environment and then independently complete the online parts of the course. Online learning could be used to supplement or replace class time. Students would also learn the same topics online that they did in class.

This is also known as hybrid learning or mixed-mode learning. However, blended-learning experiences can vary in design and execution.

The **meaning, definitions and description of blended learning** are as given below:

- ***Blended learning*** is an approach to learning that combines face-to-face and online learning experiences. Ideally, each (both online and offline) will complement the other by using its particular strength.
- Oxford Dictionary Definition of ***Blended learning*** is a style of education in which students learn via electronic and online media as well as traditional face-to-face teaching.
- ***Blended learning*** is an approach to education that combines online educational materials and opportunities for interaction online with traditional place-based classroom methods. It requires the physical presence of both teacher and student, with some elements of student control over time, place, path or pace.

In other words, blended learning is a term applied to the practice of providing instruction and learning experiences through some combination of both face-to-face and technology-mediated learning. During the technology-mediated components of these learning experiences, students are not required to be physically together in one place but may be connected digitally through online communities. For example, one blended learning course could involve students attending a class taught by a teacher in a traditional classroom setting while also completing online components of the course independently, outside of the classroom, on an online learning platform.

TYPES OF BLENDED LEARNING

Blended learning strategies vary according to the discipline, academic level, student characteristics, expected learning outcomes, course content, technology, learning spaces, etc. It involves a student-centred approach to the learning design. There are different ways of classification for blended learning. However, the common and most practical 12 different types of blended learning are described below:

1. **Station Rotation Blended Learning:** Station rotation blended learning is a model that allows students to rotate through stations on a fixed schedule, where at least one of the stations is an online learning station. This model is most common in elementary schools because teachers are already familiar with rotating in centres and stations. It is primarily characterized by the fixed schedule that guides the 'blending'.
2. **Lab Rotation Blended Learning**: The lab rotation model of blended learning is similar to 'Station Rotation', in which students are rotated on a fixed schedule in a dedicated computer lab, which allow for flexible scheduling arrangements with faculty to make use of existing computer labs. It is primarily characterized by the use of institute's computer labs in new ways.
3. **Remote Blended Learning (also referred to as Enriched Virtual Blended Learning):** In enriched virtual blended learning, the student's focus is on completing online coursework while only meeting with the teacher intermittently/as-needed. This approach differs from the flipped classroom model in the balance of online to face-to-face instructional time. In an enriched virtual blended learning model, students would not see/work with/learn from a teacher on a daily basis face-to-face but would in a flipped setting. It is primarily characterized by students completing coursework remotely and independently.

4. **Flex Blended Learning:** The 'Flex' is included in types of blended learning, and its model is one in which a course or subject in which online learning is the backbone of student learning, even if it directs students to offline activities at times. It is primarily characterized by its versatility to meet the needs of a variety of formal and informal learning processes (schools, organizations, homeschooling, etc.).
5. **The Flipped Classroom Blended Learning:** Perhaps the most widely known version of blended learning, a 'Flipped Classroom' is one where students are introduced to content, provided with learning resources and then they learn by their own before they come to discuss the topic/subject matter in classroom in brief to clear doubts and get complete understanding of the topic. In this method, active learning is promoted along with retaining the traditional test of teaching–learning process.
6. **Individual Rotation Blended Learning:** The individual rotation model allows students to rotate through stations but on individual schedules set by a teacher or software algorithm. Unlike other rotation models, students do not necessarily rotate to every station; they rotate only to the activities scheduled on their playlists. It is primarily characterized by the personalization of student learning as determined by individual schedules that have the chance to better meet the needs of each student.
7. **Project-Based Blended Learning:** Blended project-based learning is a model in which the student uses both online learning either in the form of courses or self-directed access and face-to-face instruction and collaboration to design, iterate and publish project-based learning assignments, products and related artefacts. It is primarily characterized by the use of online resources to support project-based learning.
8. **Self-Directed Blended Learning:** Self-directed blended learning allows students to combine online and face-to-face learning in order to lead their own personal inquiry, meet formal learning goals and connect with mentors both digitally and physically. The role of the online learning teacher and the physical teacher changes as the learning is self-directed. No formal online courses are required. It is primarily characterized by the exchange and facilitation of traditional academic work in order to facilitate student-centred inquiry.
9. **Inside-Out Blended Learning:** Inside-out blended learning is designed to help students finish and end up beyond the physical classroom. But they still need and can benefit from the unique strengths of both physical space and digital space. It is defined by student movement between physical and digital spaces.
10. **Outside-In Blended Learning:** Blended learning in outside-in is designed to start in nonacademic digital and physical environments but end inside a classroom. It is primarily characterized by student movement between digital and physical spaces; the potential authenticity of student work.
11. **Supplemental Blended Learning:** The model offers students the option of completing entirely online learning as a supplement to their daily face-to-face learning or to complete entirely face-to-face learning experiences to augment online learning. The big idea here is supplementing critical learning objectives are met entirely in one space while the opposite space provides the student with specific supplementing experiences that the other did not or could not provide.
12. **Mastery-Based Blended Learning:** Students alternate between face-to-face and online learning (activities assessments projects, etc.), based on the achievement of mastery-based learning goals.

The design of assessment is essential in mastery-based learning experiences. The ability to use both face-to-face and digital assessment tools can be either powerful or complex depending on the mindset of the learning designer.

ELEMENTS OF BLENDED LEARNING SYSTEM

Fig. 3.16 presents a diagram that outlines all the components of the blended learning system framework. There are six elements in the system, all with their own subsystems. These six elements are:

1 **Learners**: The role of learners changes, or adapts, as learners engage for the first time or in new ways with the elements in the system. Most important is the well-researched change from passive to active learner. This is key to the support and training of lifelong learners, a characteristic identified as important in 21st-century society.
2. **Teachers**: The role of teachers is also new in blended environments and will coevolve with students as both engage with and adapt to each other and the other four elements in the system. The teachers will be identified by new labels, such as facilitators, mentors, advisors and moderators.

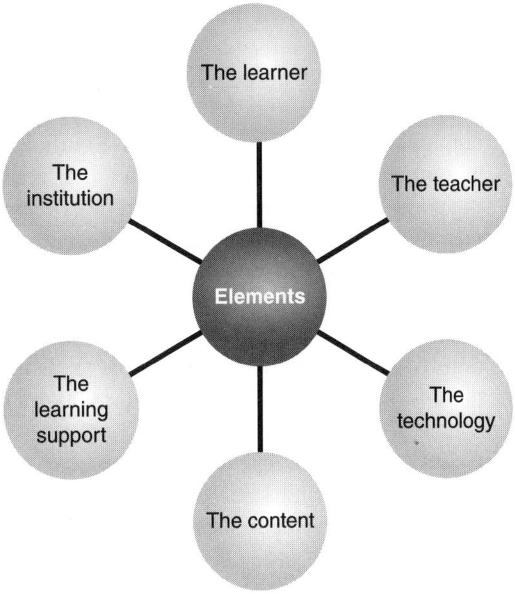

Figure 3.16

Elements of blended learning.

3. **Content:** Subject matter is still an important influence on the delivery of learning. Content refers to subject matter and the material elements used to engage learners in the process of mastering that subject. The interactive, dynamic, media-rich materials available online create opportunities for teachers and learners to add content before, during and even after the course experience. The dynamic between the learner, the teacher, the technology, the learning support and the institution impacts the choice and use of content.
4. **Technology:** Technology in general terms refers to any equipment or mechanism that extends the human capacity to get things done, the creation and use of technical means and their interrelation with life. In this theoretical framework, the technology has to be seen as part of the system of blended learning, one that includes all elements working in relation to each other.
5. **Learners Support**: Helping learners master the content and become competent learners has to be part of their education. Support can involve technology troubleshooting, material access and learning to communicate effectively online, as well as all the other usual support around understanding content and assignments.
6. **Institution:** Just as classroom-based learning requires buildings, desks, lighting and other accessories of brick-and-mortar institutions, blended learning requires technological infrastructure.

PREREQUISITES OF BLENDED LEARNING

Building an effective blended learning classroom requires careful planning and preparation. The following best practices are helpful in creating a successful blended classroom environment:

1. **A Comprehensive Learning Management System:** A comprehensive learning management system (LMS) is a prerequisite for creating an immersive learning environment. It should serve as

a central repository of information (i.e. course material, assignments, web resources, etc.) open for access and use to all students.

2. **A Well-Defined Course Outline:** At the very outset, teachers must prepare a definite course outline to guide learners. They must lay out course content and structure and the tools to be employed for instruction. The course outline should include course resources, objectives, assignment details, assessments and their grading percentage. Teachers must also clearly define the parts of the material that would be covered online and those that would form part of classroom meetings. They must also clearly state hardware and software requirements.
3. **Clear Learning Objectives:** Teachers must identify and define clear learning objectives to help students understand what they can expect from a course. There should be adequate clarity in establishing how to 'blend' online with the established methods of teaching. To determine course objectives, teachers must identify the skills that the learners should develop during the course; the information to be included; and the types of training tools and activities that form part of the course.
4. **Consistent Aesthetics:** The basic structure and layout of the LMS should be consistent with adequate visual and graphic elements to aid understanding. There should be uniformity in terms of the format of videos, assignments, games, etc., helping learners navigate through the course material without getting confused. This goes on to boost the overall readability and student engagement.
5. **Good Communication:** Effective communication between the teacher and students needs to be established to achieve improved learning outcomes in a blended learning programme. There should be an adequate exchange of queries and feedback with regular classroom discussions. Teachers can provide their contact information and encourage students to communicate in case of queries and concerns to establish a favourable rapport. Towards the end of a course, they can also engage learners in live or online surveys, evaluations and opinions on the quality of the course and its delivery.
6. **A Well-Trained Teacher:** A blended learning course necessitates the proper teacher training to facilitate optimal learning. They must understand student needs and accordingly design courses. Since blended classrooms can be difficult to plan and manage, teachers must also be trained in management strategies tailored for such classrooms. They must be well-versed with the technology required to execute blended learning, and thus need training on software and hardware management as well.
7. **Motivation:** Students need adequate motivation when engaging in a wide range of often shifting learning modalities, some of which may require significant skill development.
8. **Safety and Security**: Create awareness of cyber-malice and ensure security interventions against unethical learning practices, academic dishonesty, identity theft and bullying are in place.

BENEFITS OF BLENDED LEARNING

- It provides the opportunity to make a clear roadmap for students, as well as teachers can visualize and track each student's progress.
- It allows access the content from anywhere, anytime, on any device.
- It increases user engagement easily.
- It helps to get insightful reports about your learners.
- It makes easier to individualize learning modules based on competency.
- It enhances knowledge retention.

- It increases satisfaction and effectiveness.
- It enhances peer support.
- It enhances skills like relating well to others, time management, critical thinking, communication and team cooperation.
- It is also cost-efficient.

MEANING OF TEACHING

Teaching is a form of interpersonal influence aimed at changing the behavior potential of another person.

—American Educational Research Association Commission

Teaching is stimulation, guidance, direction and encouragement of learning.

—Burton

Teaching refers to activities that are designed and performed to produce change in student behavior.

—Clarke

Teaching is the means whereby the society trains the young in specific or selective environment as quickly as possible to adjust themselves to the world in which they live.

—Yoakm and Simpson

Teaching is concerned with growth and development of whole personality of the student—her mind, character and effective behavior.

—Thomas P. Green

Teaching is an arrangement and manipulation of situation in which there are gap and obstruction which an individual will seek to overcome and from which he/she will learn in the course of doing so.

—Johan Brubacher

CONCEPTS OF TEACHING

I. TRADITIONAL CONCEPT

Teaching used to be the act of imparting instructions and feeding the learner's mind with information in classroom situations. It emphasized on imparting instructions to learners in a classroom setting. In traditional classroom teaching, the teacher gives information to students or students can read from a textbooks. This method of teaching is not accepted by modern educators.

II. MODERN CONCEPT

Modern education has brought the child to the focus of the educative process. Teaching motivates the student to learn and acquire desired knowledge, skills and also desirable ways of living in the society. It is the process where the learner, teacher, curriculum and other variables are organized in a systematic and psychological way to attain some predetermined goals.

Following are some of the key views about the concept and meaning of education:

Gage's view

Teaching is a form of inter-personal influence aimed at changing the behavior potential of another person.

Ryburn's view

Teaching is a relationship which keeps the child to develop at his powers.

Brubacher's view

Teaching is an arrangement and manipulation of a situation in which there are gaps and obstructions which an individual will seek to overcome and from which he will learn in the course of doing so.

Green's view

Teaching is the task of teacher which is performed for the development of a child.

Morrison's view

Teaching is an intimate contact between a more mature personality and less mature one which is designed to further the education of the learner.

Smith's view

Teaching is a system of actions intended to produce learning.

Burton's view

Teaching is the stimulation, guidance, direction and encouragement of learning.

Hug and Duncan's view

Teaching is an activity – a unique, professional, rational human activity in which one creatively and imaginatively uses himself and his knowledge to promote the learning and welfare of others.

Sir Johan Adam's view

The teacher is maker of man.

H.G. Wells' view

Teacher is real maker of history.

NATURE OF TEACHING

Teaching has been viewed differently in different eras by different philosophers/educationists in different regions of the universe. The basic nature of teaching is discussed below:

- **Teaching is a tripolar process:** Teaching is tripolar process (Fig. 3.17). The three interconnected poles are teacher, pupil and subject matter.
- **Teaching is an interactive process:** Teaching is an interactive process. Interaction means participation of the teacher and student for mutual benefit to achieve objectives.
- **Teaching takes place at multiple levels:** There are multiple levels of teaching such as memory level, understanding level and reflective level.
- **Teaching must be planned:** Teaching is a planned activity. It is a systematic and organized process.
- **Teaching needs effective reciprocal communication:** Teaching can be made effective through the process of

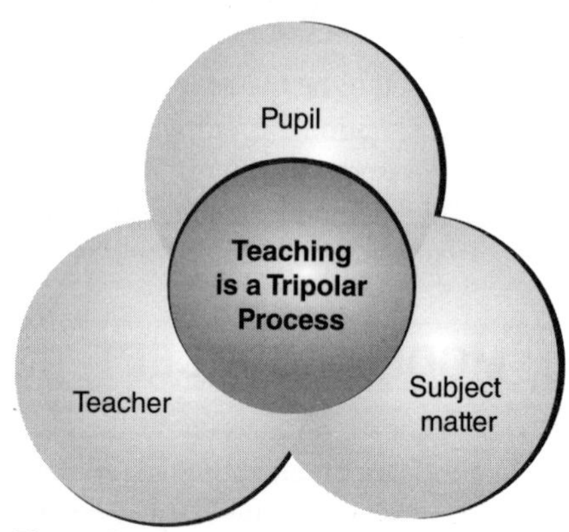

Figure 3.17

Teaching is a tripolar process.

communication. Various communication skills dominate the process of teaching as it is between two or more persons influencing each other by their ideas.

- **Teaching is the motivation to learn:** Burton considers teaching as the stimulation, guidance, direction and encouragement for learning.
- **Teaching is guidance:** Students are guided to learn the right things in the right manner and at the right time through teaching.
- **Teaching is a professional activity:** Teaching is a professional activity involving the teacher and the student resulting in student development.
- **Teaching is an art as well as science:** Teaching is a science as well as an art. The teacher has to adapt to various situations by using different techniques. Children are the raw materials the teacher has to deal with. A teacher's work is nothing less than that of an artist. Teaching has architectural functions to perform. It also involves art in the selection of proper techniques. The art of teaching is the ability to choose correct techniques at the right time.
- **Teaching helps attain information, knowledge and skills:** Teaching helps the learner attain information, knowledge of facts and skills for future use.

CHARACTERISTICS OF GOOD TEACHING

Teaching is a form of interpersonal influence aimed at changing the behaviour potential of another person and has the following main characteristics (Fig. 3.18):

- **Planned and systematic:** Good teaching is always planned and systematic. Planning involves careful selection, division and systematic revision of the subject matter.

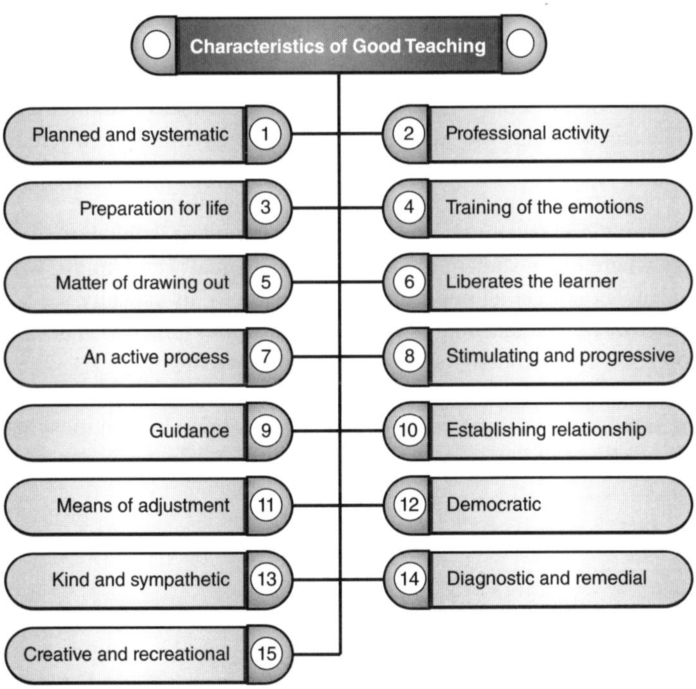

Figure 3.18

Characteristics of good teaching.

- **Professional activity:** Teaching is a professional activity involving the teacher and students and results in student development'.
- **Preparation for life activities:** Good teaching helps the child develop physically, emotionally and spiritually to enable him to participate in life activities. According to Ryburn, 'teaching is a means of preparation and helping the pupil to live his life fully at a particular stage, it is also helping him to prepare for the future'.
- **Training the emotions:** According to Ryburn, teaching should include training the child's emotions. Good teaching helps the students channelize and sublimate their emotions through activities like drama, singing, painting and games.
- **Matter of drawing out:** Good teaching is matter of drawing out rather than putting in anything. It provides suitable environment and activities for the development of a child's natural capacities.
- **Liberates the learner:** Successful teaching liberates and widens the intellectual horizon of the students. The ideal of good teaching is to liberate the student's mind from any fear he may incidentally feel and develop independence in thought and method of procedure so that he may able to solve his problems independently and work out solutions.
- **An active process:** Good teaching emphasizes the importance of active participation in learning.
- **Stimulating and progressive:** Good teaching inspires and stimulates students for independent study, self-development and self-advancement.
- **Giving guidance:** Guidance is the core of teaching. The teacher guides the students to the right path. As Burton rightly remarked, 'teaching is the stimulation, guidance, direction and encouragement of learning'.
- **Establishing relationship:** Teaching is a tripolar process comprising the teacher, students and the subject. Hence the teacher has to know:
  - The nature of students, their individual differences in terms of abilities, aptitudes, interests, achievements and emotional development.
  - Himself through his feelings for students, knowledge and method of the teaching–learning process.
  - The subject and its orderly presentation to enable the students quickly grasp it.
- **Means of adjustment:** Good teaching helps students adjust themselves to their environment in an effective manner. The teacher helps the students adjust to the environment where they live in.
- **Democratic:** Good teaching is democratic. A good teacher creates a democratic environment in the class and provides opportunities for democratic training of the students.
- **Kind and sympathetic:** Good teaching is sympathetic and kind. It is the duty of a good teacher to provide situations where every student is treated sympathetically and kindly without room for scolding. Every student should get an opportunity to develop to his capacity.
- **Diagnostic and remedial:** Good teaching is both diagnostic and remedial. The teacher knows the difficulties and problems of the students with a view to remove them.
- **Creative and recreational:** Good teaching proves to be a source of creativeness and recreation. It awakens a desire in the learners to be creative and engages them in activities that are a source of pleasure to them. According to Silverman, 'a good teacher like a doctor is one who adds creativity and inspiration to basic activity'.

PRINCIPLES OF TEACHING

Teaching principles help teachers develop an insight regarding their strengths and weaknesses and provide information pertaining to teaching like:

- Whom to teach?
- Why to teach?

- Where to teach?
- What to teach?
- How to teach?
- When to teach?

The principles of teaching are discussed under two subheadings: general and psychological principles (Fig. 3.19).

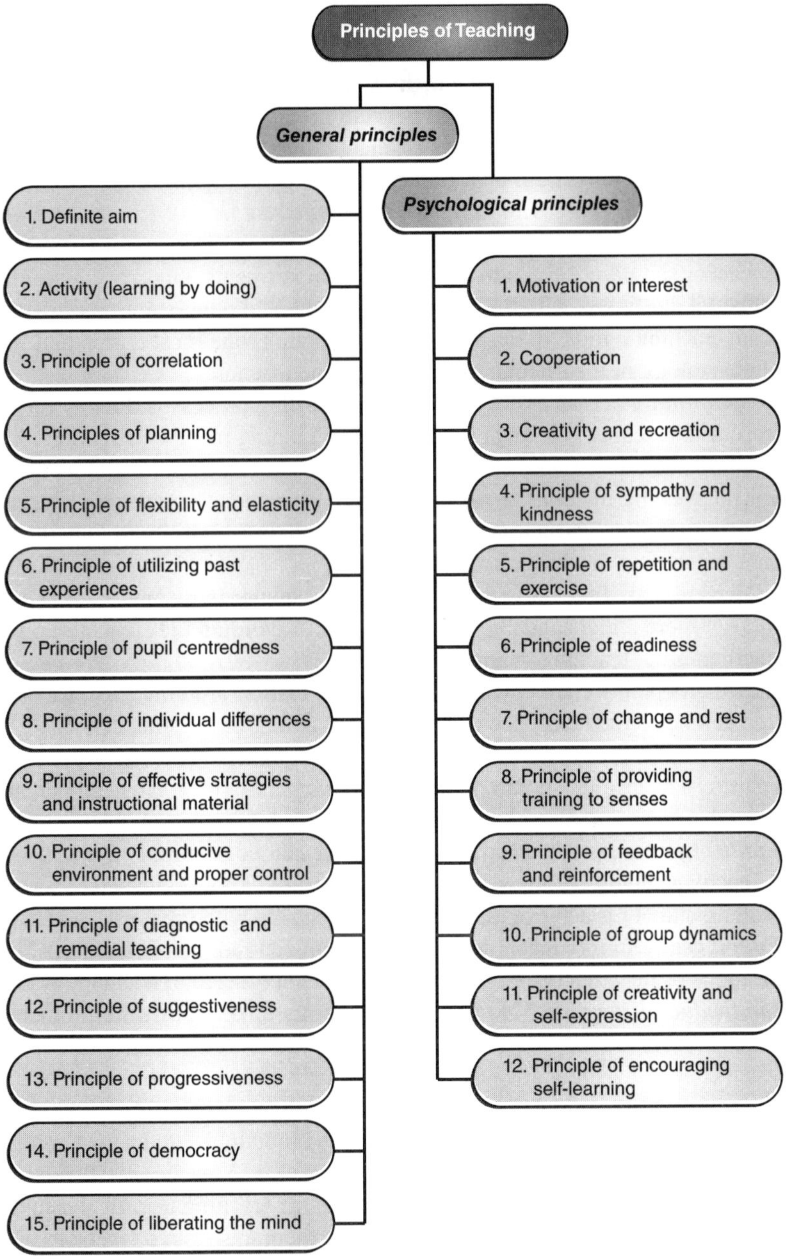

Figure 3.19

Principles of teaching.

I. GENERAL PRINCIPLES OF TEACHING

- ***Definite aim:*** Teaching should start with a definite aim that is of great help to both the teacher and the student. It makes the teaching and learning interesting, effective, precise and definite. Without definite aim, the teacher might go astray and his teaching might lack coherence and definiteness. The students do not gain much if the lesson plan is haphazardly and aimlessly planned. Without definite aim, even the best lesson would fail to achieve its objectives.
- ***Activity (learning by doing):*** Teaching is effective when students actively participate in the lesson. Learning becomes active and quicker if the student is physically as well as mentally active. Students learn through self-activity but the activity must be psychologically sound. Learning by doing removes the dullness of the lesson and puts children in life situations. The child engages himself fully and learns qualitatively as well as quantitatively. Teaching should be organized to provide the child with the maximum opportunity to learn by doing.
- ***Principle of correlation (linking with actual life and other subjects):*** Life and learning should become two poles of the same magnet; they are interdependent and cannot exist without one another. The teacher should not teach in water-tight compartments. Good teaching implies that learning must be vitally linked with the life of the learners and other subjects of their syllabus. For example, before teaching a topic in medical–surgical nursing, one must correlate it with the basic anatomy and physiology of a particular system.
- ***Principles of planning:*** The success of the teaching–learning process is directly proportional to planning. Successful teaching is always well planned. Planning involves selection, division and revision.
  - *Selection:* The teaching material should be carefully selected. The teaching material should be selected according to the instructional objectives, the teacher's ability to impart knowledge and the learner's capacity to digest the subject matter.
  - *Division:* Division makes breaking the chosen subject matter into convenient and meaningful units to make it more understandable. The technique of dividing the subject into units and subunits facilitates the teaching–learning process.
  - *Revision:* Drill and practice are essential for the assimilation of knowledge. Revision helps assimilation and helps the teacher to test the understanding of his students.
- ***Principle of flexibility and elasticity:*** Teaching should not be rigid and stereotyped. It should be flexible and elastic. The teacher should be resourceful, original, imaginative and creative enough to adapt himself to the requirements of the students and the teaching–learning situation.
- ***Principle of utilizing past experiences:*** New knowledge can be acquired on the basis of past experiences. Teaching should be linked with already acquired knowledge and experiences. It facilitates teaching and helps achieve the stipulated objectives with great ease and economy.
- ***Principle of pupil centredness:*** Teaching should be pupil centred, that is the needs, interests, abilities, aspirations of the students should be given due importance in teaching.
- ***Principle of individual differences:*** No two individuals are alike. They differ in their attitudes, abilities, interests, achievements, aims, ambitions and aspirations. Some are slow learners and some are quick learners. Good teaching always respects the individuality of students. By considering each student as a unique individual, the teacher can pay attention to individual differences and develop strategies to cater to the educational needs of the individual student.
- ***Principle of effective strategies and instructional material:*** The teacher must take care to choose appropriate strategies, devices and instructional material for teaching a particular topic/subject. For example, to teach foetal circulation, the teacher can use diagrams or live videos to make teaching more effective.

- ***Principle of conducive environment and proper control:*** Conducive environment and proper control facilitate teaching and learning. Various factors can affect the teaching–learning process, such as teacher, principal, teacher–teacher, principal–teacher and pupil–teacher relationship, group dynamics, classroom interaction, discipline, room temperature, light, ventilation, cleanliness and seating arrangement.
- ***Principle of diagnostic and remedial teaching:*** In successful teaching, it is necessary that a teacher should know the difficulties and problems of the students with a view to remove them. Successful teacher is that who is able to remove the difficulties of the students and solve their problems.
- ***Principle of suggestiveness:*** Good teaching proceeds on the basis of suggestion rather than direction. The teacher suggests activities, materials and modes of responses. Suggestions help in securing cooperation of the pupils. Good teachers give suggestions instead of giving orders.
- ***Principle of progressiveness:*** The ultimate aim of the education is overall development and progress of the child. Therefore, good teaching always strives for progressiveness of the child towards development of skills, abilities, attitude and interest in essential domain of personal and professional life.
- ***Principle of democracy:*** Each individual is entitled to equal rights. The teacher should create a democratic environment in the class. Students should not be taught with their caste, creed or religion in mind.
- ***Principle of liberating the mind:*** The ideal of good teaching is to liberate the mind of students from any fear, which he may incidentally feel and to develop independence in thought and method of procedure so that he may be able to solve his problems independently and work out solutions.

II. PSYCHOLOGICAL PRINCIPLES OF TEACHING

- ***Motivation or interest:*** Teaching is directed towards promoting learning through motivating the learner or creating an interest in learning. Motivation is the key to the success of learning. Furthermore, motivation is like a petrol engine that drives the psychological engine. The teacher should properly motivate the students by creating interesting learning situations.
- ***Cooperation:*** Teaching is a cooperative affair between the teacher and the students. Poor cooperation leads to a poor teaching–learning process.
- ***Creativity and recreation:*** Teaching is not to be continued as a routine affair but should arouse creativeness in the child. A sense of creativeness brings interest and pleasure in learning among learners, which ultimately leads to effective learning. Good teaching must strive to bring creativeness and a sense of recreation in the learners.
- ***Principle of sympathy and kindness:*** Successful teaching cannot take place in a situation that lacks sympathy and kindness with the interests and needs of the students. Students learn more when they are taught in a kind and polite manner.
- ***Principle of repetition and exercise:*** 'Practice makes a man perfect' is a well-known proverb. It applies well to the field of teaching and learning. If students are asked to repeat learning tasks, they will understand, retain and recall the subject matter more effectively.
- ***Principle of readiness:*** If students are not ready to learn, it is the teacher's duty to make them ready for learning. Teachers can choose the teaching tasks according to the student's psychology, that is their abilities, interests, attitudes, aspirations, maturation and development level.
- ***Principle of change and rest:*** Monotony fatigue and lack of attention decreases the speed of learning. Teaching–learning process followed by rest and change refreshes the mind and prepares the learners for more and effective learning.

- ***Principle of providing training to senses:*** Senses are gateways of knowledge. The power of observation, identification, discrimination, experimentation, application and generalization can be developed through proper training and functioning of the senses. The teacher should make proper arrangements for training the senses especially the senses of sight and hearing.
- ***Principle of feedback and reinforcement:*** Feedback about the progress of the student and further reinforcement are the most essential components of the teaching–learning process. Students are motivated for effective learning through timely and effective feedback and reinforcement.
- ***Principle of group dynamics:*** Group dynamics plays an important role in achievement of teaching objectives. Students tend to learn better in a group and also develop qualities of cooperation, mutual respect, sacrifice, etc. Therefore, the teacher should encourage group learning.
- ***Principle of creativity and self-expression:*** The development of the society and nation depends on creative ideas. It becomes imperative that the teacher should create situations in a classroom that inculcate creativity and self-expression in students. Usually, teachers feel happy if the students reproduce the same material in exactly the same manner. This practice can hinder a student's development and needs to be discouraged.
- ***Principle of encouraging self-learning:*** The teacher should inculcate habits of self-study, independent work and self-learning in the students by providing students with opportunities and training for this purpose.

MAXIMS OF TEACHING

The maxims of teaching may be defined as rules for presenting difficult terms and concepts to make them easy to comprehend in classroom teaching. A teacher employs some specific ways to organize teaching to make the terms and concepts communicable up to the cognition or rational process and level of learners. They are the guidelines for teaching. The maxims of teaching are very helpful in obtaining the active involvement and participation of learners in the teaching–learning process. They quicken the interest of the learners and motivate them to learn. They make students attentive to the teaching–learning process.

I. FEATURES OF MAXIMS OF TEACHING

- Maxim helps in organizing teaching–learning activities.
- It makes presentation of terms and concepts easily understandable.
- It enables teacher to make his communication for the mental level of the students.
- It is an important component of instructional procedure which is used in designing and presenting content in effective way.

II. ESSENTIAL MAXIMS OF TEACHING

Following are some of the essential maxims of teaching (Fig. 3.20):

- ***From simple to complex or easy to difficult:*** The nature of this maxim is more psychological that a child learns easy things and then proceeds towards complex things. For example, initially nursing students are taught about basic care procedures and then about complex procedures such as electrocardiogram (ECG) and central venous pressure (CVP) monitoring.

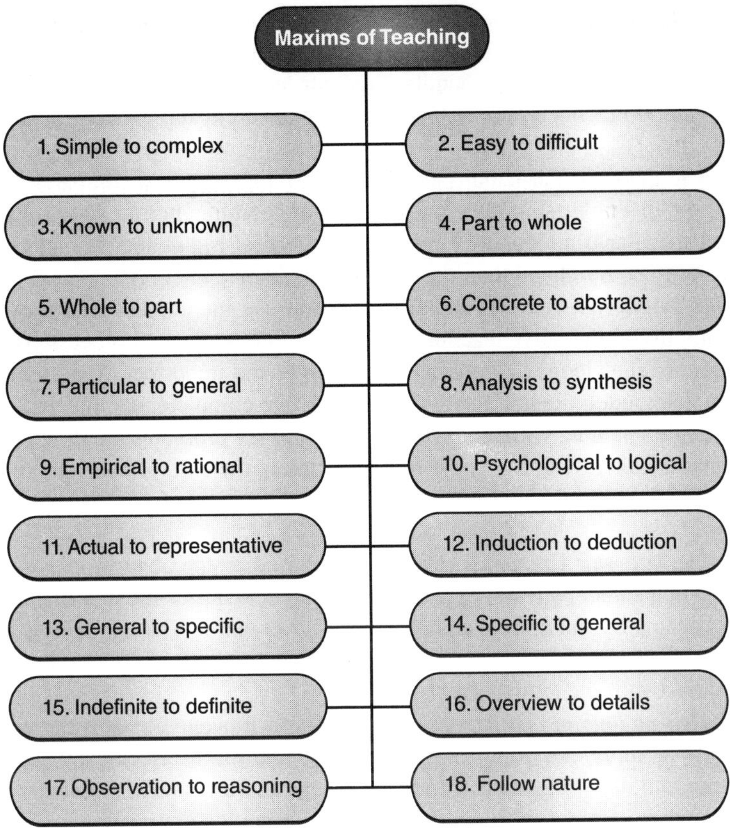

Figure 3.20

Maxims of teaching.

- ***From known to unknown:*** This maxim is based on the appreciative mass theory of learning. It assumes that student-acquired knowledge is given by linking with actuarial knowledge so the student can learn better and retain for a longer time. Students have some knowledge and teachers should enlarge this knowledge. If we link new knowledge with the old knowledge, we can make teaching clearer and effective. This maxim makes a link between the old and the new. If the teacher does not follow this maxim, then it is possible that students may be confused and may be interested in learning.
- ***From part to whole:*** B.F. Skinner gives emphasis on the part to whole maxim of teaching. He assumes that a student learns well if content is presented in small parts.
- ***From whole to part:*** According to the Gestalt school of psychology, whole is more important than parts. The whole is more motivating, understandable and effective than the study of various parts. A teacher should organize his activities in such a way that students can perceive the whole and then its parts because the whole attracts first. For example, while teaching *chambers of heart*, the teacher should show the entire heart first and then proceed with teaching the structure and functions of each part of the heart.
- ***Proceed from concrete to abstract:*** This is also a psychological rule of learning. Herbert said 'our lessons should start from the concrete and end in abstract'. A child's imagination is greatly aided

by concrete material. 'Things first and words after' is a common saying. Rousseau said, 'things, things and things'. Children cannot think in abstractions in the beginning. Young children learn first from the things they can see and handle. Students learn from perception and experience about objects. After perception, concepts which are partially concrete and partially abstract in nature are formed.

- ***From particular to general:*** Particular facts are easy to understand as compared to general facts. Particular facts and examples should be presented to the children before giving them general rules and principles. Particular is an inductive method and general is a deductive method. The process of induction is easier to comprehend than the so-called deductive one.
- ***From analysis to synthesis:*** Analysis and synthesis both are intellectual processes. This maxim is most frequently used in creative teaching. Analysis is an intellectual process. When a student comes to school, his knowledge is incomplete, indefinite and imperfect. Analysis makes the student's incomplete, indefinite and incoherent knowledge complete, definite and coherent. A teacher should begin teaching with analysis, so that complex problems are divided into systematic and comprehensible units. Synthesis must be performed in the end to make the knowledge definite and fixed. Analysis is useful for understanding and synthesis is useful for fixing this knowledge in students' minds.
- ***From empirical to rational:*** Empirical knowledge is based on the observations of students and has a significant role in a student's learning process. A student acquires most of his learning through observations. Learning by imitation is also based on observation. The activities of the teacher should be so organized that they can provide new experiences through observation and the teacher should then proceed with the logical aspect.
- ***From psychological to logical:*** The psychological approach takes into consideration student interests, abilities, aptitude, developmental level, needs and reactions. Logical approach considers the subject matter and its arrangement into logical steps and orders. An eminent writer remarked, 'logical procedure has its place in the middle of a lesson but the approach must be determined psychologically'. First, the teachers should keep in mind the selection of the subject matter to be presented. After this, the teachers should have a logical approach to arrange the matter into logical orders and steps.
- ***From actual to representative:*** The child learns more easily and quickly from actual, natural and real objects rather than from representative objects like models, charts and other aids. For example, while learning about a milk plant, an actual visit to the milk plant will make the learning more vivid and rapid rather than from a picture or model.
- ***From induction to deduction:*** Induction means drawing a conclusion from a set of examples. The process of induction calls for perception, reasoning, judgement and generalization. The teacher should proceed from induction to deduction, that is first present the principle or generalization before students and then verify the truth of this principle by applying it to particular instances. Induction discovers knowledge and deduction is the consequence of such discoveries.
- ***From general to specific:*** Explain general rules first and then specific ones. For example, while teaching paediatric nursing, the teacher explains the principles of paediatric nursing and then teaches about various disease conditions and the procedures related to child health.
- ***From specific to general:*** In certain situations, it is imperative to proceed from specific to general. For example, the role of iron in the body has to be specified before generalizing the consequences of anaemia on the body.
- ***From indefinite to definite:*** The ideas of students in initial stages are vague. These ideas should be made definite, clear, precise and systematic by adopting effective teaching methods. To make these ideas definite, the teacher can use audiovisual aids and other strategies as needed.

- ***Proceed from overview to details:*** Students can easily comprehend if the teacher proceeds from an overview to details. For example, while teaching about the instruments used for performing an endoscopy, the teacher should introduce all instruments by listing down their names before explaining their uses and the ways to handle each instrument in detail.
- ***From observation to reasoning:*** The teacher has to provide an opportunity for the students to see and notice the factors involved in a particular topic or context before explaining the reasons associated with it or eliciting reasons from the students.
- ***To follow nature:*** This maxim of teaching is based on the philosophy of naturalism. Rousseau has given the concept to follow nature. The child is the centre of educational processes. A child should be given full freedom to learn according to his own ways. The teacher's role is to observe his behaviour and learning activities. There should be one teacher and one student in an ideal situation.

REVIEW QUESTIONS

LONG-ANSWER QUESTIONS

1. Discuss the maxims of teaching.
2. Describe a lesson plan.
3. Discuss the formulation of objectives.
4. Explain problem-based learning.
5. Describe the principles and maxims of teaching.
6. Explain lesson planning.
7. What are the characteristics of learning?
8. Define learning and define its nature.
9. Differentiate between cognitive domain of learning and affective domain of learning.
10. Discuss the principles of learning.
11. Discuss the domains of learning.
12. Discuss the factors influencing learning.
13. Explain the learning process.
14. Describe the principles of teaching.
15. Discuss the dimensions and principles of classroom management.
16. Describe the essential characteristics of lesson planning.
17. Explain taxonomy of educational objectives.
18. Explain the characteristics of educational objectives.
19. Describe the characteristics of good teaching.
20. Discuss the meaning and nature of teaching.
21. Discuss characteristics of learning process.
22. Describe principles of teaching.
23. Explain characteristics of learning. Write principles and maximums of teaching.

SHORT-ANSWER QUESTIONS

1. Discuss the principles of learning.
2. What are the elements of teaching–learning process?

3. Discuss briefly peer learning.
4. Differentiate between goal and objectives.
5. List down any four qualities of educational objectives.

MULTIPLE-CHOICE QUESTIONS (MCQs)

1. Which factors help in measuring learning efficiency?
   (a) Accuracy
   (b) Speed
   (c) Retention
   (d) All of these
2. Average retention rate by a student through practising is about
   (a) 30%
   (b) 75%
   (c) 10%
   (d) 20%
3. Series of steps of learning process include
   (a) Motive of learner ... Establish goals ... Adjustment ... Behaviour change ... Behaviour stabilization
   (b) Motive of learner ... Establish goals ... Adjustment ... Behaviour stabilization ... Behaviour change
   (c) Establish goals ... Motive of learner ... Behaviour change ... Adjustment ... Behaviour stabilization
   (d) Establish goals ... Motive of learner ... Behaviour stabilization ... Behaviour change ... Adjustment
4. Elements of cooperative learning include
   (a) Face-to-face interaction and positive interdependence
   (b) Creativity and professional development
   (c) Continuity and transformation
   (d) Behavioural change and maturity
5. Role play helps to assess which domain of learning?
   (a) Cognitive
   (b) Affective
   (c) Psychomotor
   (d) All of these
6. __________ domain of learning is evaluated by formal written examinations?
   (a) Cognitive
   (b) Affective
   (c) Psychomotor
   (d) All of these
7. Doing head-to-toe examination in an OPD is an example of which domain of learning?
   (a) Affective
   (b) Psychomotor
   (c) Cognitive
   (d) All of these

8. The international poles of teaching process include
   - (a) Teacher, pupil and motivational environment
   - (b) Information, knowledge and skills
   - (c) Teacher, pupil and subject matter
   - (d) Teacher, pupil and communication system
9. Psychological principle of teaching include
   - (a) Principle of definite aim
   - (b) Principal of activity aim
   - (c) Principal of pupil centredness
   - (d) Principle of feedback and reinforcement
10. Educational objectives should be
   - (a) Attainable and realistic
   - (b) Time bound and unequivocal
   - (c) Motivational and professional
   - (d) Both (a) and (b)
11. According to the Bloom's taxonomy, educational objectives are classified into how many basic domains?
   - (a) Two
   - (b) Three
   - (c) Four
   - (d) Five
12. Characteristics of good lesson plan are
   - (a) It should be clearly written
   - (b) Simple and comprehensive
   - (c) Rigid
   - (d) Both (a) and (b)
13. Institutional objectives are also known as
   - (a) Behavioural objectives
   - (b) Departmental objectives
   - (c) Institutional objectives
   - (d) General objectives
14. The six main categories of cognitive domain of learning are
   - (a) Knowledge, comprehension, application, analysis, synthesis and evaluation
   - (b) Knowledge, comprehension, perception, mechanism, synthesis and evaluation
   - (c) Knowledge, comprehension, motivation, attitude, coordination, motivation, analysis
   - (d) None of these
15. Explaining the role of genetic factors in colorectal cancer is an example of which domain of learning?
   - (a) Cognitive
   - (b) Affective
   - (c) Psychomotor
   - (d) All of above

ANSWERS OF THE MULTIPLE-CHOICE QUESTIONS

1. (d), 2. (b), 3. (a), 4. (a), 5. (b), 6. (a), 7. (b), 8. (c), 9. (d), 10. (d), 11. (b), 12. (d), 13. (a), 14. (a), 15. (a)

FURTHER READING

Abbatt, F. R. (1992). *Teaching for better learning* (2nd ed., p. 183). Geneva: WHO.

Ahrenfelt, J., & Watkin, N. (2006). *100 ideas for essential teaching skills (continuum one hundred)*. New York, NY: Continuum.

Allen, J. D. (1986). Classroom management: Students' perspectives, goals, and strategies. *American Educational Research Journal, 23*, 437–459.

Arkoudis, S. (2006). *Teaching international students: Strategies to enhance learning. Centre for the Study of Higher Education*. Melbourne: University of Melbourne.

Baars, B. J., & Gage, N. M. (2007). *Cognition, brain, and consciousness: Introduction to cognitive neuroscience*. London, UK: Elsevier.

Baldwin, G. (2005). *The teaching-research nexus. How research informs and enhances learning and teaching in the University of Melbourne*. Melbourne: Centre for the Study of Higher Education, University of Melbourne.

Barbetta, P., Norona, K., & Bicard, D. (2005). Classroom behavior management: A dozen common mistakes and what to do instead. *Preventing School Failures, 49*(3), 11–19.

Bear, G. G. (2008). Best practices in classroom discipline. In A. Thomas, & J. Grimes (Eds.). *Best practices in school psychology V* (pp. 1403–1420). Bethesda, MD: National Association of School Psychologists.

Bear, G. G., Cavalier, A., & Manning, M. (2005). *Developing self-discipline and preventing and correcting misbehavior*. Boston, MA: Allyn & Bacon.

Berliner, D. C. (1988). Effective classroom management and instruction: A knowledge base for consultation. In J. L. Graden, J. E. Zins, & M. J. Curtis (Eds.). *Alternative educational delivery systems: Enhancing instructional options for all students*. Washington, DC: National Association of School Psychologists.

Bitterman, M. E., Menzel, R., Fietz, A., & Schäfer, S. (1983). Classical conditioning of proboscis extension in honeybees (*Apis mellifera*). *Journal of Comparative Psychology, 97*, 107–119.

Bloom, B. S. (1956). *Taxonomy of educational objectives, the classification of educational goals – Handbook I: Cognitive domain*. New York: McKay.

Brophy, J. E., & Good, T. L. (1986). Teacher behavior and student achievement. In M. C. Wittrock (Ed.). *Handbook of research on teaching* (3rd ed.). New York: Macmillan.

Candy, P. C., Crebert, G., & O'Leary, J. (1994). *Developing lifelong learners through undergraduate education*. Canberra: National Board of Employment Education and Training, AGPS.

Dave, R. (1967). *Psychomotor domain*. Berlin: International Conference of Educational Testing.

Davies, M., & Devlin, M. (2007). *Interdisciplinary higher education: Implications for teaching and learning*. Melbourne: Centre for the Study of Higher Education, University of Melbourne.

Fuchs, A. H., & Milar, K. S. (2003). Psychology as a science. In Weiner, Irving, & Donald K. Freedheim (Eds.). *Handbook of Psychology*. New York, NY: Wiley.

Gaff, J. G., & Ratcliff, J. L. (1996). *Handbook of the undergraduate curriculum*. San Francisco, CA: Jossey-Bass Publishers.

Gagne, R., & Briggs, L. (1974). *Principles of instructional design*. New York, NY: Holt, Rinehart and Winston.

Gilbert, J. J. (1983). *Educational handbook for health personnel* (6th ed.). New York, NY: WHO.

Gootman, M. E. (2008). The caring teacher's guide to discipline: Helping students learn self-control, responsibility, and respect. *Journal of School Psychology, 3*(6), 36.

Grusec, J. E., & Hastings, P. D. (2007). *Handbook of socialization: Theory and research*. New York: Guilford Press.

Harris, K. L. (2005). *Guide for reviewing assessment. Prompts and guidelines for monitoring and enhancing assessment practices*. Melbourne: Centre for the Study of Higher Education, University of Melbourne.

Harrow, A. (1972). *A taxonomy of the psychomotor domain. A guide for developing behavioral objectives*. New York: McKay.

Heidgerken, L. E. (2004). *Teaching and learning in schools of nursing* (3rd ed., pp. 123–125). New Delhi: Konark Publishers.

Hilgard, E., & Bower, G. (1966). *Theories of learning*. New York, NY: Appleton Century-Crofts.

James, R., Baldwin, G., & McInnis, C. (1999). *Which university? The factors influencing the choices of prospective undergraduates*. Canberra: AGPS.

Kauchak, D., & Eggen, P. (2008). *Introduction to teaching: Becoming a professional* (3rd ed.). Upper Saddle River, NJ: Pearson Education, Inc.

Krathwohl, D. R., Bloom, B. S., & Masia, B. B. (1973). *Taxonomy of educational objectives, the classification of educational goals. Handbook II: Affective domain*. New York: David McKay.

Laurillard, D. (1993). *Rethinking university teaching: A framework for the effective use of educational technology*. London, UK: Routledge.

Lou, C., & Walter, D. (1978). *The systematic design of instruction*. Glenview, IL: Scott, Foresman.

Marshall, M. (2001). *Discipline without stress, punishments or rewards*. Los Alamitos, CA: Piper Press.

Moskowitz, G., & Hayman, J. L., Jr. (1976). Success strategies of inner-city teachers: A year-long study. *Journal of Educational Research, 69*, 283–289.

Narang, M., & Arora, V. (2005). *Encyclopaedia of techniques of teachings* (Vol. 1, pp. 404–405). New Delhi: Anmol Publications.

Pascarella, E., & Terenzini, P. (1998). *How college affects students: Findings and insights from twenty years of research*. San Francisco, CA: Jossey Bass.

Pintrich, P. R., & De Groot, E. V. (1990). Motivational and self-regulated learning components of classroom academic performance. *Journal of Educational Psychology, 82*, 33–40.

Salsbury, D. E., & Schoenfeldt, M. (2008). *Lesson planning: A research-based model for K-12 classrooms*. Alexandria, VA: Prentice Hall.

Sandman, C. A., Wadhwa, P., Hetrick, W., Porto, M., & Peeke, H. V. S. (1997). Human fetal heart rate dishabituation between thirty and thirty-two weeks gestation. *Child Development, 68*, 1031–1040.

Seligman, M. (1970). On the generality of the laws of learning. *Psychological Review, 77*, 406–418.

Serdyukov, P., & Ryan, M. (2008). *Writing effective lesson plans: The 5-star approach*. Boston, MA: Allyn & Bacon.

Simpson, E. (1972). *The classification of educational objectives in the psychomotor domain: The psychomotor domain* (Vol. 3). Washington, DC: Gryphon House.

Skinner, C. E. (1996). *Education psychology* (4th ed., pp. 417–449). London, UK: PHI Publishers.

Skowron, J. (2006). *Powerful lesson planning: Every teachers guide to effective instruction*. Thousand Oaks, CA: Corwin Press.

Tanol, G., Johnson, L., McComas, J., & Cote, E. (2010). Responding to rule violations or rule following: A comparison of two versions of the good behavior game with kindergarten students. *Journal of School Psychology, 48*, 337–355.

Terry, W. S. (2006). *Learning and memory: Basic principles, processes, and procedures*. Boston, MA: Pearson Education, Inc.

Thompson, J. G. (2007). *First year teacher's survival guide: Ready-to-use strategies, tools & activities for meeting the challenges of each school day (J-B Ed: Survival Guides)*. San Francisco, CA: Jossey-Bass.

Thorndike, E. (1932). *The fundamentals of learning*. New York: Teachers College Press.

Thorndike, E. (1999). *Education psychology*. New York: Routledge.

Tileston, D. E. W. (2003). *What every teacher should know about instructional planning*. Thousand Oaks, CA: Corwin Press.

Tingstrom, D. H., Sterling-Turner, H. E., & Wilczynski, S. M. (2006). The good behavior game: 1969–2002. *Behavior Modification, 30*(2), 225–253.

University of Melbourne Curriculum Commission. (2006). *The Melbourne Model: Report of the Curriculum Commission*. Melbourne: University of Melbourne.

Walia, J. S. (2007). *Educational technology*. New Delhi: Ahim Paul Publishers.

Walia, J. S. (2009). *Teaching–learning process*. New Delhi: Ahim Paul Publishers.

Wolfe, S. (2006). *Your best year yet! A guide to purposeful planning and effective classroom organization (teaching strategies)*. New York: Teaching Strategies.

Wood, D. C. (1988). Habituation in Stentor produced by mechanoreceptor channel modification. *Journal of Neuroscience, 2254*(8), 112–116.

CHAPTER

Curriculum, assessment and planning

4

LEARNING OBJECTIVES

This chapter is designed to enable the reader to:

- Understand the essential qualities of a teacher and commonly used teaching styles in nursing education
- Identify types of learners and determinants of learning
- Explain the concept of emotional intelligence and motivation in teaching–learning process
- Describe meaning, types, components, approaches, factors, barriers and facilitators of curriculum development
- Exhibit skills of developing course planning, unit planning and lesson planning

KEY TERMS

ESSENTIAL QUALITIES OF A TEACHER

It is essential for a teacher to possess certain specific qualities that make them different from others to create a conducive learning environment. They must have skills of active listening, impactful communication, adaptability in every situation, empathetic approach, patience, collaboration, passion for lifelong learning, exchange of best academic practices, engaging classroom presence and values of real-world learning. These qualities are detailed below:

- **Active listener:** Listening is an art and it is a key foundation for the successful communication. It is important for a teacher to listen what is not even said and that is only possible by having quality of active listening because it provides power of wider observation and understanding the student and situation more clearly and precisely. It is generally observed that a large number of students have academic anxiety and fail to express themselves adequately. Therefore, active listening as a quality of a teacher enables them to listen to students better and provide the best solution to them. Active listening skills of a teacher also facilities them for better understanding the learners and, thereby, an effective planning of the academic activities. The active listening skills of a teacher helps to open closed doors of teacher–taught relationship, enhance mutual respect and nurtures the teaching–learning environment to the greatest heights.

- **Impactful communicator:** Skills of impactful communication is fundamental to a rubout teaching career. Most successful teachers are the most motivating communicators. Impactful communications skills help teachers to connect with everyone very effectively, motivate them and teaching–learning can be made easy and a fun. Most difficult subjects and situations can be made so easy and even enjoyable with the help of impactful communication.
- **Adaptability in every situation:** The Adaptability Quotient is a buzz word in the academic discipline today. It is believed that success of a teacher is largely determined by his adaptability skills, and it is considered more important than Intelligence Quotient and Emotional Quotient. 'Change is only constant', thus, it is essential for a teacher to have a quality to adapt to changing and evolving academic environment, such as changing leaderships, generation of students, curriculum, teaching–learning resources and teaching media and assessment methods. A teacher with skills of adaptability can gel with every situation so smoothly that they hardly can be critical about any situation, which helps them to create a most positive academic ecosystem for self and others.
- **Empathetic approach:** Being empathetic to students and treating them as an individual without judgement is a key quality of a teacher. It is essential for a teacher to be observant, attentive, positive and empathetic for effective student engagement and improved learning among them. Being empathetic not only helps teachers to understand students better but it can also facilitate teachers to consider individual differences of pupils as each student is blessed with different qualities and abilities of learning.
- **Patience**: Patience is one of the most essential quality of a good teacher in every academic situation, including working with colleagues having different working philosophy, communicating with student issues and progress to their parents and while counselling of difficult students. It is observed that patience is routinely tested being a teacher in day-to-day teaching–learning practices because the ultimate outcome of education is to bring out a better version of students, which require immense patience.
- **Focus on collaboration:** Academics and teaching is a multidisciplinary teamwork, which involves a variety of stakeholders, that is society, parents, employers, political leaders, administrators, institute heads, faculty of different departments, medical and nursing teams of the clinical units, counsellors, etc. A teacher's ability to collaborate defines the ultimate success of education processes and outcomes.
- **Passion for lifelong learning**: Learning is a continuous and constant process, which is believed to begin at the womb and only ends at the tomb. A good teacher is a lifelong learner to adapt to the evolving academic environment because change is the law of nature, and the science of teaching and learning is changing very rapidly. In the absence of continued learning, a teacher becomes rudimentary and outdated within a period of few years, especially in this era of rapid progress of science and educational technology. A good teacher needs to be updated with the latest developments in their respective fields, and that is only possible if they have the quest of lifelong learning.
- **Exchange of best academic practices**: Teaching is a scientific discipline and it requires generation of evidences related to best teaching–learning practices. Teachers are continuously engaged in testing new innovative methods of teaching, assessment, educational media and integration of technology in education. Therefore, it is essential for a good teacher to share their best practices for larger good in the field of education.
- **Engaging classroom presence**: The teachers are liked by students and appreciated for their quality and strength of engaging students in classroom or at online platforms through their sense

of humour, creative lesson plans, power point presentations, use of innovative educational media and teaching styles. An engaging teacher brings creative learning situations and experiences for learners, where learning becomes easy and interesting.
- **Value for real-world learning experiences**: Nursing education largely depends on real-life learning experiences, where a good teacher plans learning experiences in such a manner that students get more and more opportunities for real-life learning experiences. Nursing is a technical profession where graduating nurses need to take a role to provide safe care to their clients; where it is essential for nursing teachers to have value for real-world experiences for their students, so that they can produce clinical-practice ready nurses.

TEACHING STYLES

Teaching styles are connected to a teacher's educational value system and come from their educational philosophy. Teachers' teaching style is a reflection of how they teach. A teacher can improve teaching by being aware about their teaching style. The course objectives, course material and learning objectives also influence the choice of teaching styles by a teacher.

DEFINITIONS

- **A teaching style** is not just about the instructional strategies or methods used but also about the use and interpretation of certain types of rhetoric.
- **Teaching styles** are also known as teaching methods. They refer to the general principles, educational and management strategies that guide classroom instructions.

GOALS OF TEACHING STYLES

- To develop effective classroom management skills.
- To master the art of teaching and learning.
- To have high expectations.

TYPES OF TEACHING STYLES

There are many teaching styles that can be used depending on the classroom setting, the subject matter and the philosophy of education followed by the institute, teacher and students. There are a variety of teaching styles; some of the commonly used teaching styles are formal authority style, demonstrator style, facilitator style and delegator style, which are discussed in this chapter.

I. FORMAL AUTHORITY STYLE

This authoritative style of teaching follows the traditional teacher-centred approach, which is also known as the formal lecture style of teaching. This is often represented by one-way talk on a specific topic or lecture session. This method, also called 'chalk and talk', requires that students pay attention to the lecture and absorb it. Students are encouraged to take notes and pose or answer questions.

- **The authority method**, also called the lecture style, requires learners to sit down and listen to their teacher talk on a topic that has been assigned. Students then take notes and attempt to memorize what they hear.
- **Authoritative teachers** are characterized by high levels of affection, guidance and monitoring, close behavioural but low psychological control. They allow students to participate in decision-making and are consistent in their demands.

This style of teaching is not more focused on building relationships with students, nor is it as important for students to form relationships with each other. This type of teacher does not require students to be involved in class.

ADVANTAGES OF AUTHORITY STYLE OF TEACHING

- It emphasizes clear expectations and acceptable manners to do things.
- It communicates the intrinsic curiosity of a subject through their enthusiasm.
- It can be tailored to specific audiences' needs.
- It can offer a wealth of information.
- It can be shown to a large group of students.
- Professors can show how professional approach can be used to solve disciplinary problems.
- It gives the teacher full control over the learning experience.
- It appeals primarily to those who learn through listening.

DISADVANTAGES OF AUTHORITY STYLE OF TEACHING

- This results less flexible and standardized management of students and their problems.
- It does not provide feedback to instructors about student learning.
- Because there is no mechanism to ensure intellectual engagement, students can become passive, and students who are passive tend to forget information quickly.
- It assumes all students learn at the exact same rate and have the equal level of understanding.
- It is not appropriate for teaching higher levels of thinking like application, analysis and synthesis; motor skills, as well as for influencing attitudes or values.
- It is not suitable to teach complex or abstract material.
- It needs to use speakers who are effective.
- It focuses learning through listening. This can be detrimental for students who use other learning styles.

II. DEMONSTRATOR STYLE

The demonstration style is more about 'showing' and less 'telling', which is also known as coaching style of teaching. Teachers use examples, perform experiments and demonstrations, use multimedia presentations and other support materials to support explanation.

Teachers with a demonstrated teaching style tend to teach teacher-centred classes that emphasize on modelling and demonstration. This teacher is a role model, have good demonstrating skills and then act as a coach to help learners apply these skills and knowledge. The teacher acts as a role model, encouraging students to follow the same approach that they believe is most effective.

Instructors who use this style of teaching are open to learner participation and can adapt their presentation to suit different learning styles. Learners must take some responsibility for understanding what they want and asking for assistance when in doubt.

ADVANTAGES OF DEMONSTRATION METHOD OF TEACHING

- It allows to use multiple senses to make learning permanent.
- There is an active participation of teachers and learners in the teaching–learning process.
- It stimulates curiosity in learners and motivates them to take part in return demonstration.
- It is helpful in achieving psychomotor domain of learning objectives.
- It provides an opportunity to focus on direct observation and following a role model.
- Every skill, no matter how complex or simple, is easy to comprehend.

DISADVANTAGES OF DEMONSTRATION METHOD OF TEACHING

- It is good to use for only skills-related subject areas.
- Only learners are allowed to focus on the activity. However, there are limited opportunities to discuss during demonstration.
- Poor skill lab infrastructure and imitated clinical material make it challenging to use this method beyond limited areas.
- Poor economic conditions at government institutions lead to a scarcity of audiovisual aids and equipment. Teachers are not creative enough to create models to demonstrate and use these tools.
- Teachers are eager to get the syllabus completed as quickly as possible but do not put forth sincere efforts to develop model and demonstration.

III. FACILITATOR OR ACTIVITY STYLE

Facilitators or teachers focus on helping students to learn and develop critical thinking skills. The 'The facilitator teaching style' is a student-centred teaching approach that encourages critical thinking and fosters self-learning among students. This method encourages students to self-discovery as well as problem-solving skills. It can often lead to a deeper understanding into subject matter in which students are interested to learn.

Teachers that employ the facilitator teaching style tend to place a greater emphasis on activities and experiences. This teaching approach places an emphasis on the students' involvement and encourages students to take initiative in meeting learning objectives. Teachers direct and guide students by asking questions, investigating choices, recommending alternative solutions and helping them to develop criteria that will allow them to make educated judgements.

This teaching approach is effective for those who enjoy autonomous learning and can interact and collaborate with other students.

Teachers will frequently design group activities to promote active learning, student participation and problem-solving. These educators will frequently create learning settings and activities that need students to analyse and apply course knowledge in novel and creative ways.

ADVANTAGES OF FACILITATOR STYLE OF TEACHING

- It encourages students to be inquisitive and independent in learning.
- It increases long-term memory retention among students.

- It develops curiosity and analytical thinking among students.
- It builds social skills such as cooperation, delegation, negotiation and communication among students.
- It gives learner a real-life connection and experiences.
- It encourages students to express themselves freely in a learning environment.
- It promote continuous engagement of learners in the learning process.
- This teaching strategy considers individual differences of learners and promotes learning at the pace of each learner as per their choices and convenience.

DISADVANTAGES OF FACILITATOR STYLE OF TEACHING

- It can be seen to be a more expensive method of teaching.
- In this method of teaching, the teacher's role is not clearly defined.
- There is a need for extra facilities to allow for group work among students, etc.
- It is relatively time-consuming in proportion to the amount of subject matter to be covered as each individual student may have different pace of learning.
- It is not appropriate in some learning contexts.

IV. DELEGATOR OR GROUP STYLE

This style of teaching is ideal for curricula that involve or emphasize group activities. The delegator style of teaching shifts some of the responsibility of learning to the students. They are encouraged and expected to work together on projects related to the lesson themes (like science labs and debates).

Teachers are concerned with student autonomy in learning. They expect learners to work for themselves and only provide assistance when needed. The delegator style combines individual teaching styles with learning styles in one pack. Further, this allows instructors and learners to assess how they can improve their learning experience.

This teaching style involves the teacher being an active participant and working with students to guide them in the right direction. Teachers with a delegated teaching style place a lot more responsibility and control on individual students than they do on groups. The teachers with use of this style give students the opportunity to design and implement their own learning projects and act as consultants.

Learners are usually required to perform both independently and in groups. They also need to be able to stay focused and motivated on complex projects. Students who work in this setting are required to learn more than just the subject material. They must also be able to interact with others and effectively manage group situations.

The delegator approach of teaching, often known as the group method, is employed in subjects that necessitate group work, lab-based learning or peer input. To facilitate peer cooperation and student-to-student learning, the instructor functions as a delegator and would become an observer.

ADVANTAGES OF DELEGATOR STYLE OF TEACHING

- Assist learners in recognizing themselves as independent learners.
- Development of higher-level thinking and creativity among students.
- Enhancement of communication skills among students.
- Development of self-management and leadership skills among students.
- Promotion of more positive student–faculty interaction.

- Allow students to rate each other's quality during group work opportunities.
- Increase in student retention, self-esteem and responsibility.
- Exposure to and an increase in understanding of diverse perspectives among students.
- Prepare students for real-life social and employment situations.
- More flexible and creative use of instructional time by teachers.
- More learning from and with colleagues about students and about teaching and learning.
- Teachers have more energy and greater enjoyment in teaching.

DISADVANTAGES OF DELEGATOR STYLE OF TEACHING

- Loss of instructional and decision-making autonomy for teachers.
- Presence of conflict among group members (students).
- Some learners might become anxious when they have more autonomy.
- Students' unequal participation in group activity.
- Social loafing/introverts may struggle in learning and group activities.
- It is a time-consuming method of teaching.
- Individual needs of students are dominated by the needs of the group.

TYPES OF LEARNER

Every student has a learning style that suits them. This explains how they learn best and how long they can retain information. While everyone has their own learning style, most people have a particular preference. Teachers and professors create lesson plans that can be used to reach all learners in schools/colleges and classrooms. This helps teachers to address the different needs of students.

Empirical evidences have found that there is a unique learning style for each individual. Some people learn best while listening to music, while others enjoy reading silently or more drawn to writing and reading, while it is also observed that some of the learners prefer to sit in large lecture halls listening to professors and their lectures. There are various learning styles practised by different learners, and some of the commonly used learning styles are presented in this chapter, which is detailed below:

- **Kinesthetic learners:** They are the most practical types of learners and enjoy learning in a concrete manner. They learn best when they do something for themselves. They can even become anxious if they are required to study for longer periods of time. They do best when they can participate in a variety of activities and solve challenges on their own. This kind of learners can even recall their learned information during their active involvement in work, crocheting, striking the ball, tossing a coin, and other hobbies, etc. When they do things on their own, they retain more knowledge.
- **Read and write learners:** They are comfortable reading written material and enjoy writing. Study materials are a great way to learn about the subject. This type of learning is similar to the old-fashioned learning method of reading books related to a subject matter or course, revising them and then following the same process.
- **Visual or spatial learners:** These learners are able to visualize relationships and ideas, which can help them gain information. These learners take information from charts, diagrams and maps, as well as pictures and drawings. It is easier for spatial learners to retain and absorb information in a better way for longer periods of time.
- **Auditory learners:** An auditory or oral learner is someone who can best understand information when it is presented verbally. These people enjoy listening to lectures and taking part in discussions and debates to gain a better understanding of the information.

- **Natural learners:** Individual who are able to learn in any natural way can be called natural learners. The brain keeps information whether it is in a classroom, listening to lectures or watching instructional videos, participating in field trips, studying in a separate location or participating in group studies. This group of learners is most successful in capturing the information through experimentation and practical applications.
- **Linguistic learners:** This group learns best when they have a variety of linguistic skills such as reading, writing, listening and speaking. Some of their finest learning strategies include reading books, watching audio-video or class lectures, making self-note and using other learning resources. These learners are able to speak loudly and write extensively on the particular subject matter.
- **Interpersonal learners:** These are the learners who learn through relating to information. They are comfortable studying in groups and teams, as well as sharing information and exchanging ideas with each other. This type of individuals are usually excellent leaders and are good team players. They learn most effectively when they work with others. These people are most likely to be found in psychology or social science, which involves group work.
- **Intrapersonal learners:** Intrapersonal learners, in contrast to others, are learners who enjoy learning alone. These individuals usually set ambitious individual goals that sometimes fail to achieve them. In addition to external factors, these people are encouraged by internal pressures. These people can be found in many industries, including entrepreneurs, small businesses and creative fields. They prefer to work independently and are not interested in working with others and be supervised.
- **Logical or mathematical learners:** They must be able to categorize and classify things in order to comprehend a topic. They are better at understanding patterns, numbers, equations, relationships and other concepts than most people. These learners are often found in many fields, including engineering, mathematics and technical professions.
- **Musical or rhythmic learners:** These types of learners use music, rhythms or beats to learn. People learn and retain information faster when there is a background sound. This is like a musician learning how to play music by listening to various musical beats, rhythms and tones. Music is not an obstacle but a method of learning for these types of learners.

DETERMINANTS OF LEARNING

Learning is based upon some key factors that decide what changes will be caused by this experience. The key elements or the major factors that determine learning are learning needs, readiness to learn and learning style (Fig. 4.1).

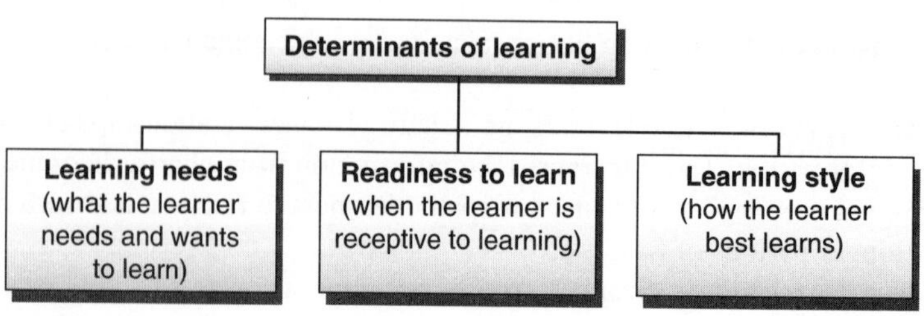

Figure 4.1

Determinants of learning.

I. LEARNING NEEDS

To determine learning deficits in cognitive, affective or psychomotor domains, educators must first identify the learning needs. The educator can then determine the best time and place for learning to occur. According to the Healthcare Education Association (1985), 'learning needs can be defined as knowledge gaps that exist between a desired level and actual performance learners'.

Furthermore, 'a learning need is simply the difference between what someone already knows and what they want to learn. These gaps can be caused by a lack in knowledge, attitude, skill, or both'.

STEPS TO ASSESS LEARNING NEEDS

These are the important steps to take when assessing learning needs:

1. ***Identify the learner:*** Who are they? Is there one audience or many? Are there multiple learners? Are their needs compatible or different? It is essential that learners are accurately identified before formal and informal education programmes can be developed.
2. ***Select the right setting:*** Trusting relationships help learners feel secure in confiding their information, feel valued, feel respected and believe that they are being taken seriously. Trusting relationships require that privacy and confidentiality are respected.
3. ***Gather data about the learner:*** After identifying the learner, the educator is able to determine the needs of the learner by looking at common issues that are of interest to the population.
4. ***Gather information from learners:*** Learners are the primary source of data for needs assessment. Let learners identify what is most important to them. Also, let them know what their learning needs are. Find out which social support systems they have access to and what type of assistance they can offer. If students are the target audience, ask them for their opinions on areas of practice or information they would like to learn more about. Learning is more enjoyable when learners are actively engaged in defining their needs and problems.
5. ***Prioritize the needs:*** It can be difficult for educators to focus on learning needs when they are dealing with multiple learning needs. Learners can set realistic and manageable learning goals by prioritizing their identified needs. It is essential that educators carefully consider the priority of needs and information to cover.
6. ***Assess educational resources' availability:*** An educator may recognize a need. However, it might not be practical to continue without the availability of proper educational resources to meet the learner's needs. In these cases, it might be more beneficial to determine the availability of educational resources and obtain the needed resources.
7. ***Determine the needs of the organization:*** This analysis offers information that represents the culture of your workplace. What are the aims, philosophy, strategic plan, purpose and values of the organization? The educator should know the requirements for performance in different categories of employees, job descriptions and organizational regulations.
8. ***Consideration of time-management issues:*** If educators expect learners to take responsibility and be actively involved in the learning process, it is important that they are allowed to give their views. Asking learners what they are interested in learning first will help to ease their fears and make it easier to move onto the next step. This method shows that educators care about what the learner believes to be important.

METHODS FOR SELECTING LEARNING NEEDS

In order to fulfil the educator role, the nurse must collect objective data as well as the learner's subjective information. Educators can use various methods to assess learner need and how they should be combined to produce realistic information. Some of the commonly used methods to assess learning needs are:

- Informal conversations
- Structured interviews
- Focus groups
- Self-administered questionnaires
- Test
- Observations
- Documentations

II. READINESS TO LEARN

After identifying learning needs, the educator can now determine the learner's willingness to get information. A learner's readiness is the ability to show an interest in learning new information that will help them to perform at their best in their job. When a learner is willing to take part in the process, receptive and open, it means they are ready to learn. The educator has the responsibility to determine whether or not learners are ready and able to learn, what they need to know and how to adapt subject matter to suit each student.

Before teaching can begin, educators need to take the time to examine four types of readiness for learning: physical readiness, experiential readiness, emotional readiness and knowledge readiness. These four factors are key readiness-related determinants of learning.

III. LEARNING STYLE

Learning styles can be used to describe the way learners collect, process, interpret, organize, make decisions and then 'store' that information for future reference. These styles can be categorized according to their sensory approaches, such as visual, aural and verbal (reading/writing), as well as kinesthetic.

Regardless of the differences in learning styles, the core idea behind them all is the same: each learner has a learning style, also known as preference. The types of readiness to learn or learners' preferences are presented in Fig. 4.2. Learners learn best when information can be presented in their preferred way. The message thus given to instructors is that 'optimal instruction requires diagnosing individuals' learning style[s] and tailoring instruction accordingly'. The learning styles are already discussed in 'types of learner' section of this chapter.

NEW GENERATION OF LEARNERS

A new generation has embraced college education. They are driven, determined achievers who rely on technology and their support network. This generation is not interested in the same teaching methods that were used 10 years ago. They have distinct learning characteristics than those of the 'Silent Generation' who were born between 1925 and 1942 and now grandparents of the Millennials. The Millennials are very different from their predecessors.

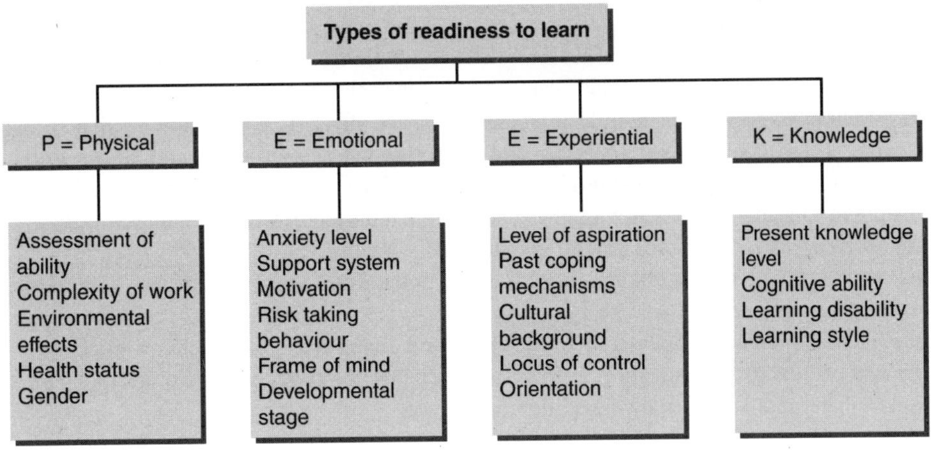

Figure 4.2

Types of readiness to learn.

CORE VALUES OF MILLENNIALS

- Confidence
- Civic duty
- Sociability
- Morality
- Diversity
- Collective active
- Pleasure learning through teamwork

THE CHARACTERISTICS OF MILLENNIAL LEARNER

- They tend to have a shorter attention span.
- They are drawn to interactive, experiential and cooperative learning.
- They are extremely comfortable with technology.
- They can perform multiple tasks.
- They are driven by immediate gratification.
- They are attracted to stimulating, informal settings.
- They value friendly and casual relationships when they are with teachers.
- They are often well-rounded.
- They are visual learners.
- They are information-hungry.
- They are confident.
- They are stressed.
- They are experimental.
- They are team-oriented.

TEACHING FOR MILLENNIALS

These are some key points educators should keep in mind as they change their teaching approach to Millennial learners. Two things to remember: long lectures are no longer effective, but technology that is focused on learning works. These could include collaborative platforms that allow papers and essays to be shared, MOOCs (massive open online courses) or Highbrow which disseminate information in small pieces, which Millennials prefer to learn. The important things teachers should keep in while teaching Millennials are:

- *Set learning objectives:* It is possible to get students to record it.
- *Make it meaningful.* Connect the lessons to culture and current events and place them in context with real-life experiences.
- *Mix the methods:* Videos, podcasts and concept charts, maps and concept charts, clickers, PowerPoint presentations with short bullets summarizing key concepts, and other tools are all available to keep the attention of the Millennial learner.
- *Give knowledge in small pieces:* Millennials will be interested for 10 minutes. Keep switching between them every 10 minutes. Let us say you have a 10-minute story, then a video and a quiz. Micro learning is worth looking into.
- *Develop collaborative environment:* Teacher can develop class blogs or wikis to accomplish this. Collaboration is also possible through social networking platforms. For example, a Facebook closed group may be created.
- *Build rapport:* It is possible to start by calling students by their first names. This can be a significant step in making a difference. The Millennials are not tolerant of authoritarians.
- *Course management systems:* It can be used for accepting and assessing assignments.

EMOTIONAL INTELLIGENCE

Emotional intelligence is comprised of two components: intelligence and emotion. Intelligence is part of the cognitive sphere, while emotions are part of the affective. Intelligence refers to the ability to acquire, apply and use knowledge and skills. The Latin word 'remove', which means to move from, is the root of emotion. However, there are six universal emotions: anger, fear, sadness, joy, surprise and happiness. Everybody feels emotions. Emotions are a valuable source of information about our relationships and behaviour as well as the human world.

DEFINITIONS

- Emotional intelligence (EI) refers to 'the ability to perceive, control, and evaluate emotions'.
- Emotional intelligence has been defined, by Peter Salovey and John Mayer, as 'the ability to monitor one's own and other people's emotions, to discriminate between different emotions and label them appropriately, and to use emotional information to guide thinking and behavior'.
- Goleman (1998) defined emotional intelligence as 'the capacity for recognizing our own feelings and those of others, for motivating ourselves, and for managing emotions well in ourselves and in our relationships'.
- Reuven Bar-On (1997) described emotional intelligence as 'an array of personal, emotional and social abilities and skills that influence one's ability to succeed in coping with environmental demands and pressures'.

PRINCIPLES OF EMOTIONAL INTELLIGENCE

Emotional intelligence is based on two fundamental principles. First, it refers to the ability to identify and comprehend emotions, both your own and those of others. The second principle is to manage and use our emotions, as well as those of others.

MODELS OF EMOTIONAL INTELLIGENCE

I. **Ability EI model**: Mayer and Salovey 1997 explained that emotions are considered useful information sources that allow one to understand and direct the social world. This model suggests that people differ in their ability to process emotions and their ability to connect emotional processing with a wider cognition. This ability manifests itself in adaptive behaviours. This model claims that emotional intelligence encompasses **four levels**, including ability to perceive emotions, to reason with emotions, to comprehend emotions and to manage them.
   - *Perceiving emotions:* Understanding emotions begins with the ability to perceive them clearly. This may include understanding nonverbal signals like facial expressions and body language.
   - *Reasoning with emotions:* Next, we use emotions to stimulate thinking and cognitive activity. Emotions are used to prioritize and respond to what is important to us. We also react emotionally to the things that grab our attention.
   - *Understanding emotions:* The emotions we perceive can have many meanings. If someone expresses anger, an observer must determine what the cause is and what it might be.
   - *Managing emotions:* It is an essential and highest level of emotional intelligence. All aspects of emotional management include managing emotions, responding appropriately, and also responding to the emotions of others.

II. **Trait EI model:** Petrides and his colleagues published the Trait EI model in 2009. The Trait EI model represents a set of emotion-related self-appraisals at earlier stages of personality. The Trait EI model is a person's view of their emotional competencies, as opposed to the ability-based model, which solely relates to real abilities.

III. **Mixed models of EI:** Daniel Goleman introduced mixed models of EI. This model defines EI as an array of skills and competencies that are essential for leadership performance. This model can be broken down into four domains:

Domains and competencies of emotional intelligence: Daniel Goleman's model identifies four domains. The original model was developed with five domains in 1998 and then redesigned with four domains in 2002. These are (1) Self-awareness, (2) Self-management, (3) Social awareness and (4) Relationship management. Each domain contains the associated competencies shown within Fig. 4.3.

- **Self-awareness:** John defines self-awareness as 'being aware both of our moods and thoughts about moods'. Goleman (2002) also describes it as the ability to understand and read emotions and identify their effects on others. Self-awareness can be described as a basic understanding about how and why we feel in a particular manner. Being aware of our own feelings makes it easier to manage them and helps to respond to others more efficiently.
- **Self-management:** Self-management, also known as self-regulation, is the ability to manage one's thoughts, feelings and actions in a way that achieves desired results. Through appropriate self-regulation, a sense of well-being, self-efficacy, confidence and connectedness to others is attainable. A self-regulating individual should be able to act and cope successfully in relationships by using his or her emotions as clues. To make this possible, it is essential to first understand self-awareness.

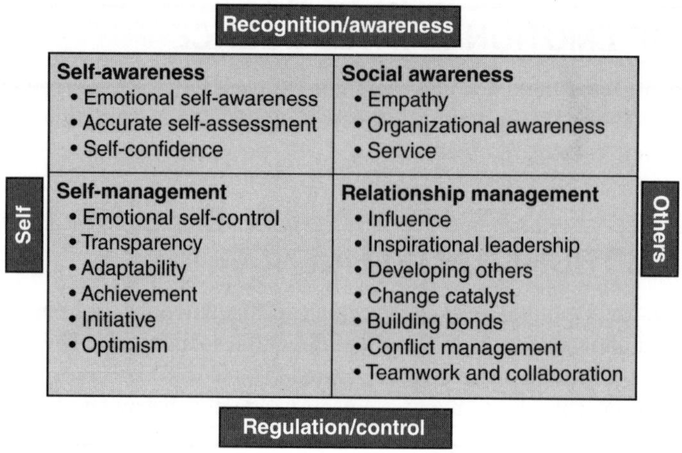

Figure 4.3

Daniel Goleman's Emotional Intelligence Quadrant.

- **Social awareness:** Social awareness refers to being able to 'read' situations and observe the emotions of others accurately. It involves sensing the thoughts and feelings of others to allow an individual to understand their perspectives, making use of his/her capacity to empathize. According to Goleman, our capacity is derived from neurons in an extensive circuitry related to the amygdala (amygdala is a core fear system in the human body). They read another person's face, speech and other nonverbal cues for emotion and help us decide how to communicate with them.
- **Relationship management:** It is the competence to perceive and consider the emotions of others in order to manage social relations. The final result, relationship management, is created by combining other three elements in this quadrant. If the other three dimensions are kept in mind, this dimension can be managed smoothly.

This can also be called 'friendliness with purpose' or 'getting desired reactions when working with others'. This is a variable trait that can change depending on the situation. There are seven competencies that fit under this dimension that all relate to relationships.

It is possible to use relationship management to influence others around you to make good decisions. We can read the reactions of others to situations and modify our responses to improve the interaction. It is important that everyone involved in this effort is genuine and not manipulated for their own benefit.

CHARACTERISTICS OF EMOTIONAL SKILLS

There are five key traits that make someone emotionally intelligent:

- **Self-awareness:** Being able to assess his capabilities realistically.
- **Self-regulation:** The ability to control emotions.
- **Motivation:** Deepest preference for achieving our goals.
- **Empathy:** Ability of understanding and identifying with other people's wants, needs or viewpoints.
- **Social skills:** Ability to resolve disputes, communicate effectively and building and maintaining connections. People with social skills have the ability to persuade, lead, negotiate, settle and coordinate for mutual benefit and teamwork.

ADVANTAGES OF EMOTIONAL INTELLIGENCE

- Emotional intelligence refers to managing own emotions well and building relationships with others. This will help one to be happier, healthier and more successful.
- Positive emotions and happy moods can open the mind and enhance creativity.
- Positive emotions enhance problem-solving abilities and aid in the identification of better responses.
- Emotionally intelligent students can effectively manage challenging circumstances and assist with negotiation and resolving disputes.
- For learning success, emotional intelligence is crucial. Administrators and educators must be emotionally intelligent.
- Research shows that students who have good social and emotional skills are more likely to be successful in learning, teaching and student achievement.
- Teachers who can recognize emotions better than less sensitive colleagues are more effective at teaching students.

MOTIVATIONAL FACTORS

Motivation is the state of mind that keeps students focused and engaged. It gives them the energy they need to accomplish their tasks. Motivation can also help to sustain activities over time. Motivation in education may have a variety of implications on students' behaviours, preferences and outcomes. Motivation, for example, can:

- Assist them to focus their attention on the tasks that must be done.
- These tasks can be completed in shorter time frames and attention is retained for longer periods.
- Avoid diversions and more successfully overcome the distractions.
- Influence students' perceptions of how tough or easy tasks are.

Motivation is what motivates pupils to do something. Without motivation, it can be difficult or impossible to complete an action.

Motivation is primarily of two types that can be correlated with academic success. These two motivations are extrinsic or intrinsic. Intrinsic motivation refers back to the ability of students to interact with the environment in order to achieve their goals. In contrast, extrinsic motivation is when people are motivated through external sources such as grades, rewards and recognition.

Motivation in teaching may have a significant influence on students' performances and outcomes. As a result, instructors who want to assist their learners succeed in school should be able to identify the factors that influence student motivation. Factors that affect the motivation of learners are person, environmental and support system, as detailed in this section.

I. PERSONAL FACTORS

The personal factors of motivation include intellectual level, learning capabilities, physical ability and emotional well-being of the learners as detailed below:

1. ***Intellectual level:*** The term refers to the individual's mental level. Success in school is generally closely related to the level of the intellect. Pupils with low intelligence often encounter serious difficulty in mastering schoolwork. Sometimes pupils do not learn because of special intellectual disabilities. In determining the effectiveness and efficiency of the learning process, it is important to consider the native capabilities of each individual.

2. ***Learning capability:*** Learning can be affected by factors such as a lack of mastery or faulty methods of studying, narrower experimental backgrounds and insufficient knowledge. If the school moves too fast and does not constantly monitor the progress of the pupil, there are many problems that can hinder their ability to master the material.
3. ***Physical ability:*** This group includes factors such as health, physical and mental development, nutrition, visual and bodily defects and glandular abnormality. It is well-known that poor health can affect motor and physical development and that malnutrition can hinder learning and physical growth.
4. ***Emotional well-being***: Personality development is influenced by one's attitude. These attitudes include enthusiasm, kindness, affection, loyalty, open-mindedness, prejudice, joy, cheerfulness and affection. Attitudes have a positive effect on learning and teaching, and the school's progress. Attitude of the learner can influence the efficiency and speed of work. Positive mental attitudes are key to learning. The factor of curiosity is closely related to the factors of reward and symbolic drive.

II. ENVIRONMENTAL FACTOR

Physical conditions needed for learning is under environmental factor. One of the factors that affect the efficiency of learning is the condition in which learning takes place. This includes the learning environment, classrooms, curricular structure, teaching methods and resources and assessments, as detailed below:

1. ***Learning environment:*** Another factor that influences motivation to learn is the school environment. The educational institute environment is defined as the set of rules and norms that influence the school's overall climate. A positive educational institute environment provides students with security and a safe environment that meets their basic needs. It also helps them build healthy social relationships.
2. ***Class and curriculum structure:*** Children thrive in order and struggle with chaos. Students feel more secure when they see that their classes are organized and have the materials and curriculum prepared in advance. Security is a basic human need. It helps learners to completely concentrate on the learning content when it is presented in an educational environment.
3. ***Teaching methods:*** Learners are more likely to be interested in educational institutes, if educators employ a variety of instructional strategies. Students will be more interested in learning if they have the opportunity to interact with different teaching methods. Also, it can be beneficial to give students the option of choosing their choices. Students in one class may have different learning styles. Therefore, teachers are more likely to be able to meet students' learning needs using different teaching methods.
4. ***Assessment:*** Regular assessment or evaluation is the key motivating factor for the students to learn. It has been generally observed that the way students learn largely depends on how exams are conducted. The standardized tests and high-quality assessment may motivate and boost achievement standards of the students.

III. SUPPORT SYSTEM

There are several support systems related factors of motivation such as teacher's behaviour and personality, parental habits and involvement, family issues and instability, and last but not least the peer relationship, which are detailed below:

i) ***Teacher's behaviour and personality***: Students who feel negative emotions like fear, disliking or fear towards their teachers can affect their perception towards the subject. An educator who exhibits favouritism towards learners or uses harsh and insulting words may have an impact on their drive to learn. However, students can be motivated to learn by encouraging, positivity, positive feedback and kindness.

ii) ***Parental habits and involvement:*** A few parenting behaviours might unintentionally influence children's desire, particularly intrinsic motivation. Some of the example are list here:

a. Displaying an interest in children's learning materials

- **i)** knowing and showing interest regarding their day
- **ii)** listening attentively
- **iii)** assisting with school-taught skills or tasks
- **iv)** attending child-parent meet
- **v)** encourage children to do their homework or preparation for examination

- **Family issues and instability:** The same as insecurity in educational institutes, a lack of security at home can have adverse effects on motivation for education.

  On average, children who live with both their parents get higher grades than those who do not. Academic performance can be affected by family conflicts and disruptions such as divorce, death of parents, frequently transferred families, separation and so on. In certain cases, educational institutes may offer additional support to students in order to address their problems.
- **Peer relationships:** With the increasing age of children, their peers' influence on them grows. Peer conflicts and problems can lead to students feeling insecure about their social standing among their classmates, which increases their level of stress and decreases their drive to learn. It is possible to avoid serious problems by keeping an eye on bullying and conflicts.

CURRICULUM PLANNING

The term curriculum has been derived from a Latin word *'Currere'* means 'to run', 'to run a course' or 'the path' that one takes up to achieve the goal. Thus, one can say that the curriculum is a pathway to achieve the educational goals. Originally, it meant the process and ways of passing the knowledge from one generation to the next. A common understanding of the curriculum is a programme of studies with specified course, leading to an academic certification, diploma or degree. However, in broader context, curriculum is anything and everything that teaches a lesson, planned or otherwise.

Pedagogically, curriculum is the description of course content, learning experiences and the course of studies to be taken up by the particular group of students to obtain a particular degree, diploma or certification. Curriculum is one of the most important components of education system, where traditionally it was subject- or content-centred, while in modern era, it is learner- or life-centred. Therefore, it is essential that curriculum must be revised from time to time based on the needs of the learner, the society and the nation.

DEFINITIONS OF CURRICULUM

The curriculum is defined differently by different authors and there is a lack of consensus on meaning of curriculum. Some of the important definitions of curriculum are as given below:

> *Curriculum is a tool in the hands of the artist (teacher) to mould his material (the pupil) in accordance with his idea in his studio (school).*
>
> **—Cunningham**

A systematic arrangement of the sum total of selected learning experiences planned by the school or a defined group of students to attain the aims of a particular educational programme.

—Florence Nightingale International Foundation

All the educational activities which are planned and guided by the school, whether they are carried out in groups or individually, inside and outside the school.

—Kerry

A curriculum is the offering of socially and scientifically valued knowledge, skills and attitudes made available to students through a variety of arrangements during the time they are at school, college or university.

—Bell

The curriculum includes all the learners' experience in or outside school that are included in a program which has been devised to help him developmentally, emotionally, socially, spiritually and morally.

—Crow and Crow

A curriculum is a plan or program of all experiences which the learner encounters under the directions of a school.

—Tanner and Tanner

Thus, a Curriculum is:

- a programme of studies.
- a course of study.
- that which is taught in educational institute.
- a set of subjects and the course content.
- a set of performance objectives and learning experiences.
- everything that in planned by an educational institute.
- a series of experiences undergone by a learner in an educational institute.
- everything that goes within the educational institute, including extra-curricular activities, guidance and interpersonal relationships.

TYPES OF CURRICULUM

It is evident from the ancient Indian literature that human being even learns in womb and thereafter through the life experiences in family, society and the formal and informal means of teaching in an educational institute. In a broader perspective, curriculum is everything through which the learner learns in this universe; thus, the types of curriculum may be the written curriculum, societal curriculum, hidden curriculum, null curriculum, phantom curriculum, concomitant curriculum and electronic curriculum. The details of each type of curriculum are given below:

- ***Written curriculum:*** It is written format of curriculum draft, which is prepared by the specially constituted curriculum committee, which is used as guidelines for providing the learning experiences for the particular group of students. It is also known as formal syllabus for a particular programme. For example, a written curriculum guidelines are prepared by the curriculum committee of Indian Nursing Council of the B.Sc. Nursing programme, which is used in the nursing colleges across India.

- ***Societal curriculum:*** The societal curriculum is an unwritten form of curriculum, which informally teaches the learner. For example, a person learns from family, friends, community, media, religious organizations, etc.
- ***Hidden curriculum:*** Each institute has varying structure, organizational design and routines in the teaching–learning process and attitude and behaviour of teachers and administrators. Therefore, learner learns spontaneously many things differently through above-mentioned factors when even they are taught with the same written content/subjects in different schools/colleges or universities. For example, same written curriculum is followed for B.Sc. Nursing in each institute in India but one can observe the difference in graduate nurses prepared in different nursing institutes because of existing hidden curriculum in the institutes.
- ***Null curriculum:*** There are certain areas/topics that are least important to be included in the written curriculum because of the changing needs and the trends, but teachers somehow convey the message to the learners that this is not an important topic in the present context that may indirectly stimulate the learner to learn about this omitted topic in written curriculum. For example, inclusion of smallpox in current curriculum of Indian medical or nursing courses may not be relevant but a message received from the teacher that it was a deadly disease of past era that does not exist in present time may stimulate the learner to learn about it.
- ***Phantom curriculum:*** The people learn many things through the messages prevalent in and through exposure of any type of media; especially the culture and subculture are learned through the media. For example, a budding Indian nurse watches a western nurse communicating with her clients in a documentary film; she may learn many things from her through the exposure of this form of media.
- ***Concomitant curriculum:*** The concomitant curriculum is an unwritten form of curriculum where learner learns what is taught or emphasized in the family milieu. The moral and ethical values and moulded behaviours are learned through family milieu.
- ***Electronic curriculum:*** The present era is the era of electronics, where in day-to-day life, every one of us communicates as well as learns through electronic means either in formal or informal ways. Many of us use Internet on a regular basis for recreational purposes or for research or personal information gathering purposes, where we get opportunity to learn many things. For example, a budding nurse learns about a new emergency drug through a post made by her friend on Facebook account and so on.

CURRICULUM DESIGN

Curriculum design looks at the overall course design, integrating material to educational goals and developing a course outline and building the course. Assessment methodologies, exercises, material, subject matter analysis and interactive activities are used to meet each learning goal.

According to Karen Schweitzer, curriculum design is a term used to describe the purposeful, deliberate and systematic organization of curriculum (instructional blocks) within a class or course'. In other words, 'it is a way for teachers to design curriculum, they identify what will be done, who will do it, and what schedule to follow'. Curriculum design has following important attributes:

- Curriculum design is purposeful
- Curriculum design is deliberate
- Curriculum design is creative
- Curriculum design operates on many levels

- Curriculum design requires compromises
- Curriculum designs can fail
- Curriculum design has stages

COMPONENTS OF CURRICULUM

Tyler says it is important to have a comprehensive theory of organization that shows which elements of curriculum are best suited to be used as organizing components. A curriculum will succeed if it is well coordinated. Although there is no agreement among experts on curricular elements, the following **four** are widely discussed**: (1) objectives, (2) content, (3) methods or learning experiences and (4) evaluation.**

These four core curricular aspects are interconnected and critical. In summation, aims, goals and objectives may be characterized as 'what is done'. The term 'subject matter/content' implies to 'what subject matter will be addressed', whereas 'learning experiences' relate to 'what instructional methodologies and resources will be employed'. Programme evaluation deals with 'what methodologies and instruments will be utilized to assess the success of the curriculum'.

Herrick and Tyler have identified five components and parts of curriculum development: (1) Situational analysis; (2) Formulation of objectives; (3) Selection of content, scope and sequence; (4) Activities, strategies and methods of teaching and (5) Evaluation.

I. SITUATIONAL ANALYSIS

Situational analysis refers to the examination of several facets of a country's emotional, political and cultural status, as well as its religious, geographical and spiritual state. This will help curriculum designers choose learning objectives, integrate learning content and identify suitable evaluation processes.

II. FORMULATION OF OBJECTIVES

The curriculum is composed of goals, objectives and aims. It outlines what is being done. It is designed to help understand the vision, the philosophy and the mission of particular programme of course. Additionally, it clearly identifies the purpose and the curriculum to be followed and explains what should be done. This element is important because it is difficult for a trip to be successful without a predecided destination.

Many times, goals are expressed using state standards. These standards can be expressed in general terms. They are then subdivided into more precise objectives. These objectives might be expressed in behavioural terms to aid in the development of learning frameworks. The goals are sometimes classified as cognitive, affective or psychomotor.

The creation of curricular objectives is influenced by four major elements: the society, the knowledge, the learner and the learning process.

III. SELECTION OF CONTENT, SCOPE AND SEQUENCE (ACTIVITIES, STRATEGIES AND METHODS OF TEACHING)

The curriculum's third element is its content. It is information that must be learned in school, college or educational institute. It is the element or medium by which the objectives can be accomplished. It refers to the knowledge or material that the learner will acquire after completion of the course. It is responsible for ensuring that curricular objectives are accomplished.

Selection of content for a topic is one of the most important considerations. The following are important considerations when choosing a subject matter:

- Society's needs and demands
- Availability of sources and resources
- International needs
- Age and level of learners
- Methods for content integration
- Availability of courses
- Qualification and availability of teaching faculty
- Scope of subject matter
- Examination pattern
- Types of society and culture

To create a solid content, it is important to have balance, articulation and sequence of learning materials.

IV. LEARNING EXPERIENCES (ACTIVITIES, STRATEGIES AND METHODS OF TEACHING)

The fourth element concerns the teaching strategies and methods or learning experiences that teachers use during teaching. It is focused with teaching–learning processes, such as teaching methods, learning experiences both within and outside the organization, learning settings and teacher's and student's material. Tyler's classic curriculum textbook characterized learning activities as follows:

The content of a course or the activities that the teacher performs are not all considered 'learning experiences'. The engagement of the learner with the external world is referred to as learning experience. The student's active behaviour is what makes learning possible.

Tyler believes that teachers have a problem selecting learning experiences that encourage active participation in order to achieve the desired learning outcomes.

Tyler also identified **five principles** that can be used **to select learning experiences**, these are:

- Students must have the chance to demonstrate the behaviour they desire during the learning experience.
- Students should feel satisfied with their learning experience.
- The learning experience must be tailored to meet the needs and abilities of the students.
- Multiple learning experiences may be necessary to meet the same goal. A wide variety of learning experiences can be better than a narrow range.
- Learning experiences should achieve multiple learning outcomes and meet more than one objective.

V. EVALUATION

Evaluation of a curriculum is the process of assigning value to it. The evaluation may be focused on the curriculum's design and content, as well as its implementation and outcomes. It evaluates the effectiveness, quality and product of the curriculum's process, programme or product.

A curriculum evaluation is not the same as a student evaluation. This is a more general term that can be used to judge the quality and effectiveness of a curriculum and to assess whether the aims or objectives have been achieved. It can also show the effectiveness of other components and strategies for teaching. Evaluation gives input to the curriculum and its components. Experts can make desired changes to the curriculum with the assistance of the evaluation phase.

APPROACHES OF CURRICULUM DESIGN

There are eight approaches to design or organize curriculum: subject-centred, student-centred, problem-centred, correlated curriculum, fusion curriculum, integrated curriculum, core curriculum and experiential curriculum, which are discussed below:

- ***Subject-centred curriculum:*** It is a type of curriculum in which the content is organized based on the subjects to be covered in a particular course. For example, the General Nursing and Midwifery (GNM) diploma, B.Sc. Nursing and M.Sc. Nursing degree curriculum prescribed by the Indian Nursing Council are the subject-centred curriculum.
- ***Student-centred curriculum:*** It is a type of curriculum in which the content is organized based on the nature, capabilities, interest, attitude and abilities of the students.
- ***Problem-centred curriculum:*** Problem-centred curriculum design is a type of learner-centred curriculum design. Problem-centred curriculum design teaches students how to see a problem and find a solution. This exposes students to real-world issues and helps them to develop skills that can be used in the real world. Problem-centred curriculum design improves the relevancy of the curriculum. It also allows students to be more creative and innovative while they learn. This type of curriculum design has a drawback that it does not consider learning styles of learners.
- ***Correlated curriculum:*** It is a type of curriculum, in which the content is organized in such a sequence that the content taught in one of the subject subsequently also helps to understand the problems in the other subject. For example, the content of microbiology is organized in such a manner that it is taught in the first semester of B.Sc. Nursing, so that students can easily understand the related topics of concurrently taught fundamentals of nursing subject, such as infections prevention, barrier nursing, medical and surgical hand washing.
- ***Fusion curriculum:*** In fusion curriculum, the two subjects are fused and are generally taught by the same instructor, such as in GNM diploma course the psychology and sociology are fused as behavioural sciences and anatomy and physiology are fused as biological sciences.
- ***Integrated curriculum:*** It is the unification of all the subjects and experiences to cover in a particular course or programme. For example, the content of anatomy-physiology, pathophysiology, pharmacology and medical-surgical nursing is organized in a manner that it had horizontal and vertical integration of subjects.
- ***Core curriculum:*** The term core curriculum, self-explanatory from the term itself, refers that the curriculum includes the core content or common to all the students and rest specialized content are differently learned by the different students. For example, advance nursing practices, nursing education, nursing research and biostatistics subjects are core or common to all the M.Sc. Nursing speciality students.
- ***Experiential curriculum:*** In the experiential curriculum, the content is organized in the form of real-life experience to teach the content through direct real-life experiences in the natural environment rather than the theoretical deliberation through classroom. For example, in the Florence Nightingale Model of curriculum of nursing, the nurses were predominantly taught through the real-life experience while working in hospital under supervision of experienced nurses; the same was followed in India before the university level nursing education era.

CURRICULUM DEVELOPMENT

The curriculum development is an ongoing process in each field of education, including nursing education, which is a scholarly and creative process to develop and design an evidence-based, context-relevant and unified curriculum. Curriculum development has different approaches. Some of the approaches are: analysing (i.e. task analysis), design (i.e. objective design), selection (i.e. selection of learning/teaching methodologies and appropriate evaluation techniques), formation (i.e. formulation of the curriculum execution committee and evaluation committee) and its review (i.e. curriculum review committee).

Curriculum development in nursing education is generally developed by the regulatory bodies such as Indian Nursing Council and/or State Nursing Council to ensure the uniformity in minimum standards of nursing and midwifery education nationally. The curriculum developed at national level also facilitates the inclusion of national health issues in curriculum and a smooth movement of nurses from one state to other or even other countries. **The curriculum process** includes the following steps (Fig. 4.4):

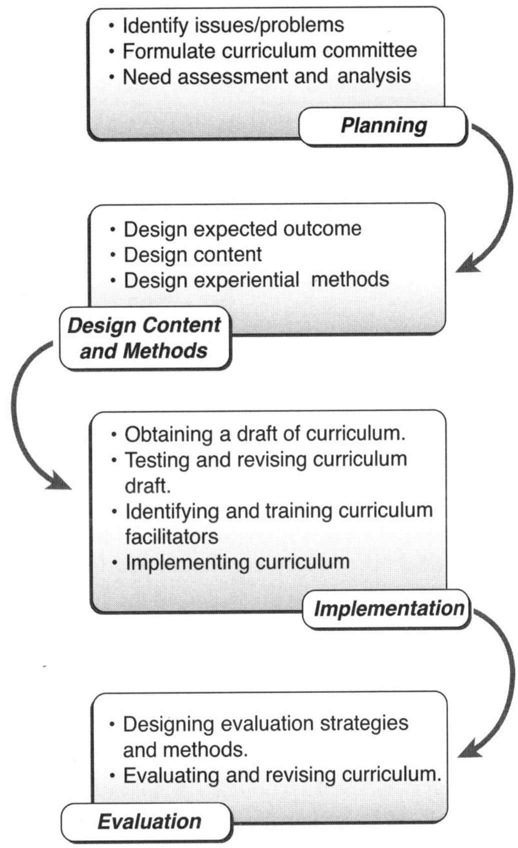

Figure 4.4

Curriculum development process.

A. PLANNING

This is the first phase of curriculum development process where issues/needs are identified for a new curriculum or in the existing curriculum; a curriculum development committee is identified and data are gathered, analysed and interpreted for need assessment and analysis for the development of particular curriculum. Through situation analysis, it is assessed that who will be the students? What will be their preentry level of education? What they have already learned before admission in a particular programme? What will be expected from the passing out graduates? And ideally what should be taught and which learning experiences are to be given during the particular course so that these students develop adequate knowledge base and skills. In addition, curriculum models are also reviewed by the curriculum committee so as to decide that based on mission, vision and philosophies of particular course/programme and national interests, which curriculum model will be most suitable for developing the curriculum for the particular programme.

The identification and formulation of curriculum committee is also a crucial decision to be made during this phase of curriculum development, where it must be ensured that members chosen for the curriculum committee should be national-level specialists, leaders, experts and researchers in the particular discipline, who have deep understanding of traditional as well as modern developments in the particular fields and are aware about the latest curriculum research findings, which are relevant for particular discipline.

B. DESIGN THE CONTENT AND METHODS

In this phase of curriculum development, the intended outcomes are stated, the relevant content is selected and experiential methods are designed. The content of the curriculum is designed based on the present and expected future trends in healthcare system, morbidity trends, education system, societal system, available teaching–learning resources, clinical facilities and prospective students. Traditionally, nursing curriculum had been the subject and semester-oriented curriculum, but recently many countries have emphasized on the module curriculum, which involves the division of curriculum in units/modules and where students are assessed at the end of each unit/module through which students earn specific credits to obtain a particular professional qualification. There are three important things to be developed in macrocurriculum: programme outcomes, content guidelines and teaching approaches, and schedules of teaching–learning during the particular programme period. The outcomes or objectives could be the programme objectives, level objectives, course objectives and unit objectives. There are three basic approaches of curriculum organization, that is organizing the curriculum by content, process and outcome. The curriculum could be a pure form of one approach or mix and match of more than any one approach of curriculum organization.

- *Content-based approach:* In this approach of curriculum organization, the focus remains on the inclusion of fundamental as well as core subjects relevant for a particular discipline. For example, including anatomy, physiology, biochemistry, psychology and sociology as fundamental subject and nursing foundations, medical-surgical nursing, child health nursing, mental health nursing as core nursing subject. The purpose of this approach is to transmit the worthwhile body of accumulated knowledge to budding students. The content-based approach is most widely used in designing the curriculum in nursing education, which start with listing the subjects to be included, followed by listing the relevant content for each subject to be included in the particular programme.
- *Process-based approach:* In this approach of curriculum organization, the focus remains towards the learner's experiences of the world of their discipline. For example, experiences of nursing, health and disease presented in the form of health problem or case studies. The purpose of this approach is to provide the learning through real-life learning experiences. This approach is based on the experiential learning theory where students develop life skills, such as problem-solving and critical thinking through direct experiences. This is a suitable approach for the programme where professionals have to be prepared in a limited time frame in which teachers help the students to search the information, analyse and interpret the problem-solving during the real-life experiences.
- *Outcome-based approach:* This approach of curriculum organization focuses on inclusion of expected competencies on the competition of particular module or course. The purpose of this curriculum organization is developing the abilities of reflection on problem and abilities to perform the tasks expected from particular professionals. This approach is very difficult to pin down the content in the terms of philosophical foundations. However, it proceeds from defining the minimum standards or outcomes to be achieved by students at the end of a particular course or degree.

I). Criteria for Selection of Content

The next most important and crucial task in this phase is selection and organization of content and learning experiences. The elements that determine the content and organization of curriculum are the educational philosophy, content, learning experiences, evaluation and outcome (Fig. 4.5).

The following criteria may be kept in mind while selecting the content and learning experiences for the particular curriculum:

- *Validity and meaningfulness:* The selected content must be meaningful for the particular programme and it must be duly validated by the experts of the particular discipline. The content also must reflect the scientific thinking and evidence-based practices. The content must focus towards fundamental knowledge rather than superficial information; it means learning the principles rather than only the facts.

- *Relevance to the social, economic, occupational, judicial, political, technical and geographic context:* The curriculum content must be socially, economically, occupationally, judicially, politically, technically and geographically relevant. In the 1980s, World Health Organization (WHO) recommended a community-based curriculum, where healthcare professionals must be initially placed for community field experience followed by long-term hospital experience so that they understand community and family dynamics before understanding the diseases and their management.
- *A balance between breadth and depth:* It is a serious dilemma in each of the course and discipline that what to teach and how much to teach and what to be left. One school of thought says that it is better to know everything but other school of thought supports that it is better to master one area rather than knowing only little about everything. The content-based approach of curriculum organization supports the ideas of covering everything though it could be only superficial but the process-based and outcome-based approaches of curriculum organization support the idea of mastering one area rather than covering everything superficially. Therefore, it is essential for the curriculum development experts to maintain balance between breadth and depth of curriculum content so that most of the essential areas are covered and mastery in essential areas is also achieved.

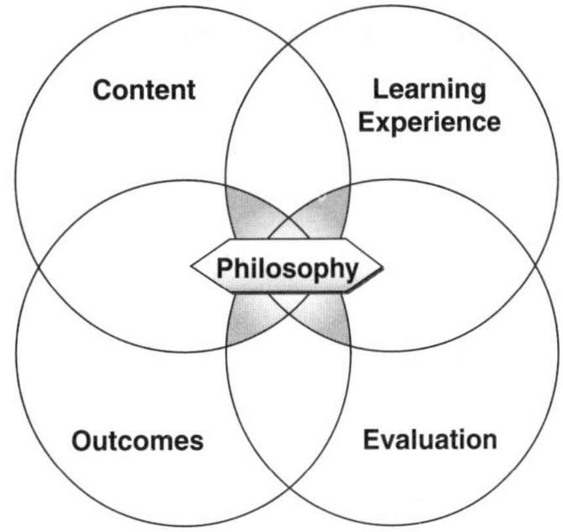

Figure 4.5

Elements determining content and organization of curriculum.

II). Principles for Organization of Content

It is essential that curriculum is a 'coherent set of course' where there is an optimum level of horizontal as well as vertical relationship of subjects/content, so that a smooth transition may be ensured from one unit/module to another and one course to another. The following criteria may be kept in mind while organizing the content and learning experiences for the particular course:

- *Principle of continuity:* The content presented in the curriculum must be in continuity so that students can experience smoothness in learning the topics. The continuity must be in terms of complexities, breadth, depth and sophistication required. To maintain the continuity in the content, the vertical and horizontal strands are used.
- *Principle of order:* Principle of learning experience is referred to the sequencing of the learning experiences and presentations of concepts. To ensure the principle of order in content organization, following teaching–learning maximums may be used:
  - *Simple to complex:* For example, teaching tables before teaching multiplications.
  - *Chronological:* First including concept and definition followed by the causes, pathophysiology, clinical manifestation, diagnostics test, treatment and nursing management.
  - *Whole to part:* Teaching complete healthcare system than teaching each part of system in detail.
  - *Part to whole:* Teaching cell, followed by tissue, organs and systems of the body.
  - *Health to illness:* Teaching physiology before the pathology.
- *Principle of integration:* It is essential to organize the content of curriculum, which is horizontally and vertically integrated to avoid the compartmentalized learning.

C. IMPLEMENTATION

After preparing the final draft of the curriculum, the curriculum is tested and revised. In this phase, the facilitators are identified and trained, who are going to facilitate the implementation of the curriculum and finally implement the curriculum in the real field. It is not easy to implement a new curriculum because of teacher's resistance to accept the change, lack of acceptance of new responsibilities due to change in curriculum and lack of knowledge and skill in implementation of new curriculum. The effective implementation of new curriculum may be ensured through facilitative leadership, training and motivation of people involved in the change process, creating conducive environment for implementation of change in curriculum, effective monitoring and support in curriculum implementation.

D. EVALUATION

This is the final phase of the curriculum development in which the evaluation strategies and methods are identified and they are utilized for evaluation of implemented curriculum. The curriculum evaluation is designed to assess logic and coherence of curriculum concepts, design, implementation and utility; in addition, fairness, objectivity, comprehensiveness, credibility, usefulness and effective communication may also be assessed. The major purpose of curriculum evaluation is to ensure the continuous improvement in the curriculum draft. The curriculum evaluation could be internal versus external, formative versus summative, holistic versus specific and high stakes versus low stakes. The evaluation process includes the following main steps:

- Defining standards against which evaluation will be done.
- Collecting the information after implementation of curriculum from different stakeholders.
- Analysing and synthesizing the results.
- Preparing the recommendations for improvement of curriculum.

FACTORS INFLUENCING CURRICULUM DEVELOPMENT

The curriculum development is influenced by many factors, such as educational psychology, educational philosophies, society, economic status, political will, scientific and technical development, available resources and capabilities, interest, attitude and abilities of students. The detail about determinants of curriculum development is given below (Fig. 4.6):

- ***Individual factors:*** The interest, attitude, abilities and capabilities of the learners are the most important factors which determine the development of the content in the curriculum. For example, the curriculum for the anatomy subject will not be similar for the Auxiliary Nurse Midwifery programme and Bachelor of Science in nursing programme.
- ***Educational philosophical factors:*** The type of educational philosophy followed for the development of the curriculum is also the important determining factor for the curriculum development. For example, the essentialism educational philosophy supports the outcome-based approach of curriculum development, whereas the realism and idealism support the content-based approach in curriculum development.
- ***Societal factors:*** The person getting education in any of the discipline ultimately has to go back and work in the society. So it is essential for the curriculum development committee to consider the social factor while developing the curriculum. It is essential to know that what particular society will be expecting from the particular group, so that content may be designed accordingly.

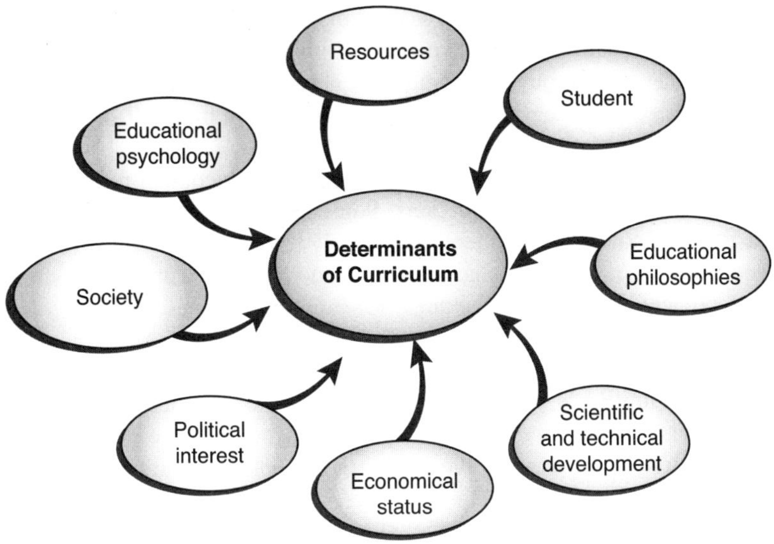

Figure 4.6

Determinants of curriculum development.

- ***Political factors:*** In any country including India, political will is very important factor for the success of any of the programme. Therefore, political interest is also a very important determinant of the curriculum development.
- ***Economic factors:*** Nothing can be possible without the availability of the finance. Therefore, curriculum development committee should consider the economic factor as one of the crucial determinant factors for the curriculum development.
- ***Scientific and technical factors:*** Scientific and technical development is the main driving force behind the development of the any of the field. Thus, scientific and technical development is also a significant determinant factor for the curriculum development for the particular discipline.
- ***Factors related to resources:*** The needs of resources are the paramount important factor in planning, implantation and evaluation of any programme. Thus, the curriculum development also largely depends on the available resources with particular organization, institute or country for the success of it. The important resource factors that may affect the curriculum development are the available teaching–learning infrastructure, faculty, teaching–learning aids and finance.

BARRIERS IN CURRICULUM DEVELOPMENT IN NURSING

Curriculum development in nursing education can encounter several barriers that can impede the process of designing and implementing effective educational programmes. Here are some common barriers in curriculum development in nursing education:

- **Limited faculty expertise**: Developing a comprehensive nursing curriculum requires faculty members with expertise in various nursing specialties and areas of practice. However, finding faculty members who possess the necessary knowledge and experience in specific domains can be challenging. This limitation can affect the depth and breadth of the curriculum, making it difficult to adequately address the diverse needs and demands of nursing education.

- **Time constraints**: Nursing faculty often have multiple responsibilities, including teaching, research, clinical practice and administrative duties. Limited time available for curriculum development can hinder the thorough exploration of new teaching methods, incorporation of evidence-based practices and integration of emerging healthcare trends. Time constraints may lead to rushed or superficial curriculum development processes.
- **Resistance to change**: Implementing curriculum changes can encounter resistance from faculty members, administrators and other stakeholders. Some faculty may be hesitant to adopt new teaching strategies, technologies or content, particularly if they have been using the same methods for an extended period. Resistance to change can impede innovation and hinder the integration of contemporary approaches into the curriculum.
- **Accreditation and regulatory requirements**: Nursing education programmes must adhere to accreditation and regulatory standards set by professional nursing organizations and regulatory bodies. Compliance with these requirements can be complex and time-consuming. It may pose challenges for curriculum developers to ensure that the curriculum meets these standards while also addressing the evolving needs of the nursing profession and the healthcare system.
- **Limited resources**: Insufficient resources, including financial, technological and material resources, can significantly impact curriculum development. Adequate funding is essential for faculty development, infrastructure enhancement, procurement of teaching materials and the incorporation of simulation and clinical learning experiences. Limited resources can hinder the implementation of an innovative and learner-centred curriculum.
- **Coordination and collaboration challenges**: Curriculum development involves collaboration among multiple stakeholders, such as faculty, administrators, clinical experts and community partners. Coordination and effective communication among these individuals and groups can be challenging, especially when they have different schedules, priorities and perspectives. Insufficient collaboration can result in a fragmented curriculum that lacks coherence and integration.
- **Dynamic healthcare environment**: The healthcare landscape is constantly evolving due to advancements in technology, changes in healthcare policies and emerging healthcare challenges. Keeping the curriculum up to date and relevant to the evolving healthcare environment can be demanding. Curriculum developers need to regularly review and update the curriculum to ensure that it prepares nursing students with the necessary knowledge and skills to address current and future healthcare needs.

FACILITATORS IN CURRICULUM DEVELOPMENT IN NURSING EDUCATION

Facilitators play a crucial role in the successful development of a nursing curriculum. They are factors or conditions that promote and support the curriculum development process. Here are some facilitators in curriculum development in nursing education:

1. **Collaboration and interdisciplinary approach**: Collaboration among various stakeholders, including nursing faculty, clinical experts, administrators and representatives from the healthcare industry, is essential for effective curriculum development. Adopting an interdisciplinary approach helps ensure that the curriculum reflects the needs and perspectives of different stakeholders, integrates diverse perspectives and prepares students for the interprofessional nature of healthcare practice.

2. **Stakeholder engagement**: Engaging stakeholders throughout the curriculum development process fosters a sense of ownership and shared responsibility. Involving nursing faculty, students, alumni, practicing nurses, employers and professional nursing organizations allows for the incorporation of diverse perspectives, expertise and experiences. This engagement helps align the curriculum with current and future healthcare needs and enhances its relevance.
3. **Clear vision and goals**: Establishing a clear vision and goals for the nursing curriculum provides a guiding framework for development. A well-defined vision and goals ensure that the curriculum is focused, coherent and aligned with the mission and values of the nursing programme and institution. It helps curriculum developers make informed decisions about content, teaching strategies and assessment methods.
4. **Evidence-based practice**: Incorporating evidence-based practice principles into curriculum development ensures that the curriculum reflects current knowledge, best practices and the latest research in nursing. Using evidence-based guidelines and research findings helps ensure that the curriculum is based on the best available evidence and prepares students to provide high-quality, evidence-based care.
5. **Faculty development and support**: Providing faculty members with ongoing professional development opportunities and support enhances their capacity to engage in curriculum development. Faculty development programmes can focus on curriculum design, pedagogy, assessment methods and incorporating emerging trends in nursing education. Supporting faculty members with dedicated time, resources and mentorship for curriculum development activities helps ensure their active participation and commitment.
6. **Continuous evaluation and feedback**: Incorporating a system for continuous evaluation and feedback allows for ongoing improvement of the nursing curriculum. Collecting data on student outcomes, course evaluations, employer feedback and societal needs helps identify areas for enhancement or modification. Regular evaluation ensures that the curriculum remains relevant, up to date and aligned with the evolving needs of the nursing profession and healthcare industry.
7. **Resources and infrastructure**: Adequate allocation of resources, including financial, human, and material resources, is essential for successful curriculum development. Sufficient resources support the development of innovative teaching strategies, investment in educational technology, creation of simulation labs and access to up-to-date teaching materials. A well-equipped infrastructure supports the implementation of the curriculum and facilitates effective teaching and learning experiences.
8. **Integration of technology**: Integrating technology into the curriculum can enhance teaching and learning experiences, engage students and prepare them for the use of technology in healthcare practices. Utilizing educational technologies, such as simulation software, virtual reality, online learning platforms and electronic health records, can facilitate active learning, skills development and critical thinking. Technology integration also aligns with the expectations and preferences of the current generation of learners.
9. **Flexibility and adaptability**: Designing a curriculum that is flexible and adaptable to changing educational and healthcare contexts is essential. A curriculum that can be easily modified or updated allows for timely incorporation of emerging trends, new research and advancements in nursing practice. Flexibility also accommodates evolving student needs, societal demands and changes in healthcare policies and technology.
10. **Diversity and inclusion**: Promoting diversity and inclusion in the curriculum development process is crucial. Recognizing and valuing diverse perspectives, experiences and cultural backgrounds contribute to a curriculum that is relevant, inclusive and sensitive to the needs of diverse populations. Incorporating content related to cultural competence, social determinants of health and health disparities helps prepare nursing students to provide equitable and culturally sensitive care.

By leveraging these facilitators, nursing education institutions can enhance the development of a robust and responsive curriculum that prepares students to meet the evolving demands of the nursing profession and provide high-quality patient care.

FORMULATION OF EDUCATIONAL OBJECTIVES

Objectives serve as a guiding path for people who move ahead; if someone is not certain of where he is going, he may end up at an unexpected place. Similarly, teaching–learning activities must begin with well-planned objectives so that the expected purposes of the planned teaching–learning activities can be efficiently achieved.

For an educational programme to be effective, the purposes and objectives are to be clearly stated so that it is easy to select the right subject content, learning experiences, clinical experiences and the right methods to evaluate student performance and the teaching–learning process. The objectives can either be teacher centred, student centred or subject content centred and must be planned keeping in mind the needs of the society, educational philosophy, values and circumstances under which students are expected to perform tasks in their life.

I. MEANING OF EDUCATIONAL OBJECTIVES

The words *aims*, *goals*, *objectives* and *targets* are often interchangeably used in relation to educational purposes. However, they are distinct and primarily the most commonly used terms for educational purposes to be achieved by students after undergoing the teaching–learning process.

> *Educational objectives are the results sought by the learner at the end of the educational program that is what the student should be able to do at the end of a learning period that they could not be beforehand.*
>
> **—J.J. Guilbert**

> *Educational objectives are the behaviors to be displayed by a learner, aims are for the teacher and the objectives are for the learners to achieve through the support and guidance of the teacher.*

> *Educational objectives are the statement of those changes in behavior that are desired as a result of specific learner and teacher activity which is a two-way process.*

II. FUNCTIONS AND IMPORTANCE OF EDUCATIONAL OBJECTIVES

The aim of education is to transfer knowledge to students and ensure their overall expected development. Crystal clear objectives are essential for the ultimate success of the teaching–learning process. Further, evaluation or assessment in the educational system will be aimless in the absence of clearly stated objectives. Therefore, before planning an educational activity, one must have clearly stated educational objectives so that the teacher and learner are clear about what needs to be done to reach at these prespecified goals. Thus, educational objectives have a significant importance in the teaching–learning process as discussed below:

- Educational objectives are essentially important in the teaching–learning process, where the teacher and the learner get clear direction about where they are expected to reach at the end of a particular teaching–learning process.

- Educational objectives also help teachers plan appropriate evaluation methods and procedures for the students so that the students can be appropriately judged (whether the students have achieved the preset goals of a particular teaching activity or not).
- They are also important to inform the teacher and students of the gap between the expected and actual number of changes that have occurred in a particular student at the end of a particular teaching–learning activity.
- Educational objectives are responsible for providing direction to the teaching–learning as well as the evaluation process in a particular educational system.
- Educational objectives also help the teacher and the learner focus on a particular teaching–learning activity to achieve the specific predetermined educational goals.
- Educational objectives also help determine the educational recourse material, infrastructure, course content and curricular and cocurricular activities to achieve specific predetermined educational goals.
- Educational objectives provide an opportunity for the teacher to effectively monitor the teaching–learning process under the light of predetermined objectives.

III. CHARACTERISTICS OF EDUCATIONAL OBJECTIVES

The well-stated objectives should be **SMART** (**S**pecific, **M**easurable, **A**ttainable, **R**ealistic and **T**ime bound) and **FOCUSED** (**F**easible, **O**bservable, **C**entred on students **U**nequivocally, **S**equentially appropriate, **E**ver relevant and **D**evelopmentally appropriate). The characteristics of the educational objectives are discussed below (Box 4.1):

- ***Specific:*** Educational objectives must be specific for a particular educational programme or learning instructions so that learners can achieve the specific goals of the educational programme or instructions.
- ***Measurable:*** Objectives must be stated in measurable terms rather than in an ambiguous nonmeasurable manner so that the teacher can evaluate the learners without any undue inconvenience. The teacher and the learner should be clear about what and how the evaluation is to be done towards the end of the programme or learning instructions.
- ***Attainable:*** Good educational objectives must be attainable within a stipulated time frame without undue wastage of time. Objectives that are too broad and require multiple cluster components to be achieved at one time may make educational objectives unattainable. Therefore, educational

BOX 4.1 CHARACTERISTICS OF EDUCATIONAL OBJECTIVES

Smart

S: Specific
M: Measurable
A: Attainable
R: Realistic
T: Time bound

Focused

F: Feasible
O: Observable
C: Centred on student
U: Unequivocal
S: Sequentially appropriate
E: Ever relevant
D: Developmentally appropriate

objectives must be planned with a single learning outcome and a narrow focus so they are attainable within a predetermined time frame.

- ***Realistic:*** Objectives must be planned keeping in mind the availability of basic resources and abilities and capabilities of the individual group of students so that they can be considered as realistic with reference to resources and individuality.
- ***Time bound:*** Well-written objectives must be time bound so that the teacher and the learner are clear about when learning has to be achieved and should motivate them do so accordingly.
- ***Feasible:*** Objectives must be feasible in terms availability of time, resources, attitude and intellectual abilities of the students.
- ***Observable:*** The educational objective must be observable so that it can be observed and evaluated effectively. If an objective is not observable, it imposes a difficulty on the observation and measurement of learning in students. Verbs such as *to list, to compute* and *to define* make the stated educational objectives observable. On the contrary, verbs such as *to know, to understand* and *to enjoy* make the educational objectives unobservable.
- ***Centred on student:*** Good educational objectives are generally student centric and focus on what the student is expected to do rather than what the teacher is expected to do.
- ***Unequivocal:*** Ambiguous language or words should not be used while writing the objectives. Simple, precise and concise statements should be used while stating the educational objectives.
- ***Sequentially appropriate:*** Educational objectives must be sequentially appropriate that is preliminarily things that are expected to be achieved should be listed first followed by the complex things that should be achieved. For example, begin with define and then proceed towards enlisting and describing the complex parts of the topic or course content.
- ***Ever relevant:*** Objectives must always be relevant to a particular subject content and individual group of students. Further, objectives must be relevant to the level of expected learning as well as other teaching–learning factors.
- ***Developmentally appropriate:*** The educational objectives must be developmentally appropriate to a particular learner. They must be customized according to the intellectual, linguistic, social and moral developmental level of the learner.

IV. TYPES OF EDUCATIONAL OBJECTIVES

A. ACCORDING TO LEVEL OF EDUCATIONAL OBJECTIVES

- *General/institutional objectives:* These objectives are known as *professional functions*, which are the statements identifying the major knowledge or skills that all students of a programme are expected to possess at the completion of their programme. They are short and relatively vague, but they clearly define what students are expected to achieve at the end of their course or programme.
- *Intermediate objectives:* These objectives are also known as *departmental objectives* or *professional activities*. Intermediate objectives are a set of statements identifying the skills expected to be acquired by a group of students while studying in a particular department/division of their course or programme. However, these intermediate or departmental objectives must be consistent with institutional or general objectives of a particular programme.
- *Instructional objectives or specific objectives:* Instructional objectives are also known as *behavioural objectives* or *learning objectives* and are basically statements which clearly describe an anticipated learning outcome. They are brief and precise statements which clearly identify the

basic skill or competence expected to be demonstrated by a group of students on the completion of a specific teaching–learning instructions.

B. ACCORDING TO TAXONOMY OF EDUCATIONAL OBJECTIVES

- *Cognitive domain objectives:* The cognitive domain objectives (Bloom, 1956) involve knowledge and development of intellectual skills. This includes the recall or recognition of specific facts, procedural patterns and concepts that serve in the development of intellectual abilities and skills. There are six major categories: knowledge, comprehension, application, analysis, synthesis and evaluation, starting from the simplest behaviour to the most complex. The categories can be thought of as degrees of difficulty. The first ones must normally be mastered before the next one can take place.
- *Affective domain objectives:* The affective domain objectives (Krathwohl, Bloom and Masia, 1973) include the manner in which we deal with things emotionally, such as feelings, values, appreciation, enthusiasms, motivations and attitudes. The five major categories are receiving phenomenon, responding to phenomenon, valuing, organizing and internalizing values (characterizing), from the simplest behaviour to the most complex.
- *Psychomotor domain objectives:* The psychomotor domain objectives (Simpson, 1972) include physical movement, coordination and the use of the motor-skill areas. The development of these skills requires practice and is measured in terms of speed, precision, distance, procedures or techniques in execution. The seven major categories are perception, set, guide response, mechanism, complex overt response, adaptation and organization, from the simplest behaviour to the most complex.

V. TAXONOMY OF EDUCATIONAL OBJECTIVES

The taxonomy for the educational objectives points out that they are concerned with intended behaviour or the behaviour to be learned by students rather than the actual behaviour learned from an educational objective (Bloom, 1956). In other words, taxonomy means 'a set of classification principles or structure and domains simply means category'.

Bloom's taxonomy divides educational objectives into three domains: cognitive, affective and psychomotor. Within these domains, learning at higher levels is dependent on having attained the prerequisite knowledge and skills at lower levels. The goal of Bloom's taxonomy is to motivate educators to focus on all three domains creating a more holistic form of education.

Bloom initially focused on the cognitive domain and later his colleagues published on affective domain. However, the details of the psychomotor domain were published by other authors later. The major categories in each domain are discussed below (Fig. 4.7).

I. COGNITIVE DOMAIN OF EDUCATIONAL OBJECTIVES

The aspects of the cognitive domain revolve around knowledge, comprehension and critical thinking on a particular topic. This domain focuses on thinking skills. Traditional education tends to emphasize on skills in this domain, particularly the lower-order objectives. There are six levels in the cognitive domain, moving from the lowest order processes to the highest as discussed in Fig. 4.8 and Table 4.1.

II. AFFECTIVE DOMAIN OF EDUCATIONAL OBJECTIVES

The aspects in the affective domain describe the way people react emotionally and their ability to feel another living thing's pain or joy. Affective objectives typically target the awareness and growth in

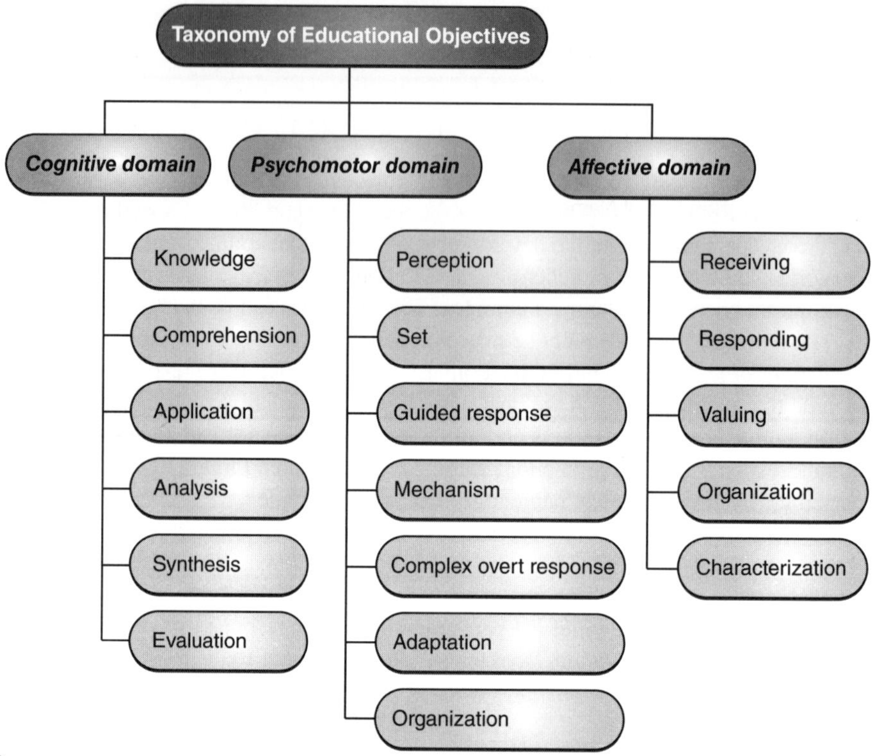

Figure 4.7

Educational objectives, based on Bloom's taxonomy.

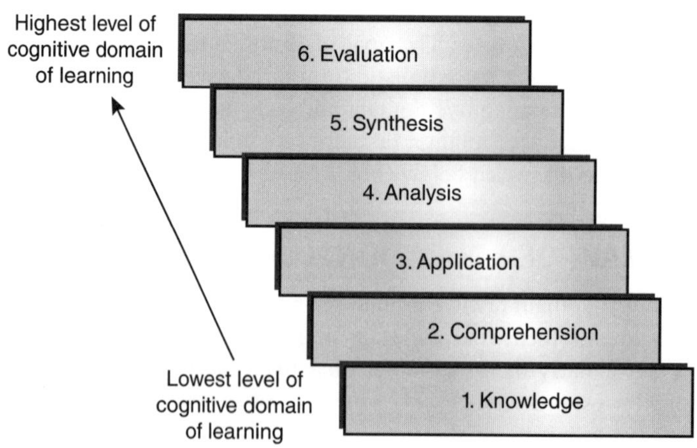

Figure 4.8

Categories of cognitive domain of the educational objectives.

Table 4.1 Description of Categories in Cognitive Domain With Relevant Examples and Active Verbs

Categories with Description	Examples of Educational Objective	Commonly Used Action Verbs
1. Knowledge: Remembering terms, facts and details without necessarily understanding the concept.	List the names of the bones in axial skeletal system Name the part of small intestine	Defines, describes, identifies, labels, lists, matches, names, outlines, recalls, recognizes, reproduces, selects, states
2. Comprehension: Understand the meaning, translation, interpolation and interpretation of instructions and problems. State a problem in one's own words.	Distinguishes the male and female reproductive system Explain the role of genetics factors in colorectal cancer	Comprehends, converts, defends, distinguishes, estimates, explains, extends, generalizes, gives an example, infers, interprets, paraphrases, predicts, rewrites, summarizes, translates
3. Application: Use a concept in a new situation or unprompted use of an abstraction. Applies what was learned in the classroom into novel situations in the work place.	Applies the formula to calculate the daily protein requirement of a healthy adult person Construct a conceptual model using Roy's adaptation model	Applies, changes, computes, constructs, demonstrates, discovers, manipulates, modifies, operates, predicts, prepares, produces, relates, shows, solves, uses
4. Analysis: Separates material or concepts into component parts so that its organizational structure may be understood. Distinguishes between facts and inferences.	Troubleshoot a piece of equipment by using logical deduction Recognize logical fallacies in reasoning	Analyses, breaks down, compares, contrasts, diagrams, deconstructs, differentiates, discriminates, distinguishes, identifies, illustrates, infers, outlines, relates, selects, separates
5. Synthesis: Builds a structure or pattern from diverse elements. Put parts together to form a whole, with emphasis on creating a new meaning or structure.	Design a procedure manual for critical care unit Plan a staff requirement for a newly opened 20 bedded surgical unit	Categorizes, combines, compiles, composes, creates, devises, designs, explains, generates, modifies, organizes, plans, rearranges, reconstructs, relates, reorganizes, revises, rewrites, summarizes, tells, writes
6. Evaluation: Make judgements about the value of ideas or materials.	Select a most practical solution for reduction in prevalence of bedsores in neurological unit Justify the new planned budget for a nursing college library	Appraises, compares, concludes, contrasts, criticizes, critiques, defends, describes, discriminates, evaluates, explains, interprets, justifies, relates, summarizes, supports

attitudes, emotion, motivation and feelings. There are five levels in the affective domain, moving from the lowest order processes to the highest as discussed in Fig. 4.9 and Table 4.2.

III. PSYCHOMOTOR DOMAIN OF EDUCATIONAL OBJECTIVES

The psychomotor domain describes about obtaining the skills or abilities to carry out physical tasks such as the skill of a nurse in catheterizing a patient or operating a mechanical ventilator. Psychomotor educational objectives usually focus on the expected changes in skills of an individual. Bloom and his colleagues did not offer subcategories of the psychomotor objectives, but other authors (Dave, 1967; Simpson, 1972; Harrow, 1972) later created the exhaustive subcategories of the psychomotor domain. Simpson's proposed subcategories are as discussed in Fig. 4.10 and Table 4.3.

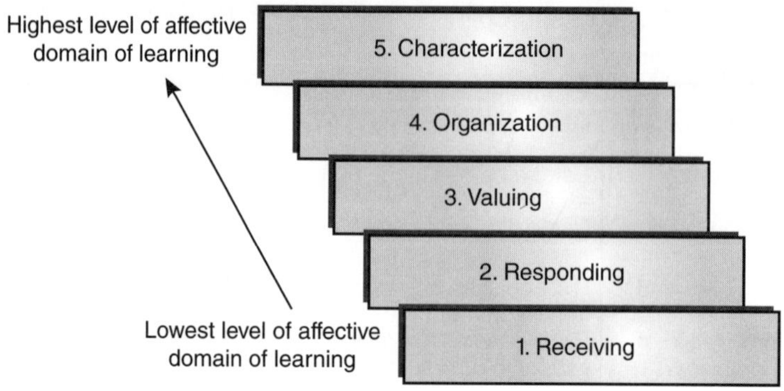

Figure 4.9

Categories of affective domain of the educational objectives.

Table 4.2 Description of Categories in Affective Domain With Relevant Examples and Active Verbs

Categories With Description	Examples of Educational Objective	Commonly Used Action Verbs
1. Receiving phenomena: Awareness, willingness to hear, selected attention.	Listen to others with respect Listen for and remember the name of newly introduced people	Asks, chooses, describes, follows, gives, holds, identifies, locates, names, points to, selects, sits, erects, replies, uses
2. Responding to phenomena: Active participation on the part of the learners. Attends and reacts to a particular phenomenon. Learning outcomes may emphasize compliance in responding, willingness to respond or satisfaction in responding (motivation).	Participates in class discussions Questions new ideals, concepts, models, etc. in order to fully understand them	Answers, assists, aids, complies, conforms, discusses, greets, helps, labels, performs, practises, presents, reads, recites, reports, selects, tells, writes
3. Valuing: The worth or value a person attaches to a particular object, phenomenon or behaviour. This ranges from simple acceptance to the more complex state of commitment. Valuing is based on the internalization of a set of specified values, while clues to these values are expressed in the learner's overt behaviour and are often identifiable.	Demonstrates belief in the democratic process Is sensitive towards individual and cultural differences (value diversity)	Completes, demonstrates, differentiates, explains, follows, forms, initiates, invites, joins, justifies, proposes, reads, reports, selects, shares, studies, works
4. Organization: Organizes values into priorities by contrasting different values, resolving conflicts between them and creating a unique value system. The emphasis is on comparing, relating and synthesizing values.	Explains the role of systematic planning in solving problems Accepts professional ethical standards	Adheres, alters, arranges, combines, compares, completes, defends, explains, formulates, generalizes, identifies, integrates, modifies, orders, organizes, prepares, relates, synthesizes
5. Internalizing values (characterization): Has a value system that controls their behaviour. The behaviour is pervasive, consistent, predictable, and most importantly, characteristic of the learner. Instructional objectives are concerned with the student's general patterns of adjustment (personal, social and emotional).	Cooperates in group activities Displays a professional commitment to ethical practice on a daily basis	Acts, discriminates, displays, influences, listens, modifies, performs, practices, proposes, qualifies, questions, revises, serves, solves, verifies

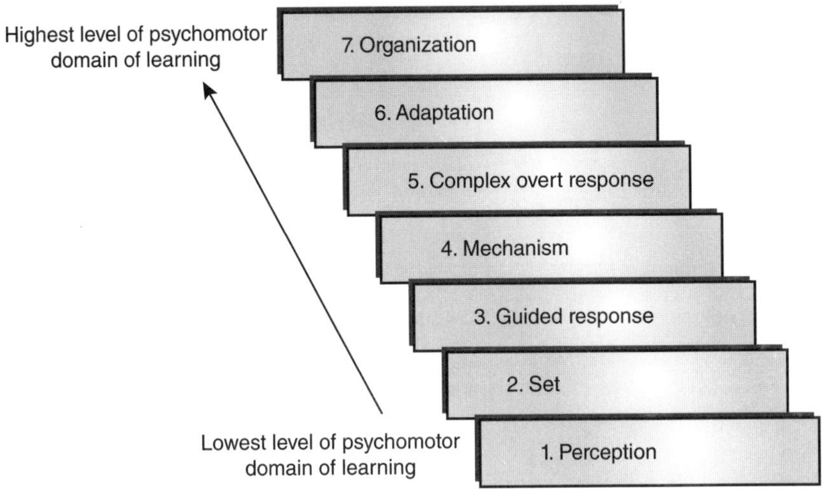

Figure 4.10

Categories of psychomotor domain of the educational objectives.

Table 4.3 Description of Categories in Psychomotor Domain With Relevant Examples and Active Verbs

Categories With Description	Examples of Educational Objective	Commonly Used Action Verbs
1. Perception: The ability to use sensory cues to guide motor activity. This ranges from sensory stimulation, through cue selection, to translation.	Detects nonverbal communication cues Adjusts drop rate based on the CVP readings of the patients	Chooses, describes, detects, differentiates, distinguishes, identifies, isolates, relates, selects
2. Set: Readiness to act. It includes mental, physical and emotional sets. These three sets are dispositions that predetermine a person's response to different situations (sometimes called *mindsets*).	Recognize one's abilities and limitations Shows desire to learn a new process	Begins, displays, explains, moves, proceeds, reacts, shows, states, volunteers
3. Guided response: The early stages in learning a complex skill that includes imitation and trial and error. Adequacy of performance is achieved by practising.	Follows instructions to build a model Responds hand signals of instructor while learning to operate a mechanical ventilator	Copies, traces, follows, reacts, reproduces, responds
4. Mechanism: This is the intermediate stage in learning a complex skill. Learned responses have become habitual and the movements can be performed with some confidence and proficiency.	Use a personal computer Operate a mechanical ventilator	Assembles, calibrates, constructs, dismantles, displays, fastens, fixes, grinds, heats, manipulates, measures, mends, mixes, organizes, sketches
5. Complex overt response: The skilful performance of motor acts that involve complex movement patterns. Proficiency is indicated by a quick, accurate and highly coordinated performance, requiring a minimum of energy. This category includes performing without hesitation and automatic performance. For example, players often utter sounds of satisfaction or expletives as soon as they hit a tennis ball or throw a football because they can tell by the feel of the act what the result will produce.	Operates a computer quickly and accurately Displays competence in performing wound dressing	Assembles, builds, calibrates, constructs, dismantles, displays, fastens, fixes, grinds, heats, manipulates, measures, mends, mixes, organizes, sketches NOTE: The keywords are the same as mechanism but will have adverbs or adjectives that indicate that the performance is quicker, better, more accurate, etc.

Continued

Table 4.3 Description of Categories in Psychomotor Domain With Relevant Examples and Active Verbs—cont'd

Categories With Description	Examples of Educational Objective	Commonly Used Action Verbs
6. Adaptation: Skills are well developed and the individual can modify movement patterns to fit special requirements.	Responds effectively to unexpected experiences such as emergency shock case	Adapts, alters, changes, rearranges, reorganizes, revises, varies
7. Organization: Creating new movement patterns to fit a particular situation or specific problem. Learning outcomes emphasize creativity based upon highly developed skills.	Constructs a new nursing theory Develops a new and comprehensive training programming for critical care nurses	Arranges, builds, combines, composes, constructs, creates, designs, initiate, makes, originates

ACTION VERBS USED FOR WRITING OBJECTIVES

The actions verbs suggested in Tables 4.4–4.6 should be used for writing objectives in each domain. However, some of these verbs cannot be measured or are redundant and known as *nonfunctional verbs*. They should be *avoided* when writing objectives (Box 4.2).

Table 4.4 Active Verbs Used for Writing Objectives in Cognitive Domain

Knowledge	Comprehension	Application	Analysis	Synthesis	Evaluation
Count	Associate	Add	Analyse	Categorize	Appraise
Define	Compute	Apply	Arrange	Combine	Assess
Describe	Convert	Calculate	Breakdown	Compile	Compare
Draw	Defend	Change	Combine	Compose	Conclude
Identify	Discuss	Classify	Design	Create	Contrast
Labels	Distinguish	Complete	Detect	Drive	Criticize
List	Estimate	Compute	Develop	Design	Critique
Match	Explain	Demonstrate	Diagram	Devise	Determine
Name	Extend	Discover	Differentiate	Explain	Grade
Outlines	Extrapolate	Divide	Discriminate	Generate	Interpret
Point out	Generalize	Examine	Illustrate	Integrate	Judge
Quote	Give examples	Graph	Infer	Modify	Justify
Read	Infer	Interpolate	Outline	Order	Measure
Recite	Paraphrase	Manipulate	Relate	Organize	Rank
Recognize	Predict	Modify	Select	Plan	Rate
Record	Rewrite	Operate	Separate	Prescribe	Support
Repeat	Summarize	Prepare	Subdivide	Propose	Test
Reproduces		Produce	Utilize	Rearrange	
Selects		Show		Reconstruct	
State		Solve		Reorganize	
Write		Subtract		Revise	
		Translate		Summarize	
		Use		Specify	

Table 4.5 Active Verbs Used for Writing Objectives in Affective Domain

Receiving	Responding	Valuing	Organizing	Characterization by Value
Accept	Agree	Adopt	Anticipate	Act
Acknowledge	Allow	Aid	Collaborate	Administer
Attend (to)	Answer	Care (for)	Consider	Advance
Follow	Ask	Complete	Consult	Advocate
Listen	Assist	Compliment	Coordinator	Challenge
Meet	Choose	Contribute	Design	Change
Observe	Communicate	Delay	Direct	Commit (to)
Receive	Comply	Encourage	Establish	Counsel
	Confront	Endorse	Facilitate	Criticize
	Cooperate	Enforce	Follow	Debate
	Demonstrate	Evaluate	Though	Defend
	Describe	Expedite	Investigate	Disagree
	Discuss	Foster	Judge	Dispute
	Display	Guide	Head	Empathize
	Exhibit	Initiate	Manage	Endeavour
	Follow	Interact	Modify	Enhance
	Give	Join	Organize	Excuse
	Help	Justify	Plan	Forgive
	Identify	Maintain	Qualify	Influence
	Locate	Monitor	Recommend	Motivate
	Notify	Praise	Raise	Negotiate
	Obey	Present	Simplify	Object
	Offer	Propose	Specify	Persist
	Participate (in)	Query	Submit	Praise
	Practice	React	Synthesize	Prompt
	Present	Respect	Test	Reject
	Read	Seek	Vary	Seek
	Reply	Share	Weight	Strive
	Report	Study		
	Respond	Subscribe		
	Select	Suggest		
		Support		
		Uphold		

Table 4.6 Active Verbs Used for Writing Objectives in Psychomotor Domain

Absorb	Cool	Fill	Manoeuvre	Start	Stopper
Add	Correct	Filter	Manipulate	Read	Store
Adsorb	Count	Fractionate	Mark	Record	Suspend
Adjust	Create	Frame	Macerate	Release	Take
Aliquot	Crush	Freeze	Measure	Remove	Test
Apply	Cut	Grade	Mix	Replace	Thaw
Aspirate	Decant	Grasp	Moisten	Resuspend	Thread

Continued

Table 4.6 Active Verbs Used for Writing Objectives in Psychomotor Domain —cont'd

Assemble	Demonstrate	Grind	Mount	Retest	Tilt
Balance	Describe	Group	Pack	Rinse	Time
Bind	Design	Guide	Palpate	Roll	Tip
Blend	Dialyse	Handle	Participate	Rotate	Titrate
Build	Differentiate	Heat	Perform	Save	Trim
Calculate	Dilute	Observe	Pick	Scan	Touch
Calibrate	Discard	Obtain	Pipet	Score	Transfer
Centrifuge	Dismantle	Open	Place	Screen	Troubleshoot
Change	Dispense	Hemolyse	Plate	Seal	Turn
Choose	Dispose	Identify	Plot	Select	Type
Classify	Dissect	Illustrate	Position	Sensitize	Use
Clean	Dissolve	Incubate	Pour	Separate	Utilize
Collate	Drain	Inject	Prepare	Set	View
Collect	Draw	Input	Press	Sever	Warm
Combine	Dry	Insert	Process	Shake	Wash
Connect	Elute	Invert	Produce	Sharpen	Watch
Construct	Employ	Investigate	Programme	Ship	Weigh
Control	Estimate	Isolate	Pull	Siphon	Withdraw
Combine	Evacuate	Label	Puncture	Spin	Wipe
Confirm	Examine	Locate	Push	Spread	Wrap
Connect	Expel	Localize	Squeeze	Stick	
Construct	Operate	Maintain	Stain	Stir	
Control	Fasten	Make	Standardize	Stop	

BOX 4.2 ACTION VERBS COMMONLY AVOIDED WHEN WRITING OBJECTIVES

Able to	Familiar with	Learns
Appreciation for	Shows interest in	Memorizes
Awareness of	Knows	Understands
Capable of	Has knowledge of	Will be able to
Comprehend		
Conscious of		

COURSE PLANNING

Course planning is a fundamental process in education that involves designing and organizing a structured learning experience for students. It encompasses the careful selection of content, instructional strategies, assessments and resources to achieve specific learning objectives. Course planning ensures that educators create a cohesive and effective curriculum that promotes student engagement, learning and achievement.

Course planning in nursing education is a systematic process that involves designing and organizing individual courses within a nursing curriculum. It is a critical step in creating an effective learning experience for nursing students, ensuring that they acquire the necessary knowledge, skills and competencies to become competent healthcare professionals.

DEFINITIONS

- Oermann and Gaberson (2006): Course planning is 'the process of developing a plan for a specific course that includes the course objectives, content, activities, and assessments'.
- Bevis and Shelly (2013): Course planning is 'the process of designing a course that will meet the needs of the students and the objectives of the program'.
- Nursing Education Perspectives (2014): Course planning is 'the process of developing a course that is aligned with the program's mission, goals, and objectives'.

These definitions all emphasize the importance of planning a course that is both student-centred and aligned with the programme's goals. Course planning should be a collaborative process that involves input from faculties, students and clinical experts. It is important to consider the needs of the students, the resources available and the demands of the profession when planning a course.

PURPOSES OF COURSE PLAN

The purposes of a course plan in education are multifaceted and serve as a guide for teachers in delivering effective instruction and facilitating student learning. Here are some key purposes of a course plan:

i. Curriculum alignment with educational standards and guidelines.
ii. Clear articulation of course goals and learning objectives.
iii. Sequential organization of course content and topics.
iv. Guidance for selecting instructional strategies and resources.
v. Structured framework for assessment and evaluation.
vi. Facilitation of student engagement and active learning.
vii. Alignment with students' prior knowledge and future learning.
viii. Support for differentiation and addressing diverse learner needs.
ix. Promotion of coherence and continuity across instructional units.
x. Documentation of instructional plans for communication and accountability.
xi. Basis for reflection and continuous improvement in teaching practices.

COMPONENTS OF COURSE PLAN

When developing a course plan in nursing education, several key components should be considered to ensure a comprehensive and effective learning experience. The content of a course plan typically includes:

1. **Course information:** Provide basic information about the course, including the course title, code, credit hours, prerequisites and corequisites.
2. **Course description:** Offer a brief description of the course, highlighting the main topics, concepts and skills that will be covered.
3. **Course objectives:** Clearly state the specific learning objectives that students are expected to achieve by the end of the course. These objectives should be measurable and aligned with programme goals.

4. **Course outline or syllabus:** Present a detailed outline of the course, breaking down the content into units, modules or topics. Include the estimated time for each topic and any recommended readings or resources.
5. **Teaching methods and strategies:** Describe the instructional strategies and methods that will be employed to deliver the course content. This may include lectures, discussions, case studies, simulations, group projects, laboratory exercises, clinical experiences or online activities.
6. **Content coverage:** Specify the content areas that will be covered in the course, highlighting the essential nursing concepts, theories, principles and practice standards. Provide a breakdown of the content by units or modules.
7. **Learning resources:** Identify the resources, materials and references that will support student learning. This may include textbooks, articles, websites, multimedia resources, simulation tools, laboratory equipment or software applications.
8. **Assessments and grading criteria:** Outline the assessment methods and criteria that will be used to evaluate student learning. Specify the types of assessments, such as quizzes, exams, papers, presentations, skills demonstrations, clinical evaluations or projects. Clarify the grading criteria and weighting for each assessment.
9. **Course schedule:** Provide a schedule or timeline that indicates the sequence of topics, dates for assignments, assessments and any important milestones or deadlines.
10. **Student support and policies:** Communicate the available student support services, such as tutoring, academic advising or online resources. Additionally, outline any relevant course policies, including attendance, late submission, academic integrity or accommodations for students with disabilities.
11. **Professional standards and ethics:** Emphasize the professional standards, ethics and codes of conduct that students are expected to adhere to during the course. Reinforce the importance of professionalism, communication skills and ethical decision-making in nursing practice.
12. **Recommended learning strategies:** Provide guidance on effective learning strategies and study techniques that can help students succeed in the course. Encourage active participation, self-directed learning and peer collaboration.

It is important to note that the content of a course plan may vary depending on the specific nursing programme, educational institution and the level of the course (e.g. introductory, intermediate, advanced). The above components serve as a general guideline to ensure a well-structured and comprehensive course plan in nursing education.

STEPS OF COURSE PLAN

The process of creating a course plan involves several key steps to ensure a well-structured and effective learning experience. Here are the steps typically involved in course planning:

1. **Identify learning goals and objectives**: Determine the desired learning outcomes for the course and specify clear, measurable objectives that align with these goals.
2. **Define course content**: Determine the key concepts, theories and topics that need to be covered in the course to achieve the learning objectives. Consider the depth and breadth of the content based on the course level and duration.
3. **Select instructional strategies**: Choose appropriate instructional methods and strategies that support the learning objectives and engage students. This may include lectures, discussions, case studies, group work, simulations or hands-on activities.

4. **Develop assessment methods**: Design assessments that align with the learning objectives and provide opportunities for students to demonstrate their understanding and application of the course content. Consider a variety of assessment methods, such as quizzes, exams, projects, presentations or reflective journals.
5. **Sequence and structure the course**: Determine the logical sequence and structure of the course, including the order in which topics will be taught and the duration of each instructional component. Consider any prerequisites or corequisites required for the course and ensure that the course builds upon previously learned content. Develop a course schedule that provides sufficient time for instruction, practice, assessments and student interaction.
6. **Gather learning resources**: Identify and gather the necessary resources, including textbooks, readings, online materials, multimedia resources or laboratory equipment, to support student learning and supplement the course content.
7. **Incorporate technology**: Integrate technology tools and resources that enhance the learning experience and facilitate student engagement. Consider the use of learning management systems, online collaboration platforms, simulations or multimedia presentations.
8. **Incorporate student support**: Identify any necessary support services or resources that can assist students in their learning journey. This may include academic support, tutoring services, library resources or access to faculty or teaching assistants.
9. **Establish course policies**: Clearly communicate any course policies, such as attendance requirements, grading criteria, late submission policies or academic integrity guidelines. Ensure that students are aware of the expectations and standards for the course.
10. **Review and revise**: Regularly review and revise the course plan based on feedback from students, assessment results and reflection on teaching and learning practices. Make necessary adjustments to improve the course and enhance student learning outcomes.
11. **Implement and evaluate**: Implement the course plan and monitor student progress throughout the course. Collect feedback from students and use assessment data to evaluate the effectiveness of the course plan in achieving the desired learning outcomes.

PRINCIPLES OF COURSE PLANNING

The principles of course planning serve as guiding principles for educators when developing and designing a course. These principles ensure that the course is well-structured, meaningful and aligned with the desired learning outcomes. Here are some key principles of course planning:

i. Align course objectives with programme goals and desired learning outcomes.
ii. Select and organize relevant content based on essential nursing concepts, theories and practice standards.
iii. Choose instructional strategies that promote active learning, critical thinking and application of knowledge.
iv. Design assessments that align with course objectives and measure student learning effectively.
v. Incorporate a variety of teaching methods, such as lectures, discussions, case studies, simulations and clinical experiences.
vi. Integrate technology and educational resources to enhance teaching and learning experiences.
vii. Ensure a logical sequence and structure of the course, considering prerequisites and corequisites.
viii. Provide student support mechanisms, such as tutoring, library resources and academic advising.
ix. Regularly evaluate and revise the course based on feedback from students, colleagues and stakeholders.
x. Foster a supportive and inclusive learning environment that values diversity and cultural competence.

xi. Allocate sufficient time for instruction, practice, assessments and student interaction.
xii. Incorporate evidence-based practices and current research findings into the course design.
xiii. Promote interdisciplinary collaboration and integration of healthcare concepts and practices.
xiv. Foster professional values, ethics and standards in nursing education.
xv. Engage students in self-reflection and metacognitive processes to enhance their learning experience.
xvi. Promote lifelong learning and the development of critical thinking skills necessary for nursing practice.

ROLE OF A TEACHER IN COURSE PLAN

The role of a teacher in course planning is crucial in ensuring the effective design and delivery of a course. Some key roles of a teacher in course planning include:

i. Developing clear and measurable learning objectives for the course.
ii. Selecting and organizing the content to be covered in the course.
iii. Choosing appropriate instructional strategies and methods to deliver the content effectively.
iv. Designing and implementing assessments to measure student learning outcomes.
v. Creating a structured course schedule and timeline.
vi. Providing guidance and support to students throughout the learning process.
vii. Adapting the course plan to meet the needs and abilities of diverse learners.
viii. Incorporating technology and educational resources to enhance teaching and learning.
ix. Creating a positive and inclusive learning environment.
x. Facilitating active learning and student engagement.
xi. Monitoring student progress and providing timely feedback.
xii. Assessing and adjusting the course plan based on student performance and feedback.
xiii. Encouraging critical thinking, problem-solving and application of knowledge.
xiv. Fostering collaborative learning and peer interaction.
xv. Promoting professionalism, ethics and adherence to nursing standards.
xvi. Keeping up to date with current research and best practices in nursing education.
xvii. Reflecting on teaching strategies and continuously improving the course plan.
xviii. Communicating course expectations and policies to students.
xix. Collaborating with colleagues and stakeholders to ensure alignment with programme goals.
xx. Providing additional support and resources to students as needed.
xxi. Encouraging self-directed learning and metacognitive skills.
xxii. Cultivating a passion for lifelong learning in students.

BENEFITS OF COURSE PLAN

1. **Clarity and focus**: A well-developed course plan provides clear learning objectives, content and assessment criteria, ensuring that students have a clear understanding of what is expected of them. It helps maintain focus and alignment between the instructional activities and the desired learning outcomes.
2. **Consistency and coherence**: A course plan ensures consistency and coherence in the delivery of content and instructional strategies throughout the course. It helps educators maintain a structured and organized approach, promoting a cohesive learning experience for students.

3. **Alignment with programme goals**: A course plan helps ensure that individual courses align with the broader goals of the nursing programme. It ensures that the curriculum is well-rounded and covers the essential knowledge, skills and competencies required for nursing practice.
4. **Student engagement and learning**: A thoughtfully designed course plan employs various instructional strategies and assessments to engage students actively in the learning process. It promotes critical thinking, problem-solving and application of knowledge, enhancing student learning outcomes.
5. **Time management**: A course plan allows for effective time management by allocating sufficient time for instruction, practice and assessments. It helps educators plan and deliver the course content within the given time frame, ensuring that all essential topics are covered adequately.
6. **Assessment alignment**: A course plan facilitates alignment between the learning objectives and the assessments used to evaluate student understanding. It ensures that assessments measure the intended learning outcomes and provide valuable feedback to students on their progress.

LIMITATIONS OF COURSE PLAN

1. **Rigidity and lack of flexibility**: A course plan, if too rigid, may limit the ability to adapt and adjust the instructional strategies or content based on the evolving needs of students or changes in healthcare practice. It may not allow for timely integration of emerging trends or current research findings.
2. **Student variability**: Each student is unique in terms of their learning styles, backgrounds and prior knowledge. A course plan may not fully account for the individual needs and preferences of all students, requiring educators to make adjustments or provide additional support as necessary.
3. **Limited scope**: A course plan focuses on the specific content and objectives of an individual course, which may restrict the integration of interdisciplinary or holistic approaches to nursing practice. It may not fully capture the interconnections and complexities of healthcare delivery.
4. **Time constraints**: Developing a comprehensive course plan requires significant time and effort from educators. The need to cover a wide range of content within a limited time frame may result in a packed curriculum, leaving little room for in-depth exploration or student-led inquiry.
5. **External factors**: Course plans may be affected by external factors, such as changes in accreditation standards, healthcare policies or resource availability. Educators may need to revise or update course plans periodically to adapt to these external factors.

It is important for educators to be aware of these limitations and work towards mitigating them by incorporating flexibility, student-centred approaches and ongoing evaluation and feedback mechanisms within the course planning process.

UNIT PLAN

The unit plan aims to provide nursing educators with a structured framework for designing and implementing effective instructional activities to enhance clinical competence among nursing students. Nursing education plays a vital role in preparing future healthcare professionals to provide safe and effective patient care. By utilizing this unit plan, educators can guide students in acquiring the necessary knowledge, skills and attitudes to excel in the clinical setting.

DEFINITIONS

- Oermann and Gaberson (2006): A unit plan is 'a detailed outline of the content, activities, and assessments that will be covered in a unit of study'.
- Bevis and Shelly (2013): A unit plan is 'a roadmap for teaching a specific unit of content'.
- Nursing Education Perspectives (2014): A unit plan is 'a tool that helps teachers organize and deliver instruction'.

PURPOSES OF UNIT PLAN

The unit plan in nursing education serves several important purposes, aiming to facilitate effective teaching and learning experiences for nursing students. Here are some key purposes of a unit plan in nursing education:

i. Provides a structured framework for organizing instructional activities and content.
ii. Aligns learning objectives with instructional activities to promote focused learning.
iii. Integrates various content areas and instructional strategies coherently.
iv. Supports differentiated instruction to meet diverse learning needs.
v. Guides the design of assessments and evaluations to measure student learning.
vi. Facilitates time management and resource allocation.
vii. Enhances collaboration and communication among educators and students.
viii. Supports ongoing professional development for nursing educators.

COMPONENTS OF A UNIT PLAN

The components of a unit plan can vary depending on the specific educational context and the preferences of the teacher. However, here are some common components that are typically included in a unit plan:

- ***Unit title:*** A concise and descriptive title that represents the focus or theme of the unit.
- ***Unit overview/objectives:*** A brief summary of the unit's purpose, goals and desired learning outcomes. It outlines what students will know, understand and be able to do by the end of the unit.
- ***Standards or learning outcomes:*** Specific educational standards, learning outcomes or competencies that the unit aims to address or achieve.
- ***Preassessment:*** Diagnostic or preassessment strategies to gather information about students' prior knowledge, skills and misconceptions related to the unit topic. This helps inform instruction and differentiate learning experiences.
- ***Instructional strategies:*** Detailed descriptions of the teaching methods, approaches and activities that will be used to deliver the content and engage students. This may include lectures, discussions, group work, hands-on activities, multimedia resources and technology integration.

- ***Resources and materials:*** A list of instructional resources, materials, textbooks, websites, multimedia or other relevant materials that will be used during the unit. This ensures that necessary resources are gathered and readily available for effective instruction.
- ***Assessment and evaluation:*** Description of assessment methods, including formative and summative assessments, quizzes, tests, projects or presentations that will be used to measure student understanding and progress throughout the unit. It also includes criteria for evaluating student work and determining levels of achievement.
- ***Differentiation and adaptation:*** Strategies and modifications to address diverse learner needs, such as accommodations for students with special needs, English language learners or gifted students. This ensures inclusivity and supports all students' access to the content and achievement of the learning objectives.
- ***Instructional timeline:*** A timeline or schedule that outlines the sequence and duration of instructional activities and assessments across the unit. It helps teachers manage instructional time effectively and ensures appropriate pacing.
- ***Reflection and next steps:*** A section for teachers to reflect on the effectiveness of the unit, identify areas for improvement and consider adjustments for future instruction. This promotes ongoing professional growth and enhances instructional practices.

STEPS OF UNIT PLAN

The steps involved in creating a unit plan in nursing education may vary depending on individual preferences and institutional requirements. However, here is a general outline of the steps involved:

1. **Identify learning objectives**: Determine the specific learning objectives that align with the unit's content and desired outcomes. These objectives should be measurable and reflect the knowledge, skills and attitudes students are expected to achieve.
2. **Select content and resources**: Identify the key content areas and resources that will be covered in the unit. Consider textbooks, reference materials, online resources, multimedia and any other relevant sources that support student learning.
3. **Design instructional activities**: Develop a variety of instructional activities that engage students and facilitate their understanding of the content. This may include lectures, group discussions, case studies, simulations, laboratory exercises and hands-on practice.
4. **Plan assessments**: Determine the assessment methods that will be used to evaluate student learning and achievement of the learning objectives. This may include quizzes, exams, practical skills assessments, written assignments or presentations.
5. **Sequence the learning activities**: Arrange the instructional activities in a logical sequence, considering the progression of content complexity and the prerequisites for each activity. Ensure that the activities build upon each other and lead to the achievement of the learning objectives.
6. **Determine timing and duration**: Estimate the time required for each instructional activity and allocate the appropriate duration within the unit plan. Consider the total length of the unit and any scheduling constraints.
7. **Consider differentiation and student engagement**: Incorporate strategies to accommodate diverse learning needs and engage students. This may include providing options for individual or group work, incorporating multimedia resources and addressing different learning styles.

8. **Develop assessments and rubrics**: Create assessment tools, such as rubrics or scoring guidelines, that align with the learning objectives and provide clear expectations for student performance. Ensure that the assessments accurately measure student achievement.
9. **Integrate technology and resources**: Identify opportunities to integrate technology tools and resources that enhance student learning and engagement. This may include online platforms, educational apps, virtual simulations or multimedia presentations.
10. **Review and revise**: Conduct a thorough review of the unit plan to ensure alignment of content, objectives, instructional activities and assessments. Revise as necessary to improve clarity, coherence and effectiveness.
11. **Implement and reflect**: Implement the unit plan in the classroom or clinical setting, making any adjustments as needed. After completion, reflect on the effectiveness of the plan and student learning outcomes, using feedback to inform future revisions and improvements.

Remember that flexibility is essential, and adjustments may be needed during the implementation of the unit plan based on student feedback and assessment results. Regular reflection and revision of the unit plan contribute to continuous improvement in nursing education.

PRINCIPLES OF UNIT PLAN

When developing a unit plan in nursing education, several principles can guide the process and ensure effective teaching and learning experiences. Here are some key principles to consider:

- ***Alignment with learning objectives:*** Ensure that all components of the unit plan, including content, instructional activities and assessments, are aligned with the stated learning objectives. This alignment promotes a clear focus on desired student outcomes and facilitates meaningful and purposeful learning.
- ***Active learning and engagement:*** Incorporate instructional strategies that promote active learning and student engagement. Encourage students to participate actively in discussions, problem-solving activities, case studies, simulations and hands-on experiences to foster deeper understanding and critical thinking.
- ***Constructivist approach:*** Embrace a constructivist approach to learning, where students actively construct their knowledge and understanding through interactions with the content and their peers. Provide opportunities for students to explore, question and reflect on their learning experiences.
- ***Differentiated instruction:*** Recognize and accommodate the diverse learning needs and styles of students through differentiated instruction. Provide various avenues for learning, such as visual aids, auditory resources, hands-on activities and collaborative group work, to cater to different learning preferences.
- ***Integration of theory and practice:*** Facilitate the integration of theoretical knowledge with clinical practice. Connect the concepts and content covered in the unit to real-world healthcare scenarios, encouraging students to apply their knowledge and skills in authentic contexts.
- ***Formative assessment:*** Implement formative assessments throughout the unit to monitor student progress and provide timely feedback. Use a variety of assessment methods, such as quizzes, class discussions, skill demonstrations and self-assessments, to inform instruction and guide student learning.
- ***Authentic and meaningful assessments:*** Design authentic assessments that closely resemble real-world nursing situations. Assess students' ability to apply knowledge, critical thinking and clinical reasoning skills through case studies, simulations, clinical scenarios or reflective journals.

- ***Integration of technology:*** Utilize technology effectively to enhance teaching and learning experiences. Incorporate digital resources, educational apps, interactive simulations, online discussion boards and electronic health record systems to engage students and promote active learning.
- ***Collaboration and interprofessional education:*** Promote collaboration among students and interdisciplinary healthcare teams. Design activities that encourage teamwork, communication and an understanding of each professional's role in delivering patient-centred care.
- ***Reflective practice:*** Encourage students to engage in reflective practice, encouraging them to think critically about their learning experiences, identify areas for improvement and set goals for further development. Foster an environment that values self-reflection and continuous learning.

By following these principles, nursing educators can create unit plans that foster student engagement, critical thinking and the integration of theory and practice, ultimately preparing students for successful nursing careers.

ROLE OF A TEACHER IN UNIT PLAN

The role of a teacher in a unit plan is crucial in guiding and facilitating the teaching and learning process. Here are some key roles that a teacher plays in the context of a unit plan:

1. **Unit designer**: The teacher designs the unit plan, determining the content, learning objectives, instructional activities and assessments that align with the curriculum and educational standards. The teacher ensures that the unit plan addresses the specific needs and goals of the nursing education programme.
2. **Facilitator of learning**: The teacher takes on the role of a facilitator, guiding students through the learning process. They create a supportive and engaging learning environment, encouraging student participation, fostering discussions and promoting critical thinking and problem-solving skills.
3. **Instructional designer**: The teacher designs and organizes instructional activities that support the achievement of learning objectives. They select appropriate teaching strategies, resources and technologies to effectively deliver the content and engage students in active learning.
4. **Knowledge expert**: The teacher serves as a subject matter expert, possessing in-depth knowledge of the content being taught. They provide accurate and up-to-date information, clarify concepts and answer students' questions to ensure a comprehensive understanding of the subject matter.
5. **Learning facilitator**: The teacher supports individualized learning by recognizing and addressing the diverse needs and learning styles of students. They differentiate instruction, provide additional resources or support when necessary and create opportunities for student collaboration and peer learning.
6. **Assessor of learning**: The teacher designs and administers assessments to evaluate student learning and progress. They provide feedback and guidance on students' performance, identify areas for improvement and adjust instructional strategies based on the assessment results.
7. **Mentor and guide**: The teacher acts as a mentor and guide, offering support, encouragement and guidance to students throughout the unit. They facilitate discussions, provide mentoring sessions and offer academic and professional advice to help students succeed in their learning journey.
8. **Classroom manager**: The teacher manages the learning environment, ensuring that it is conducive to learning, organized and safe. They establish and enforce classroom rules and expectations, manage time effectively and maintain discipline to create a positive and respectful learning atmosphere.

9. **Reflective practitioner**: The teacher engages in continuous reflection and professional development. They evaluate the effectiveness of the unit plan, instructional strategies and assessment methods. They seek opportunities to improve their teaching practices, stay updated with current trends and research in nursing education and adapt their approach based on student feedback and outcomes.

BENEFITS OF UNIT PLAN

1. **Coherence and organization**: Unit plan provides a structured and organized framework for teaching and learning. It ensures that the content, activities and assessments are aligned and logically sequenced, promoting a coherent and meaningful learning experience for students.
2. **Clear learning objectives**: Unit plan helps teachers define clear learning objectives for each unit. This clarity enables both teachers and students to understand the desired outcomes and focus their efforts on achieving them.
3. **Effective resource management**: Unit plan allows teachers to effectively manage resources such as time, materials and instructional aids. By outlining the sequence and duration of activities, teachers can allocate resources efficiently and optimize learning opportunities.
4. **Differentiated instruction**: Unit plan facilitates the incorporation of differentiated instruction strategies to meet the diverse learning needs of students. Teachers can design activities and assessments that cater to various learning styles, abilities and interests, enhancing student engagement and understanding.
5. **Assessment alignment**: Unit plan ensures that assessments are aligned with the learning objectives and instructional activities. This alignment helps measure student progress and provides feedback to guide instruction and support student learning.
6. **Increased student engagement**: Well-designed unit plans with varied instructional activities can increase student engagement and motivation. By incorporating interactive and hands-on learning experiences, teachers can stimulate student curiosity and active participation.
7. **Continuous improvement**: Unit plan allows teachers to reflect on their teaching strategies, content choices and assessment methods. This reflection promotes ongoing professional growth and enables teachers to refine their instructional practices over time.

LIMITATIONS OF UNIT PLAN

1. **Time constraints**: Developing comprehensive unit plans requires a significant amount of time and effort. Teachers may struggle to find sufficient time for thorough planning, especially when faced with heavy workloads and other professional responsibilities.
2. **Rigidity**: Unit plans, once created, can sometimes become rigid and inflexible. This can restrict teachers from adapting or modifying the plan to meet the specific needs and interests of their students as they arise throughout the unit.
3. **Lack of individualization**: Unit plans are typically designed to address the needs of the entire class as a whole. This may result in limited individualization for students with diverse learning styles, abilities or needs. Teachers must be mindful of incorporating differentiation strategies to ensure all students are appropriately challenged and supported.
4. **Limited contextualization**: Unit plans may not always fully consider the unique contextual factors, such as the local community, culture or current events. Failure to incorporate these factors can result in a less relevant and meaningful learning experience for students.

5. **External influences**: The implementation of unit plans can be influenced by external factors beyond the teacher's control, such as interruptions due to school events, changes in the schedule or unexpected circumstances. These factors may disrupt the continuity and flow of the planned unit.
6. **Assessment limitations**: Unit plans may not always allow for comprehensive or in-depth assessment of all aspects of student learning. Teachers must carefully select and design assessments that align with the unit's objectives while being mindful of time constraints and other practical considerations.
7. **Curriculum constraints**: Unit plans need to align with the broader curriculum and educational standards, which may impose limitations on the content, scope or sequencing of the units. Teachers must navigate these constraints while ensuring the unit plan adequately covers the required curriculum.

It is important for teachers to be aware of these limitations and strive to address them through ongoing reflection, professional development and adaptation of their unit plans to meet the specific needs of their students and the context in which they teach.

LESSON PLANNING

Lesson planning is an important activity of daily teaching. The lesson plan might include the main points to be covered in the lesson activities for the students to do, questions related to the topic being taught and some form of assessment for the realization of stipulated instructional objectives. It indicates clearly what has already been done, what the students are to do, how the students are to be engaged in various activities and what activities are to be pursued. Lesson planning is the heart of effective teaching. The teacher has to consider the following points while lesson planning:

- Define broader objectives of the subject.
- Define classroom objectives of the lesson.
- Organize the subject matter to be covered to achieve the stipulated objectives.
- Decide on the way of presenting the subject matter, teaching strategies and tactics, and classroom interaction and management.
- Provide appropriate provision for evaluation and feedback.

I. DEFINITIONS OF LESSON PLAN

Lesson plan is the title given to a statement of achievement to be realized and specific meanings by which these are to be attained as a result of the activities engaged during the period.

—**N.L. Bossing**

Daily lesson planning involves defining the objectives, selecting and arranging the subject matter and determining the method of procedure.

—**Bining and Bining**

A lesson plan is a teaching outline of the important points of lesson arranged in which they are to be presented. It may include objectives, points to be made, questions to be asked, references to materials, assignments etc.

—**Carter V. Good**

II. FUNCTIONS OF A LESSON PLAN

- It ensures a definite objective for the day's work and a clear visualization of that objective.
- Lesson planning helps for adequate and appropriate use of resources in an efficient way.
- It keeps the teacher on track to ensure steady progress and a definite outcome of teaching and learning procedures.
- It helps clarify ideas about what, how, where and when and whom to teach.
- Lesson plan directs the teaching–learning process and procedures in the right direction.
- Helps review the subject matter and gives up-to-date knowledge.
- It helps the teacher delimit the teaching.
- When it is planned well, a student's interest can be maintained.
- It provides guidelines for the teacher about classroom instructions.
- It provides sensible framework for a teacher to be taught.
- It provides confidence, self-reliance ease and freedom to teacher in teaching.

III. SIGNIFICANCE AND IMPORTANCE OF A LESSON PLAN

- In a teaching education programme, the lesson plan provides guidelines to students and the teacher during their teaching–learning practices.
- It helps in achieving the definite objectives.
- It makes teaching systematic, orderly and economical.
- It helps teachers overcome feelings of nervousness and insecurity and gives them confidence to face the class.
- It links new knowledge with previous knowledge acquired by a student.
- It prepares pivotal questions and illustrations.
- It enables the teacher evaluate his work as the lesson proceeds.
- It helps the teacher use a wider variety of teaching materials and learning activities in the classroom through a wider acquaintance with resources.
- It also helps the teacher plan the teaching–learning process per the availability and accessibility of resource materials.

IV. PREREQUISITES OF A LESSON PLAN

- ***Knowledge and mastery of subject matter:*** The teacher must be a master of his subject. He should have thorough knowledge of the subject matter, materials and activities to be used.
- ***Knowledge of student psychology:*** The teacher must have knowledge of child psychology, that is the teacher should know the standard and individuality of the students and present the subject matter accordingly.
- ***Knowledge of methods and techniques:*** The teacher should be conversant with the methods and techniques of teaching.
- ***Knowledge of aims:*** The teacher should have a basic understanding of the aims and objectives of education. He should have the ability and skills to write objectives in behavioural terms and a knowledge of various teaching skills.
- ***Knowledge about the student's interests, traits and abilities:*** The teacher must have adequate knowledge about the interests, traits and abilities of an individual student. This helps the teacher have an individual customized lesson plan for a specific group of the students.

- ***Teacher's competence:*** Teacher must have an ability to construct better lesson plans within a short time. In addition, he/she must have the ability to make constructive preparation for cooperative planning of activities with students.
- ***Selection and organization of subject matter:*** Teaching–learning activities, illustrative material, assignment and evaluation for students, references and bibliography must be planned by the teacher well in advance so that the lesson can be planned and executed in an effective manner.
    - ***Learning activities:*** The teacher chooses the learning activities. They should be varied sufficiently to allow for individual differences in the group.
    - ***Teaching activities:*** The teaching techniques that are objective-oriented and cost-effective directly help the teacher to obtain the educational objectives.
    - ***Type of illustrative materials:*** Audiovisual aids and instruction media.
    - ***Assignments:*** The plan should use assignments to project the immediate work to the next situation.
    - ***Evaluation:*** Some type of evaluation should be planned for each lesson.
    - ***References and bibliography:*** The teacher will have ready references and bibliography to be used indirectly in student assignments.

V. ESSENTIAL CHARACTERISTICS OF A GOOD LESSON PLAN

The essential characteristics of a lesson are discussed below and may also be seen in Box 4.3.

- ***Clearly written:*** Lesson plans must preferably be in a written form. It must be appropriately written and depict who will be taught, who will teach, when will it be taught, where the class will be taken, what will be taught, why it will be taught, how it will be taught and what should be expected from students after the lesson.
- ***Definite aim and objectives:*** A good lesson plan must have clearly defined aim and objectives that very clearly specify the purpose of the lesson and the purpose of each activity included in the lesson plan.
- ***Extension of existing knowledge:*** The topic of a lesson plan should be planned in a consecutive sequence of the previously taught topics or existing knowledge for better understanding of the topic. It should not be a repetition nor an isolated topic plan.
- ***Simple and comprehensive:*** Each lesson plan must be simple, lucid, concise and precise and must include all activities that are expected to be carried out by a teacher in classroom during the teaching–learning process comprehensively.
- ***Flexible plan:*** A planned lesson must not be rigid; it must be flexible to adopt the changes expected to arise in specific classroom situations. A flexible lesson plan facilities the teacher adapt to specific incidental situations in the classroom.

BOX 4.3 ESSENTIAL CHARACTERISTICS OF A GOOD LESSON PLAN

- Clearly written
- Definite aim and objectives
- Extension of existing knowledge
- Simple and comprehensive
- Flexible
- Ensures active teaching–learning process
- Division with essence of wholesomeness
- Individualized and customized
- Feasibility and significance
- Proceed from general to specific
- Completeness
- Inclusion of summary, recapitalization, bibliography and student assignment

- ***Ensure active teaching–learning process:*** A good lesson plan ensures active participation of both the teacher and the student for effective achievement of educational objectives. A passive lesson plan fails to motivate the teacher and/or the student for an effective teaching–learning activity outcome.
- ***Division with essence of wholesomeness:*** A lesson plan must be divided into subsections for better presentation; however, its wholesomeness must not be distorted. A logical sequence and efficient cohesion of the subsections of the lesson may help in the preservation of the lesson plan's wholesomeness.
- ***Individualized and customized:*** The content of the lesson plan should be designed according to the needs, interests, abilities and level of the students. This individualized and customized approach helps the teacher achieve the expected aim of a lesson plan.
- ***Feasibility and significance:*** A lesson plan must be planned in a manner that it is feasible in terms of time and available resources. It must be as practical as possible without overestimations in a hypothetical manner. In addition, a lesson plan must have significance to a particular group of students because nonsignificant topics fail to create interest in learners as well as the teacher. Therefore, the teaching–learning activity may not be fruitful without the significance of a lesson/topic.
- ***Proceed from general to specific:*** A lesson plan must be planned such that it proceeds from general or basic knowledge to specific knowledge so students can easily understand the lesson.
- ***Completeness:*** A good lesson plan must be complete in itself without leaving any essential component like topic of the lesson, general and specific objectives, content, teacher–student activity and methods of presentation, audiovisual aids, question to be asked for students, summary, recapitalized and assignment for the students.
- ***Inclusion of summary, recapitalization, bibliography and student assignment:*** In addition to a basic introductory plan and body of the lesson, the lesson plan must include the summary, recapitalization, bibliography and student assignment.

VI. STEPS OF LESSON PLANNING

- ***Preparation or introduction:*** Exploration of the student's knowledge helps to lead them on to the lesson. The teacher needs to prepare the students to receive new knowledge.
- ***Presentation:*** The aim of the lesson should be clearly stated before presentation of the subject matter, which helps both the teacher and students have common pursuit.
- ***Comparison or association:*** Quote examples and associate facts with two examples so that learners can understand easily and arrive at generalizations on their own.
- ***Generalizations:*** The knowledge presented by the teacher should be thought-provoking, innovating and stimulating to assist the students generalize the situation.
- ***Application:*** The students should be able to make use of the knowledge acquired and test the validity of the generalization arrived at in theory. It has to apply in the clinical field to make learning more permanent and worthwhile.
- ***Recapitulation:*** The teacher has to ask suitable, stimulating and pivotal questions on the topic. The answer will give feedback to the teacher regarding the efficacy of the method of teaching and he can decide whether or not clarification is needed.

VII. TYPE OF APPROACHES TO LESSON PLANNING

Several educational philosophers have suggested a few lesson planning approaches. Some essential approaches of lesson planning have been discussed in the following sections (such as Herbertian approach of lesson planning, Bloom's evaluation approach of lesson planning, Gloverian approach of lesson planning and RCEM approach of lesson planning).

A. HERBERTIAN APPROACH

J.F. Herbart, a German philosopher advocated lesson planning using the following five steps:

i) ***Preparation:*** Preparing means the preparation of the learner's mind to receive new knowledge. Preparation of the learner involves two steps:

  a. Previous knowledge testing: Through testing previous knowledge, the teacher becomes familiar with what pupils already know relevant to the topic.

  b. Announcement of the aim: An aim will automatically emerge if the lesson has been effectively introduced. The aim should be clear, concise and free from unknown words. J. Welton said, 'To know where the pupils are and where they should try to be are the first two essentials of the teaching'.

ii) ***Presentation:*** It involves a good deal of intellectual activity on the part of the students. A teacher is to put himself into the students' shoes to present things to them. Selected subject matter should be presented according to the needs, interests, abilities and developmental level of the students.

iii) ***Comparison and abstraction:*** Association is linking new ideas with the old ones and with one another into a system. The selected examples or facts are presented before the students and they are asked to carefully observe and compare them with another set of facts to arrive at some conclusion.

iv) ***Generalization:*** Comparison and association helps students find a certain conclusion that enables them to frame general laws, principles or formulas. The teacher's function is to enable the students to draw out the generalization from relevant data.

v) ***Application:*** Knowledge that is not used will soon fade away from consciousness. Knowledge is power, but it is only when the mind can apply it to practical situation.

Merits

- Avoids unnecessary repetition in teaching.
- Simple and easy approach.
- Logical and psychological.
- Used in achieving the cognitive objective of teaching.
- Assists in making the teaching systematic.

Demerits

- Highly dominated by the teacher.
- More stress on teaching rather than on learning.
- Does not consider the learning structure in organizing teaching activities.
- Specific objectives are not written in behavioural terms.
- Teaching activities are less meaningful and practical.

B. BLOOM'S EVALUATION APPROACH ON LESSON PLANNING

B.S. Bloom believed that the teaching–learning process must be objective centric. He considered education as a tripolar process (Fig. 4.11). The three pools are educational objectives, learning experiences and learning outcome or change in the student's behaviour. The major features of this approach of lesson planning are as follows:

- Teaching–learning activity is learning objective based rather than content based.

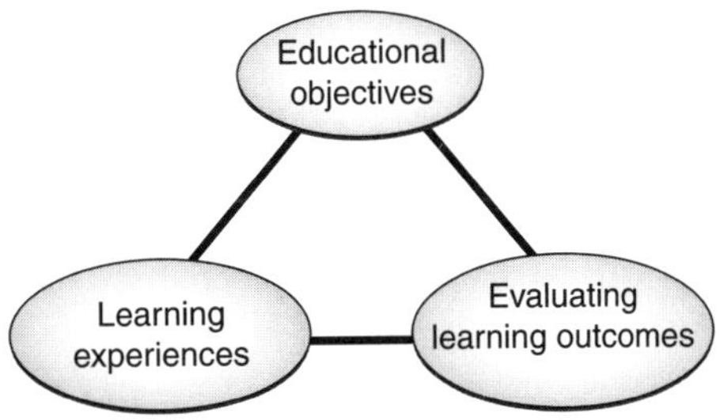

Figure 4.11

Bloom's major features of lesson planning.

- The expected outcome of the teaching–learning activity is an overall change in behaviour of the student rather than learning-specific content.
- The outcome of learning is measured based on predetermined learning objectives, including cognitive, affective and psychomotor learning objective outcome.

Merits

- The objectives are written in behavioural terms.
- The teaching activities are related to learning structures.
- It makes the teaching purposeful and objective-centred.
- It is based on psychological and scientific principles.

Demerits

- Gives rise to rigid and mechanical planning which lacks flexibility.
- Does not provide an opportunity for creativity among students.
- It is a highly structured approach and imposes a high demand on the teacher and the student during the teaching–learning process.

C. RCEM APPROACH

RCEM approach was developed by Indian educationists at the Regional College of Education, Mysore, and therefore known as *RCEM approach*. This approach has its roots in the system approach and has defined three main steps of the teaching–learning process: input, process and output.

- ***Input:*** It includes the identification of objectives. They are also known as expected behavioural outcomes. Input further resembles the preparation steps of the Herbarin approach where the teacher tries to know what students know and what they are expected to know.
- ***Process:*** The main focus of the process is to create the learning situation. It implies the interaction of teacher and students. It includes teacher and student activities, teaching strategies and audiovisual aids and techniques of motivation.
- ***Output:*** It is the evaluation phase of the lesson plan. We get desirable behavioural changes among students through the output. These are the real learning outcomes.

Merits

- It is an indigenous method; therefore, more suitable for local teaching–learning pursuits.
- Learning objectives are formulated in the form of measurable student abilities and rational processes.
- The teaching–learning scenario, methods, materials and audiovisual aids are clearly defined.
- This model of teaching can be used for basic as well as advanced learning.
- Theoretical knowledge of teaching concepts can be applied.
- The evaluation aspect of a lesson plan is efficiently and adequately clarified.

Demerits

- Writing lesson plans using this approach is a cumbersome task.
- This method is not considered practical as it is time-consuming.
- There is limited understanding and utilization of this method.

VIII. STRATEGIES FOR EFFECTIVE IMPLEMENTATION OF THE LESSON PLAN

A good, planned lesson can only be considered effective if it implemented in an efficient manner. Some suggested strategies for effective implementation of a planned lesson are as follows:

- The lesson plan must be efficiently written, prepared and designed with a complete sense of confidence.
- The presenter or teacher must be clear about the aim and objectives of the lesson plan. In addition, the presenter must have thorough command on the subject content planned to be delivered to a group of students.
- Use of audiovisual aids must be well planned, judicious and efficient. It is said that the right audiovisual aid at the right time and right place by the right person for the right individuals should be used.
- Efficient classroom management is very important for effective implementation of the lesson plan. It must be ensured that the classroom is well ventilated, clean, of optimum temperature and the students are comfortably seated.
- Introduction of the lesson must create interest in the students and they must be well motivated to receive the subject content. This introduction usually takes about the first 5 minutes of the total 45 minutes of class time.
- It is essential to use the right methods of teaching ensuring the active involvement of students and charge their brains to receive and retain the subject content.
- There must be careful use of blackboard and other audiovisual methods. It must be ensured that the content presented on a blackboard or using other audiovisual aids is legible, clear, concise, attractive, lucid and large enough for students to visualize without undue discomfort.
- Questions planned and presented in a lesson plan must be definite, clear, stimulating and thought-provoking.
- Content must be delivered in a simple language with a clear and audible voice with complete sense of confidence and using relevant real-life examples to promote understanding of the subject content.
- Provide enough time to the students for clarifying their doubts. Confusing content must be clarified and reinforced with simple and relevant examples.
- Individual student attention while taking and giving regular feedback on the understating of subject content is very essential for effective implementation of the lesson plan.
- Efficient time management, appropriate recapitalization of the subject matter and relevant thought-provoking questioning and continuous feedback are key aspects of effective implementation of the lesson plan.
- End recapitalization, discussion of reference, bibliography and further reading and expected students exercise assignments are also considered to be important in the success of a lesson plan.

IX. FORMAT OF A LESSON PLAN

An effective lesson must have the following format (refer to a detailed lesson plan in Appendix A).

I. **Cover page:** This page must include topic of lesson, date of submission, name of supervisor and name and details of the presenting teacher.

II. First page: This page must include the following basic information:

Basic Lesson Plan Information

- Subject : Communication and Education Technology
- Name of topic : Assessment of learning needs
- Name of student's teacher : Ms Jasveen Kaur
- Name of supervisor : Dr Suresh K. Sharma
- Date of teaching : ___________
- Time of teaching : ___________
- Venue of teaching : Lecturer Theater No. 3
- Group : B.Sc. (N) 2nd year students
- Size of group : 25
- Method of teaching : Lecture cum discussion
- Duration : ___ minutes
- AV aids : PowerPoint Presentation

Previous knowledge: The group has some knowledge about the topic: Assessment of learning needs.

General objective: At the end of the class, students will be able to acquire knowledge about assessment of learning needs.

Specific objectives: At the end of teaching, students will be able to

- Define various terms related to assessment of learning needs.
- Explain about historical perspective.
- Enlist types of assessment.
- Enumerate principles of assessment for learning.
- Describe purposes of conducting assessment of learning needs.

III. Main body of lesson plan:

S. No.	Time	Contributory Objective	Content Matter	Teaching–Learning Activities	
				AV Aids	Evaluation

IV. Appendix of lesson plan: This includes giving the assignment to students and recommending further reading, writing the bibliography and references.

LONG-ANSWER QUESTIONS

1. Discuss the essential qualities of a good teacher.
2. Explain different styles of teaching.
3. Enlist the different types of learner and describe delegator type of teaching in detail.
4. Describe determinants of learning.
5. Explain emotional intelligence and mention its uses in teaching and learning.
6. Define curriculum and describe types of curriculum and components and approaches of curriculum development.

7. Describe curriculum development process.
8. Describe essential characteristics of lesson planning.
9. Discuss the role of teacher in course planning.

SHORT-ANSWER QUESTIONS

1. Enlist qualities of a good teacher.
2. List down the advantages of authoritative teaching style.
3. Enlist the types of learners.
4. Mention steps to assess learning needs.
5. Discuss models of emotional intelligence.
6. Describe Daniel Goleman's Emotional Intelligence Quadrant.
7. State types of curriculum.
8. Define lesson planning.
9. Enlist factors influencing curriculum development

MULTIPLE-CHOICE QUESTIONS (MCQs)

1. Which of the following terms refer to a learner who prefers to process information through listening and verbal communication?
   (a) Visual learner
   (b) Auditory learner
   (c) Kinesthetic learner
   (d) Reflective learner
2. A student who learns best through hands-on activities and physical movement is categorized as a
   (a) Visual learner
   (b) Auditory learner
   (c) Kinesthetic learner
   (d) Reflective learner
3. The curriculum in nursing education is designed to
   (a) Train nurses in basic patient care skills
   (b) Provide theoretical knowledge only
   (c) Prepare nurses for advanced research roles
   (d) Develop nursing knowledge, skills and professional attributes
4. The purpose of incorporating evidence-based practice (EBP) in the nursing curriculum is to
   (a) Teach students about historical nursing practices
   (b) Promote critical thinking and decision-making skills
   (c) Focus on personal experiences and opinions
   (d) Emphasize theoretical concepts over practical application
5. The nursing curriculum is regularly updated to
   (a) Keep up with the latest trends in healthcare technology
   (b) Increase the length of the programme
   (c) Reduce the amount of clinical practice hours
   (d) Standardize nursing education globally

6. Which of the following best describes the approach of the demonstrator teaching style?
   (a) Instructor-centred
   (b) Student-centred
   (c) Theory-focused
   (d) Exam-oriented
7. One potential limitation of the demonstrator teaching style in nursing education is
   (a) It may not cater to diverse learning preferences and styles
   (b) It requires extensive technological resources and equipment
   (c) It can lead to reduced instructor–student interaction
   (d) It may not effectively prepare students for standardized exams
8. Which of the following best describes the approach of the delegator teaching style?
   (a) Instructor-centred
   (b) Student-centred
   (c) Theory-focused
   (d) Exam-oriented
9. Which of the following activities is most aligned with the delegator teaching style in nursing education?
   (a) Delivering a traditional lecture with PowerPoint slides
   (b) Facilitating small group case studies and problem-solving
   (c) Assigning textbook readings and quizzes for self-study
   (d) Demonstrating clinical procedures and techniques
10. The formal authority teaching style in nursing education is characterized by
   (a) Encouraging student autonomy and decision-making
   (b) Promoting active learning through discussions and activities
   (c) Emphasizing the instructor's power and control over the classroom
   (d) Facilitating collaborative learning and peer interactions
11. Which of the following activities is most aligned with the formal authority teaching style in nursing education?
   (a) Engaging students in small group problem-solving activities
   (b) Assigning research projects and presentations
   (c) Delivering a traditional lecture with minimal student interaction
   (d) Facilitating case studies and real-life scenarios
12. One way to assess emotional intelligence in nursing education is through
   (a) Written exams and quizzes
   (b) Clinical competency evaluations
   (c) Self-assessment and reflection exercises
   (d) Research projects and publications
13. Understanding learning styles in nursing education can contribute to
   (a) Increased student satisfaction and motivation
   (b) Decreased student diversity and inclusivity
   (c) Standardization of teaching approaches and content
   (d) Reduction in the need for continuing education and professional development
14. Which of the following components is typically included in a course plan in nursing education?
   (a) Course objectives and learning outcomes
   (b) Faculty qualifications and experience
   (c) Textbook recommendations for students
   (d) Individual student evaluation and assessment methods

15. The timeline or schedule in a unit plan in nursing education outlines
- **(a)** The duration of the entire nursing programme
- **(b)** The specific dates and times for each class session within the unit
- **(c)** The order and sequence of topics and activities throughout the unit
- **(d)** The deadlines for submission of assignments and exams within the unit

ANSWERS TO THE MULTIPLE-CHOICE QUESTIONS

1. (b), 2. (c), 3. (d), 4. (b), 5. (a), 6. (a), 7. (a), 8. (b), 9. (b), 10. (c), 11. (c), 12. (c), 13. (a), 14. (a), 15. (b)

FURTHER READING

Alavi, N. M., Nabizadeh-Gharghozar, Z., & Ajorpaz, N. M. (2022). The barriers and facilitators of developing clinical competence among master's graduates of gerontological nursing: A qualitative descriptive study. *BMC Medical Education*, *22*(1), 500.

Barsade, S. G. (2002). The ripple effect: Emotional contagion and its influence on group behavior. *Administrative Science Quarterly*, *47*, 644–675.

Chakma, D. (2019). *Meaning and principles of curriculum construction.* https://myeducation2019.wordpress.com/2019/03/12/meaning-andprinciples-of-curriculum-construction/

Dash, N. R., Guraya, S. Y., Al Bataineh, M. T., Abdalla, M. E., Yusoff, M. S. B., Al-Qahtani, M. F., ... Mukhtar, W. N. O. (2020). Preferred teaching styles of medical faculty: An international multi-center study. *BMC Medical Education*, *20*(1), 480.

den Hertog, R., & Boshuizen, H. P. (2022). Learning professional knowledge: Bachelor nursing students' experiences in learning and knowledge quality outcomes in a competence-based curriculum. *Vocations and Learning*, *15*(1), 21–47.

Factors influencing students motivation to learn in Bahauddin Zakariya University, Multan (Pakistan). https://www.researchgate.net/publication/313289542_Factors_Influencing_Students_Motivation_to_Learn_in_Bahauddin_Zakariya_University_Multan_Pakistan. Accessed November 13, 2021.

Ford, J. H., II., Robinson, J. M., & Wise, M. E. (2016). Adaptation of the Grasha Riechman student learning style Survey and teaching style inventory to assess individual teaching and learning styles in a quality improvement collaborative. *BMC Medical Education*, *16*(1), 252.

Goleman, D. (1998). Working with Emotional Intelligence. London: Bloomsbury Publishers.

Goleman, D., Boyatzis, R., & McKee, A. (2002). *Primal leadership: Realizing the power of emotional intelligence.* Boston: Harvard Business School.

Grasha, A. F. (1994). A matter of style: The teacher as expert, formal authority, personal model, facilitator and delegator. *College Teaching*, *42*, 142–149.

Grasha, A. F. (1996). Teaching with style: A practical guide to enhancing learning by understanding teaching and learning styles (p. 372). Alliance Publishers, Cognitive styles.

Grasha, A. F. (2003). The dynamics of one-on-one teaching. *The Social Studies*, *94*(4), 179–187.

https://downloads.lww.com/wolterskluwer_vitalstream_com/sample-content/9780781783422_ABMP/samples/Williams_Ch01_001-024.pdf

https://resilienteducator.com/classroom-resources/5-types-of-classroom-teaching-styles/

https://www.acc.edu.au/blog/students-suit-different-styles/

Jones, B. (2023). *Course plan for English class.* https://www.example.com/course-plan/

Li-fang, Z. (2011). Teaching styles and conceptions of effective teachers: Tibetan and Han Chinese academics compared. *Learning and Individual Differences*, *21*(5), 619–623.

Mayer, J. D., & Salovey, P. (1997). What is emotional intelligence? In P. Salovey & D. Sluyter (Eds.), *Emotional development and emotional intelligence: Implications for educators* (pp. 3–31). New York: Basic Books.

Petrides, K. V. (2015). Ability and Trait Emotional Intelligence. In T. Chamorro-Premuzic, S. von Stumm, & A. Furnham (Eds.), *The Wiley-Blackwell handbook of individual differences* (pp. 656–678). London: John Wiley & Sons.

Salovey, P., & Grewal, D. (2005). The Science of Emotional Intelligence. *Current Directions in Psychological Science*, *14*(6), 6.

Schweitzer, K. (2020). *Curriculum design: Definition, purpose and types*. ThoughtCo. thoughtco.com/curriculum-design-definition-4154176

Sezer, H., & Şahin, H. (2021). Faculty development program for coaching in nursing education: A curriculum development process study. *Nurse Education in Practice*, *55*, 103165.

Smith, J. (2023). *Unit plan for science class*. https://www.example.com/unit-plan/

Tanveer, M. A., Shabbir, M. F., Ammar, M., Polla, S. I., & Aslam, H. D. (2012). Influence of teachers in students motivation in management sciences studies. *American Journal of Scientific Research*, *67*, 76–87.

The millennial student: A new generation of learners. https://www.researchgate.net/publication/228343335_The_Millennial_Student_A_New_Generation_of_Learners. Accessed November 11, 2021.

Vaughn, L., & Baker, R. (2001). Teaching in the medical setting: Balancing teaching styles, learning styles and teaching methods. *Medical Teacher*, *23*(6), 610–612.

Xiao, L., & Men, Y. (2022). Nursing teaching curriculum setting by introducing postcompetency model under the vision of internet informatization. *Contrast Media & Molecular Imaging*, *2022*, 6164614.

CHAPTER

Methods of teaching

5

LEARNING OBJECTIVES

This chapter is designed to enable the reader to:

- Define and classify teaching methods
- Describe the purposes, processes, advantages and disadvantages of lecture method, demonstration, group discussion, seminar, symposium, one-to-one interaction, team-based learning, peer-sharing, case study analysis, journaling, debate, gaming, interprofessional education and panel discussion as methods of teaching
- Discuss the concept, purposes, processes, advantages and disadvantages of role-play, project method, field trip, workshop, exhibition as method of teaching
- Explain the concept, principles, processes, merits and demerits of CAL, problem-based learning, self-directed learning and problem solving as method of teaching–learning
- Demonstrate the skills in planning and implementation of micro-teaching
- Describe details about clinical learning environment, factor influencing selection of clinical learning experiences, practical model, characteristics of effective clinical teacher, writing clinical learning outcomes and practical competencies
- Appreciate the concept, purposes, principles and processes of clinical nursing teaching methods, such as patient assignment, clinical conference, clinical presentation, bedside clinics, case study, simulation, nursing rounds, concept mapping, questioning in clinical teaching and process recording

KEY TERMS

INTRODUCTION

Good teaching is the main criterion of an effective teacher. Every individual is unique and so different teachers adopt different methods and strategies of teaching. The main objective of teaching is to bring about desired changes in the attitude and behaviour of the learner. The selection of the teaching methods depends upon the nature of a task, learning objectives, learner's abilities and student's entering behaviour. Teaching methods, teaching skill and technical competency affect students' learning. Learning the art of teaching is necessary to give systematic attention to methods as well as a mastery over the subject matter.

CLASSROOM MANAGEMENT

The principal is the head of an institution and a classteacher is the head of a class. Institutional management comes under the preview of the head of the institution but classroom management is the ultimate responsibility of the classteacher. The classteacher is expected to manage his class. Academic success of an institution principally depends on efficient class management by a competent classteacher. A teacher must possess some core qualities for efficient management of a class such as general academic proficiency, professional and managerial efficiency and positive personality traits.

DEFINITIONS OF CLASSROOM MANAGEMENT

Classroom management is an organizational function in which tasks are performed in a variety of settings, resulting in the inculcation of certain values such as human respect, personal integrity, self-direction and group cohesion etc.

—Johanson and Brooks

Classroom management is a system of action and activities are managed in classroom to induce learning through teacher–taught relationship. Teacher and students are the basic components for managing classroom activities.

(Operational meaning)

DIMENSIONS OF CLASSROOM MANAGEMENT

In behavioural terms, classroom management can be classified in four different dimensions: physical or environmental dimension, psychological dimension, ethical dimension, and social and cultural dimension of classroom management (Fig. 5.1).

- ***Physical/environmental dimension:*** Physical or environmental dimension of classroom management includes light and ventilation of the classroom, seating arrangement for students,

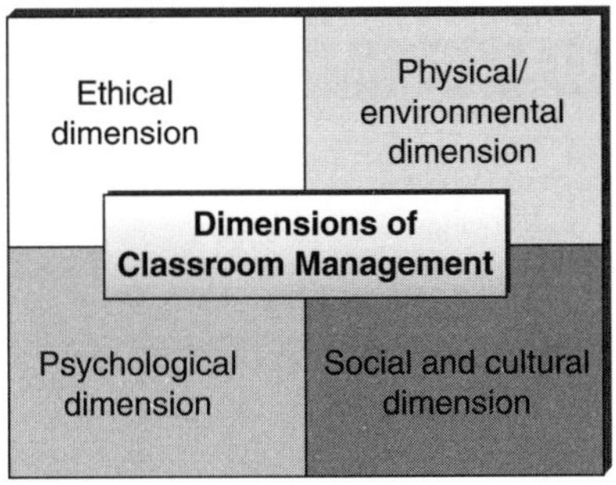

Figure 5.1

Dimensions of classroom management.

availability and functioning of blackboard and/or other audiovisual facilities in classroom, offering aesthetic academic environment inside and/or outside classroom. A teacher as a classroom manager should ensure the optimum and efficient management of these physical or environment facilities/services which are essential for overall learning in the students.

- ***Psychological dimension:*** Psychological dimension of classroom management is considered similar to software of the computer; without its presence mere hardware (physical/environmental dimension) is of no use and vice versa. Psychological classroom management includes infusion of motivation in students to promote the learning process. Motivation could be infused verbally or nonverbally through continuous feedback, behavioural reinforcement and positive encouragement in students. Psychological dimension of classroom management plays a pivotal role in the overall management of a classroom.
- ***Social and cultural dimension:*** A classroom is a miniature replica of an institution as well as of the society. The new society is shaped in the classroom through its desirable social and cultural environment. Classroom management involves the relationship of social and cultural environment in its overall management which depends on certain factors such as the teacher–taught relationship, relationship among students, relationship among teachers, relationship between teachers and the head of the institution. A teacher must know the background of his students and their entering behaviour, learning activities and interests.
- ***Ethical dimension:*** The ethical dimension of classroom management is concerned with feelings, attitudes, values and ethical aspects of students. A teacher is the manager of the class and an ideal to his students. He should look like and behave like a teacher. Further, the teacher should maintain classroom code and conduct which should be value-based or ethics-oriented.

PRINCIPLES OF THE CLASSROOM MANAGEMENT

Classroom management can primarily be governed by general as well as specific principles discussed below (Box 5.1).

GENERAL PRINCIPLES OF CLASSROOM MANAGEMENT

General principles can be learned and practised systematically. The general principles can be applied in several situations and provide a strong base to the teachers to manage vivid classroom management

BOX 5.1 PRINCIPLES OF CLASSROOM MANAGEMENT

I. *General principles of classroom management*
  - Self-control and role model approach of teacher
  - Understanding and acceptance of student uniqueness
  - Realistic and practical goals of teaching–learning
  - Exercising the productive teaching–learning activities
  - Understanding student's interest and ability

II. *Specific principles of classroom management*
  - Appropriate planning of classroom management
  - Encouragement of students
  - Giving responsibility to learners
  - Minimum disruption of teaching–learning activities
  - Clear guidelines of rules for students
  - Reward and punishment for student's activities
  - Conducive learning environment

related problems. Some of the assumptions related to general principles of the classroom management are as follows:

- *Self-control and role model:* Teachers must follow the principle of self-control and be a role model to the students. This provides a sense of confidence and trust to the students towards their teachers and institution as a whole and effective classroom management can be ensured.
- *Understanding and acceptance:* Teachers must ensure that they understand the individual differences of each student and accept them as they are. This will not only prevent biasness in teachers towards students but also provide each student with an equal opportunity to be a part of the class. This will also promote decreased psychological stress and decreased dissatisfaction in students and ultimately better classroom management.
- *Realistic and practical goals:* Teachers must plan realistic achievable educational goals for their students so undue psychological pressure in students can be avoided and the classroom can be efficiently managed.
- *Productive teaching–learning activities:* Teachers must ensure that learning experiences planned for the students are productive in nature so that classroom academics can be fruitful.
- *Student's interests and ability:* Teaching and learning activities must be planned on the principles of student's interests and abilities so that the teaching–learning environment can be goal-achieving in nature.

SPECIFIC PRINCIPLES OF CLASSROOM MANAGEMENT

Specific principles of classroom management can be adapted and used in certain specific situations and can be very helpful for overall classroom management. These are discussed below:

- *Planning:* Plan independent activities as well as organized lessons so students can be motivated to achieve their educational goals.
- *Encouragement:* Encourage effort and cues and reinforce positive and appropriate behaviour so students can be motivated for learning.
- *Responsibility:* Let students assume independent responsibility so they can develop a sense of responsibility and accountability towards their own education.

- *Minimum disruption:* Teachers must ensure that there is minimal disruption in natural learning among the students so they can have uninterrupted natural learning.
- *Clear rules:* The rules established for the students must be crystal clear so that ambiguity can be avoided and following rules and their implementation becomes easy.
- *Reward and punishment:* Students must be rewarded for their behaviour so they can be reinforced for repeating positive behaviour and discouraged from negative behaviour.
- *Conducive learning environment:* It is believed that the environment influences a person more than anything else. Therefore, a conducive teaching–learning environment can help a classteacher achieve the expected positive behaviour in students.

CLASSROOM MANAGEMENT PROBLEMS

- ***Inadequate light and ventilation:*** Effective classroom work can take place only in a congenial classroom atmosphere that includes adequate light and ventilation, temperature, furniture and seats. Inadequate light and ventilation can create problems for the student. It has an adverse effect on their learning as well as health.
- ***Inadequate furniture and lack of conducive seating environment:*** In the absence of proper seating arrangements, the students find themselves uneasy and uncomfortable. They do not feel like working wholeheartedly. They find it difficult to concentrate on learning in the class.
- ***Overcrowded classrooms:*** It is not possible for the teacher to teach effectively in a fully packed classroom. The teacher cannot give individual attention to all students. Therefore, the number of students in a class should not exceed more than 50.
- ***Inadequate apparatus:*** In an overcrowded class, it is difficult to provide adequate equipment to all students affecting their learning.
- ***Lack of routine:*** Breaking a routine creates confusion, chaos, disorder and indiscipline in the class. Routine should be followed in taking roll-calls, performing practicals, entering or leaving the classroom and other activities.
  The noise of one class disturbs students sitting in other classrooms. This can affect their studies.
- ***Problems of indiscipline:*** Absenteeism among teachers and the taught can also affect classroom teaching.
- ***Poor teacher–taught interpersonal relationship:*** In ancient times, there was a strong teacher–pupil relationship; however, with the present changing cultural values, there is a lack of teacher–taught relationship these days that ultimately affects the teaching–learning outcome in an institution.

STRATEGIES FOR CLASSROOM MANAGEMENT

- ***Promotion of rhythm in teaching–learning activities:*** Rhythm should be introduced in every teaching–learning activity. It guarantees smoothness in the sequence of movements. Routine is essential to rhythm. A chaotic, confusing, disturbing and insecure class is one where routines have been neglected and the sequence of activities has not been followed.
- ***Enhancing healthy classroom customs and traditions:*** The teacher should develop class traditions in the class. He should encourage the students to play their role well with a sense of responsibility.

It will help maintain self-discipline and ensure respect for college authority, self-progress, love for orderliness and development of good character.

- ***Promote positivity in teacher's behaviour:*** The teacher's verbal and nonverbal behaviour significantly influences student behaviour. The teacher's high character, high moral alertness, courage, practice, love and humility, his love and affection for students, his sense of humour, optimistic and democratic outlook, sympathy and wisdom, justice and impartiality, his resourcefulness, originality, confidence and his emotional and social health can positively influence student behaviour.
- ***Infuse motivation in students:*** The teaching–learning process is ineffective without proper motivation. The following techniques can be used for motivating students:
  - Goal, ideal and purposeful events
  - Knowledge of results or progress
  - Use of reward or punishment
  - Active participation
  - Use of competition
  - Cooperation
  - Evaluation
  - Audiovisual aids
  - Teacher–pupil relationship
- ***Encouraging pupil's participation:*** The teacher should encourage students to take part in daily activities and cocurricular activities that suit their interests, abilities and other potentialities such as discussions and declamations. Student participation may also be sought in the following programmes:
  - Development of lessons
  - Activity methods
  - Cocurricular activities

ROLE OF A TEACHER IN CLASSROOM MANAGEMENT

A teacher plays a pivotal role in classroom management because he is the central component of classroom management and has the authority, responsibility and accountability to manage a class. He plays variety of roles such as teacher, manager, philosopher, guide, researcher and leader. Efficient classroom management demands strong interpersonal relationship skills in a teacher, where he/she needs to build strong interpersonal relationship with students, colleagues, head of the institution and even parents of students and society as a whole. The main roles of the teacher in classroom management are as follows (Fig. 5.2):

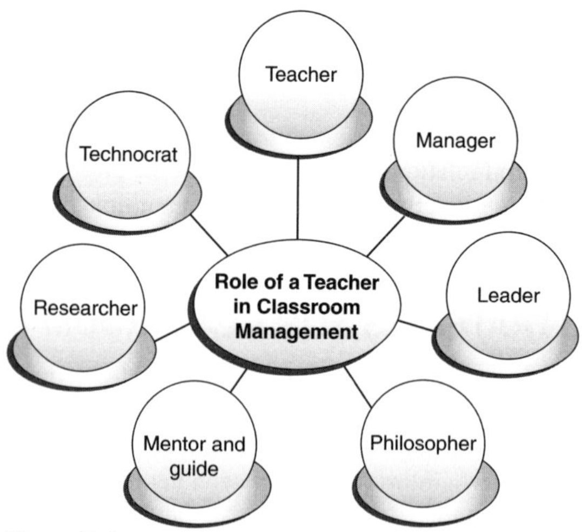

Figure 5.2

Role of the teacher in classroom management.

- ***Teacher:*** The core aim of classroom management is to achieve the expected outcome of the particular teaching–learning process. Therefore, the primary role of the teacher in classroom management is functioning efficiently as a teacher.

- ***Manager:*** Classroom management demands managerial skills from teachers. They are expected to perform responsibilities of planning, organizing, supervising, directing, coordinating and controlling the teaching–learning process.
- ***Leader:*** The teacher is expected to lead the class as a classroom manager for its overall functioning and taking desired messages to higher authorities and convincing them with the expected demands.
- ***Philosopher:*** The teacher is expected to have a strong hold and mastery over the subject content that has to be delivered to students. In addition, a teacher is expected to teach moral values, ethics and discipline to the students.
- ***Mentor and guide:*** Each of us requires a mentor or guide to help us choose the right path in life. Students also require a mentor or guide to help them take the right decisions for learning activities. Therefore, a teacher is expected to perform the role of a mentor or guide for a particular group of students to solve their personal as well as teaching–learning related problems.
- ***Researcher:*** Solutions for problems are generated through research. A teacher also faces a lot of problems related to classroom management that can be easily solved by generating evidence-based solutions generated through action research. Therefore, a teacher must act as researcher to generate the empirical solutions for classroom management related problems.
- ***Technocrat:*** Advancement in science and technology has offered a wide range of technologically sophisticated audiovisual aids to the educational institutions. A teacher must be technologically skilled to operate and manage these technologically sophisticated audiovisual aids as and when required.

CLASSROOM COMMUNICATION

Classroom communication is the process of exchanging information and ideas between teachers and students. It is a two-way process, and both parties need to be able to effectively communicate in order for learning to take place. Effective classroom communication is essential for creating an engaging and productive learning environment. It involves establishing clear expectations, promoting open and respectful dialogue, utilizing various forms of communication (verbal, nonverbal and written) and integrating technology to support learning. By fostering effective communication, educators can enhance student understanding, participation and overall academic success.

Classroom communication in nursing education is a critical component of preparing future nurses for their professional roles. Effective communication in the nursing classroom is vital for promoting understanding, developing critical thinking skills, fostering collaboration and preparing students for effective patient interactions.

DEFINITIONS

- Classroom communication in nursing refers to the exchange of information, ideas and feedback between nursing educators and students within the classroom setting of a nursing education programme.
- Classroom communication in nursing is the process of exchanging information and ideas between nursing students and their instructors.

METHODS OF CLASSROOM COMMUNICATION IN NURSING

The best method of classroom communication will vary depending on the topic being taught, the learning objectives and the needs of the students. However, by using a variety of methods, instructors can create a classroom environment that is conducive to learning and that helps students to develop the communication skills they need to be successful in their careers. Some of the most common methods include:

1. ***Lectures:*** Lectures are a traditional method of classroom communication in which nursing educators deliver content and information to students. Through verbal communication, educators provide explanations, present concepts and share knowledge related to nursing theory, practice and patient care. Lectures often incorporate visual aids, such as slides or multimedia presentations, to enhance understanding and engagement.
2. ***Discussions:*** Classroom discussions encourage active participation and critical thinking among nursing students. Educators facilitate discussions by asking open-ended questions, encouraging students to share their perspectives and fostering dialogue and debate. Discussions provide opportunities for students to analyse nursing concepts, apply theory to practice and explore different viewpoints.
3. ***Case studies:*** Case studies involve the analysis and discussion of realistic patient scenarios. Nursing students are presented with a patient's health condition, and they work collaboratively to assess the situation, identify nursing diagnoses and develop appropriate care plans. Case studies encourage critical thinking, problem solving and decision-making skills of nursing students in a practical context.
4. ***Simulations:*** Simulations simulate real-life clinical scenarios in a controlled environment. They allow nursing students to practice their clinical skills, decision-making and communication in a safe and supportive setting. Simulations can involve role-playing as patients, colleagues or healthcare team members, allowing students to experience different perspectives and develop effective communication strategies.
5. ***Group work and collaborative learning:*** Group work promotes collaboration and teamwork among nursing students. Educators assign students to small groups to work on projects, presentations or problem-solving activities. Group work encourages active engagement, effective communication and the sharing of knowledge and skills among peers.
6. ***Technology-mediated communication:*** With advancements in technology, classroom communication in nursing has expanded to include various technological tools. Educators use online platforms, video conferencing, virtual simulations and multimedia resources to facilitate communication and engagement in the classroom. Technology-mediated communication allows for interactive discussions, remote learning and the integration of multimedia content to enhance learning experiences.
7. ***Written communication:*** Written communication is essential in nursing education. It includes assignments, written exams, documentation and written feedback. Through written communication, educators provide instructions, assess students' understanding of nursing concepts and offer constructive feedback on their written work.
8. ***Active listening and questioning:*** Active listening and effective questioning techniques are important elements of classroom communication in nursing. Educators actively listen to students' questions, comments and concerns and respond appropriately to foster understanding and engagement. Educators also use probing questions to stimulate critical thinking, encourage reflection and deepen students' understanding of nursing concepts.

BENEFITS OF EFFECTIVE CLASSROOM COMMUNICATION IN NURSING

Effective classroom communication is a vital part of nursing education. It allows students to learn from each other, from their instructors and from the clinical experiences they have. There are many benefits to classroom communication in nursing, including:

1. ***Increased knowledge:*** Classroom communication allows students to share their knowledge and learn from each other. This can help them to gain a deeper understanding of the material they are learning.
2. ***Improved critical thinking:*** Classroom communication can help students to develop their critical thinking skills. When they are asked to explain their thinking, they are forced to think more deeply about the material.
3. ***Enhanced problem-solving skills:*** Classroom communication can help students to develop their problem-solving skills. When they are asked to work together to solve problems, they learn to collaborate and to think outside the box.
4. ***Improved teamwork skills:*** Classroom communication can help students to develop their teamwork skills. When they are working together to achieve a common goal, they learn to communicate effectively and to work together towards a common purpose.
5. ***Increased confidence:*** Classroom communication can help students to increase their confidence. When they are able to share their ideas and thoughts in a safe and supportive environment, they begin to believe in themselves and their abilities.
6. ***Cultural competence:*** Classroom communication exposes students to diverse perspectives and cultures. By engaging in discussions and sharing experiences, students develop cultural competence, learning to communicate effectively with individuals from different backgrounds and respecting cultural diversity in healthcare settings.
7. ***Professionalism development:*** Classroom communication contributes to the development of professionalism in nursing. Students learn how to communicate respectfully, ethically and empathetically with patients, families and healthcare professionals. They gain insights into ethical decision-making, cultural sensitivity and maintaining professional boundaries.

CHALLENGES OF EFFECTIVE CLASSROOM COMMUNICATION IN NURSING

There are also some challenges to classroom communication in nursing, including:

1. ***Difficult to participate:*** Some students may find it difficult to participate in classroom discussions. This may be due to shyness, anxiety or a lack of confidence.
2. ***Difficult to understand:*** Some students may find it difficult to understand the material that is being discussed in class. This may be due to a language barrier, a learning disability or a lack of prior knowledge.
3. ***Difficult to stay focused:*** Some students may find it difficult to stay focused during class discussions. This may be due to fatigue, distractions or a lack of interest in the material.
4. ***Technological challenges:*** Incorporating technology in the classroom can enhance communication, but it can also present challenges such as technical glitches, limited access to technology resources or difficulty in effectively integrating technology into teaching methods.
5. ***Diversity in student population:*** Nursing classrooms often consist of students from diverse backgrounds, including varying ages, cultures and experiences. Navigating these differences and ensuring inclusive communication can be a challenge for educators.

6. ***Engaging all students:*** Ensuring active participation and engagement from all students can be challenging, as some may be hesitant to contribute or may feel overshadowed by more vocal classmates. Creating an inclusive environment that encourages all students to share their perspectives is crucial.

STRATEGIES TO OVERCOME CHALLENGES OF EFFECTIVE CLASSROOM COMMUNICATION IN NURSING

Effective classroom communication in nursing is essential for creating a conducive learning environment and preparing future nurses for their professional roles. Here are some tips for enhancing classroom communication in nursing:

1. ***Be clear and concise:*** While speaking, make sure that message is clear and easy to understand. Avoid using jargon or technical terms that students and others may not be familiar with.
2. ***Be respectful:*** Even when we disagree with someone, it is important to be respectful of their opinion. Avoid name-calling, insults or other personal attacks.
3. ***Be open to feedback:*** Be willing to listen to feedback from students and others. This will help to improve communication skills.
4. ***Be active in class discussions:*** Participate in class discussions by asking questions, sharing thoughts and contributing to the conversation.
5. ***Encourage student participation:*** Create an inclusive classroom environment where students feel comfortable and encouraged to participate.
6. ***Use technology effectively:*** Incorporate technology tools and resources to enhance classroom communication. Utilize online discussion boards, virtual simulations, multimedia presentations and educational apps to promote engagement and active learning.
7. ***Be prepared:*** Come to class prepared by reading the assigned readings and taking notes. This will help to participate more effectively in class discussions.
8. ***Be organized:*** Keep notes organized so that it can be easily located when required.
9. ***Be patient:*** It takes time to develop effective communication skills. Be patient with self, students and other colleagues as communication skills develop gradually.
10. ***Make eye contact:*** Eye contact shows that attention is being paid and interested in what the other person is saying.
11. ***Nod your head:*** Nodding head shows that one is following along and understanding what the other person is saying.
12. ***Smile:*** Smiling shows gesture of friendliness and approachability.
13. ***Use open body language:*** Crossing arms or legs signifies and give an impression of being closed off and unapproachable. Instead, try to sit with arms and legs uncrossed and your body facing the other person.
14. ***Be aware of tone of voice:*** Tone of voice can convey a lot of information, even if one is not saying anything. Be careful not to use a harsh or condescending tone of voice.

INFORMATION AND COMMUNICATION TECHNOLOGY IN EDUCATION

Information and Communication Technology (ICT) has revolutionized education by transforming the way we learn, teach and interact within educational environments. ICT encompasses a wide range of technologies, such as computers, the internet, digital devices, software applications and online platforms, that have profoundly impacted every level of education, from primary schools to universities.

ICT has significantly transformed the field of nursing education, revolutionizing the way students learn and preparing them for the dynamic healthcare industry. ICT encompasses various technological tools and platforms that enhance the learning experience, foster collaboration and promote the acquisition of essential nursing knowledge and skills. From e-learning platforms and virtual simulations to teleconferencing and mobile learning, ICT has become an integral part of nursing education, empowering students to engage with educational resources, connect with peers and experts and gain hands-on experience in a virtual environment.

DEFINITIONS

- The World Bank defines ICT as 'the combination of hardware, software, networks, and media for the collection, storage, processing, transmission, and presentation of information (voice, data, text, images)'.
- ICT in nursing education refers to the integration and utilization of digital technologies and communication tools to enhance the teaching, learning and practice of nursing.
- ICT refers to the use of technology, digital tools and communication systems to facilitate the collection, storage, retrieval, processing and sharing of information in nursing education.

COMPONENTS OF INFORMATION AND COMMUNICATION TECHNOLOGY

ICT is a broad term that encompasses a wide range of technologies. The specific components of ICT that are used in a particular setting will vary depending on the needs of the users. The components of ICT include:

- ***Hardware:*** This is the physical equipment that is used to create and use ICT. Examples of hardware include computers, printers, scanners and mobile devices.
- ***Software:*** This is the code that is used to run on hardware. Examples of software include operating systems, word processors and web browsers.
- ***Data:*** This is the information that is stored on hardware or transmitted over networks. Examples of data include text, images, audio and video.
- ***Networks:*** These are the connections that allow hardware to communicate with each other. Examples of networks include the internet, intranets and extranets.
- ***People:*** These are the users of ICT. People use ICT to create, store, retrieve, transmit and manipulate data.

BENEFITS OF USING INFORMATION AND COMMUNICATION TECHNOLOGY IN NURSING EDUCATION

The use of ICT in nursing education offers several significant benefits, enhancing the learning experience for students and preparing them for the challenges of modern healthcare. Some key benefits of using ICT in nursing education include:

1. ***Access to a wealth of resources:*** ICT provides nursing students with access to a vast range of educational resources, including e-books, online databases, medical/nursing journals and

multimedia materials. This allows students to explore up-to-date information, research findings and best practices, expanding their knowledge and promoting evidence-based practice.

2. ***Interactive and engaging learning experiences:*** ICT offers interactive learning experiences through multimedia resources, virtual simulations and educational software. These tools engage students in active learning, enabling them to visualize complex concepts, practice clinical skills in a virtual environment and enhance critical thinking and decision-making abilities.
3. ***Flexibility and self-paced learning:*** ICT enables flexible learning options, allowing nursing students to access educational materials and participate in online modules at their own convenience. This flexibility accommodates different learning styles and helps students manage their time effectively, especially for those balancing education with work or other responsibilities.
4. ***Collaboration and communication:*** ICT fosters collaboration and communication among nursing students, faculty and experts. Online discussion forums, video conferencing and collaborative tools enable students to share knowledge, engage in group projects and interact with experts and peers from different geographical locations. This promotes teamwork, cultural diversity and a sense of community in nursing education.
5. ***Virtual patient simulations:*** ICT facilitates the use of virtual simulations, providing nursing students with opportunities to practice clinical skills and decision-making in a safe and controlled environment. These simulations can replicate diverse patient scenarios, allowing students to apply theoretical knowledge, develop critical thinking skills and gain confidence before engaging in real patient care.
6. ***Accessible and inclusive learning:*** ICT helps overcome geographical barriers, making education accessible to students in remote areas or those with limited physical mobility. It also promotes inclusivity by catering to diverse learning needs, such as providing alternative formats for materials, accommodating students with disabilities and offering multilingual resources.
7. ***Real-world preparation:*** By incorporating ICT, nursing education prepares students for the digital advancements and technologies they will encounter in their professional careers. Familiarity with electronic health records, telehealth and other digital tools ensures graduates are equipped with the necessary skills to navigate the modern healthcare environment.
8. ***Lifelong learning and professional development:*** ICT supports lifelong learning in nursing by offering continuing education opportunities, online certification programmes and access to professional communities. Nurses can stay updated on the latest research, advancements and best practices through online platforms, webinars and virtual conferences.

CHALLENGES OF USING INFORMATION AND COMMUNICATION TECHNOLOGY IN NURSING EDUCATION

While ICT offers numerous benefits in nursing education, its implementation also presents certain challenges. Some of the challenges associated with using ICT in nursing education include:

1. ***Technological barriers:*** Implementing ICT requires adequate infrastructure, including reliable internet access, updated hardware and software and technical support. Insufficient resources and outdated technology can hinder effective integration and usage of ICT in nursing education.
2. ***Digital literacy and skills gap:*** Not all nursing students may possess the necessary digital literacy skills to effectively utilize ICT tools and platforms. Training and support may be required to ensure students can navigate digital resources, software applications and online learning platforms confidently.
3. ***Resistance to change:*** Integrating ICT may encounter resistance from faculty members, administrators or even students who are accustomed to traditional teaching methods. Overcoming

resistance to change and encouraging adoption of new technologies may require faculty development programmes and a supportive institutional culture.

4. ***Privacy and security concerns:*** ICT involves the collection and storage of sensitive information, including patient data and student records. Ensuring data privacy, security and compliance with healthcare regulations presents challenges, requiring robust security measures, encryption and protocols for handling confidential information.
5. ***Equity and access disparities:*** Access to ICT tools and resources may not be equitable, especially in resource-limited settings or areas with limited internet connectivity. This can create a digital divide, exacerbating disparities in education and limiting equal opportunities for all nursing students.
6. ***Cost concern:*** ICT infrastructure and software require regular maintenance, updates and troubleshooting. This can pose challenges in terms of financial resources, technical expertise and ensuring uninterrupted access to technology for both faculty and students.
7. ***Training and support:*** Proper training and ongoing support for faculty and students are crucial to maximize the benefits of ICT. Adequate training programmes and resources should be provided to ensure users are proficient in utilizing ICT tools, platforms and applications effectively.

METHOD OF TEACHING

The way or style of the presentation of content in a classroom is called *teaching method.* M. Varma has presented a broad meaning of the term *teaching method.* According to him, content matter is important for determining the teaching method. Teaching methods are classified under three domains: telling method, showing method and doing method (Fig. 5.3).

According to Burton, teaching method is the stimulation, guidance, direction and encouragement of learning.

Teaching method is a broad and general term. It covers both teaching strategies and tactics of teaching. Teaching strategy includes two main concepts, that is a generalized plan for a lesson that includes structure and the desired learner behaviour in terms of objectives to be achieved. Teaching tactics, according to E. Stones and E. Moris, are the influencing behaviour of the teacher in the instructional situation to achieve objectives. Tactics may range from nonverbal cues to verbal instructions and the teacher's behaviour. For example, the strategy includes content matter and objectives to be achieved in the lecture method of teaching.

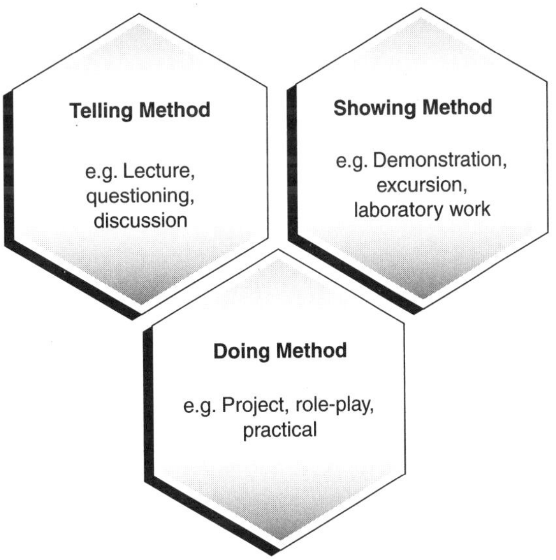

Figure 5.3
Domains of teaching methods.

LECTURE METHOD

The lecture method is the oldest method of teaching based on the philosophy of idealism and is an autocratic style of teaching. In this method, the teacher is more active while students are passive listeners.

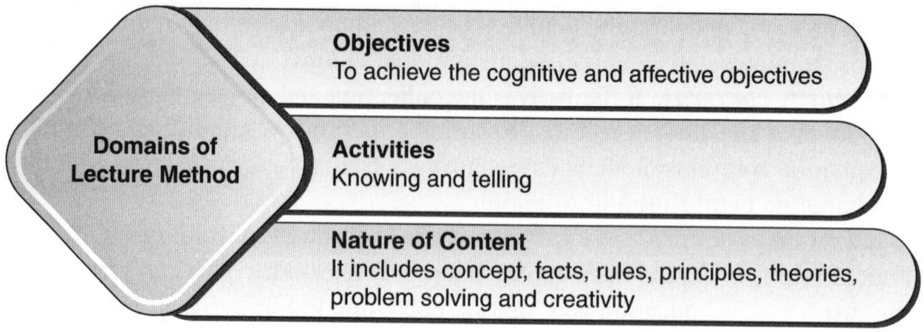

Figure 5.4

Domains of lecturer method.

BOX 5.2 FACTORS CONSIDERED WHILE PLANNING THE LECTURE METHOD

Related to Students	Related to Teacher	Related to Environment
Learner's • Capability and ability • Interest and attitude • Cognitive level • Previous knowledge • Type of programme, e.g. ANM, GNM, B.Sc. (N), M.Sc. (N), etc.	*Teacher's* • Knowledge and mastery over the subject matter • Teaching tactics include voice, gestures, eye contact and manners • Teacher–learner relationship • Preparation of lecture before presentation • Purpose or reason to be taught	• Time of the day, e.g. morning lecture seems superior to afternoon lectures for recall information • Duration and length, i.e. lecture more than 40 minutes can reduce the absorption and assimilation power of students • Use of audiovisual aids • Good light facility

This method is centred on the presentation of content and does not consider the learner's abilities, interests and personality. The purpose of this method is to achieve cognitive and affective objectives. The main focus of this method is on the presentation of content as a whole. The teacher talks continuously to the class, and students learn better through listening. This method consists of several special components or domains to be considered (Fig. 5.4). Moreover, several factors related to student, teacher and environment must be considered as depicted in Box 5.2 while planning this method.

Lecture method is the teaching procedure comprising the presentation of content, clarification of doubts and explanation of facts, principles and relationships.

I. PURPOSES OF THE LECTURE METHOD

The main purposes of the lecture method are:

- To stimulate thinking in students.
- To develop concentration in students.
- To achieve a very high order of cognitive objectives.
- To influence learners to inculcate the habits of listening and learning.
- To introduce new content in the classroom.
- To correlate subjects with other subjects.
- To develop problem solving on a factual basis.

II. COMPONENTS OF THE LECTURE METHOD

Lecture as a teaching method includes the following components:

A. INTRODUCTION TO THE LECTURE

This is the first component of an effective lecture, and the student's perception and interest depend on this stage. It usually lasts 3–5 minutes. The teacher should provide a general idea and framework for the lecture's content in this stage so that students get familiar with the ongoing topic. It helps the teacher capture the student's attention and stimulate their interest. During the introduction of the lecture, the teacher must ensure the following:

- The teacher should establish good rapport with students. The teacher's tactics and personality should generate interest in students. Establishing friendly communication to provide a positive learning so that students feel comfortable is important.
- In the first meeting with students, teachers should introduce themselves by using an 'ice breaker' and maintain a consistent and affectionate relationship with students so that the students feel comfortable while approaching the teacher.
- Teachers should assess the students' preexisting knowledge. They should not simply announce the topic. To maintain interest, teachers should disclose the topic in the form of a story, situation or picture or question. For example, a nurse educator may begin a lecture on ventilators while showing pictures of patients on ventilators in the ICU.
- The teacher should relate the student's goals and interest with the topic of lecture. A lecture may also be introduced by describing how it will help the students succeed in their education and careers.
- The teacher should clarify the objectives and purposes of a lecture and describe how it is organized.
- The teacher should introduce the topic by raising some related issues for student participation.

B. THE BODY OF THE LECTURE

The body of the lecture covers the content in an organized way. Since this component is allotted the greatest amount of time in a classroom, it includes many more teaching procedures than in introduction and conclusion. The body lays emphasis on the presentation of the content. The teacher is more active, while students are relatively passive participants. The teacher uses question–answer techniques to keep students attentive in class. Teacher controls and plans all student activities. The teacher generally uses maxims of teaching to make the students understand the concept using various examples, situations, etc.

C. CONCLUSION

Conclusion helps the teacher summarize and re-emphasize the key points of the lecture and also get feedback from the students. The teacher can motivate the students to ask questions by focusing their mind to specific points. Students can also clarify their doubts and raise questions at this stage.

ADVANTAGES OF THE LECTURE METHOD

- This method develops concentration in students.
- It is an economical teaching strategy. Large subject content may be taught in a relatively small duration.

- Teaching activities are dominated by the teacher.
- It provides current information from many sources.
- It provides a summary or synthesis of information from different sources.

DISADVANTAGES OF THE LECTURE METHOD

- The lecturer method lends little emphasis on problem solving, decision-making, analytical thinking or transfer of learning.
- It is not conducive to meeting students' individual needs.
- This method brings with it the problems of limited attention span on the part of the learners.
- The lecture does not allow the instructor estimate student understanding easily as the material is covered.

GROUP DISCUSSION

Group discussion is an effective method of teaching and considered a learner-centric approach of the teaching–learning process. In a group discussion, a number of learners interact face-to-face to achieve specific educational objectives. It provides wider interaction among the members of a group and is useful when long-term compliance is involved. Common forms of group discussion are classroom discussions, seminar symposiums and panel discussions and conferences.

Group discussion is a cooperative, problem-solving activity, which seeks a consensus regarding the solution of a problem.

Group discussion can be defined as three or more participants who have an agreed topic to discuss and share their views in all the aspects and submit/present their views in the form of report to bigger gathering.

I. PURPOSES OF GROUP DISCUSSION

- It provides an opportunity for sharing information among the members of a group.
- Members get an opportunity to attend group consortium to gain and share knowledge necessary to achieve specific educational objectives.
- It develops the skills of group development, group cohesiveness and group socialization in group members under the leadership of teacher.
- A variety of information may be learned in a short time, when a number of people in a group share their own experience and knowledge with others.

II. GUIDELINES TO CONDUCT A GROUP DISCUSSION

A group discussion conducted in an efficient manner using the following guidelines may be one of the best teaching methods because of its richness of vivid content and the ability to get long-lasting memory.

- There must be adequate and effective planning of the topic of discussion, educational objectives to be achieved and environment for group discussion.

- Plenty of time and motivation must be provided to students for preparation on the topic of discussion.
- Group leader and each member should be well aware of their moral and professional responsibilities during group discussion.
- The teacher opens the discussion session with a brief introduction of the topic with specific objectives. This is followed by students who are invited to express their ideas and viewpoints about the topic of discussion.
- During discussion, the teacher assumes the role of the mentor and leader, and students are facilitated to share their viewpoints. Overtalkative students are discouraged, and passive students are motivated to participate in the discussion.
- One student from the group is asked to record the proceedings of the discussion.
- During the discussion, the teacher intervenes in case of argumentative and ambiguous discussions and clarifies doubts when required.
- At the end of the discussion, the teacher summarizes the discussion and concludes with a comprehensive note of carry home messages and words of encouragement for the participants.

ADVANTAGES OF GROUP DISCUSSION

- Each group member actively participates in achieving the educational objectives.
- It boosts the self-esteem and morale of students when their viewpoints are accepted and given due regard.
- It helps the students develop a problem-solving approach while working in a group.
- It also offers group members an opportunity to express their viewpoints and ideas in full freedom.
- Individuals in a group develop social skills and feelings of team activity.

DISADVANTAGES OF GROUP DISCUSSION

- Group discussions are generally time-consuming and are usually not completed in the scheduled time.
- Some members in a group may dominate and some may only be passive listeners.
- Group discussion may not be a very effective method for large groups.
- Adequate preparation is required by each member to have a fruitful discussion; else the discussion may remain polarized.
- Equal participation of group members may not be possible in a group discussion.

MICRO-TEACHING

The idea of micro-teaching originated for the first time at Stanford University, United States, when an experimental project on the identification of teaching skills was in progress under the guidance and supervision of faculty members. The team of experts was assigned the development of testing and evaluation tools to measure the attainment of teaching skills. A research worker was investigating the utility of video tape recorders in the development of technical teaching skills. This instrument could be used for recording class interaction and behaviours of the trainees vividly and accurately, which led to the development of a systematic and accurate method of providing feedback to teacher trainees. All the steps of the micro-teaching technique, that is *Teach → Feedback → Re-plan → Re-teach → Re-feedback*, were formulated. The term *micro-teaching* was coined for this method of developing teaching skills in 1963. Since then this technique has been widely used in almost all colleges and universities. It is being used with great emphasis in all teacher training programmes for developing teaching skills and competencies in teacher trainees.

Micro-teaching is a teacher training technique that helps the teacher trainee to master the teaching skills. It requires the teacher trainee to:

- Teach a single concept of content.
- Use a specified teaching skill.
- Teach for a short time.
- Teach to a very small number of students.

In this way the teacher trainee practices the teaching skill in terms of definable, observable, measurable and controllable form with repeated cycles till he attains a mastery in the use of that skill.

I. ASSUMPTIONS OF MICRO-TEACHING

From the foregoing discussion about the concept of micro-teaching, the basic assumption on which it is based is the premise that teaching can be analysed into various teaching skills that can be practised and evaluated.

- Micro-teaching seems to be based on Skinner's theory of operant condition. This theory is the very basis of feedback session. Skinner's theory of shaping a successive approximation can be applied to explain the acquisition of new patterns of behaviour in the *teach → feedback → re-teach* pattern in micro-teaching.
- Teaching is a complex process but can be analysed into simple skills.
- Teaching skills can be practised one by one up to the mastery level under specific and simplified situations.
- Appropriate feedback, if systematically given, proves very significant for obtaining a mastery level in each skill.
- When all skills have been mastered, taken one by one, they can be integrated for real classroom teaching.
- Skill training can be conveniently transferred from a simulated teaching situation to the actual classroom teaching situation.
- Teaching skill is the set of behaviours or acts of the teacher that facilitate students' learning.
- Teaching is observable, definable, measurable and demonstrable and can be developed through training.
- Micro-teaching is a teacher training technique that plays a significant role in developing teaching skills in student teachers.
- The procedure of micro-teaching involves the following steps: *Plan → Teach → Feedback → Re-plan → Re-teach → Re-feedback*. These steps are repeated till the student teacher attains mastery in the use of the skill.
- The micro-teaching cycle consists of all the essential steps of basic teaching.
- For practising teaching skills, the setting of micro-teaching involves:
    - A single skill for practice.
    - One concept of content for teaching.
    - A class of 5–10 students.
    - 5–10 minutes of practice time.
- Systematic use of feedback plays a significant role in the acquisition of the skill up to the mastery level.
- After the acquisition of the core skills, it is possible to integrate them for effective teaching in actual classroom situations.

II. BENEFITS OF MICRO-TEACHING

- Visual feedback (through watching a recorded lesson) has been found to provide one of the most effective means of evaluating teaching strengths and identifying areas of improvement.
- Micro-teaching enables both intrinsic (self-assessment) and extrinsic (peer-review) assessment of teaching behaviours.
- Through micro-teaching, one can seek to identify and improve these observable teaching skills and behaviours. Some such skills and observable teaching behaviours include:
  - Oral presentation skills (voice modulation and articulation, enthusiasm, gestures, nonverbal cues, clarity of explanations and examples)
  - Organization skills (structure of lessons, strong opening and closing, good transitions between sections, clear learning objectives, effective use of time and good pacing)
  - Relating to the student (speaker engages audience, material is audience-appropriate, effective questioning and use of real-life examples)
  - Effective use of teaching aids (handouts, blackboard, presentation software, overhead transparencies, props and charts, etc.).
- Aside from helping to identify teaching skills to be improved as well as teaching strengths, micro-teaching sessions can also provide an opportunity for the following:
  - Practising a part of a lecture or running an activity or explaining a procedure before you have to deliver a course or demonstrate a lab for the first time.
  - Practising a guest lecture you have been asked to deliver in someone else's course.
  - Practising a job talk before you visit a campus when applying for jobs.
  - Practising public speaking skills before you address students for the first time.
  - Polishing your questioning techniques or your opening and closing skills, if you are already an experienced instructor.

III. STEPS OF MICRO-TEACHING

It is also known as the *micro-teaching cycle* and includes the following six steps (Fig. 5.5):

A. PLAN

- This involves the selection of the topic and related content of a nature in which the use of components of the skill under practice may be made easily and conveniently.
- The topic is analysed into different activities of the teacher and the students.
- The activities are planned in a logical sequence such that the maximum application of the components of a skill is possible.

B. TEACH

- This involves the attempts of the teacher trainee to use the components of the skill in suitable situations in the process of teaching–learning per his or her planning of activities.
- If the situation is different and not as visualized in the planning of the activities, the teacher should modify his or her behaviour as per the demand of the situation in the class.
- The teacher should have the courage and confidence to handle the situations arising in the class effectively.

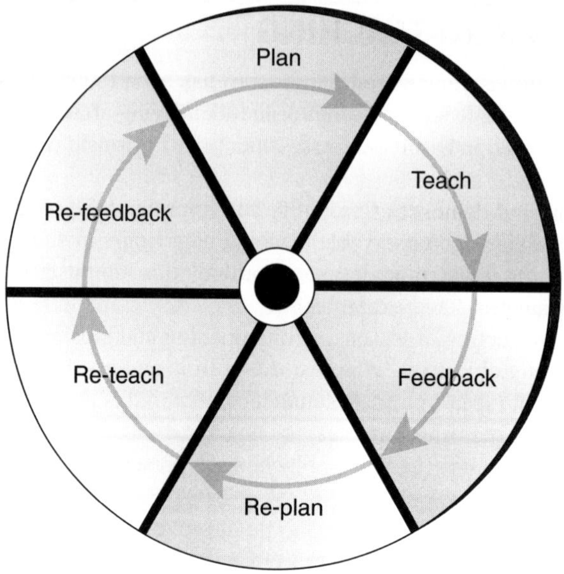

Figure 5.5

Micro-teaching cycle.

C. FEEDBACK

- This term refers to giving information to the teacher trainee about his performance.
- The information includes the points of strength as well as weakness relating to his or her performance.
- This helps the teacher trainee improve his or her performance in the desired direction.

D. RE-PLAN

The teacher trainee re-plans his lesson incorporating the points of strength and removing the points not skilfully handled during teaching in the previous attempt either on the same topic or on another topic suiting the teacher trainee for improvement.

E. RE-TEACH

- This involves teaching the same group of students if the topic is changed or a different group of students if the topic is the same.
- This is done to remove boredom or monotony in the students.
- The teacher trainee teaches the class with renewed courage and confidence to perform better than the previous attempt.

F. RE-FEEDBACK

This is the most important component of micro-teaching for behaviour modification of the teacher trainee in the desired direction in each and every skill practice.

IV. PHASES OF MICRO-TEACHING

There are three phases of the micro-teaching procedure and they are (Fig. 5.6):

- ***Knowledge acquisition phase:*** In this phase, the teacher trainee learns about the skill and its components through discussion, illustrations and demonstration of the skill given by the expert. He learns about the purpose of the skill and the condition under which it proves useful in the teaching–learning process. The teacher trainee's analysis of the skill into components leads to various types of behaviours to be practised. The teacher trainee tries to gain the skill from the demonstration given by the expert. He discusses and clarifies each and every aspect of the skill.
- ***Skill acquisition phase:*** On the basis of the demonstration presented by the expert, the teacher trainee plans a micro-lesson for practicing the demonstrated skill. He practices the teaching skill through the micro-teaching cycle and continues his efforts till he attains the mastery level. The feedback component of micro-teaching contributes significantly towards the mastery level acquisition of the skill. On the basis of the performance of teacher trainee in teaching, feedback is provided for the purpose of change in behaviour of the teacher trainee in the desired direction. These skills are called *core skills* because of their extensive use in classroom teaching. The specifications of these skills are given in Box 5.3.
- ***Transfer phase of micro-teaching:*** After attaining mastery and command over each of the skills, the teacher trainee integrates all these skills and transfers to actual classroom teaching during this transfer phase.

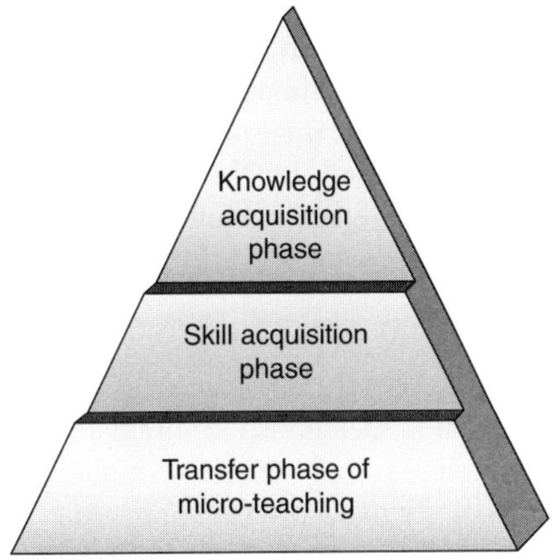

Figure 5.6

Phases of micro-teaching.

BOX 5.3 TEACHING SKILLS AND THEIR SPECIFICATIONS

Skill	Components
1. Probing questions	Prompting, seeking further information, redirection, focusing, increasing critical awareness
2. Explaining	Clarity, continuity, relevance to content using beginning and concluding statements, covering essential points
3. Illustrating with examples	Simple, relevant and interesting examples and use of appropriate media
4. Stimulus variation	Body movements, gestures, changes in speech pattern, changes in style of interaction, pausing, focusing, oral–visual switching
5. Reinforcement	Use of words and statements of praise, accepting and using students' ideas, repeating and rephrasing, extra vertical cues, use of pleasant and approving gestures and expressions, writing students' answers on the blackboard
6. Classroom management	Call students by names, make norms of classroom behaviour, attending behaviour reinforced, clarity of direction, check nonattending behaviour, keep students in eye span, check inappropriate behaviour immediately
7. Use of blackboard	Legible, neat and adequate with reference to content covered

V. ORGANIZATION OF THE MICRO-TEACHING SESSION

- It is not easy and workable to get actual students practice the skill because of administrative reasons so a simulated class of peers has been found suitable and useful for this purpose. How to organize the micro-teaching cycle for 10 teacher trainees who have come prepared with planned micro-lessons for the practice of a particular skill? Allot roll numbers to teacher trainees from 1 to 10 and prepare the following plan (Box 5.4).

DEMONSTRATION

A teaching method is the stimulation, guidance, direction and encouragement for learning. It inculcates the desire to work with the maximum efficiency one is capable of. The demonstration method is of utmost importance in the teaching of nursing. It teaches by exhibition and explanation and provides opportunities to students to apply their acquired knowledge and skill practically. This method utilizes the patient's bedside as a live teaching field for demonstrations of a variety of nursing care situations. A creative teacher knows how to use the demonstration method to modify concepts and skills and to maximize possibilities for transfer of learning so that students can use previously acquired knowledge in new contexts.

Demonstration can be defined as visualized explanation of facts, concepts and procedures. It trains, explains the students in the art of careful observation.

I. PURPOSES OF DEMONSTRATION

- To show the learner how to perform certain psychomotor skills. The learner must reproduce the behaviour of demonstration exactly.
- To show why things occur. The behaviour is intended only as a strategy to aid the learner's understanding of a concept or principle.

SPECIAL PURPOSES IN NURSING

- Teaches new procedures either at bedside in a ward or in the nursing laboratory on simulators.

BOX 5.4 ORGANIZATION MATRIX OF A MICRO-TEACHING SESSION

Teacher (Roll No.)	Students (Roll No.)	Supervisor (Roll No.)	Feedback (Roll No.)	Re-plan (Roll No.)
1	3, 4, 5, 6, 7, 8, 9, 10	2	–	–
3	5, 6, 7, 8, 9, 10	4	2 to 1	–
5	2, 7, 8, 9, 10	6	4 to 3	1
7	1, 2, 4, 9, 10	8	6 to 5	3
9	1, 2, 3, 4, 6	10	8 to 7	5
2	3, 4, 6, 5, 8	1	10 to 9	7
4	5, 6, 7, 8, 10	3	1 to 2	9
6	1, 7, 8, 9, 10	5	3 to 4	2
8	1, 2, 3, 9, 10	7	5 to 6	4
10	1, 2, 3, 4, 5	9	7 to 8	6

- Applies the knowledge of underlying scientific principles to nursing care situations.
- Teaches the uses, functioning and care of new equipment.
- Teaches the application of observation techniques and skills to nursing situations.
- Teaches maintenance of health and preventive healthcare measures to patients and family.

II. CHARACTERISTICS OF DEMONSTRATION

- The demonstrator should understand the entire procedure before attempting to perform.
- All equipment needed should be assembled before demonstration.
- A positive approach should be used.
- Knowledge about the procedure should be given to students.
- The setting for a demonstration should be as real to life as possible.

III. COMPONENTS/STEPS TO DEMONSTRATING

The main components and steps of the demonstration method are as follows.

A. BEFORE DEMONSTRATION

- Formulate behavioural objectives.
- Perform skill analysis and determine the sequence.
- Assess entry behaviour of learners and determine prerequisites.
- Formulate the lesson plan for demonstration.

B. DURING DEMONSTRATION

- State the objectives to the learner.
- Motivate learners by explaining why the skill is required.
- Demonstrate the complete skill at a normal speed.
- Demonstrate each partial skill slowly, in the correct sequence.
- Obtain feedback by questioning and observation of nonverbal behaviour.
- Avoid the use of negative examples and variations in technique.

C. AFTER DEMONSTRATION

- Provide immediate supervised practice with adequate time allowance.
- Make the environment psychologically safe by providing a friendly atmosphere and constructive criticism.
- Discuss the points for improvement and provide constructive criticism and feedback.

IV. RESPONSIBILITIES OF TEACHERS AND STUDENTS IN THE DEMONSTRATION METHOD

The detailed responsibilities of teachers and students in the demonstration method may be seen from Box 5.5.

BOX 5.5 RESPONSIBILITIES OF TEACHERS AND STUDENTS IN DEMONSTRATION METHOD

Teacher's responsibilities

- Time demonstration in accordance with student's background of knowledge and readiness for practice of new knowledge.
- Arrange for demonstration to be as similar to the actual situation as possible.
- Provide students with advance information regarding activity to be demonstrated.
- Arrange physical settings for demonstration so all observers feel comfortable and can see the demonstration.
- Explain the purpose of activity, results desired and equipment to be used.
- Proceed with each step of activity in a logical sequence.
- State the scientific principles underlying the steps of an activity.

Student's responsibilities

- Familiarize self with objectives for demonstration.
- Follow the steps being demonstrated along with written information.
- Identify how the activity can be modified to meet the patient's individual needs.
- Ask for clarification of points that were not understood.
- Translate the observation of demonstration into return performance.
- Evaluate self-regarding growth and the areas where help is needed.
- Seek opportunities to build on newly gained knowledge and skills in application to other areas.

ADVANTAGES OF DEMONSTRATION

- It provides an opportunity for observational learning.
- It commands interest by using concrete illustrations. Students can not only hear the explanation but also see the process.
- It has a universal appeal because it is understandable to all.
- It is adaptable to both group and individual teaching.
- Return demonstration by the student under the supervision of the teacher provides the opportunity for well-directed practice before the students use the procedure on the ward.
- Questioning forms an important part of demonstration to get feedback from students about their understanding and assimilation.
- Important points and terms are mentioned on the chalkboard. The chalkboard should be behind the teacher and in front of students.
- It activates several senses and increases learning.
- It correlates theory with practice.
- It has a particular reference to student demonstration of procedures already learned.
- It serves as a strong motivational force for students.
- Student's interest is maintained throughout demonstration.

DISADVANTAGES OF DEMONSTRATION

- Only a small group of students can be included in a demonstration.
- Keeps the students in a passive situation.
- Involves a high cost in terms of personnel and time required.
- Difficulty in repeating demonstrations to acquire competence.

SIMULATION

Simulation is a newer pedagogical approach that has recently got much of popularity because it facilitates to provide the learning experiences in the controlled environment that enhances the patient safety and students' confidence and comfort. Simulation is role-playing where the process of teaching is displayed artificially and an effort to practice some important skills is made. The teacher and students simulate an actual life situation or a person's actual role.

As defined in Wikipedia, 'Simulation is the imitation of the operation of a real-world process or system over time. The act of simulating something first requires that a model be developed; this model represents the key characteristics or behaviors/functions of the selected physical or abstract system or process'.

Simulation as a method of clinical teaching is rapidly recognized as an effective method to supplement and enhance clinical learning in nursing education. Simulation is a method of clinical teaching where real-life clinical scenarios are simulated for leaning and practicing new clinical skills without involving real patients. The level and sophistication of simulation vary from simple skill training model to computerized full body mannequins with all possible control and responses, which are as close to real patients. The emerging research evidence has proven the importance of simulations in nursing education. However, it must be integrated into curriculum in such a way that there is clarity on transition of clinical skill learnt through simulation to the real patients.

Recently, use of simulation in nursing education has increased because of (1) increased awareness about availability and usefulness of simulators in nursing education; (2) shortage of clinical facilities for real patient care experiences for the nursing students; (3) decreasing cost of simulators; (4) increased felt need of patient safety and (5) support of empirical evidences about usefulness of simulators in skill building among nurses.

I. TYPES OF SIMULATORS

Based on the simulator's ability to be realistic as close to the real patient and its ability to simulate the real patient scenario, the simulators may be classified into three broad categories: low fidelity, moderate fidelity and high fidelity. The term fidelity is used for simulator to describe the extent of accuracy of system being used to produce the clinical scenario as close as to the real one.

- ***Low-fidelity simulators:*** The low-fidelity simulators are static, lack the realism, vitality and they just structurally resemble to the actual part or whole body. For example, foam-made intramuscular model or a patient care dummy.
- ***Moderate-fidelity simulator:*** Moderate-fidelity simulators are relatively more complex than low-fidelity simulators, where learner may get feedback from the simulator. They may also provide limited opportunity to experience airway, breathing, chest movements, pulse, breath or heart sounds, etc. but will not be as sophisticated as high-fidelity simulators. An example of this is a feedback-oriented basic life support mannequin.
- ***High-fidelity simulator:*** High-fidelity simulator may produce the most realistic simulated patient experiences. They have the ability to react as close as to real patient, when the students are interacting or practicing the nursing procedures. In addition, nursing faculty also has opportunity to control the different scenarios using remote computer device. They cosmetically also look and give feel of as real as an actual patient. An example of this is advanced level Advanced Cardiac Life Support (ACLS) simulator. The high-fidelity simulators are relatively more expensive than the moderate and low-fidelity simulators. These simulators do have the facility of simultaneous video recording, which is useful in debriefing conference to give feedback to the students.

II. PRINCIPLES OF SIMULATION

- The simulators are representative of the real patients and then make decisions in response to their assessment of the setting they find themselves in.
- The experiences simulated are consequences that relate to their decisions and general performance.
- Monitoring the results of their actions to reflect upon the relationship between their own decisions and the resultant consequences.

III. PURPOSES OF SIMULATION

- Enables the learner to learn directly from simulated experiences which are as close to as real one.
- Promotes a high level of skills and critical thinking.
- Develops in the students an understanding of the problems that may be encountered in real situation and ability of decision-making.
- Enables the individual to empathize with the real-life situations.
- Provides feedback to the learners on the consequences of actions and decision made.
- Motivates the students by making real-life situations exciting and interesting.
- Enables teachers and learners to assess the realism of the situation by uncovering misconceptions.

IV. MODES OF SIMULATION

There are a variety of ways to simulate the clinical environment as discussed below:

- ***Full-body mannequins:*** These simulators physically look like a patient; however, the complexity of full-body simulators varies from just being physically like a patient to be a sophisticated electronically controlled simulator, which has the ability to provide most of the physiological or pathological responses when remotely controlled through computer device.
- ***Part-task trainers:*** The part-task trainers are the models that are primarily used for practising technical nursing skills, for example a gluteal intramuscular injection model or airway trainer model or an intravenous arm. These models are available as a specific part rather than the full body, which make them more cost-effective and easy to handle and store.
- ***Simulated patients:*** They are popularly known as 'patient actors' or 'standardized patients'; they are also called as clinical teaching associates who are especially trained to behave like a particular patient to create an artificial clinical scenario. They are especially used for the situations that are sensitive in nature or require a real individual vital signs monitoring, physical examination, breast examination, etc.
- ***Computer-generated simulators:*** The computer-generated simulators may be as simple as a computer program, which demonstrates the steps of equipment functioning, for example a mechanical ventilator. They may be as complex as a three-dimensional virtual clinical environment, where student gets an opportunity to virtually interact with virtual patient and healthcare team.
- ***Hybrid simulators:*** They are the combination of standardized patient and the part-task trainer to make clinical learning more real. For example, a gravid uterus is worn by a simulated or standardized patient, where students may have more close to realist experience of the clinical skills, communication skills and professional behaviour. The specific electronic devices, such as a modified stethoscope, may be used to create the desired physiological or pathological responses such as adventitious respiratory sounds or abnormal heart sounds.

ADVANTAGES OF SIMULATION

- Simulation establishes a setting where theory and practice can be combined.
- Simulation requires the teacher to be an active participant in the process.
- Patient safety can be ensured. The decisions are made and carried out without physical or psychological harm to real patients.
- It is possible to have a very good control over clinical teaching environment.
- Simulation is a teaching technique that motivates and involves students. It changes teacher behaviour and introduces novelty in the whole learning process. The level of freshness and novelty is maintained throughout the learning session.
- Students are not expected to identify the group time and follow it. Every student is expected to have experiences that are different from the usual laboratory type experiences common to all.
- It stimulates the students for the acquisition of purposeful activities and they feel keenly interested.
- It removes the student–teacher polarization. Simulations are self-monitoring. Participants recognize their aim progress by various feedback methods. Students are involved in decision-making. They observe their own evaluation of these consequences, which influence their future actions. Personal tensions in the teaching situation are likely to be reduced by the process of self-monitoring. The teacher's role may be as an interpreter of the simulation and as a guide, but he does not have to pose as an expert or as a judge.
- It develops decision-making skills into action. It develops various skills in students in an increasing order or difficulty.
- It provides an integrated view and is a vehicle for free interdisciplinary communication.
- It provides dynamic framework.
- Simulation works to bridge the gap between unreal and real. Students enact real situations and learning becomes more interesting and lively than purely theoretical.

DISADVANTAGES OF SIMULATION

- It is not possible to simulate each and every scenario in all subjects of the curriculum.
- Inadequately designed simulated scenario may convey the unintended message to the learners.
- Simulators may not provide some of the realistic clinical presentations, such as sweating, skin colours, which lead to the habit of ignoring these presentations in real-life situations.
- In simulations, generally, shortcuts are used, such as not obtaining consent, using safety precautions, lack of complete communication, use of opened IV fluid, expired drugs and not wearing gloves, leading to a habit of unsafe behaviour/practice in real-life clinical settings.
- It is also a problem in simulation that students get habitual of artificial communication rather than realistic communication skills.
- Simulation cannot be conveniently used in the case of isolated simpler tasks because mechanism is too difficult for them to follow.
- It requires a lot of preparation on the part of teachers; very few teachers are prepared to take up the extra work which is required to make this technique as a success.
- Learning is a serious activity which is highly individualized and needs concentration on the part of the learner. Simulation reduces the seriousness of learning.
- It has difficulty in using analytic approach.
- Many simulators are needed sometimes, which may not be practically possible sometimes.

SYMPOSIUM

Symposium technique is a type of discussion where two or more speakers talk for 10–20 minutes, develop individual approaches or solutions to a problem or present aspects of a policy, process or programme. This is a technique of higher learning. It is an instructional technique that is used to achieve higher cognitive and effective objectives.

This technique is also an essential method of teaching and learning. It is useful to achieve high cognitive and effective functioning. This method helps to make a decision about a particular problem or solve the problem. It can help all the students improve their learning skills.

The word *symposium* has several dictionary meanings. Plato used this term for *good dialogue* to present views towards God. Another meaning of the term is intellectual recreation or enjoyment. The main purpose of a symposium is to provide an understanding to students or listeners on the theme or problem specifically to develop certain values and feelings.

Symposium is defined as a teaching technique that serves as an excellent method for informing the audiences, crystallizing their opinion and preparing them for arriving at decision regarding a particular issue or a topic.

I. PURPOSES OF SYMPOSIUM

- To identify and understand various aspects of the theme and problems.
- To develop the ability to come to a decision and provide judgement regarding a problem.
- To develop values and feelings regarding a problem.
- To enable the listeners form policies regarding a theme or problem.
- To provide understanding to the students or listeners on a theme or problem to specifically develop certain values and feelings.
- To investigate a problem from several points of view.
- To boost students' abilities to speak in the group.
- To encourage the students to study independently.

II. CHARACTERISTICS OF SYMPOSIUM

- It provides broad understanding of a topic or problem.
- The listener is provided with an opportunity to take decisions about a problem.
- It is used in higher classes for specific themes and problems.
- It develops feelings of cooperation and adjustment.
- The objectives of synthesis and evaluation are achieved by employing the symposium technique.
- It provides different views on the topic of the symposium.

III. PRINCIPLES OF SYMPOSIUM

- The speeches may be persuasive, argumentative and informative.
- Original presentation is objective and accurate.
- Summary to be always included at conclusion.
- Each speech proceeds without interruption.

- The chairman of the symposium introduces the topic, suggests its importance and sometimes indicates the general approaches.
- All members of the symposium performing group can sit in a straight line behind the table, or in adjoining chairs with the chairman in the middle or to one side of the speakers.
- The symposium presents two conflicting points of view, the reading arrangement can separate the speakers on the platform to indicate differences in opinion or to preserve peace.

IV. GUIDELINES FOR CONDUCTING SYMPOSIUM

- All members of the performing group can sit in a straight line behind a table or in adjoining chairs with the chairman in the middle or to one side of the speakers.
- The chairman of the symposium introduces the topic and suggests something of its importance.
- Two or more speakers talk from 10 to 20 minutes. The speech may be persuasive, argumentative, informative or evocative. Each speech proceeds without interruption.
- The speeches are followed by questions or comments from the audience as in the panel form.

ADVANTAGES OF SYMPOSIUM

- It is suited to a large group or classes.
- This method can be frequently used to present broad topics for discussion at conventions and organization of meetings.
- Organization is good as speeches are prepared beforehand.
- It gives deeper insight into the topic.
- It directs the students to continuous independent study.
- This method can be used in political meetings.

DISADVANTAGES OF SYMPOSIUM

- It provides inadequate opportunity for all students to participate actively.
- The speech is limited to 15–20 minutes.
- It has limited audience participation.
- Questions and answers limited to only 3–4 minutes.
- It has possibility of overlapping of subjects.
- The chairman has no control over the speakers as they have full freedom to prepare the theme for discussion. They can present any aspect of the theme or problem.
- There is a probability of repetition of content. The different aspects of the theme are not prepared separately. It creates difficulty of understanding for the listeners.
- The different aspects of the theme are not presented simultaneously. Therefore, the listeners are not able to understand the theme correctly.
- The listeners remain passive in the symposium because they are not given an opportunity to seek clarification and put questions in between the symposium.

PANEL DISCUSSION

All techniques of higher learning require discussion among the participants. The discussion provides equal opportunities in the instructional situation to every participant. This technique was used by Harry

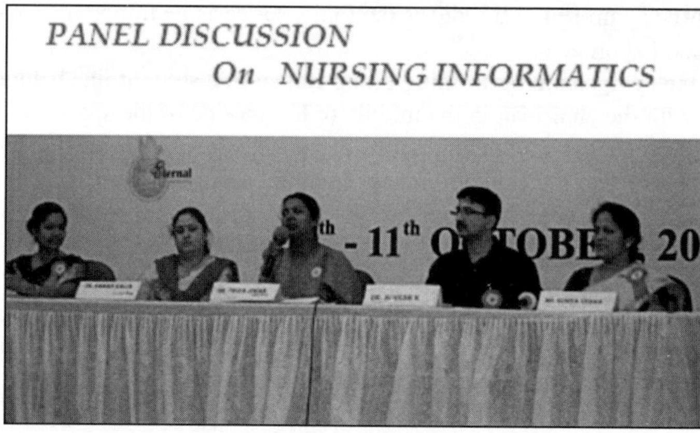

Figure 5.7

Panel discussion on nursing informatics.

A. Ober Street for the first time in 1929. The purpose of the panel is to make use of a small group discussion for the benefit of a large group. Fig. 5.7 depicts a panel discussion in process on the topic of nursing informatics where a group of nursing experts in the presence of a moderator/chairperson are carrying out the discussion in front of a large group of audience.

> *Panel is a discussion in which a few persons carry out a conversation in front of an audience.*
>
> *The panel discussion is a method of teaching in which four to six or eight persons or students discuss the assigned topic/issue/problem creatively among themselves in front of an audience which may be too large.*

I. PURPOSES OF PANEL DISCUSSION

- To provide information and new facts.
- To analyse the current problem from different angles.
- To identify the values.
- To organize for mental recreation.
- To influence the audience to an open-minded attitude and respect for other's opinion.
- When handled intelligently and creatively, the panel discussion stimulates thought and discussion and clarifies thinking.

II. TYPES OF PANEL DISCUSSION

A. PUBLIC PANEL DISCUSSION

This type of panel discussion is organized for the common-man problems. Generally, the public panel discussion is organized through television programmes. The main objectives achieved by this type of panel discussion are:

- To provide factual information regarding current problems.
- To determine social values.
- To recreate the common man.

B. EDUCATIONAL PANEL DISCUSSION

It is used in educational institutes to provide factual and conceptual knowledge and clarification of certain theories and principles. The main objectives achieved through this type of panel discussion are:

- To provide factual and conceptual knowledge.
- To raise awareness of theories and principles.
- To provide solutions for certain problems.

III. GUIDELINES FOR CONDUCTING PANEL DISCUSSION

The following guidelines must be kept in mind while organizing and conducting panel discussions:

- Identify or help participants identify an issue or topic that involves an important conflict in values and interests. The issue or topic may be set forth as a topical question, a hypothetical incident, a student experience or an actual case.
- Select panellists who are well informed and have specific points of view regarding the issue or topic. A panel discussion that includes 3–5 panellists is usually most workable.
- Select a leader or chairperson/moderator of the panel discussion.
- Decide on the format of the panel discussion.
- There should be a rehearsal before the actual panel discussion.

IV. ORGANIZING THE PANEL DISCUSSION

- The panel discussion consists of the chairperson/moderator, the panellists and the audience.
- The panel consists of 4–8 panellists along with a chairperson or moderator seated in a semicircle facing the audience. The chairman or moderator is generally seated in the middle of the panellists.
- The chairperson or moderator should be selected carefully because success of the panel depends on his/her leadership.
- The chairperson must keep the discussion to the subject and see that all members of the panel get an equal opportunity to express their views.
- Further, the chairperson should act as a neutral referee and begin the panel discussion by exploring the whole proceedings.
- The members of the panel are first introduced by name and background of experience. The topic is announced and the limit of discussion is stated.
- The chairperson may start the procedure rolling by making a comment or by directing a question to a particular person.
- The panel discussion should provide a natural setting in which the audience will have the opportunity to ask questions, evaluate replies and make constructive contributions.
- The chairperson coordinates the discussion and makes sure the discussion is carried on in a conversational way.
- The chairperson clarifies an issue or misconception and may also introduce another thought so that the subject is fully covered. Then he/she summarizes the main points presented by the speakers and invites the audience to contribute and ask questions.
- Finally the chairperson sums up the discussion.

ADVANTAGES OF PANEL DISCUSSION

- Different points of views on the subject are presented by experts.
- The quick exchange of facts, opinions, etc. helps develop critical attitude and better judgement.
- Students learn to discuss a topic in conversational form in a small group in front of a large group.

DISADVANTAGES OF PANEL DISCUSSION

- It requires more time for planning, organizing and presentation.
- The discussion may be vague and superficial if the panel members lack mastery.
- The effectiveness of the method depends on:
  - The competency and preparation of the panel members.
  - The competency and leading abilities of the chairperson.
  - Planning, organizing and conducting the panel discussion.

SEMINAR

Seminar is a controlled type of discussion. It is a method of teaching where the student's ability to solve problems is increased by way of rational thinking and reasoning. It can be a motivating strategy in nursing, where a learner presents a paper on some aspects of nursing and then participates in a discussion with the group. A seminar can be used in all fields, particularly in colleges or schools to supplement the student learning after they have acquired specific information and experience.

In general, the seminar consists of a scientific approach to the study of a selected problem. It involves a discussion of the problem using a small group of students and a teacher who is an expert in the field of study. The seminar differs from other group discussion methods because of its specific features, that is in-depth library research and literature review on presenting problem, systematic writing of seminar report under guidance of teacher or expert and presentation of the report, followed by discussion of the report by the group participants for further analysis, evaluation and drawing conclusions and recommendations. The best distinct feature of the seminar is expert or teacher's significant contribution in planning, presentation and evaluation of teaching–learning activity. A seminar may be a single problem for study by the total group, a problem shared by several group members or individual subproblems studied by each member and presented as part of the total problem. The nature of the seminar method usually requires a series of sessions for completion of study of the problem.

Seminar is one of the techniques of discussion for small groups, a small group is one in which face to face relationship among participants is there.

Seminars are simply a group of people coming together for the discussion and learning of specific techniques and topics. Usually there are several keynote speakers within each seminar, and these speakers are usually experts in their own fields or topics.

I. SEMINAR AS A METHOD OF TEACHING

- Seminar is a form of a class organization that utilizes a scientific approach for the analysis of a problem chosen for discussion.
- It is an organized, guided discussion with a focus on the discovery of new relationships by the participating individuals. It differs from intellectual initiative. The student's role is active in contrast to the relatively passive role assumed in a lecture.

- The objective of a seminar is to give students the opportunity to participate in methods of scientific analysis and research procedures. Students are expected to do considerable library research and when feasible obtain primary sources of data.
- A seminar group is mainly concerned with academic matters rather than individual students and commonly involves the reading of an essay or paper by one group member followed by a discussion by the total group on the topic.
- It is a discussion method of teaching where an informal group of 10–15 students (not more than 25) participate to solve problems in a scientific approach and analysis. Generally, the duration of a seminar should not be more than 1–2 hours.
- This method gives students the opportunity to participate in methods of scientific analysis and research procedures.
- Students are expected to do considerable library research, and if feasible, obtain primary sources of data. Data are analysed, critically evaluated and conclusion reached under the directions of the teacher.
- The teacher should help the students select, formulate and resolve the most significant student problems and suggest the available sources of information.
- As the seminar progresses, the students assume increased responsibilities for preparing the problems and conducting the discussion.

II. CHARACTERISTICS OF THE SEMINAR

- Teacher is the leader (students can also function as leaders in certain selected situations).
- The group generally consists of 10–15 participants.
- An ideal seminar lasts for 1–2 hours. The topic is initially presented by the presenter followed by group discussion.
- The leader should keep the discussion within limits so the focus of discussion can be mentioned.
- In student seminars, students present their data in an informal way under the leadership of the teacher, followed by a teacher-monitored discussion.
- Care should be taken to avoid stereotypes.
- All members take part in discussion in an informal but orderly manner.
- The chairman should be skilled in encouraging timid participants.
- A student secretary may record the problems that came up and the solutions given to them.

III. ORGANIZING A SEMINAR

The establishment of an environment that contributes to the purpose of the seminar is very important and requires a skilled teacher. A motivating learning situation that is not too highly organized or too relaxed is essential. The teacher usually guides the seminar; however, students may carry out this function under the guidance of a teacher. The teacher may decide to be the leader or may delegate leadership to the group.

The basic guidelines for organizing a seminar are:

- To define the purpose of the seminar.
- To relate the topic of seminar and discussion to the main concept or the objectives to be attained.
- To direct and focus the discussion on the topic.
- To help students express their ideas.
- To keep the discussion at a high level of interest so that the students listen attentively to those contributing ideas.

- To plan comments and questions that relate to the subject and also help guide the discussion.
- To set time limitations for each person's contribution.
- To guard against monopoly of the discussion by any member of the seminar.
- To plan for a summary at intervals during the discussion and also at the end and relate the ideas expressed to the purpose of discussion.
- To have the discussion recorded either by a student as a recording secretary or by tape recording.
- To plan for teacher and student self-evaluation of the progress made towards the immediate objectives.

IV. ROLE OF TEACHER IN THE SEMINAR

- Select the topic (giving reasonable time for preparation).
- Remain in the background at the seminar but sit where the whole group can be seen.
- Prepare to help out in the initial stages of using this method in case of long silences.
- See that no essential points are overlooked and that gross inaccuracies are corrected (preferably by another member of the class).
- See that all members have a share in the discussion and that irrelevant discussion is avoided.

ADVANTAGES OF SEMINAR

- Role of the student is active; it presupposes that the student has background knowledge.
- If properly conducted, the seminar teaches the method of scientific analysis and techniques of research.
- The group as a whole and individual students try to solve problems.
- Exchange of facts and attempts to crystallize group opinion that is sound and workable.
- By participation in the solution of problems, the students develop problem-solving skills.
- By participation in the solution of problems, the students becomes more articulate and develop a more critical point of view and a more organized, scientific approach towards the issue.
- A seminar helps in self-learning and promotes independent thinking.
- Ability to see and solve our own problems is increased because personal difficulties can be compared to those of the group.
- Skilfully directed, the seminar promotes group spirit and cooperativeness.

DISADVANTAGES OF SEMINAR

- It is quite a time-consuming process.
- It cannot be applied to new students.
- Timid students cannot improve.
- If subject knowledge is poor, unnecessary discussions arise.
- The approach to problems extends to students' professional and personal activities.

SCIENTIFIC WORKSHOP

The word *workshop* is related to any area that provides both space and tools required for the manufacture and repair of goods. Similarly, in educational workshops, experts provide knowledge and skills to deal with problems. It is a teaching method organized to develop the psychomotor aspects of the learner regarding the practices of new innovations in education, where persons are trained to use new practices in their teaching–learning process.

> *Workshop is a meeting during which experienced people in responsible positions come together with experts and consultants to find solutions for the problems that cropped up in the course of their work and they have had difficulty in dealing with on their own. It is a large group discussion method.*

> *Workshop is defined as assembled group of 10–25 persons who share a common interest or problem. They meet together to improve their individual skill of a subject through intensive study, research, practice and discussion.*

I. ESSENTIAL FEATURES OF WORKSHOP

- Complete active involvement by the participants.
- The whole point of attention is to work and learn from practical experiences.
- Participants may have to work as reporters or a leader.
- Workshop offers each member an opportunity to make his own contribution.

II. PRINCIPLES OF WORKSHOP

- Allowing the participants to prepare and select objectives to be reached will increase the participant's motivation.
- Giving the participant an active role will make teaching more effective.
- Improve a person's attitude towards other people.
- Learn better human relations.
- Every individual has worth and contributes to the common goals.
- Cooperation is a technique and a way of life that is superior to competition and is a primary factor to be allowed.

III. OBJECTIVES OF THE WORKSHOP

An educational process has two aspects: *theoretical and practical.* The objective of a workshop is to achieve higher cognitive objectives and develop psychomotor skills (Box 5.6).

BOX 5.6 OBJECTIVES OF THE WORKSHOP

Cognitive Objectives

- To learn the new innovations and practices of education.
- To solve problems in the area of teaching education.
- To provide a broad understanding of a topic and theme.
- To provide a rationalized and philosophical background for instructional and teaching situation.

Psychomotor Objectives

- To put people in a situation where they will evaluate their own efforts.
- To develop the proficiency for planning and organizing teaching and instructional activities.
- To provide an opportunity for personal growth through accepting and working towards a goal held in common with others.

IV. PREPARATION OF A WORKSHOP

The success of a workshop will depend largely on the way it is planned and on the arrangements made before the opening session. The following activities have to be carried out (Fig. 5.8):

- ***Opening a file:*** A suitable system might be a loose leaf with the following subdivisions: budget, workshop sitting arrangements, selection of participants, documentation and equipment checklist, publicity press and evaluation.
- ***Formulation of aims and objectives:*** Aims and objectives of the workshop should be formulated for the participants as well as the organizers. At the first stage of the workshop, theoretical aspects are discussed by experts on the theme of the workshop.
- ***Arrangement of funds:*** The whole programme and schedule is prepared by the organizer. He has to arrange for the funds needed for boarding and lodging facilities for participants as well as experts.
- ***Choosing the date and place:*** For the first day of the workshop, a nonworking day is usually selected. Ensure that at least one working day precedes the opening of the workshop. While selecting a place, it should be kept in mind that the place should enable the participants to take part in all activities without interruption.
- ***Identifying the experts or resource persons:*** In organizing a workshop, resource persons play an important role in providing theoretical and practical aspects of the theme. They provide guidance to participants at every stage and train them to perform the task effectively.
- ***Selection of participants:*** The participants should be keen or interested in the theme of the workshop. Number of participants, type of participants and voluntary participation should be specified.
- ***Identifying the sponsors:*** People in administrative positions should be represented as committees that will be called on to apply the selection criteria defined earlier.
- ***Working language:*** The workshop is usually carried out in a national language or preferred one.
- ***Invitation to the participants:*** A personal letter should be sent to the participants selected with the following points:
  - Aims of the workshop
  - What is implied by the workshop
  - Working methods of the workshop
  - Theme of the workshop

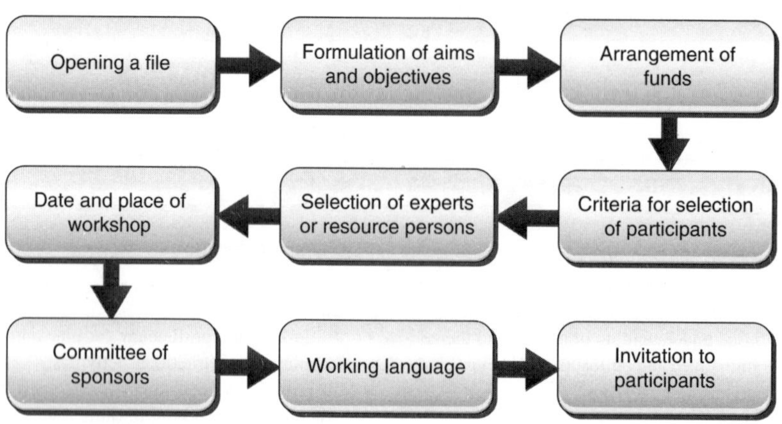

Figure 5.8

Steps in preparation of a workshop.

V. OUTCOMES OF THE WORKSHOP

- Widening specified knowledge
- Professional and personal growth
- Friendships, team spirit and human relations

EXHIBITION

Many times in the school, a department of the school or a class puts up their work for showing it to people outside the school and such a show is called *exhibition*. The pieces of work done by students for an exhibition are called *exhibit*.

I. BASIC CHARACTERISTICS OF EXHIBITION

- The exhibition should have a central theme with a few subthemes to focus attention on a particular concept.
- The exhibits should be clean and properly labelled.
- The concepts of contrast in colour and size should be used for laying out the exhibitions.
- The exhibits should be placed so that most visitors can see them.
- The place and exhibits should be well lighted.
- Both motion and sound should be utilized to capture the attention and interest of visitors.
- The exhibition should have some exhibits with operative mechanisms such as switches and handles to be operated by visitors.
- The exhibition should include a lot of demonstrations as they involve the students and the visitors deeply.
- The exhibition should be able to relate various subject areas to provide integrated learning.

ADVANTAGES OF EXHIBITION

- Exhibitions inspire the students to learn by doing things themselves and get a sense of involvement.
- They give students a sense of accomplishment and achievement.
- They develop social skills of communication, cooperation and coordination.
- They foster better school community relations and make community members conscious about the school.
- They couple information with pleasure.
- They foster creativity in students.

DISADVANTAGES OF EXHIBITION

- It requires thorough preparation.
- It is a time-consuming process.
- It requires a large amount of funds or budget.

ROLE-PLAY

Role-playing is the spontaneous acting out of a clearly defined situation by two or more persons for subsequent discussion by the whole class. Role-playing is a teaching method where a group of participants act out the assigned role to deliver the content of topic to be taught to the participants. In a role-playing group, the members play the assigned role the way they think the character would act in reality which helps in arousing feelings and elicit emotional responses in learners where cognitive and affective domain learning may be achieved.

According to Karen S. Kesten, role-plays using the SBAR (**S**ituation, **B**ackground, **A**ssessment and **R**ecommendation) technique are helpful to improve observed communication skills in senior nursing students. Skilled communication and respectful interaction between the healthcare team members are critical to achieve optimization of quality patient care outcomes. Patients in the care of clinically expert professionals suffer medical errors with alarming frequency. The Joint Commission on National Patient Safety Goals strives to improve the effectiveness of communication in caregivers by recommending the implementation of standardized tools known as SBAR. The findings suggest that role-play may have a place in teaching communication skills in nursing schools as well as continuing education and training in hospitals and other healthcare settings. Interdisciplinary communication training may provide even more effective learning.

Role-playing is an educational method in which people spontaneously act out problems of human relations and analyze the enactment with the help of other role players and observers.

Role-playing is a discussion technique that makes it possible to get maximum participation of a group through acting out an example of some problem or idea under discussion.

Role-play is a spontaneous acting out of roles in the context of human situations. It is a part of two broad methods: sociodrama and psychodrama. Both sociodrama and psychodrama require not only players but also an audience that helps the players interpret their roles.

Sociodrama: It deals with the interactions of people with other individuals or groups like mother, nurse and leader. It always involves situations of more than one person and deals with problems related to a majority of the group.

Psychodrama: It is practised in a group setting, mainly concerned with the unique needs and problems of a particular individual. It should not be attempted except under the guidance of a trained therapist. The audience identifying with roles in a role-playing or critical observation brings about much greater learning than simply passive watching.

I. PURPOSES OF ROLE-PLAY

- To present interpersonal problems.
- To provide emotional and affective stimulus for solving problems.
- To provide awareness about social and psychological issues.
- To develop a situation for an analysis.
- To prevent alternative courses of action.
- To prepare for meeting future situations.
- To develop an understanding of others points of view.
- To convey information to develop specific skills.

II. PRINCIPLES OF ROLE-PLAY

- As a teaching technique, role-play is based on the philosophy that meanings are in people and not in words or symbols. If the philosophy is accurate, we must first of all share the meanings, then clarify our understanding of each other's meanings, and finally, if necessary, change our meanings.
- In the language of phenomenological psychology, this has to do with changing the self-concept. The self-concept is best changed through direct involvement in a realistic and life-related problem situation rather than through hearing about such situations from others.
- Creating teaching situations that can lead to change of self-concept requires a distinct organizational pattern.
- It should be flexible.
- It should be a stimulant to think and should not be an escape from the discipline of learning.
- There is no single best method of selecting the characters; the group may do the assigning.
- It requires rehearsal as an important feature to produce effective outcome and for audience to help players interpret their roles.
- It should be done for a brief period so that the attention of audience may be captured effectively.
- Enough time should be allowed for discussion and analysis of the situation.
- It evaluates the teacher and participants through discussion or follow-up as to specific individual behaviour or sequence of group actions.

III. STEPS IN ROLE-PLAY

The following main steps must be followed while carrying out a role-play.

A. PLANNING PHASE

During this phase, the following components must be ensured:

- *Select a problem for role-play*
    - The group leader recognizes a problem that can be used effectively and suggests it to the group.
    - The group can list problems on the blackboard and decide which problem they want to work out.
- *Set up the role-play scene*
    - The group should come to a clear agreement on the chief objectives to be realized in role planning.
    - The group working with the leader must determine:
        - What characters are to be involved.
        - The attitudes and personality of the characters.
        - The setting of the story.
        - The point at which the story should begin.
    - The leader may brief the players on the situation they have decided they want to portray. The leader may arbitrarily assign individuals to take the various roles or members may volunteer to play the different roles.
- *Getting underway in role-play*
    - The role takers usually go out of the room and are given a few minutes to warm up or to get a feeling of the roles they are about to play. Specific names, other than their own, should be used to help them get into their roles.

   - The role-players should attempt to express the attitudes the group has assigned to the various characters as well as achieve the goals decided upon.
   - The story grows out of natural reactions of the characters enacted in role-playing.
   - Those members not involved in the actual role-playing act as observers. They may be assigned to watch particular role-players or to look for important clues that come out of role-playing.
- *Cutting the content and making role-play comprehensive*
   - The leader may cut at a point where enough action has already occurred to provide a basis for discussion.
   - The leader may get immediate reaction of role-players. How they felt in their roles and how they responded to other responses in the scene.
   - The leader may use the role name of each person in the discussion so that the player does not feel he is being evaluated.
   - When role-players succeed in really projecting themselves into the roles assigned to them, they usually give valuable insight into the problem and provide additional material for discussion.

B. IMPLEMENTATION AND EVALUATION PHASE

The role-play is carried out to convey particular content to the audience and discussion is stimulated.

- *The audience observers*
   - The comments of the audience observers constitute the heart of role-playing as a discussion technique. It may consider:
      - How did the group think the role was handled?
      - What were the good points of the action?
      - What were the poor points or omissions?
- *Role-playing observers*
   - This might be played by different people so that there might be a comparison of the behaviours of different people.
- *Summarize phase*
   - The leader sums up to the group chief points or principles which have come out in role-playing and the comments of the observers that follow.
   - The comments on specific problems should be taken under consideration.
- *Cautions in use of role-playing*
   - Use role-play only when it will be useful and not just for the sake of doing it.
   - Be careful about interpersonal relationships within the group.
   - If there is a popular role, give it to a person with enough status in the group to carry it successfully. If necessary, the leader might play it to spare the feelings of others.
   - Avoid uncovering deep seated personal problems that require professional help.

ADVANTAGES OF ROLE-PLAY

- Develop real communication skills in leadership, interviewing and social interaction and obtain constructive feedback from peers. For example, learning how to put another case, how to listen, how to lead a discussion and how to be a member of the team responsible for patient care.
- Develop sensitivity to another's feelings by having the opportunity to put oneself in another's place, by noting there is a difference between what a person says and what a person does and develop empathy and understanding.

- Develop skills in group problem solving. For example, the group works as a whole to develop concerns for the group, develop the situation, identify critical issues and come to some mutual agreement.
- Develop an ability to observe and analyse situations. For example, discussion following role planning provides the opportunity to identify critical issues, suggest alternatives to deal with a situation and to appraise the actor's concept of role.
- Practice selected behaviours in a real-life situation without the stress of making a mistake. A person is more appropriate to permit true feelings to be expressed when it is a safe role. For example, the student is exposed to reaching to and having others react to her pointing up strengths and weakness with dramatic impact retained, but she is working with others in a similar situation.
- In a teaching–learning situation, role-play provides the opportunity to:
  - Note individual student needs by observing and analysing student needs in a simulated real-life situation.
  - Assist the students in meeting their own needs by either giving them or encouraging group members to give them on the spot suggestions.
  - Encourage independent thinking and action by stepping aside or giving indirect guidance as emphasis is on the students helping themselves.

DISADVANTAGES OF ROLE-PLAY

- Role-playing is a means, not an end.
- It requires expert guidance and leadership.
- Participants may sometimes feel threatened.
- It is used as an education technique, not as a therapeutic one, strongly dependent on student's imagination.
- It is time-consuming in developing group readiness, should not be used when time constraints are present.
- It is limited only by the teacher's ingenuity and realistic use.

PROJECT METHOD

The project method has been recognized as a teaching technique since many years; it has its primary inception in the field of agriculture sciences where students carried out some planned creative activities in a natural environment or a planned work field to produce certain products. Later it was used in vocational education programmes. The essential characteristics of the project method are planned activity of the individual and production of tangible results.

This method is a teaching method where students learn to work individually or in a group to achieve preplanned learning objectives. William H. Kilpatrick viewed the project method as a vivid educational activity where several types of learning activities included enhancing the learning over already learned behaviour or knowledge. He also emphasized on the importance of the learner's activity and attitude while working in an environment rather than just considering the educational objectives to be achieved. Therefore, true creative thinking and true mental activity is essential to the project method and ultimately there will be a production of some physical or mental products and acquisition of the ability to handle real-life problems.

- According to Prof. Ballard, 'a project is a bit of real life that has been imparted into the school, further in project method, learning by living; this life has spontaneity, purpose, significance and interest, freedom'.

- According to William Kilpatrick, 'project method is a whole-hearted, purposeful activity proceeding in a social environment'.
- According to Stevenson, 'a project method is a problematic act carried to completion in its natural setting'.
- Stevenson also mentioned that to be a project method, the learning activity must be:
  - Problematic in nature.
  - Aimed at a definite, attainable goal.
  - Purposeful, natural and lifelike in its procedure to attain the goal.
  - Directed and planned by the student.
  - Practical in nature with an emphasis on a single, resulting in a concrete achievement. The undertaking must be complete in itself and the goal must be definite and objectively measurable.
- Project method involves all types of mental and manipulative activities according to the purpose and objectives by which the learning activities are unified and shaped.

I. CHARACTERISTICS OF A GOOD PROJECT METHOD

- The method aims at teaching the learner to get the best out of life.
- An attempt to use experience, trust and the best master whose lessons are unforgettable.
- The project method gives an opportunity for self-expression.
- The experiments of the project method want to reset the whole curriculum and break all barriers of the subject matter.
- The project matter proposes the whole sequence of activities involved in complete understanding.
- A project can be a large unit of appreciational learning or of attitude development that increases motor skills and technical knowledge.
- A project is a play activity and learners are engaged in carrying out the activity.
- The project method is a complete surrender to the learner's point of view.
- In the project method, the procedure of the school is liable to be determined by the technique of a workshop because the individual learns much better from his own activity than by constant instruction.
- An attempt is made to establish a positive relation with life.
- The project method lends itself naturally to group work.
- It is a large unit plan of teaching.
- The method seeks to have individuals see and understand life in its unity.

II. TYPES OF PROJECTS

According to William Kilpatrick, project method is classified in the following four categories (Fig. 5.9):

- ***Projector type:*** Projects where students are getting to something like building a house or a garden or planning to execute a model of a textile factory are called *projector type projects*.
- ***Consumer type:*** Projects where students set and enjoy the direct experience with their future expected consumers. *For example*, a master level community health nursing student may be given a consumer type

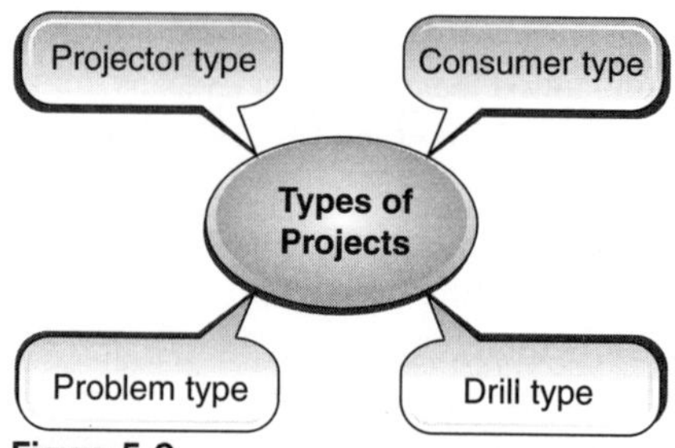

Figure 5.9

Types of projects used as a teaching method.

project to carry out the home visits and make the assessment of most common primary health problems of elderly residing in urban communities and suggest the best possible solution for the identified problems based on locally available resources. In such a project, nursing student will get direct experience and will enjoy working with his future expected consumers of his services.
- ***Problem type:*** Projects where a solution to a problem is to be found out.
- ***Drill type:*** The drill type projects involve an activity that aims at acquiring greater skill. *For example*, a nursing student may be given a project to obtain competency skills in specific nursing procedures such as mouth care, back care, enema administration, intramuscular injection, suctioning and so on.

III. ESSENTIALS OF A GOOD PROJECT

- The project should stress present and future values and experiences that supplement and extend rather than duplicate learning acquired outside the school.
- The projects must have a bearing on a great number of subjects and the knowledge acquired through it may be applied in a variety of ways.
- The project should be timely.
- The project should be challenging.
- The project should be feasible.

IV. ORGANIZING A PROJECT

- The teacher must exercise guidance in the selection of a project.
- Whole-hearted acceptance of the project, almost every student must be secured if the teacher wants to ensure its success.
- Good planning should be done by the students beforehand. It may be in the form of a drawing or a list of steps to be followed, materials to be used, a picture to be prepared or other specific indications of what is to be done.
- The project is an activity to accomplish certain purposes.
- Sufficient preparations must be made to avoid interruptions and delays later.
- During the execution of the project, the teacher should carefully supervise the students in manipulative skills to prevent a waste of materials and to guard against accidents.
- The relation between chalked-out plans and the developing project should be constantly checked.
- The evaluation of a project should be done by both—the students and the teacher.

V. THE ROLE OF TEACHER IN THE PROJECT METHOD

- The teacher has to skilfully guide in the selection.
- The student has to be given help when required.
- The teacher should be good prompter.
- The relations of the teacher and students should be much closer and informal than in ordinary classroom teaching.
- The teacher is like a friend with rich and mature experience.
- The teacher acts as a director, that is the teacher's psychological knowledge must be thorough and specific.

- The teacher must be a keen observer and a true sympathizer.
- The teacher should be a store house of information and knowledge.

ADVANTAGES OF THE PROJECT METHOD

- It follows the psychological laws of learning:
  - Law of readiness.
  - Law of exercise.
  - Law of effect.
- It gives freedom to the students.
- It suited to the psychological concept of maturation.
- It drives social values.
- It trains for social adjustments.
- It saves children from insincerity and superficiality.
- It trains for a democratic way of life.
- It promotes learning through practical problem solving.
- It helps the students and teachers grow. The student stimulated by and encouraged in his exploration of many materials will ultimately approach other areas of learning in a similar manner. The teacher will grow in his or her understanding of a child's creative developments.
- It confers on school work a much needed sense of reality.
- It sets up an intrinsic standard of evaluation.
- It leads to satisfaction of completing the whole task.
- It is economical; the students take more interest and learn in the shortest possible time.
- It is ideal for science work, handicrafts and practical geography and dramatic work literature.

DISADVANTAGES OF THE PROJECT METHOD

- The role of communication is subordinated to the glorification of active learning.
- The practical difficulties of covering a syllabus rule out the project method as the basis of teaching in most schools.
- It is time-consuming and limited by availability and cost of materials.
- It is most valuable in students with lesser academic interest, for it provides an opportunity for the practical enthusiast.
- It leaves gaps in student knowledge.
- It may be too ambitious: beyond a student's capacity.
- Opportunity for the correlation with the academic subjects is extremely limited.
- In this method instructions are more planned; therefore, it may disturb the regular instructional schedule.
- It involves difficulty to ensure any kind of systematic progress in instructions.
- A complete reorganization of the school is needed for a new teacher.
- Children may ignore maxims, working from simple to complex.
- Time-bound projects are introduced artificially and may require more than necessary help.
- Projects may be adopted or abandoned at will.
- The project approach often results in an incomplete mastery of the tools of learning, which are essential to student education later.

FIELD TRIP

An educational trip is defined as an educational procedure by which the students obtain first-hand information by observing places, objects, phenomena and processes in their natural setting to further learning.

I. PURPOSES OF FIELD TRIP

The main purposes of the field trip are:

- To provide real-life situations for first-hand information.
- To supplement classroom instruction, to secure definite information for a specific lesson.
- To serve as a preview of a lesson and gather instructional material.
- To verify previous information, class discussion and conclusion of individual experiments.
- To create situational teaching for cultivating observation, keenness and discovery.
- To serve as a means to develop positive attitudes, values and specific skills.

II. GUIDELINES FOR USING FIELD TRIP AS A TEACHING METHOD

- The field trip must be planned to meet specific educational objectives rather than merely a picnic activity.
- Plan the field trip with a specific checklist such as prior permissions, arrangement of transpiration, booking boarding facility, parental notification and safety and emergency arrangements.
- Plan a schedule and route plan for the field trip. Further, identify a main leader of the group and subleaders of the small groups.
- Assign different responsibilities to different individuals and make every individual understand the overall schedule and route plan of the field trip.
- Have a list of all the candidates, contact numbers of the people in case of an emergency or special needs.
- During a field trip, individuals must be provided with opportunities to achieve educational objectives of the field trip.
- Post the field trip, a review and presentation along with a report must be made to the institutional head and other target group of the institution.

ADVANTAGES OF FIELD TRIP

- Classroom experiences could be further enriched with field trip experiences.
- Field trips provide the opportunity for learners to get first-hand information from natural settings.
- The monotony and boredom of classroom teaching may be supplemented with natural, interesting and exciting teaching methods.
- Field trips give natural stimulation that motivates and makes learners interactive and creative.
- Field trips help the learners learn things very quickly and remember them for a longer period.
- They provide an opportunity to solve the individual's problems by interacting with a group in a natural setting.

SELF-DIRECTED LEARNING

Gibbons (2002) stated, 'self-directed learning is any increase in knowledge, skill, accomplishment, or personal development that an individual selects and brings about by his or her own efforts using any method in any circumstances at any time'.

Knowles (1975) defines self-directed learning as 'a process in which individual take the initiative, with or without the help of other, to diagnose their learning need, formulate learning goals, identify resources for learning, select and implement learning strategies, and evaluate learning outcomes'.

I. SKILLS FOR SELF-DIRECTED LEARNING

Skills particularly important in successful self-directed learning are as follows (Fig. 5.10):

- Goal-oriented skills
- Information-processing skills
- Competency and aptitude skills
- Decision-making skills
- Self-awareness
- Self-confidence
- Inner direction
- Achievement motivated

II. PRINCIPLES OF SELF-DIRECTED LEARNING

The basic principles of self-directed learning as a method of teaching:

- Self-directed learning should be congruent with lifelong, natural and individual learning drives.
- It should be adapted to the maturation, transformations and transitions experienced by students.
- It should be concerned with all aspects of a full life.
- It should employ a full range of human capacities, including senses, emotion and action as well as intellects.
- The self-directed learning activities should be conducted in settings suited to their development.

III. PROCESS OF SELF-DIRECTED LEARNING

Knowles has given the five-step model for the process of self-directed learning. His five-step model of self-directed learning is illustrated in Fig. 5.11.

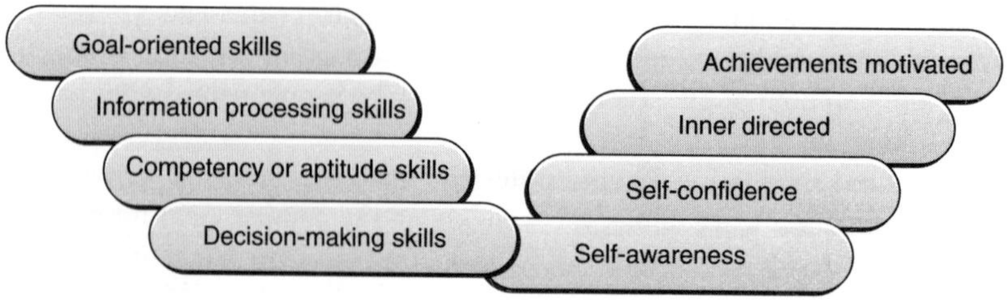

Figure 5.10

Skills for self-directed learning.

IV. ROLE OF TEACHER IN SELF-DIRECTED LEARNING

The principal responsibilities of a teacher using self-directed learning as a method of teaching are:

- To teach inquiry skills, decision-making, personal developments and self-evaluation of work.
- To help learners develop positive attitudes and feelings of independence related to learning.
- To help learners acquire the needs and assessment techniques necessary to discover what objectives they should set.
- To help the learners identify the starting point for a learning project and understand the relevant modes of examination and reporting.
- To create a partnership with the learner by negotiating a learning contact for goals, strategies and evaluation criteria.
- To make sure that learners are aware of the objectives, learning strategies, resources and evaluation criteria once they are decided.
- To teach inquiry skills, decision-making, personal development and self-evaluation of work.
- To act as advocates for educationally underserved populations to facilitate their access to resources.
- To help match resources to the needs of the learners.
- To help learners locate resources.
- To encourage critical thinking skills.
- To create an atmosphere of openness and trust to promote better performance.

ADVANTAGES OF SELF-DIRECTED LEARNING

- Self-directed learning allows learners to be more effective learners.
- It helps the learner develop a sense of responsibility.
- It can encourage students to develop their own rules and leadership patterns.
- It helps the learners to be motivated and persistent, independent, self-disciplined, self-confident and goal-oriented.

DISADVANTAGES OF SELF-DIRECTED LEARNING

- Learners can easily be distracted by their own needs, assumptions, values and misperceptions.

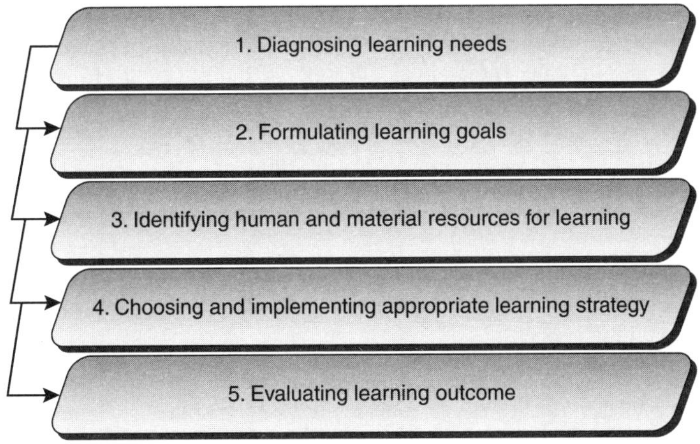

Figure 5.11

Process of self-directed learning.

- Research has shown that some adults are unable to engage in self-directed learning because they lack independence, confidence or resources.
- Self-directed learning needs to be combined with other learning methods for content to be fully learned.

COMPUTER-ASSISTED LEARNING

The word *computer* is derived from the word *compute*, which means to calculate justifying its usefulness. A computer is an electronic machine, which works under the control of a stored program, automatically accepting processing of data to producing designed results. Computer-assisted learning (CAL) is also known as *computer-assisted* instruction (CAI).

CAI or learning refers to the introduction or remediation presented on a computer. Many educational computer programs are available online from computer stores and textbook companies. They enhance the teacher's instruction in several ways.

CAL or CAI facilitates access to information with infinite patience, accuracy and provides an opportunity to all learners. It provides complete individualizing instruction.

CAI mechanizes human brain and human beings are converted into machines.

I. TYPES OF COMPUTER-ASSISTED LEARNING

- *Logo:* This system was developed by Feurzing and Papart. Logo is a simple programming language, which can be taught to children. The program provides instructions that can be used to produce pictures on an oscilloscope or make a little mechanical robot. The children who learn logo make up their own programs to draw flowers or faces or generate designs on the screen.
- *Stimulation:* This language enables students to mount an experiment in a symbolic form.
- *Controlled learning:* Controlled learning involves the use of interesting adaptive strategies. It includes both drill and practice. Drill and practice programmes are supplementary to the regular curriculum followed by the classroom teacher.

II. COMPUTER-ASSISTED WRITING INSTRUCTIONS

A computer program for writing helps students with developing ideas, organizing, outlining and brainstorming. A template provides the framework and reduces the physical effort spent on writing so that students can pay attention to organization and content.

COMPUTER PROGRAMS FOR WRITING

- *Word prediction*
  - Speech: Specific programs that identify words students use repeatedly; when a student types the first few letters, the program lists the frequently used words that start with those letters.
  - Speeds up the typing process.
- *Speech-to-text*
  - Students speak into a microphone and the program types the words.
  - Program must be 'trained' to the student's word pronunciation and speech style.
  - Students must be taught how to use the program.
  - Increased speed from voice to text.

- *Text-to-speech*
  - Students can hear what they have typed to check if it says what they want it to say.
  - Good for editing.
- *Spellchecker*
  - Helps students identify misspelled words.
  - Automatically corrects words if the teacher sets the program that way.

III. EXPERTS NEEDED IN COMPUTER-ASSISTED LEARNING

- Computer engineer
- Lesson writer
- System operator

IV. ROLE OF A TEACHER IN COMPUTER-ASSISTED LEARNING

- The teacher will be liberated from his routine duty.
- CAI can complete the language data accurately and rapidly.

DISADVANTAGES OF COMPUTER-ASSISTED LEARNING

- Inadequate training of teachers and inadequacy of instructional material.
- The computer fails to appreciate students' emotions. The warm emotional climate created by the teacher in classroom interaction with the students is lacking in CAL.
- CAL fails to develop essential features of language competency.
- CAL is a mechanical approach to education.
- The peripheral equipment puts constraints in the ways a student can interact with the computer.

APPLICATION OF COMPUTERS IN NURSING

The main areas for the application of computers in nursing are as follows.

I. EDUCATION

- Knowledge of computers can be applied to prepare slides in MS PowerPoint on the topics to be taught to students.
- Knowledge of multimedia helps the nursing teachers and students teach effectively.
- Education through internet and CAL has simplified education in nursing schools.
- A computer aids in learning and instructions:
  - By providing information and instructions.
  - By asking questions.
  - By doing difficult calculations.
  - By being tireless and repetitive.
  - By simulated process.
  - By selecting the right speed for providing information to individual learners.

II. ADMINISTRATION

- Preparing records of nursing students by lecturers and nursing superintendent.
- Preparing and maintaining records of assessment and results.
- Preparing duty rosters that saves time.
- Preparing drafts of a plan annually, monthly and weekly.

III. HOSPITAL

- Computers keep records of patient's health status during hospital stay and OPD.
- Hospital information management system (HIMS) helps to have access to the patient treatment chart, operation list or anaesthetic record; this is possible with computer knowledge.
- Computer helps nurses manage routine documents in a fraction of a time, which may otherwise take up a lot of time manually.
- It increases productivity of nurses.
- Other functions in hospitals, that is automatic generation of reminder letters, determination of milestones, are performed with the help of appropriate software.

FEATURES OF HIMS

- Data are retrieved quickly and easily.
- Entry of data is easy.
- It has a high degree of security of data.
- Data validation is stringent.

BENEFITS OF HIMS

- Improvement in the doctor's productivity.
- Reduced patient waiting time.
- Eliminating wastage of stationary.
- Prompt medical attention.
- Accuracy and timeliness of data.
- Eliminating any possibility of mixing of blood samples.
- Authorization check and accuracy of billing.
- Prompt issue of medication for patients.
- Maintaining inventory of medication.
- Safe recording of data and saving the time that has to be spent in the medical record department.
- Carrying legal value.
- Prescribing diet from the ward through a computer.
- Giving secret code to prevent manipulation for security reasons.
- Blood bank module for donor registration and certification helps make referrals within the hospital, prepare duty rosters, OT scheduling, diagnostic appointments and patient records.

IV. RESEARCH WORK

- Computers are used to get information on the research works being carried out via the internet.
- They help support research findings with other research that has been carried out.
- Knowledge of computers helps nurses increase their productivity and provide the best patient-centred care. A knowledge of computers reduces the time taken to for documentation which usually takes time when done manually.

ONE-TO-ONE INTERACTION

One-to-one interaction in education is a teaching method in which a teacher works with one student at a time. One-to-one interaction in education refers to a teaching and learning approach where a teacher or educator engages directly with an individual student. It involves a focused and personalized interaction between the teacher and the student, allowing for tailored instruction, feedback and support to meet the specific needs, abilities and learning style of the student.

In the context of nursing education, one-to-one interaction is a highly effective method that focuses on individualized instruction and personalized learning experiences between a nurse educator and a nursing student. This approach recognizes the unique needs, strengths and learning styles of each student, allowing for tailored instruction and support. By engaging in direct and intimate interactions, the educator can provide targeted guidance, mentorship and feedback, which are crucial for the development of competent and compassionate nursing professionals.

DEFINITIONS

- One-to-one interaction in nursing education refers to a teaching and learning approach where a nurse educator engages directly with an individual nursing student in a personalized and intimate manner.

EXAMPLE OF ONE-TO-ONE TEACHING

Here are some examples of how one-to-one teaching can be used in nursing education:

- ***Teaching a student how to give an injection:*** The nurse educator can demonstrate the procedure and then have the student practice on a mannequin. The nurse educator can provide feedback and answer any questions the student has.
- ***Teaching a student how to change a dressing:*** The nurse educator can show the student how to clean the wound, apply a new dressing and secure it in place. The nurse educator can answer any questions the student has and make sure the student feels comfortable with the procedure.

COMPONENTS OF THE ONE-TO-ONE TEACHING METHOD

The one-to-one teaching method in nursing education encompasses several key elements or components that contribute to its effectiveness. These elements focus on providing personalized and tailored instruction to individual nursing students. Here are some essential components of the one-to-one teaching method in nursing education:

1. ***Individualized learning plans:*** One-to-one teaching in nursing education involves developing individualized learning plans for each student. The educator assesses the student's knowledge, skills and learning needs and designs a plan that addresses their specific areas for growth and development. This personalized approach ensures that the instruction is tailored to the student's unique requirements.
2. ***Personalized instruction:*** In one-to-one teaching, the educator delivers instruction in a personalized manner, considering the student's learning style, pace and preferences. They adapt their teaching strategies to accommodate the individual student, ensuring that the content is comprehensible and engaging. This personalized instruction helps to maximize the student's understanding and retention of the nursing concepts.
3. ***Ongoing assessment and feedback:*** Regular and ongoing assessment is a crucial component of one-to-one teaching in nursing education. The educator continually evaluates the student's progress, identifies strengths and areas for improvement and provides timely feedback. This feedback helps the student to monitor their performance, make adjustments and further enhance their learning outcomes.
4. ***Mentorship and guidance:*** The one-to-one teaching method in nursing education often includes a mentorship relationship between the educator and the student. The educator serves as a mentor, offering guidance, support and professional insights. They share their expertise, experiences and wisdom to help the student develop their nursing skills and professional identity.
5. ***Clinical practice and skill development:*** The one-to-one teaching method emphasizes clinical practice and skill development. The educator provides opportunities for the student to apply theoretical knowledge in real-world scenarios. They guide the student in developing their clinical skills, such as patient assessment, medication administration and nursing interventions. Through hands-on practice, the student gains confidence and proficiency in their nursing skills.
6. ***Individualized resources and support:*** The educator provides individualized learning resources and support to the nursing student. These resources may include textbooks, articles, research papers, online modules and additional references. The educator also offers individualized support, answering questions, clarifying concepts and providing further explanations as needed.
7. ***Reflective practice:*** Reflective practice is a fundamental component of one-to-one teaching in nursing education. The educator encourages the student to reflect on their learning experiences, clinical practice and professional growth. Through reflective discussions, the student develops self-awareness, critical thinking skills and the ability to identify areas for improvement in their nursing practice.
8. ***Collaboration and communication:*** One-to-one teaching fosters collaboration and open communication between the educator and the student. They engage in discussions, exchange ideas and explore nursing concepts together. This collaborative approach enhances the student's understanding, encourages active participation and facilitates a supportive learning environment.

BENEFITS OF ONE-TO-ONE INSTRUCTION IN NURSING EDUCATION

1. ***Personalized learning:*** One-to-one instruction allows for personalized learning experiences tailored to the individual needs and learning styles of nursing students. This customized approach enhances understanding, engagement and knowledge retention.

2. ***Individualized feedback:*** With one-to-one instruction, educators can provide immediate and specific feedback to students, addressing their strengths and areas for improvement. This feedback promotes student growth, self-reflection and continuous learning.
3. ***Enhanced mentorship:*** One-to-one instruction fosters strong mentorship relationships between educators and students. This mentorship provides guidance, support and professional development opportunities, nurturing the student's growth as a nursing professional.
4. ***Targeted remediation:*** Students who require additional support or have specific learning challenges can benefit greatly from one-to-one instruction. Educators can identify individual learning gaps and provide targeted remediation to help students overcome difficulties and achieve academic success.
5. ***Clinical competence development:*** One-to-one instruction allows for focused clinical practice and skill development. Educators can provide hands-on guidance and mentorship, helping students develop clinical competence, critical thinking skills and confidence in their nursing abilities.

CHALLENGES OF ONE-TO-ONE INSTRUCTION IN NURSING EDUCATION

1. ***Resource intensiveness:*** One-to-one instruction demands more resources, including time and personnel, compared to traditional classroom settings. The availability of qualified educators and the need for individualized attention can pose challenges in terms of resource allocation.
2. ***Limited scalability:*** One-to-one instruction may not be easily scalable to accommodate a large number of students, particularly in programmes with high student-to-faculty ratios. It may be challenging to maintain the same level of personalized attention and support with a large cohort of students.
3. ***Time constraints:*** One-to-one instruction requires dedicated time and scheduling to ensure sufficient interaction between educators and students. Balancing this individualized instruction with other educational responsibilities can be demanding for educators.
4. ***Student engagement and motivation:*** While one-to-one instruction can enhance student engagement, it relies on the active participation and motivation of students. Some students may require additional support or encouragement to fully engage in the individualized learning process.

TEAM-BASED LEARNING

Team-based learning (TBL) is an educational approach that promotes active learning and collaboration among students. It is a structured method that encourages students to work together in teams to solve problems, engage in discussions and apply their knowledge to real-world scenarios. TBL was developed by Dr. Larry Michaelsen in the late 1970s and has gained popularity in various educational settings.

TBL has become popular and is a preferred teaching method in nursing education in many institutions. It is an active learning and teaching strategy where students have an active role in their learning. Further, it is a method where the instructor facilitates learning, not lecture from the front of the room. TBL is also a very structured teaching strategy based on cognitive learning theory.

DEFINITIONS OF TEAM-BASED LEARNING

- 'Team-based learning (TBL) is an active learning strategy that involves students working together in teams to learn and apply concepts. TBL is a four-phase process: preparation, readiness assurance process (RAP), application activities, and peer evaluation'. (Dolowitz, 2020).
- 'Team-based learning (TBL) is a student-centered instructional method in which small groups of students work together to learn and apply concepts. TBL is based on the principles of cognitive learning theory and is designed to promote active learning, critical thinking, and teamwork'. (Michaelsen et al., 2004).
- 'Team-based learning (TBL) is an active learning strategy that involves students working together in small teams to learn and apply concepts. TBL is designed to promote student engagement, critical thinking, and teamwork'. (Smith & Jones, 2016)

  These definitions all highlight the key features of TBL, which include:
  - ***Active learning:*** TBL is a student-centred approach that encourages students to be actively involved in their learning.
  - ***Small group learning:*** TBL is designed to be implemented in small groups of students, which allows for more collaboration and interaction.
  - ***Application of concepts:*** TBL requires students to apply the concepts they have learned to real-world problems.
  - ***Peer evaluation:*** TBL includes a peer evaluation component, which allows students to provide feedback to each other on their learning.

ELEMENTS OF TEAM-BASED LEARNING

When implementing TBL in nursing education, the essential elements are as follows:

1. ***Team formation:*** In nursing education, teams are typically formed with a diverse mix of students, including those from different nursing specialties or levels of experience. This diversity promotes collaboration and exposes students to different perspectives and areas of expertise within the nursing profession.
2. ***Application of nursing concepts:*** TBL in nursing education focuses on applying nursing concepts and skills to real-world scenarios. Application activities may involve analysing patient case studies, simulating clinical situations or developing care plans. These activities strengthen critical thinking and clinical reasoning skills.
3. ***Preclass preparation:*** Students engage in preclass preparation, which may include reading nursing literature, reviewing relevant guidelines or watching instructional videos. This prepares them with foundational knowledge and enables more focused discussions and application activities during the class session.
4. ***Clinical decision-making:*** TBL in nursing education emphasizes the development of clinical decision-making skills. Students work together in teams to analyse complex patient situations, identify priorities and determine appropriate nursing interventions. This encourages students to think critically and make evidence-based decisions.
5. ***Patient safety and communication:*** TBL provides opportunities for students to enhance their communication skills and learn about patient safety practices. Collaborative discussions within teams promote effective communication and teamwork, emphasizing the importance of clear and accurate information exchange to ensure patient safety.
6. ***Reflection and ethical considerations:*** TBL in nursing education incorporates opportunities for students to reflect on ethical issues and ethical decision-making in nursing practice. Teams may

engage in discussions about ethical dilemmas, explore different perspectives and develop ethical frameworks for nursing care.

7. ***Assessment and evaluation:*** Assessments in TBL for nursing education may include both individual and team components. Individual assessments can measure students' understanding of nursing concepts, while team assessments evaluate teamwork skills, communication and application of knowledge to patient scenarios. Peer evaluations can also be utilized to provide feedback on individual and team performance.
8. ***Faculty facilitation:*** In TBL for nursing education, faculty members serve as facilitators and clinical experts. They guide team discussions, provide clarification on nursing concepts and facilitate debriefing sessions. Faculty members also ensure that the TBL activities align with the learning objectives of the nursing curriculum.

PHASES OF TEAM-BASED LEARNING

TBL is an active learning strategy that involves students working together in teams to learn and apply concepts. TBL is a four-phase process:

1. ***Preparation:*** In the preparation phase, students are given readings or other materials to prepare for the lesson. They are also given a set of readiness assurance questions (RAQs) to answer individually. The RAQs are designed to assess students' understanding of the material that will be covered in the lesson.
2. ***Readiness assurance process (RAP):*** In the RAP, students take a quiz on the RAQs. Students who do not pass the RAP are required to complete additional work before they can participate in the application activities.
3. ***Application activities:*** In the application activities, students work in teams to solve problems or answer questions related to the material that has been covered. The application activities are designed to give students the opportunity to apply the concepts they have learned to real-world problems.
4. ***Peer evaluation:*** At the end of the lesson, students are asked to evaluate their teammates. This feedback is used to help students identify their strengths and weaknesses as learners.

BENEFITS OF TEAM-BASED LEARNING IN NURSING EDUCATION

TBL has been shown to be an effective teaching method in nursing education. It has been shown to improve student learning outcomes, such as knowledge, critical thinking skills and clinical reasoning skills. TBL has also been shown to increase student satisfaction with their learning. Here are some of the benefits of using TBL:

- ***Improved student learning outcomes:*** TBL has been shown to improve student learning outcomes in a variety of subjects, including math, science, health sciences including nursing and business.
- ***Increased student engagement:*** TBL is a student-centred approach that encourages students to be actively involved in their learning.
- ***Enhanced critical thinking skills:*** TBL requires students to apply the concepts they have learned to real-world problems, which helps them to develop critical thinking skills.
- ***Improved teamwork skills:*** TBL requires students to work collaboratively in teams, which helps them to develop teamwork skills.

- ***Accountability and responsibility:*** TBL instils a sense of accountability and responsibility among nursing students. Each team member's contributions are valued, and students are accountable for their preparation, active participation and collaborative efforts.
- ***Peer learning and support:*** TBL provides opportunities for peer learning and support. Nursing students can exchange knowledge, share experiences and learn from each other's insights. Peer learning fosters a supportive learning community, enhances teamwork and strengthens understanding through explanations and discussions among team members.
- ***Application of knowledge:*** TBL facilitates the application of theoretical nursing knowledge to practical situations. By analysing patient cases, engaging in simulations or conducting role-plays, students practice clinical reasoning, decision-making and critical thinking skills.

CHALLENGES OF TEAM-BASED LEARNING IN NURSING EDUCATION

- ***Requires careful planning and preparation:*** TBL requires instructors to carefully plan and prepare for each lesson. This includes creating RAQs, developing application activities and creating a peer evaluation rubric.
- ***Time management:*** TBL can be more time-consuming than traditional lecture-based teaching methods. This is because instructors need to spend time planning and preparing for each lesson, and students need to spend time working in teams and completing application activities.
- ***Requires a skilled instructor:*** TBL requires instructors who are skilled in facilitating active learning and providing feedback to students.
- ***Assessment and evaluation:*** Assessing individual and team performance in TBL can be complex. Developing fair and reliable assessment methods to evaluate both individual understanding and teamwork skills can pose challenges.

PROBLEM-BASED LEARNING

Problem-based learning is a student-centric instructional strategy where students collaboratively solve problems and reflect on their experiences. It is an inquiry-based method of instruction that guides students to solutions of real-world problems through cooperative group work and builds critical thinking skills.

- According to D.J. Boud (1985), 'the principal idea behind problem-based learning is that the starting point should be a problem, a query, or a puzzle that the learner wishes to solve'.
- According to John Dewey (1916), 'a careful inspection of methods which are permanently successful in formal education. Problem based learning will reveal that they depend for their efficiency upon the fact that they go back to the type of situation which causes reflection out of school in ordinary life. They give pupils something to do, not something to learn; and if the doing is of such a nature as to demand thinking naturally results'.

Problem-based learning is a process of acquiring understanding, knowledge, skills and attitudes in the context of an unfamiliar situation and applying this learning to that situation. Problem-based learning includes the following components:

- Nonlecture format with the teacher as a facilitator.
- The presentation of real-world situation or problems that expand on previous learning.
- Student group work and discussion.
- Student-directed solution of the problem.

Problem-based learning is guided by a constructivist framework that emphasizes problem solving should occur in the same environment as the problem, the presence of a problem is what starts and guides the learning process and determines how the problem is solved, and knowledge is expanded through group discussion and collaboration.

I. USE OF PROBLEM-BASED LEARNING

Problem-based learning is introduced and continued for many reasons including:

- Acquiring subject matter knowledge.
- Motivating students to learn.
- Helping students with retention.
- Developing students' thinking skills.
- Developing students' key skills relevant to employment such as interpersonal communication skills.
- Fostering professional competence and confidence together with professional identity.
- Mirroring the interdisciplinary team process graduates will use in work and research.
- Facilitating students how to learn.
- Encouraging students to integrate knowledge from different subjects, disciplines and sources.
- Linking theory and practice.
- Having a sense of belonging and friendship.
- Having a sense of fun while learning.
- Expressing in operational form a philosophy of learning that is student-centric and problem focused.

II. COMMON FEATURES OF PROBLEM-BASED LEARNING

The main features of problem-based learning are:

- Learning is initiated by a problem.
- Problems are based on complex, real-world situations.
- All information needed to solve the problem is not given initially.
- Students identify, find and use appropriate resources.
- Students work in a permanent group.
- Learning is active, integrated, cumulative and connected.

III. PROCESS OF PROBLEM-BASED LEARNING

The main steps in the process of problem-based learning are (Fig. 5.12):

- Presentation of problem.
- Organize ideas and prior knowledge.
- Pose questions.
- Assign responsibilities for questions and discuss resources.
- Research questions, summarize and analyse findings.
- Reconvene and report on research.
- Integrate new information and refine questions.
- Resolution of problem.

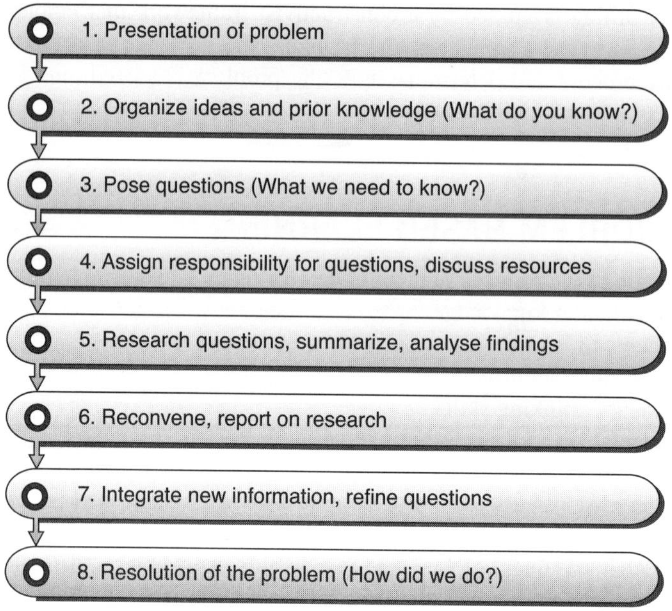

Figure 5.12

Steps of the problem-based learning process.

IV. THE PROBLEM-BASED LEARNING CYCLE

Problem-based learning consists of the following steps (Fig. 5.13):

Kenneth J. Oja conducted a study on using problem-based learning in the clinical setting to improve nursing students' critical thinking. In today's arena, new graduate nurses are exposed to increasingly demanding and complex acute care environments that require an ability to effectively think and reason to provide quality patient care. So there is a need to demonstrate critical thinking skills to the new graduate students. Problem-based learning is a method of education designed to encourage critical thinking. The studies reviewed a positive relationship between problem-based learning and improved critical thinking in nursing students.

ADVANTAGES OF PROBLEM-BASED LEARNING

- Relates to real world and motivate students.
- Requires decision-making or judgements.
- A multipage and multistage process.
- Designed for group solving.
- Poses open-ended initial questions that encourage the discussion.
- Incorporates course content, objectives, higher-order thinking and other skills.

PROBLEM SOLVING AS A METHOD OF TEACHING

There is a prevailing idea that education provides us with a knowledge base that enables us to deal with life's problems in our professional work and in everyday life. Problem solving requires an integrated use

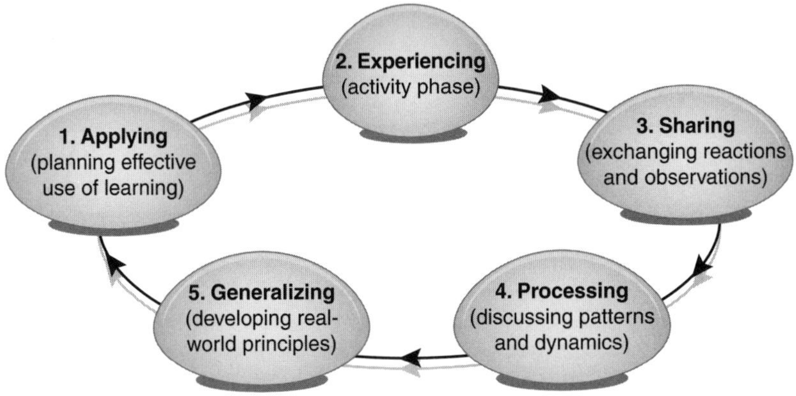

Figure 5.13

Steps of the problem-based cycle.

of thinking skills which produce novel solutions from limited information. Problem solving forms a part of thinking. It occurs if an artificial intelligence system does not know how to proceed from a given state to a desired goal state. It is a part of the larger problem process that includes problem finding and shaping.

> *The problem solving is a process of overcoming difficulties that appears to interfere with the attainment of goal. It is a procedure of making adjustment in spite of interferences.*
>
> **—Skinner**

> *Problem solving is a method of organization of subject matter in such a way that it can be dealt with through the study of problems encountered.*

I. PURPOSES OF PROBLEM SOLVING

The main proposes of problem solving as a method of teaching are:

- To train the student in the act of reasoning.
- To give practical knowledge.
- To discover new knowledge.
- To solve a puzzling problem.
- To improve student knowledge.
- To help overcome the obstacles or inferences in the attainment of objectives.
- To help in an individual's as well as society's progress.

II. ESSENTIAL FEATURES OF PROBLEM SOLVING

The main features of problem solving as a method of teaching are:

- The problem should be meaningful, interesting and worthwhile.
- It should have correlation with life.
- It should arise out of the real needs of students.
- Students must possess some background knowledge of the problem.
- The problem should be clearly defined.
- The solution of the problem should be found out by the students under the guidance of the teacher.

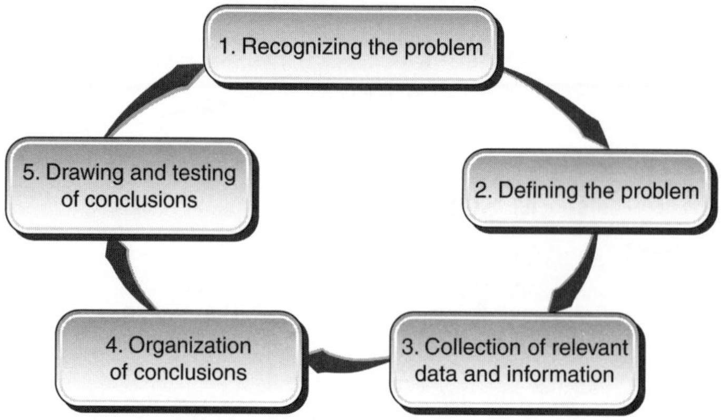

Figure 5.14

Steps in problem solving.

III. STEPS IN PROBLEM SOLVING

The main steps followed in the problem-solving process are (Fig. 5.14):

- Recognizing the problem.
- Defining the problem.
- Collecting relevant data and information.
- Organizing conclusion.
- Drawing and testing conclusion.

IV. METHODS/APPROACHES TO PROBLEM SOLVING

- ***Inductive method:*** The inductive method is a method of development. The student is led to discover the truth about him. It includes:
  - Observation of the given material.
  - Discrimination and analysis noting differences and similarities.
  - Classification.
  - Abstraction and generalization.
  - Application or verification.
- ***Deductive method:*** In the deductive method rules, generalizations and principles are provided to students and they are asked to verify them with the help of particular examples.
- ***Combination of deductive and inductive method:*** Induction is followed by deduction and deduction is followed by induction. According to Miller, induction is the making of the tools of thought and deduction is the using of tools.

V. ROLE OF TEACHER IN PROBLEM SOLVING

The major roles of a teacher in problem solving as a method of teaching are:

- To get the students to define the problem clearly.
- To aid them to keep the problem in mind.

- To get them to make suggestions by encouraging them.
- To give them time to evaluate each suggestion carefully.
- To give them time to organize material.
- To set up an atmosphere of freedom in the class.

ADVANTAGES OF PROBLEM SOLVING

- Improves problem-solving abilities.
- Is student-centric rather than teacher-centric.
- Is an activity of collaboration.
- Helps in the development of constructivism.
- Allows for multiple intelligence development.
- Offers opportunity of extended time frames.
- Provides a deeper understanding of knowledge.
- Other advantages of problem solving as a method of teaching:
  - It helps in developing good study habits.
  - It affords opportunities for participation in social activities.
  - The students learn to be self-dependent.
  - Discussions help develop the power of expressions of students.
  - It provides opportunities to the teachers to know their students in detail.
  - Students learn facts that are meaningful and have been discovered by their own efforts.
  - It helps in the maintenance of discipline.
  - Learning becomes more interesting in place of dread.
  - It gives the power of critical judgement.
  - It helps verify an option.
  - It satisfies curiosity.
  - It helps learn how to act in a new situation.

DISADVANTAGES OF PROBLEM SOLVING

- Problem solving involves mental activity only. There is less body activity.
- There is a lack of suitable references and source books for students.
- It involves a lot of time and teachers find it difficult to cover the prescribed syllabus.
- Problem-solving methods need very capable teachers to provide effective guidance.

CLINICAL TEACHING METHODS

Nurses need learning in three domains, that is cognitive, affective and psychomotor. However, psychomotor domain of learning is most essential in nursing discipline because nurses need to have hands-on skills to provide best quality nursing care to their patients or clients. Therefore, it is essential for nurse educators to provide clinical teaching through most robust and advanced methods, so that nursing students can swiftly learn the real-life clinical knowledge and clinical skills.

According to Schweer (1972), 'clinical teaching is a vehicle that provides students with the opportunity to translate basic theoretical knowledge into the learning of a variety of intellectual and psychomotor skills needed to provide patient centred quality nursing care'.

BOX 5.7 RESPONSIBILITIES AND QUALITIES OF A CLINICAL TEACHER

I. *Responsibilities of clinical teacher*
 1. Plan and implement the clinical learning experiences through most effective methods of clinical teaching.
 2. Plan and prepare required clinical area and needed resources for effective clinical experiences.
 3. Orient the new group of students to the clinical environment to promote their adaptation to the new clinical setting.
 4. Facilitate in arranging all the essential resources required for the clinical learning.
 5. Demonstrating clinical nursing skills and motivating the students to carryout return demonstrations to ensure that they have acquired the required clinical learning.
 6. Helping the students to gradually become independent in performing the learned clinical knowledge and skills.
 7. Assessing the students to ensure that they have achieved optimum level of desired learning in the particular clinical field/area.
 8. Keep himself/herself updated with most advanced and effective methods of clinical teaching.

II. *Qualities of a good clinical teacher*
 1. Available, approachable and nonthreatening.
 2. Resourceful.
 3. Clinically competent.
 4. Nonjudgemental.
 5. Enthusiastic and passionate in clinical teaching and learning.
 6. Empathetic and tolerant.
 7. Three *'A'* for qualities of clinical teacher are
    - Ability (attitude, knowledge and clinical skills).
    - Availability (physical presence of teacher in clinical setting/bedside).
    - Affability (approachable, affectionate, gentle, gracious and friendly).

Clinical teaching is a time-bound process in which the teacher and the student create a partnership within a shared environment in such a way that the teacher's primary operational frame of reference is maintained as the legitimate means for affecting the student's behaviour towards intended purposes.

A teacher's core activity in the clinical setting is clinical instruction and guidance. The teacher must guide, support, stimulate and facilitate learning. He/she can facilitate learning by designing appropriate activity in appropriate setting and allowing the student to experience that learning. The main responsibilities and qualities of a clinical teacher are presented in Box 5.7.

I. TYPES OF CLINICAL TEACHING METHODS

The brief description of types of clinical teaching methods are presented in Box. 5.8.

II. GUIDELINES FOR SELECTION OF CLINICAL TEACHING METHODS

The selected method for the clinical teaching must be in:

- Concurrence with the educational objectives and desired behavioural changes of the learner.
- Accordance with the principles of teaching and learning.
- Accordance with the capacity and capabilities of the learner.
- Accordance with the availability of resources.
- Accordance with the teacher's ability to use it effectively and creatively.

BOX 5.8 TYPES OF CLINICAL TEACHING METHODS

Type of Clinical Teaching Method	Concept/Meaning
1. Patient assignment	Patient assignment is a clinical teaching method commonly used in nursing education to provide students with hands-on learning experiences in healthcare settings. It involves assigning nursing students to care for specific patients under the supervision of a registered nurse or clinical instructor. This method allows students to apply their theoretical knowledge and develop essential clinical skills while caring for real patients in various healthcare settings, such as hospitals, clinics or long-term care facilities.
2. Clinical conference	Clinical conferences are also widely used as a teaching method in nursing education. They offer an interactive and case-based approach to enhance critical thinking, clinical judgement and problem-solving skills among nursing students and practising nurses.
3. Clinical presentation	Clinical presentation is an effective method of teaching in nursing that involves the direct observation and analysis of patient cases or clinical scenarios. It is a dynamic and interactive approach that brings real-world clinical situations into the educational setting, allowing nursing students to apply their knowledge, develop critical thinking skills and enhance their clinical decision-making abilities.
4. Bedside clinics	Bedside clinic, also known as bedside teaching, is a method of teaching in healthcare, including nursing, that involves direct observation and instruction at the patient's bedside. It is a valuable educational approach that allows students to learn in the actual clinical setting and interact with patients under the guidance of experienced healthcare professionals.
5. Case study	Case study is in-depth study and analysis of progress of a patient with specific disease, who received nursing care for an extended period ranging between 7 and 10 days. In the case study, students get an opportunity to understand the effects of particular nursing interventions on specific nursing problems/diagnoses.
6. Bedside nursing clinics	Bedside nursing clinic is a method of clinical teaching, which is also called as bedside teaching where a small group of students are taught about a disease condition or nursing care practices directly on a real patient at bedside, which provides rich opportunity of visual, auditory, tactile and olfactory experiences.
7. Nursing rounds	Nursing rounds are a structured process in which healthcare professionals, primarily nurses, come together to review and discuss patient cases, coordinate care and facilitate interdisciplinary collaboration. These rounds are typically conducted in a healthcare facility, such as a hospital or clinic, and involve primarily group of nurses but sometimes may involve other healthcare team members, including doctors, specialists and students from different disciplines.
8. Concept mapping	Concept mapping is a powerful clinical teaching method that involves the creation of visual representations to organize and link key concepts, ideas and relationships. It is a valuable tool for promoting critical thinking, knowledge integration and deep understanding among nursing students. Concept mapping enables students to visually represent complex information, identify patterns and develop a comprehensive view of a particular topic or patient case.
9. Questioning in clinical teaching	Questioning in clinical teaching is particularly important in nursing education, as it plays a vital role in developing the critical thinking and clinical decision-making skills necessary for safe and effective patient care.
10. Process recording	Process recording is a method of clinical teaching in which students get an opportunity to directly interact with patient in the supervision of clinical faculty where he/she gets a chance to obtain skills of communication, history taking, critical thinking and recording of interaction.
11. Field visits	Field visit is defined as a planned activity to take the students out of classroom for an observation of particular place, persons, organization or situation to obtain first-hand experiences.

CLINICAL LEARNING ENVIRONMENT

A clinical learning environment (CLE) refers to the physical, social and psychological setting where healthcare professionals, such as medical students, nursing students and other allied health professionals, acquire and develop their clinical skills and knowledge. It can be a hospital, clinic or other healthcare setting. The CLE is important because it provides students with the opportunity to apply their theoretical knowledge to practice, acquire clinical skills and develop problem-solving and clinical reasoning skills. It serves as a crucial component of professional education and plays a vital role in shaping future healthcare providers.

Creating a positive and conducive CLE requires collaboration between educational institutions, healthcare organizations and healthcare professionals. It necessitates a commitment to continuous improvement, innovation and adaptation to evolving healthcare practices and technologies.

DEFINITIONS

- The clinical learning environment is the setting in which health professions students learn and practice clinical skills. (Griffiths, 2008)
- The clinical learning environment is the interactive network of forces that influences clinical learning outcomes. (Dunn & Hansford, 2005)
- The clinical learning environment is the physical, social, and cultural context in which health professions students learn and practice clinical skills. (Roff & McAleer, 2001)

These definitions all emphasize the importance of the CLE in the development of health professions students' clinical skills and knowledge. The CLE can have a significant impact on students' learning, and it is important to create a positive and supportive environment that encourages students to learn and grow.

FACTOR CONTRIBUTING CLINICAL LEARNING ENVIRONMENT

A positive CLE is essential for nursing students to learn and develop the skills they need to be successful in their careers. By providing students with a safe, supportive and learning-focused environment, clinical instructors can help students to develop the skills and knowledge they need to be effective nurses. In nursing education, several factors contribute to creating a positive and effective CLE. These factors include:

1. **The quality of the clinical setting:** The clinical setting should be a safe and supportive environment where students can learn and practice their skills. The setting should also be well-equipped with the resources that students need to learn.
2. **The availability of qualified clinical instructors:** Clinical instructors should be qualified and experienced nurses, who can provide students with the guidance and support they need to learn. Instructors should also be able to create a positive and supportive learning environment.
3. **Collaborative interprofessional learning**: Collaboration with other healthcare professionals, such as physicians, pharmacists and therapists, enhances nursing students' understanding of interdisciplinary teamwork and the holistic nature of patient care.
4. **Simulated learning experiences**: Simulation-based learning provides a safe and controlled environment for nursing students to practice clinical skills, critical thinking and decision-making. Simulated scenarios allow students to gain confidence, learn from mistakes and apply their knowledge in realistic patient care situations.
5. **Meaningful clinical assignments**: Assigning nursing students to clinical placements that align with their educational goals and learning needs enhances their engagement and learning

experience. Well-planned clinical assignments expose students to a variety of patient populations, healthcare settings and nursing specialties.

6. **The opportunity for hands-on learning:** Students need the opportunity to practice their skills in a real-world setting. The clinical setting should provide students with opportunities to care for patients and to practice a variety of nursing skills.
7. **The availability of feedback:** Students need regular feedback on their performance in the clinical setting. Feedback should be constructive and helpful, and it should be provided in a timely manner.
8. **The support of the nursing faculty:** The nursing faculty should provide students with support and guidance throughout the clinical experience. Faculty members should be available to answer questions and to provide support when needed.

By considering all of these factors, clinical instructors can create a positive and supportive learning environment that will help students to succeed in their nursing education.

BENEFITS OF CLINICAL LEARNING ENVIRONMENT

1. **Hands-on experience:** CLEs provide healthcare professionals and students with the opportunity to apply their theoretical knowledge in real-life situations. They gain practical experience in performing procedures, interacting with patients and managing complex cases, which helps build clinical competence.
2. **Opportunity to learn from experienced nurses**: Clinical instructors are experienced nurses who can provide students with guidance and support. They can also help students to develop their clinical skills and knowledge.
3. **Patient interaction and communication skills:** Working directly with patients in a clinical setting enhances healthcare professionals' ability to communicate effectively, develop empathy and build rapport. They learn how to address patients' concerns, provide education and deliver patient-centred care.
4. **Interprofessional collaboration:** CLEs often involve collaboration with professionals from different healthcare disciplines. This fosters teamwork, promotes a holistic approach to patient care and improves communication and collaboration skills across professions.
5. **Professional networking:** Clinical settings provide opportunities to network and establish professional connections with experienced healthcare providers. Students and professionals can learn from their mentors and preceptors, potentially leading to future career opportunities and mentorship.
6. **Exposure to diverse patient populations:** CLEs expose healthcare professionals and students to a wide range of patients with diverse backgrounds, medical conditions and cultural beliefs. This exposure enhances cultural competence and the ability to provide individualized care.
7. **Decision-making and critical thinking skills:** Working in clinical settings challenges healthcare professionals and students to think critically, make quick decisions and solve problems in real-time. This improves their analytical skills and prepares them for handling complex and urgent situations.

CHALLENGES OF CLINICAL LEARNING ENVIRONMENT

1. **Limited resources:** Clinical settings may have limitations in terms of equipment, facilities and patient availability, which can hinder the breadth and depth of learning experiences. Students and professionals may not always have access to the latest technology or exposure to rare or specialized cases.

2. **Emotional and psychological demands:** CLEs can be emotionally challenging, as healthcare professionals and students may encounter patients with serious illnesses, difficult emotional situations or end-of-life care. This can lead to emotional stress and burnout if proper support and coping mechanisms are not in place.
3. **Variation in clinical experiences:** CLEs can vary in terms of patient populations, healthcare settings and experiences available to learners. Some learners may have limited exposure to certain specialties or patient populations, which can impact the breadth and depth of their learning experiences.
4. **Ethical dilemmas and professional challenges:** Clinical settings present ethical dilemmas and professional challenges that require healthcare professionals and students to navigate complex situations. Balancing patient autonomy, confidentiality and ethical decision-making can be demanding and require ongoing reflection and guidance.
5. **Lack of experience**: Nursing students often lack the experience and knowledge to care for complex patients. This can lead to feelings of inadequacy and frustration.
6. **Lack of support**: Clinical instructors are often busy with their own work and may not have the time to provide students with the support they need. This can lead to feelings of isolation and loneliness.

Overall, while CLEs offer invaluable opportunities for hands-on experience, patient interaction and professional development, it is essential to address the challenges to ensure optimal learning experiences and support the well-being of healthcare professionals and students. Effective mentorship, resources, support systems and a focus on work-life balance can help mitigate these challenges and create a positive and enriching CLE.

FACTORS INFLUENCING SELECTION OF CLINICAL LEARNING EXPERIENCES

The selection of clinical learning experiences for nursing students is influenced by several factors that are specific to their education and training. These factors include:

1. **Educational objectives and curriculum:** The clinical learning experiences should align with the educational objectives and curriculum of the nursing programme. The experiences selected should provide opportunities for students to achieve the required clinical competencies, apply theoretical knowledge and develop nursing skills relevant to their specific programme.
2. **Accreditation and regulatory requirements:** Nursing education programmes must adhere to accreditation and regulatory requirements set by nursing boards or governing bodies. These requirements specify the types and duration of clinical experiences needed for nursing students to meet educational standards and eligibility for licensure.
3. **Specialty focus:** Nursing programmes may have specific specialty areas or tracks, such as medical-surgical, paediatrics, obstetrics, mental health or community health. The selection of clinical experiences should reflect the chosen specialty or area of focus and provide students with opportunities to gain hands-on experience in their intended nursing field.
4. **Availability of clinical sites:** The availability of clinical sites is a crucial factor in selecting clinical learning experiences for nursing students. Educational institutions must establish partnerships with healthcare facilities to secure clinical placements. The number and diversity of available clinical sites determine the range of experiences that can be offered to students.
5. **Scope of practice and level of proficiency:** The clinical experiences should match the students' scope of practice and level of proficiency. As students progress through their nursing programme, the complexity and autonomy of their clinical experiences should increase to reflect their advancing skills and competencies.

6. **Patient population and diversity:** It is important for nursing students to have exposure to a diverse range of patient populations, including different age groups, cultural backgrounds and health conditions. Clinical experiences should offer opportunities to work with patients across the lifespan and from various socioeconomic backgrounds to enhance students' cultural competence and patient-centred care skills.
7. **Faculty expertise and resources:** The expertise and availability of nursing faculty members and preceptors play a role in selecting clinical experiences. Faculty members with specialized knowledge and skills may guide the selection of experiences to ensure optimal learning opportunities for nursing students.
8. **Collaborative opportunities:** Nursing is a collaborative profession, and clinical experiences that provide opportunities for interprofessional collaboration and teamwork are highly valued. Experiences in multidisciplinary healthcare settings or collaborations with professionals from different healthcare disciplines enhance students' understanding of teamwork and interdisciplinary care.
9. **Community needs and public health:** Nursing programmes often emphasize community health and public health initiatives. The selection of clinical experiences may prioritize community-based healthcare settings or focus on addressing specific health issues or public health priorities in the local community.
10. **Learner preferences and feedback:** Nursing students' preferences and feedback should be taken into consideration when selecting clinical experiences. Understanding their interests, goals and unique learning needs can help tailor experiences that promote engagement and satisfaction.

By considering these factors, nursing education programmes can strategically select clinical learning experiences that provide students with diverse and relevant opportunities to develop their nursing skills, knowledge and professional competencies in preparation for their future nursing careers.

PRACTICAL MODEL

Practical Model, also known as the practical teaching method or experiential learning, is a highly effective approach used in the field of nursing. It focuses on providing hands-on experiences and real-life scenarios to enhance the learning process for nursing students and professionals. This approach recognizes the importance of active participation, critical thinking and practical application of knowledge in preparing nurses for their clinical practice.

In the Practical Model, nursing students are actively involved in various clinical activities, allowing them to develop and refine their nursing skills. They engage in authentic patient encounters, simulations, case studies and interactive activities that mirror the challenges and complexities of real-life healthcare settings. This method creates a dynamic learning environment that encourages active learning, problem solving and collaboration.

DEFINITIONS

- 'The Practical Model is a problem-based approach to clinical teaching that focuses on the development of critical thinking skills and the ability to apply theoretical knowledge to real-world situations'. (Bevis and O'Rourke, 2006)
- 'The Practical Model is a student-centered approach to clinical teaching that emphasizes the development of clinical reasoning skills and the ability to make independent judgments in clinical situations'. (Tanner, 2009)

- 'The Practical Model is a process-oriented approach to clinical teaching that focuses on the development of clinical expertise through the acquisition of tacit knowledge'. (Benner, 2010)

No matter how it is defined, the Practical Model is a valuable tool for helping nursing students develop the skills and knowledge they need to be successful in clinical practice.

COMPONENTS OF THE PRACTICAL MODEL IN NURSING EDUCATION

The Practical Model is a student-centred approach to clinical teaching that emphasizes the development of clinical reasoning skills and the ability to make independent judgements in clinical situations. The model is based on the following components:

1. **Preparation**: Prior to the clinical experience, students are given an opportunity to review the theoretical content related to the patient population they will be working with. This helps to ensure that students have a foundation of knowledge to draw from when they are in the clinical setting.
2. **Reflection**: Throughout the clinical experience, students are encouraged to reflect on their experiences and to identify what they learned. This helps students to make sense of their experiences and to develop their own clinical reasoning skills.
3. **Feedback:** Students receive regular feedback from their clinical instructors. This feedback helps students to identify their strengths and weaknesses and to make improvements in their clinical skills.
4. **Evaluation**: Students are evaluated on their clinical performance at the end of the clinical experience. This evaluation helps to ensure that students have met the learning objectives for the clinical experience.

The Practical Model is a comprehensive approach to clinical teaching that can help students develop the skills and knowledge they need to be successful in clinical practice.

Here are some **examples of how the Practical Model can be used in clinical teaching**:

- **Preparation**: Prior to a clinical experience, students can be given a case study to read. The case study should describe a patient with a specific health condition. Students can then be asked to answer questions about the case study, such as:
  What are the patient's symptoms?
  What are the possible diagnoses?
  What are the treatment options?
  What are the nursing interventions for each treatment option?
- **Reflection**: During a clinical experience, students can be asked to reflect on their experiences in a journal. Students can be asked to write about what they learned, what they found challenging and what they would do differently next time.
- **Feedback**: Clinical instructors can provide students with feedback on their clinical performance throughout the clinical experience. This feedback can be given verbally or in writing. Feedback should be specific and constructive. It should help students to identify their strengths and weaknesses and to make improvements in their clinical skills.
- **Evaluation**: At the end of a clinical experience, students can be evaluated on their clinical performance. This evaluation can be done through a written exam, a skills check or a combination of both. The evaluation should be fair and consistent. It should measure students' ability to apply their theoretical knowledge to real-world clinical situations.

BENEFITS OF THE PRACTICAL MODEL IN NURSING EDUCATION

1. **Enhanced clinical competence:** The Practical Model allows nursing students to gain hands-on experience and develop their clinical skills. By actively participating in patient care activities, they become more confident and competent in performing nursing procedures and interventions.
2. **Application of theoretical knowledge:** The Practical Model helps bridge the gap between theory and practice by providing opportunities for nursing students to apply their theoretical knowledge in real-life scenarios. This promotes a deeper understanding of nursing concepts and their practical application.
3. **Critical thinking development:** Through the Practical Model, nursing students are exposed to complex clinical situations that require critical thinking and problem solving. They learn to analyse information, make sound clinical judgements and develop effective nursing interventions.
4. **Interdisciplinary collaboration:** The Practical Model often involves working with healthcare professionals from different disciplines. Nursing students learn the importance of teamwork, effective communication and collaboration in delivering patient-centred care.
5. **Professionalism and ethical decision-making:** Nursing students encounter ethical dilemmas and challenging situations during their practical experiences. The Practical Model provides a platform for students to develop their professionalism and ethical decision-making skills, ensuring they uphold the highest standards of patient care.

CHALLENGES OF THE PRACTICAL MODEL IN NURSING EDUCATION

1. **Limited availability of clinical placements**: Securing appropriate and sufficient clinical placements for nursing students can be challenging. There may be limitations in terms of the number of available clinical sites and the variety of patient populations and healthcare settings that students can experience.
2. **Time constraints**: The Practical Model often requires a significant time commitment from both students and faculty. Balancing clinical experiences with classroom learning and other academic responsibilities can be demanding for nursing students. Faculty members may also face challenges in managing and coordinating practical experiences for large groups of students.
3. **Safety concerns**: Patient safety is of utmost importance in nursing education. The Practical Model involves students directly providing patient care, which can present risks if proper supervision, guidance and safety protocols are not in place. Ensuring that students are adequately prepared and supported to deliver safe care is essential.
4. **Integration of theory and practice**: It can be challenging to seamlessly integrate theoretical knowledge with practical experiences. Nursing students may struggle to connect classroom learning to real-life patient care situations, which requires effective teaching strategies and support from faculty members.
5. **Evaluation and assessment**: Assessing students' performance in the Practical Model can be complex. It requires comprehensive evaluation methods to capture the development of both clinical skills and critical thinking abilities. Faculty members need to design appropriate assessment tools and provide timely and constructive feedback to nursing students.

CHARACTERISTICS OF AN EFFECTIVE CLINICAL TEACHER

Effective clinical teachers are those who can effectively facilitate student learning in a clinical setting. They are able to create a safe and supportive learning environment, provide clear and concise instructions and provide constructive feedback. Here are some of the characteristics of effective clinical teachers:

- **Expertise:** An effective clinical teacher possesses a high level of expertise in their field of practice. They have a deep understanding of the subject matter and keep their knowledge and skills up to date.
- **Clear communication:** Effective clinical teachers have strong communication skills and can clearly convey information to students. They use appropriate language, provide explanations in a concise manner and actively listen to students' questions and concerns.
- **Adaptability:** Effective clinical teachers are flexible and adaptable to the diverse needs of their students. They can adjust their teaching strategies to accommodate different learning styles and adapt to varying clinical settings or patient populations.
- **Approachability and supportiveness:** Effective clinical teachers create a supportive and approachable learning environment. They foster open communication, encourage questions and provide constructive feedback to help students learn and grow.
- **Role modelling:** Effective clinical teachers serve as positive role models for students. They demonstrate professionalism, ethical behaviour and compassionate patient care. They exhibit a strong work ethic, empathy and respect for all members of the healthcare team.
- **Motivation**: Effective clinical teachers are able to motivate and inspire students to learn. They are able to create a positive and supportive learning environment, and they are able to challenge students to reach their full potential.
- **Patient-centred focus:** Effective clinical teachers emphasize the importance of patient-centred care. They teach students to prioritize patients' needs and preferences, involve them in decision-making and consider their holistic well-being.
- **Critical thinking and problem-solving skills**: Effective clinical teachers promote critical thinking and problem-solving skills in their students. They encourage students to analyse complex situations, consider evidence-based practice and make sound clinical judgements.
- **Mentorship and guidance skills:** Effective clinical teachers provide mentorship and guidance to students. They offer support, encouragement and opportunities for professional growth. They help students set goals, reflect on their experiences and develop their clinical competencies.
- **Organizational skills**: Effective clinical teachers are able to organize and manage their time effectively. They are able to plan and implement clinical activities, and they are able to keep track of student progress.
- **Evaluation and feedback skills:** Effective clinical teachers provide timely and constructive feedback to students. They assess students' performance objectively, identify areas for improvement and offer guidance on how to enhance their clinical skills and knowledge.
- **Lifelong learning:** Effective clinical teachers demonstrate a commitment to lifelong learning. They engage in continuous professional development, stay updated with current evidence-based practices and model the importance of ongoing learning to their students.

In addition to these characteristics, effective clinical teachers are also patient, enthusiastic and committed to their students' success. They are able to create a positive and supportive learning environment where students feel comfortable asking questions and making mistakes. They are also able to provide constructive feedback that helps students to improve their skills and knowledge.

WRITING CLINICAL LEARNING OUTCOMES/PRACTICAL COMPETENCIES

Clinical learning outcomes and practical competencies are essential components of healthcare education and training programmes. These outcomes and competencies define the knowledge, skills and attitudes that students should acquire during their clinical training to become competent healthcare professionals.

Clinical learning outcomes are specific goals that describe what students are expected to achieve by the end of their clinical training. These outcomes provide a clear direction and focus for students and educators, ensuring that the learning experience is purposeful and aligned with the desired competencies.

Practical competencies, on the other hand, refer to the specific abilities and skills that students need to develop to effectively perform tasks and responsibilities within their chosen healthcare field. These competencies are practical in nature and directly applicable to real-world patient care scenarios.

DEFINITIONS

- 'Clinical learning outcomes are the specific skills, knowledge, and attitudes that nursing students are expected to demonstrate in the clinical setting. They are typically derived from the nursing curriculum and are aligned with the professional nursing standards'. (Oermann & Gaberson, 2021)
- 'Clinical expertise is the ability to make sound clinical judgments in complex and uncertain situations. It is developed over time through experience and reflection'. (Benner, 2010)
- 'Clinical competencies are the skills and abilities that nurses need to provide safe and effective care. They are typically assessed through a combination of clinical performance, written exams, and other assessments'. (Tanner, 2009)

It is important to note that there is no one-size-fits-all definition, as the specific outcomes/competencies will vary depending on the nursing programme and the clinical setting.

Here are some examples of clinical learning outcomes/practical competencies that are commonly assessed in nursing education:

- *Communication skills:* The ability to communicate effectively with patients, families and other healthcare professionals.
- *Assessment skills:* The ability to collect and interpret patient data.
- *Planning skills:* The ability to develop and implement a plan of care for patients.
- *Implementation skills:* The ability to provide safe and effective care to patients.
- *Evaluation skills:* The ability to assess the effectiveness of care and make necessary adjustments.

GUIDELINES TO WRITE CLINICAL LEARNING OUTCOMES/ PRACTICAL COMPETENCIES

- Begin by clearly identifying the desired knowledge, skills and attitudes that nursing students should acquire during their clinical training.
- Use action verbs that describe observable and measurable behaviours to specify what students should be able to do.
- Ensure that the clinical learning outcomes/practical competencies align with professional standards and guidelines.

- Keep the outcomes/practical competencies concise and focused, avoiding excessive detail.
- Use specific language to clearly define the expected performance levels and criteria for achievement.
- Consider the context and scope of nursing practice, taking into account different healthcare settings and patient populations.
- Involve stakeholders such as faculty members, clinical preceptors and nursing professionals to gather input and ensure the relevance and comprehensiveness of the outcomes/practical competencies.
- Balance specificity and flexibility to allow for adaptability to evolving healthcare needs.
- Provide a logical progression of learning outcomes/practical competencies, building upon foundational knowledge and skills.
- Consider the integration of theoretical knowledge and practical application to promote the synthesis of knowledge and skills.
- Align the outcomes/practical competencies with the programme's curriculum, instructional strategies and assessment methods.
- Regularly review and update the clinical learning outcomes/practical competencies to stay current with changes in healthcare practice and standards.
- Clearly communicate the clinical learning outcomes/practical competencies to students, faculty and other stakeholders to ensure a shared understanding and facilitate the learning process.

Remember, these guidelines are intended to provide a starting point for writing clinical learning outcomes/practical competencies in nursing education. It is important to adapt them to the specific context and requirements of your nursing programme, considering the unique needs of your students and the healthcare landscape in which they will practice.

BENEFITS OF WRITING CLINICAL LEARNING OUTCOMES/ PRACTICAL COMPETENCIES

1. **Clarity and focus**: Writing clear and specific clinical learning outcomes/practical competencies helps provide clarity and focus for nursing education programmes. It ensures that educators and students have a shared understanding of the expected knowledge, skills and attitudes to be achieved.
2. **Alignment with professional standards**: Clinical learning outcomes/practical competencies are often aligned with professional standards and guidelines set by nursing regulatory bodies. By aligning education outcomes with these standards, nursing programmes ensure that graduates are well-prepared to meet the professional expectations of the nursing profession.
3. **Guidance for curriculum development**: Clear clinical learning outcomes/practical competencies serve as a guide for curriculum development in nursing education. They assist educators in selecting appropriate learning experiences, instructional strategies and assessment methods that align with the desired outcomes.
4. **Assessment and evaluation**: Well-defined clinical learning outcomes/practical competencies provide a basis for assessing and evaluating student performance. Educators can develop assessment tools and rubrics to measure the achievement of specific competencies, ensuring that students are progressing and meeting the desired learning outcomes.
5. **Student motivation and engagement**: Clearly defined clinical learning outcomes/practical competencies help students understand the relevance and purpose of their education. This can enhance their motivation and engagement in the learning process, as they have a clear understanding of what they are working towards and why it is important.

CHALLENGES IN WRITING CLINICAL LEARNING OUTCOMES/ PRACTICAL COMPETENCIES

1. **Balancing specificity and flexibility**: Striking the right balance between specific and flexible clinical learning outcomes/practical competencies can be challenging. While specific outcomes provide clarity, they may limit the adaptability of the curriculum to evolving healthcare needs. Finding the right level of specificity that allows for flexibility is crucial.
2. **Alignment with evolving healthcare landscape**: The healthcare landscape is constantly evolving, with new technologies, evidence-based practices and healthcare delivery models emerging. Writing clinical learning outcomes/practical competencies that remain relevant and adaptable to these changes can be a challenge for nursing educators.
3. **Resource limitations**: Developing and implementing educational programmes that align with comprehensive clinical learning outcomes/practical competencies can require significant resources, including faculty expertise, time and financial support. Limited resources can pose challenges in adequately addressing and assessing all desired competencies.
4. **Standardization across programmes**: Ensuring consistency and standardization in clinical learning outcomes/practical competencies across different nursing programmes can be challenging. Different educational institutions may have varying interpretations and priorities, which can impact the comparability of nursing graduates' competencies.
5. **Evaluation and measurement**: Assessing student achievement of clinical learning outcomes/ practical competencies can be complex. Developing valid and reliable assessment methods that capture the desired competencies requires careful planning, faculty training and ongoing evaluation to ensure the accuracy and consistency of assessments.

Despite these challenges, the benefits of writing clinical learning outcomes/practical competencies in nursing education outweigh the difficulties. With careful consideration and collaboration among educators, regulatory bodies and healthcare stakeholders, nursing programmes can develop meaningful and relevant clinical learning outcomes/practical competencies that prepare graduates for successful nursing careers.

CLINICAL TEACHING STRATEGIES

Clinical teaching, supervision and mentorship requires special strategies. There are numerous clinical teaching strategies such as patient assignment, clinical conference, clinical presentation, bedside clinics, case study/care study, nursing rounds, concept mapping, project, debate, game, role-play, simulation, problem-based learning, questioning, written assignment and process recording, which are discussed in this section.

PATIENT ASSIGNMENT

Patient assignment is a clinical teaching method commonly used in nursing education to provide students with hands-on learning experiences in healthcare settings. It involves assigning nursing students to care for specific patients under the supervision of a registered nurse or clinical instructor. This method allows students to apply their theoretical knowledge and develop essential clinical skills while caring for real patients in various healthcare settings, such as hospitals, clinics or long-term care facilities.

DEFINITIONS

- Bevis and Oermann (1999) define patient assignment as 'the process of assigning patients to students for clinical instruction'.
- Tanner (2000) defines patient assignment as 'the process of matching students with patients for the purpose of providing care and learning'.
- Henderson (2001) defines patient assignment as 'the process of assigning students to patients for the purpose of providing care and learning, under the supervision of a registered nurse'.

These definitions all emphasize the importance of patient assignment as a clinical teaching method in nursing. Patient assignment allows students to apply their theoretical knowledge to real-world situations and to develop their clinical skills under the supervision of a registered nurse.

FACTORS INFLUENCE PATIENT ASSIGNMENT IN CLINICAL TEACHING

Several factors can influence patient assignment in clinical teaching. These factors need to be considered to ensure an optimal learning experience for students while maintaining patient safety and quality of care. Some of the key factors include:

1. **Educational level**: The educational level of the students is an important factor in patient assignment. Students at different stages of their education may have varying levels of knowledge, skills and competencies. Assigning patients that align with the students' educational level allows for appropriate learning opportunities and challenges that match their capabilities.
2. **Learning objectives**: The specific learning objectives of the clinical course or rotation play a crucial role in patient assignment. The objectives may focus on specific skills, procedures or clinical conditions. Patients should be selected in a way that aligns with the learning objectives, providing students with the necessary exposure and opportunities to achieve those objectives.
3. **Patient complexity and acuity**: The complexity and acuity of patients' healthcare needs are important considerations. Students should be assigned patients whose conditions and care requirements match their educational level and learning objectives. Assigning patients with a range of complexity ensures that students are exposed to diverse clinical situations and challenges, enabling them to develop a comprehensive understanding of patient care.
4. **Clinical setting**: The clinical setting or healthcare facility can impact patient assignment. Different settings, such as hospitals, clinics or long-term care facilities, offer distinct patient populations and care environments. Students may benefit from exposure to a variety of settings to gain a broader understanding of healthcare delivery.
5. **Clinical instructor expertise**: The expertise and experience of the clinical instructors or preceptors involved in the teaching process can influence patient assignment. Assigning patients that align with the instructors' areas of expertise allows for effective guidance, supervision and mentorship. Instructors with specialized knowledge can facilitate students' learning and provide valuable insights and support.
6. **Patient preferences and consent**: Patient preferences and consent should be considered when assigning patients to students. Some patients may have preferences regarding the involvement of students in their care. Respecting patient autonomy and preferences is crucial, and assignments should be made in collaboration with patients and their families, ensuring they understand the educational nature of the student's involvement.

7. **Ethical and legal considerations**: Ethical and legal considerations play a vital role in patient assignment. Students must adhere to professional codes of ethics and patient confidentiality. Assignments should comply with institutional policies, privacy regulations and any applicable legal requirements.

BENEFITS OF PATIENT ASSIGNMENT

1. **Practical application of knowledge:** Patient assignment allows students to apply their theoretical knowledge in real-world clinical scenarios. They have the opportunity to observe and participate in patient care, translating textbook concepts into practical skills and interventions.
2. **Skill development:** Working with assigned patients helps students develop and refine their clinical skills. They gain hands-on experience in performing assessments, administering medications, conducting procedures and managing patient care. This enhances their technical competencies and confidence in delivering safe and effective care.
3. **Critical thinking and decision-making:** Patient assignment promotes critical thinking and clinical reasoning. Students must analyse patient data, prioritize needs and make decisions about appropriate interventions. This cultivates their ability to think critically, solve problems and make evidence-based decisions in complex clinical situations.
4. **Interpersonal communication:** Through patient assignment, students develop effective communication and interpersonal skills. They learn to interact with patients, families and healthcare team members, improving their ability to convey information, actively listen and provide emotional support. This enhances their capacity to establish therapeutic relationships and deliver patient-centred care.
5. **Interdisciplinary collaboration:** Patient assignment exposes students to interdisciplinary collaboration. They work alongside other healthcare professionals, fostering teamwork, mutual respect and understanding of various roles and responsibilities. This promotes effective communication, shared decision-making and an appreciation for the holistic nature of patient care.

CHALLENGES OF PATIENT ASSIGNMENT

1. **Patient safety:** Ensuring patient safety is paramount when assigning students to patients. There is a risk of errors or inadequate care if students are not adequately supervised or if assignments are beyond their competency level. Close monitoring and supervision by clinical instructors are essential to mitigate this challenge.
2. **Patient privacy and confidentiality:** Respecting patient privacy and maintaining confidentiality can be challenging when assigning students to patients. Students must understand and adhere to ethical and legal standards regarding patient information. Proper training and clear guidelines are necessary to address this challenge.
3. **Limited resources:** Availability of appropriate patients, clinical sites and resources can be a constraint in patient assignment. It may be challenging to match students with specific patient conditions or to provide a diverse range of clinical experiences. Optimizing the utilization of available resources and ensuring equitable access to learning opportunities can help overcome this challenge.
4. **Patient preferences and consent:** Patient preferences regarding student involvement in their care can vary. Some patients may decline or have reservations about student participation. Respecting

patient autonomy and preferences while ensuring students have adequate learning opportunities can be challenging. Clear communication, patient education and informed consent processes are essential to manage this challenge.

Addressing these challenges requires effective communication, collaboration and ongoing evaluation among nursing faculty, clinical instructors and healthcare facility staff. Clear guidelines, supervision and support systems help ensure patient safety, ethical practice and meaningful learning experiences for students.

CLINICAL CONFERENCE

A clinical conference is a teaching method commonly used in medical education to enhance clinical reasoning and decision-making skills among healthcare professionals, including physicians, residents and medical and nursing students. It provides a platform for interactive discussions and learning from real patient cases.

Clinical conferences are also widely used as a teaching method in nursing education. They offer an interactive and case-based approach to enhance critical thinking, clinical judgement and problem-solving skills among nursing students and practising nurses.

DEFINITIONS

There are many different definitions of clinical conference as a teaching method in nursing. However, most authors agree that it is a group discussion led by a faculty member in which students share their experiences and learn from each other. Here are some definitions of clinical conference from different authors:

- 'A clinical conference is a group discussion led by a faculty member in which students share their experiences and learn from each other'. (Werner-McCullough & L'Orange, 1985)
- 'A clinical conference is a teaching method in which students discuss their clinical experiences with a faculty member'. (American Nurses Association, 2010)
- 'A clinical conference is a forum for students to share their clinical experiences, learn from each other, and receive feedback from a faculty member'. (National League for Nursing, 2013)

PURPOSES

i. Clinical conferences serve several important purposes in nursing education. These purposes are designed to enhance the learning experience, develop critical thinking skills and prepare nursing students for real-world nursing practice. Here are some key purposes of clinical conferences in nursing education:

ii. **Integration of theory and practice**: Clinical conferences provide a platform for nursing students to bridge the gap between theoretical knowledge gained in the classroom and its application in clinical settings. By analysing real patient cases, students can apply their theoretical knowledge to practical situations, facilitating the integration of theory and practice.

iii. **Critical thinking and clinical reasoning**: Clinical conferences stimulate critical thinking and clinical reasoning skills in nursing students. Through case discussions, students learn to analyse and interpret patient data, identify relevant nursing diagnoses and develop appropriate nursing interventions. This process helps students develop sound judgement and make evidence-based decisions in clinical practice.

- iv. **Problem solving and decision-making**: Nursing is a profession that requires effective problem-solving and decision-making skills. Clinical conferences provide nursing students with opportunities to analyse complex patient scenarios, consider alternative approaches and make informed decisions regarding patient care. By engaging in case discussions, students develop their problem-solving abilities and gain confidence in their decision-making skills.
- v. **Collaboration and interdisciplinary teamwork**: Nursing is a collaborative profession that often involves working with a multidisciplinary healthcare team. Clinical conferences promote collaboration and interdisciplinary teamwork by providing a platform for students to interact with other healthcare professionals, such as physicians, pharmacists and therapists. Students learn to appreciate different perspectives, communicate effectively and contribute to a collaborative healthcare environment.
- vi. **Application of evidence-based practice**: Clinical conferences foster the application of evidence-based practice in nursing. Students are encouraged to critically evaluate research evidence, guidelines and best practices relevant to the presented cases. This promotes the integration of current knowledge into nursing care and prepares students to provide evidence-based, high-quality care to their patients.
- vii. **Reflective practice and self-assessment**: Clinical conferences encourage nursing students to engage in reflective practice and self-assessment. Through case discussions, students can reflect on their clinical experiences, identify strengths and areas for improvement and enhance their self-awareness as developing professionals. This self-reflection contributes to ongoing personal and professional growth.
- viii. **Professional development and networking**: Clinical conferences offer nursing students opportunities for professional development and networking. They allow students to interact with experienced nursing professionals, engage in mentorship relationships and establish connections within the nursing community. Attending conferences can broaden students' perspectives, expose them to new ideas and innovations and inspire lifelong learning.

Overall, clinical conferences in nursing education serve the various purpose and are vital in preparing nursing students to become competent and confident professionals in the dynamic healthcare field.

STEPS TO ORGANIZE CLINICAL CONFERENCE

Using a clinical conference as a teaching method in nursing can be an effective way to engage students and enhance their learning experience. Here are the steps involved in implementing a clinical conference as a teaching method in nursing:

1. **Identify the learning objectives**: Determine the specific learning objectives you want to achieve through the clinical conference. These objectives should align with the curriculum and focus on developing critical thinking, clinical reasoning and evidence-based practice skills among nursing students.
2. **Select a relevant patient case**: Choose a patient case that is appropriate for the learning objectives and the level of the students. The case should be complex enough to challenge students and encourage critical thinking. Ensure that the case is de-identified and respects patient confidentiality.
3. **Prepare the case presentation**: Gather relevant patient information, including medical history, physical examination findings, laboratory results and imaging studies. Organize the information in a coherent and structured manner to facilitate case presentation during the conference.
4. **Introduce the case to the students**: Begin the clinical conference by introducing the patient case to the students. Provide a brief overview of the patient's background, presenting symptoms

and relevant clinical findings. Emphasize the importance of active participation and engagement throughout the conference.

5. **Facilitate case-based discussion**: Encourage students to discuss the case and ask questions. Guide the discussion by asking open-ended questions that promote critical thinking and encourage students to consider different perspectives. Allow students to share their thoughts, propose differential diagnoses and discuss potential nursing interventions.
6. **Integrate evidence-based practice**: Incorporate evidence-based practice principles into the clinical conference. Encourage students to critically appraise relevant research literature, guidelines and best practices. Discuss how the evidence can be applied to the patient case and guide nursing interventions.
7. **Foster collaborative learning**: Promote collaboration and teamwork among the students during the conference. Encourage students to work together, share their knowledge and experiences and learn from each other. Facilitate discussions that allow students to appreciate the contributions of different nursing specialties and the importance of interdisciplinary collaboration.
8. **Reflect on the learning experience**: Conclude the clinical conference by facilitating a reflective discussion. Encourage students to reflect on what they have learned, identify gaps in their knowledge or skills and set goals for further learning. Provide an opportunity for students to share their insights, challenges and personal growth resulting from the clinical conference.
9. **Follow-up and assessment**: Provide resources, references or additional learning materials related to the case or topics discussed during the clinical conference. Assess student learning through quizzes, case-based assignments or reflective journaling to ensure that the desired learning outcomes have been achieved.

BENEFITS OF CLINICAL CONFERENCES

1. Promotes active learning and engagement among nursing students.
2. Enhances critical thinking and clinical reasoning skills.
3. Encourages evidence-based practice and integration of research findings.
4. Fosters interdisciplinary collaboration and teamwork.
5. Provides opportunities for students to learn from real patient cases.
6. Facilitates networking and professional development within the nursing community.

LIMITATIONS OF CLINICAL CONFERENCES

1. Requires adequate time and resources for planning and organization.
2. May not accommodate a large number of students or participants.
3. Limited opportunity for individualized instruction or personalized feedback.
4. Relies heavily on the expertise and availability of speakers and presenters.
5. Challenges in maintaining confidentiality and privacy when discussing patient cases.

CLINICAL PRESENTATION

Clinical presentation is a method of teaching that involves the direct observation and explanation of patient cases or clinical scenarios. It is commonly used in medical and healthcare education to enhance students' clinical skills, knowledge and decision-making abilities.

Clinical presentation is an effective method of teaching in nursing that involves the direct observation and analysis of patient cases or clinical scenarios. It is a dynamic and interactive approach that brings real-world clinical situations into the educational setting, allowing nursing students to apply their knowledge, develop critical thinking skills and enhance their clinical decision-making abilities.

DEFINITIONS

- Werner-McCullough and L'Orange (1985) define clinical presentation as 'a group discussion led by a faculty member in which students share their experiences and learn from each other'.
- American Nurses Association (2010) defines clinical presentation as 'a teaching method in which students discuss their clinical experiences with a faculty member'.
- National League for Nursing (2013) defines clinical presentation as 'a forum for students to share their clinical experiences, learn from each other, and receive feedback from a faculty member'.

These definitions all emphasize the importance of students sharing their clinical experiences in a group setting. This allows students to learn from each other, to receive feedback from a faculty member and to develop critical thinking skills.

PURPOSES

Clinical presentation as a method of teaching in nursing serves several important purposes. Here are the key purposes and objectives of using clinical presentation as a teaching method in nursing:

1. **Application of theoretical knowledge**: Clinical presentations allow nursing students to apply their theoretical knowledge to real-life patient scenarios. It helps them bridge the gap between classroom learning and clinical practice by demonstrating how nursing concepts and theories are utilized in the care of actual patients.
2. **Development of critical thinking skills**: Clinical presentations stimulate critical thinking among nursing students. They are encouraged to analyse and interpret patient data, identify relevant nursing diagnoses and formulate appropriate nursing interventions. This process enhances their ability to think critically and make sound clinical judgements.
3. **Integration of clinical reasoning**: By presenting complex patient cases, clinical presentations promote the integration of clinical reasoning skills. Nursing students learn to consider multiple factors, evaluate evidence and make informed decisions about patient care. They develop the ability to prioritize and address the unique needs of each patient.
4. **Enhancement of communication skills**: Clinical presentations provide opportunities for nursing students to practice their communication skills. They learn to present patient cases effectively, articulate their thoughts and engage in discussions with peers and instructors. This improves their ability to communicate and collaborate with healthcare team members and patients.
5. **Exposure to diverse patient populations**: Through clinical presentations, nursing students are exposed to a variety of patient cases representing diverse populations. This exposure enhances their cultural competency and understanding of the unique challenges faced by different patient groups. It promotes sensitivity and adaptability in providing patient-centred care.
6. **Promotion of evidence-based practice**: Clinical presentations emphasize the use of evidence-based practice in nursing. Students learn to critically evaluate research findings, guidelines and best practices and apply this knowledge to make informed decisions about patient care. They develop skills in accessing and utilizing relevant evidence to guide their practice.

7. **Exploration of ethical considerations**: Clinical presentations often include ethical dilemmas or challenging ethical situations. This allows nursing students to explore ethical considerations in patient care, such as autonomy, beneficence and justice. It encourages them to reflect on ethical decision-making and develop a strong ethical foundation in their nursing practice.
8. **Engagement and motivation**: Clinical presentations capture the attention and interest of nursing students. The use of real patient cases and interactive discussions promotes engagement and motivation for learning. It provides a dynamic and practical learning experience that fosters curiosity and lifelong learning among nursing students.

By fulfilling these purposes, clinical presentations as a teaching method in nursing contribute to the development of competent, compassionate and evidence-based nursing professionals who are well-prepared to meet the challenges of the healthcare setting.

STEPS TO ORGANIZE CLINICAL PRESENTATION

Organizing a clinical presentation as a method of teaching in nursing involves careful planning and preparation to ensure its effectiveness. Here are the key steps to consider when organizing a clinical presentation:

1. **Determine the learning objectives**: Clearly define the specific learning objectives you want to achieve through the clinical presentation. These objectives should align with the curriculum and focus on the development of critical thinking, clinical reasoning and application of theoretical knowledge.
2. **Select appropriate patient cases**: Choose patient cases that are relevant to the learning objectives and reflect the level of the nursing students. The cases should be diverse and representative of different health conditions, age groups and cultural backgrounds. Ensure that patient privacy and confidentiality are maintained by de-identifying the cases.
3. **Gather relevant clinical data**: Collect all relevant clinical data related to the selected patient cases. This may include medical history, physical examination findings, laboratory results, diagnostic tests and imaging studies. Organize the data in a structured and coherent manner to present it effectively during the clinical presentation.
4. **Prepare presentation materials**: Develop presentation materials that effectively convey the patient cases and relevant clinical information. This may include PowerPoint slides, handouts or multimedia resources. Ensure that the presentation materials are clear, concise and visually appealing to facilitate understanding and engagement.
5. **Engage participants in active learning**: Plan interactive activities and discussions to engage the nursing students during the clinical presentation. Encourage them to actively participate, ask questions and share their thoughts and perspectives on the presented cases. Use case-based questions and scenarios to stimulate critical thinking and clinical reasoning.
6. **Facilitate group discussions**: Allocate sufficient time for group discussions to allow nursing students to analyse and discuss the patient cases. Guide the discussions by asking thought-provoking questions, facilitating peer-to-peer learning and providing clarification when needed. Encourage students to share their insights, experiences and potential nursing interventions.
7. **Integrate evidence-based practice**: Emphasize the importance of evidence-based practice during the clinical presentation. Encourage nursing students to critically evaluate research evidence, guidelines and best practices related to the presented cases. Discuss how evidence can inform nursing interventions and decision-making in patient care.
8. **Provide resources and references**: Share relevant resources and references with the nursing students to support their learning and further exploration of the presented topics. This may include journal articles, textbooks, websites or clinical guidelines. Ensure that the resources are credible, up-to-date and accessible to the students.

9. **Evaluate and provide feedback**: Assess the effectiveness of the clinical presentation and gather feedback from the nursing students. This can be done through surveys, quizzes or reflective exercises. Use the feedback to identify areas for improvement and make adjustments to future clinical presentations.

By following these steps, you can effectively organize a clinical presentation as a method of teaching in nursing. This will create a stimulating and engaging learning experience for nursing students, facilitating their development of critical thinking, clinical reasoning and application of theoretical knowledge in patient care.

BENEFITS OF CLINICAL PRESENTATION

i. Real-world relevance and application of theoretical knowledge.
ii. Active learning and student engagement.
iii. Development of critical thinking skills.
iv. Integration of knowledge and skills.
v. Promotion of collaboration and communication among students.
vi. Exposure to diverse patient cases and populations.

LIMITATIONS OF CLINICAL PRESENTATION

i. Time-consuming in terms of case selection, data gathering and presentation preparation.
ii. Limited opportunity for individualized instruction and personalized feedback.
iii. Reliance on the availability and expertise of presenters.
iv. Challenges in maintaining patient privacy and confidentiality.

BEDSIDE CLINIC

All clinical teaching methods aim to enhance patient care and provide students with knowledge about the clinical or hospital environment. One such method is bedside teaching. During bedside clinics, we discuss nursing care specific to individual patients, applying principles and practices to real-life scenarios. This approach helps improve learners' observation, communication and interviewing skills.

Bedside clinic, also known as bedside teaching, is a method of teaching in healthcare, including nursing, that involves direct observation and instruction at the patient's bedside. It is a valuable educational approach that allows students to learn in the actual clinical setting and interact with patients under the guidance of experienced healthcare professionals.

DEFINITIONS

- Somodra defines bedside clinic as 'a clinical teaching method where nursing supervisor/tutor meet with their subordinates or nursing students in order to carry out nursing instruction in presence of the patient at the bedside. It is a teaching in the presence of the patient'.
- JaypeeDigital defines bedside clinic as 'a process in which a clinical teacher and a group of learners sees a patient, elicits or verifies physical signs, discusses provisional diagnosis, diagnostic or therapeutic options in the clinical setting'.

- Nursing Education Perspectives defines bedside clinic as 'a teaching method in which students are paired with a clinical instructor to provide care for a patient. The instructor and student discuss the patient's care plan, assess the patient's condition, and implement interventions. Bedside clinics provide students with the opportunity to apply their knowledge to real-world situations and to develop their critical thinking skills'.

Bedside clinic is a valuable teaching method that can help nursing students to develop the skills and knowledge they need to provide safe and effective care to patients. It is a hands-on learning experience that allows students to see how the theories they learn in the classroom are applied in practice. Bedside clinic can also help students to develop their communication, critical thinking and problem-solving skills.

PURPOSES

Bedside clinics in nursing education serve several important purposes. Here are the key purposes and objectives of utilizing bedside clinics:

1. **Application of theoretical knowledge**: Bedside clinics provide nursing students with the opportunity to apply their theoretical knowledge in a practical and clinical setting. They can observe and apply nursing concepts, principles and skills learned in the classroom to real patient care situations.
2. **Development of clinical assessment skills**: Bedside clinics allow nursing students to practice and develop their clinical assessment skills. They can observe and assess patients' physical conditions, vital signs and other relevant clinical indicators. This helps students become proficient in conducting thorough and accurate patient assessments.
3. **Integration of clinical skills**: Bedside clinics facilitate the integration of clinical skills in nursing practice. Students can directly perform nursing interventions, such as medication administration, wound care or patient hygiene, under the supervision of experienced instructors or preceptors.
4. **Observation of clinical decision-making**: Nursing students can observe and learn from the clinical decision-making process during bedside clinics. They can witness how experienced nurses and healthcare professionals assess patient conditions, develop care plans and make critical decisions to ensure optimal patient outcomes.
5. **Interprofessional collaboration**: Bedside clinics provide opportunities for nursing students to engage in interprofessional collaboration. They can work alongside other healthcare professionals, such as physicians, pharmacists and therapists, to understand the collaborative nature of patient care and the importance of effective teamwork.
6. **Communication and patient interaction**: Bedside clinics promote communication and patient interaction skills in nursing students. They have the chance to communicate directly with patients, families and healthcare team members, enhancing their ability to establish therapeutic relationships, provide patient-centred care and effectively convey information.
7. **Ethical considerations**: Bedside clinics expose nursing students to ethical dilemmas and discussions related to patient care. They learn to navigate ethical considerations, respect patient autonomy and uphold confidentiality and privacy principles in healthcare practice.
8. **Professional development and confidence-building**: Bedside clinics contribute to the professional development of nursing students. They gain confidence in their clinical skills, develop professionalism and build self-assurance in their ability to provide safe and competent nursing care.
9. **Reflective practice and continuous learning**: Bedside clinics encourage nursing students to engage in reflective practice and continuous learning. They can reflect on their observations,

experiences and interactions with patients, identifying areas for improvement and further professional growth.

STEPS TO ORGANIZE BEDSIDE CLINICS

Organizing bedside clinics in nursing education requires careful planning and coordination to ensure a meaningful and effective learning experience. Here are the key steps to consider when organizing bedside clinics:

1. **Identify learning objectives**: Clearly define the specific learning objectives you want to achieve through the bedside clinics. These objectives should align with the curriculum and focus on the development of clinical assessment skills, integration of theoretical knowledge and promotion of interprofessional collaboration.
2. **Select appropriate clinical settings**: Choose clinical settings, such as hospital units or healthcare facilities, where nursing students can have access to a diverse patient population and opportunities for hands-on learning. Consider the availability of patients with varying health conditions and the ability to maintain patient privacy and confidentiality.
3. **Coordinate with healthcare professionals**: Collaborate with healthcare professionals, such as nurses, physicians or clinical instructors, to ensure their involvement and support in conducting the bedside clinics. Inform them about the purpose and objectives of the sessions and discuss their roles and responsibilities during the clinics.
4. **Schedule and logistics**: Determine the schedule and logistics of the bedside clinics, including the duration, frequency and number of nursing students per session. Consider factors such as the availability of patients, staffing considerations and the availability of instructors or preceptors.
5. **Prepare student materials**: Develop educational materials for nursing students to support their learning during the bedside clinics. This may include case studies, patient assessment tools, relevant guidelines and reference materials. Ensure that the materials are easily accessible and aligned with the learning objectives.
6. **Preparing patients and obtaining consent**: Communicate with patients and obtain their informed consent for nursing students to participate in the bedside clinics. Explain the purpose of the clinics, ensure patient privacy and confidentiality and address any concerns or questions they may have. Respect patient autonomy and their right to decline participation.
7. **Orientation and preclinic briefing**: Conduct an orientation session or preclinic briefing for nursing students before the bedside clinics. Provide an overview of the learning objectives, expectations and guidelines for professional conduct. Review essential clinical skills, assessment techniques and communication strategies to prepare students for the clinical setting.
8. **Facilitate the bedside clinics**: During the bedside clinics, facilitate student learning by guiding them through patient assessments, encouraging active participation and promoting discussion and reflection. Foster interprofessional collaboration by involving other healthcare professionals and encouraging teamwork.
9. **Debriefing and reflection**: After each bedside clinic session, facilitate a debriefing session to allow students to reflect on their experiences, share insights and discuss the clinical decision-making process. Encourage students to reflect on their performance, identify areas for improvement and apply lessons learned in future patient care encounters.
10. **Evaluation and feedback**: Evaluate the effectiveness of the bedside clinics and gather feedback from nursing students and healthcare professionals. Use this feedback to identify strengths, areas for improvement and make necessary adjustments to enhance future bedside clinic sessions.

BENEFITS OF BEDSIDE CLINICS

i. Promote real-world application of theoretical knowledge.
ii. Enhance hands-on learning experience.
iii. Development of observation and critical thinking skills.
iv. Promotion of interprofessional collaboration.
v. Improved patient interaction and communication skills.
vi. Integration of skills and knowledge.
vii. Exposure to ethical considerations in patient care.

LIMITATIONS OF BEDSIDE CLINICS

i. Limited availability of appropriate patients.
ii. Time constraints in managing patient assessments and discussions.
iii. Maintaining patient privacy and confidentiality.
iv. Variation in the complexity of patient cases.
v. Dependence on instructor availability and expertise.
vi. Challenges in providing individualized instruction and feedback.

CASE STUDY/CARE STUDY

Nursing case study is the blueprint of nursing care rendered by a nursing student to a selected patient, for a particular period by following nursing process approach, with an intention to develop comprehensive nursing care abilities.

I. PURPOSES OF CASE STUDY

- It provides an opportunity to the student to learn nursing skills using the problem-solving approach.
- Students learn to identify and define a patient's problem.
- It trains the students to locate, gather and process the information required to solve the patient's problem.
- It develops a sense of accomplishment from providing individualized comprehensive care.
- It helps the student solve the patient's problems by critical and reflective thinking.
- It emphasizes the facts that the patient is an individual personality with unique problems.
- It accentuates the health and social aspects of nursing.
- It points out the relationship and cooperation of the various agencies interested in the patient's problems and welfare such as social service and public health nursing.

II. PRINCIPLES OF CASE STUDY

- The students should be able to make their nursing care study on a patient for whose nursing care they are responsible for.
- The selection of patients can be done by coordination between the clinical instructor and students.
- With the help of a case study, the student should be able to study the patient's state of health and self-help abilities, his cultural background, his economic level, hobbies and interests, as an understanding of all these factors will contribute to the patient's welfare.

- The first part of the study should be concerned with information and facts about the patient, his disease condition and his social and personal history, and how this knowledge is applied in providing nursing care to the patient.
- The second part of the nursing study takes in the responsibilities and the activities the nursing student will be concerned with in giving complete comprehensive nursing care to the patient.
- It should emphasize on the individual needs of a patient and how they are met.
- Special emphasis should be made on patient learning.
- If outpatient experience and home nursing is included in the study, it helps in better evaluation of the patient's recovery and his ability to maintain healthy health habits.
- It should serve as an excellent tool to demonstrate nursing skills, scientific knowledge and sociological or psychological insight into the problems of the patient.
- It should encourage critical evaluation of solutions presented by others. The student is presented with the whole situation so that she may visualize it completely.

III. FORMS AND PRESENTATION OF CASE STUDY

- Written
- Verbal/oral

ADVANTAGES OF CASE STUDY

Written Case Study

- It provides for individual differences of the student.
- It provides an opportunity for self-expression in writing.
- It provides experience in organizing and writing a paper in a scientific manner.
- It provides a source of material for future reference.

Oral Case Study

- It provides an opportunity for the instructor to direct student thinking into new channels and to correct errors of information.
- It serves as a basis for better personal understanding and relationship between the instructor and the student.
- It is time-saving and does not require lengthy recopying of the notes to acceptable forms.
- It offers an opportunity for a public-speaking experience.
- If discussion is invited after presentation, the case becomes cooperative and everyone involved benefits from the study. This is a source of motivation to the student because she shares the benefits of her study with other students.
- The student feels the thrill of achievement in presenting her study to others.

DISADVANTAGES OF CASE STUDY

Written Case Study

- It gives no opportunity to branch out and incorporate new ideas once the study is completed.
- It requires a great deal of time to rewrite to an acceptable form.

Oral Case Study

- It does not offer an opportunity for writing and other creative expressions, since only notes are used for the presentation.
- It leaves no records that may be kept for future reference as it is used generally.

NURSING ROUNDS

Nurses and nursing students acquire knowledge through various methods, including courses, accredited programmes, seminars, conferences and independent study. However, one highly effective approach is their involvement in dedicated nursing rounds. These rounds cater to learners at all stages, whether they are preregistration students or experienced professionals.

Nursing rounds are a structured process in which healthcare professionals, primarily nurses, come together to review and discuss patient cases, coordinate care and facilitate interdisciplinary collaboration. These rounds are typically conducted in a healthcare facility, such as a hospital or clinic, and involve various members of the healthcare team, including nurses, doctors, specialists and students from different disciplines.

DEFINITIONS

- Barker and Young define nursing rounds as 'a teaching and learning method in which a group of students and a clinical instructor visit a number of patients together. The instructor discusses the patients' conditions with the students and answers any questions they may have'.
- Bevis defines nursing rounds as 'a group discussion of patient care that occurs at the bedside. It is a time for students to learn from the instructor and from each other about the care of individual patients'.
- Tanner defines nursing rounds as 'a teaching method that allows students to learn about the overall management of a patient's care. The instructor discusses the patient's condition, the plan of care, and the patient's progress with the students'.

Nursing rounds are a valuable teaching method that can help nursing students to develop the skills and knowledge they need to provide safe and effective care to patients. It is a group-oriented learning experience that allows students to learn from the instructor and from each other. Nursing rounds can also help students to develop their communication, critical thinking and problem-solving skills.

DIFFERENCES BETWEEN BEDSIDE CLINIC AND NURSING ROUNDS

Bedside clinic and nursing rounds are both teaching methods used in nursing education. However, there are some key differences between the two methods. Here is a table that summarizes the key differences between bedside clinic and nursing rounds:

Features	Bedside Clinic	Nursing Rounds
Purpose	Apply theoretical knowledge and clinical skills at the patient's bedside.	Review and discuss patient cases, coordinate care and facilitate interdisciplinary collaboration.

Features	Bedside Clinic	Nursing Rounds
Setting	Patient's hospital room or clinical setting	Conference room or designated meeting area
Participants	Nursing students, instructors/preceptors and the patient	Nurses, doctors, specialists, students from different disciplines and healthcare team members
Focus	Specific nursing care needs of individual patients	Comprehensive review of patient cases, interdisciplinary care coordination and planning
Time and structure	More flexible in timing and structure, tailored to patient and student needs	Follows a structured schedule with a predefined agenda or checklist
Primary activity	Direct observation and interaction with the patient, applying nursing principles and skills	Discussion among healthcare professionals, review of patient cases, interdisciplinary coordination

PURPOSES

The purposes of nursing rounds as a teaching method in healthcare are:

1. **Comprehensive patient care**: Nursing rounds facilitate a holistic approach to patient care by allowing healthcare professionals to discuss and review all aspects of a patient's condition, including assessments, treatment plans and progress. The primary purpose is to ensure coordinated and high-quality care for patients.
2. **Interdisciplinary collaboration**: Nursing rounds provide a platform for interdisciplinary collaboration, allowing nurses, doctors, specialists and other healthcare professionals to come together and share their expertise, perspectives and insights. This collaboration promotes effective communication and teamwork, leading to improved patient outcomes.
3. **Learning opportunities for students**: Nursing rounds offer valuable learning experiences for nursing students, giving them the chance to observe and participate in real-life patient care discussions. Students can learn from experienced professionals, deepen their understanding of clinical decision-making and enhance their critical thinking skills.
4. **Application of theoretical knowledge**: Nursing rounds bridge the gap between theoretical knowledge and its application in clinical practice. They provide an opportunity for nurses and other healthcare professionals to apply their theoretical knowledge, guidelines and evidence-based practices in real patient scenarios, thereby enhancing their clinical competence.
5. **Skill development**: Nursing rounds foster the development of essential skills in nursing practice, such as patient assessment, communication and care planning. By actively participating in the rounds, nurses can refine their skills, receive feedback and enhance their ability to deliver safe and effective patient care.
6. **Professional growth and knowledge sharing**: Nursing rounds facilitate knowledge sharing and professional growth among healthcare professionals. They allow for the exchange of experiences, best practices and updates on evidence-based guidelines, contributing to the continuous learning and development of the nursing workforce.
7. **Quality improvement and patient safety**: Through nursing rounds, healthcare professionals can identify areas for improvement in patient care, discuss strategies to enhance patient safety and implement quality improvement initiatives. The focus on collaborative decision-making and evidence-based practices helps ensure the delivery of safe and effective care.

TYPES OF NURSING ROUNDS

There are several types of nursing rounds, each with its own purpose and benefits.

1. **Clinical rounds:** These are the most common type of nursing rounds. They involve a group of nurses, led by a physician, who visit patients to assess their condition and discuss their care plan. Clinical rounds are an opportunity for nurses to learn from the physician and to collaborate on patient care.
2. **Teaching rounds:** These rounds are led by a nurse educator and are designed to teach nursing students about patient care. Teaching rounds typically involve a group of students and a nurse educator who visit patients and discuss their condition, the plan of care and the students' learning objectives.
3. **Multidisciplinary rounds:** These rounds involve a team of healthcare professionals, including nurses, physicians, social workers and dietitians, who visit patients to discuss their care plan and to coordinate services. Multidisciplinary rounds are an opportunity for healthcare professionals to share information and to develop a plan of care that meets the patient's needs.
4. **Family rounds:** These rounds involve the patient's family and the healthcare team. They are an opportunity for the family to learn about the patient's condition, the plan of care and the patient's rights. Family rounds can help to improve communication between the family and the healthcare team and to promote patient-centred care.

STEPS TO ORGANIZE NURSING ROUNDS

Organizing nursing rounds as a teaching method involves several steps to ensure effective implementation. Here are the steps to organize nursing rounds:

1. **Identify objectives**: Clearly define the objectives and learning outcomes of the nursing rounds. Determine what specific skills, knowledge or competencies you want participants to gain from the experience.
2. **Establish a schedule**: Determine the frequency and timing of nursing rounds. Consider the availability of healthcare professionals, including nurses, doctors and specialists and ensure that the schedule aligns with their clinical duties.
3. **Select patient cases**: Choose patient cases that are relevant and representative of various healthcare scenarios. Consider cases that provide opportunities for learning and discussions on different aspects of patient care.
4. **Invite participants**: Communicate with the healthcare team members, including nurses, doctors, specialists and students, to invite them to participate in the nursing rounds. Ensure that all relevant team members are aware of the schedule and objectives.
5. **Prepare materials**: Gather relevant patient information, including medical history, assessments, progress notes and treatment plans. Compile these materials into a concise and organized format that can be easily shared with participants during the nursing rounds.
6. **Facilitate discussions**: During the nursing rounds, facilitate open and constructive discussions among the participants. Encourage active participation and the exchange of ideas, perspectives and experiences related to patient care. Maintain a supportive and respectful learning environment.
7. **Promote interdisciplinary collaboration**: Emphasize the importance of interdisciplinary collaboration during the nursing rounds. Encourage participants from different disciplines to share their expertise, ask questions and contribute to the care planning process. Foster effective communication and teamwork among the healthcare team members.

8. **Provide guidance and feedback**: As the facilitator of the nursing rounds, provide guidance and feedback to participants. Clarify concepts, answer questions and ensure that discussions stay focused on the learning objectives. Offer constructive feedback to enhance participants' knowledge and skills.
9. **Reflect and evaluate**: After each nursing round, take time to reflect on the session and evaluate its effectiveness. Gather feedback from participants to identify areas of improvement and make necessary adjustments for future rounds.
10. **Continuously improve**: Use the feedback and insights gained from each nursing round to enhance future sessions. Continuously refine the organization, structure and content of the nursing rounds to optimize the learning experience for participants.

BENEFITS OF NURSING ROUNDS

i. Interdisciplinary collaboration and teamwork.
ii. Real-life application of theoretical knowledge.
iii. Skill development, including critical thinking and decision-making.
iv. Enhanced understanding of patient care and holistic approach.
v. Opportunities for professional growth and knowledge sharing.

CHALLENGES OF NURSING ROUNDS

i. Time constraints in organizing and conducting rounds.
ii. Availability and coordination of healthcare professionals.
iii. Maintaining patient privacy and confidentiality.
iv. Variation in complexity of patient cases and learning opportunities.
v. Balancing the needs of learners with patient care responsibilities.

CONCEPT MAPPING

A concept map is a visual representation of knowledge. It is a way to show the relationships between different concepts. Concept maps can be used to help students learn new material, to organize their thoughts and to solve problems. Concept maps are made up of nodes and links. Nodes are boxes or circles that represent concepts. Links are lines that connect the nodes and show the relationships between the concepts. The relationships between concepts can be shown using words, arrows or symbols.

Concept mapping is a powerful clinical teaching method that involves the creation of visual representations to organize and link key concepts, ideas and relationships. It is a valuable tool for promoting critical thinking, knowledge integration and deep understanding among nursing students. Concept mapping enables students to visually represent complex information, identify patterns and develop a comprehensive view of a particular topic or patient case.

DEFINITIONS

- Daley (2010) describes concept maps as 'a graphic tool for organising and representing knowledge'.

- Twelve tips for teaching with concept maps in medical education (2013) defines concept mapping as an instructional strategy for individual and group learning that involves integration of knowledge and creation of meaning by relating concepts.
- Concept map as a teaching and learning tool for medical students (2022) states that concept maps are graphical representations of a given concept.

These definitions all emphasize the use of concept maps to represent knowledge, organize information and promote critical thinking. Concept maps can be used in a variety of clinical teaching settings, including:

- **Preclinical education**: Concept maps can be used to help students learn basic medical concepts. For example, students could create concept maps to illustrate the pathophysiology of a disease or the steps involved in a surgical procedure.
- **Clinical rotations**: Concept maps can be used to help students learn about the clinical presentation of diseases and the management of patients. For example, students could create concept maps to illustrate the signs and symptoms of a particular disease or the different treatment options available.
- **Continuing medical education**: Concept maps can be used to help practising clinicians stay up to date on the latest medical knowledge. For example, clinicians could create concept maps to illustrate the latest research on a particular disease or the latest treatment guidelines.

ELEMENTS OF CONCEPT MAPPING

Concept mapping as a clinical teaching method typically includes several key elements to effectively facilitate learning and understanding. Here are the essential elements of concept mapping in clinical teaching:

1. **Central theme or focus:** Concept mapping begins with identifying a central theme or focus. This could be a specific patient case, a clinical condition, a nursing concept or a healthcare process. The central theme serves as the anchor for the concept map and provides the context for organizing related concepts.
2. **Concepts and nodes:** Concepts are the main ideas or elements related to the central theme. Each concept is represented as a node or box in the concept map. Concepts can include signs and symptoms, nursing interventions, assessments, patient outcomes or any other relevant information related to the central theme.
3. **Links and relationships:** Links or connectors are used to illustrate the relationships between concepts. These connections demonstrate how the concepts are related, such as cause-and-effect relationships, associations or hierarchical structures. The links can be labelled to provide further clarification of the relationship.
4. **Hierarchical structure:** Concept maps often include a hierarchical structure that shows the organization and subordination of concepts. Key concepts or main ideas are placed closer to the central theme, while supporting concepts branch out from them. This hierarchical arrangement helps to create a logical flow and structure within the concept map.
5. **Cross-links and interconnections:** Cross-links or interconnections are connections between concepts that are not directly related but have some relevance or impact on each other. These cross-links highlight the interdependencies and interactions between different aspects of the central theme. They encourage students to consider the broader context and explore the comprehensive nature of the topic.
6. **Examples and illustrations:** Including specific examples, case studies or illustrations within the concept map can enhance understanding and application. These examples provide real-life context,

making the concepts more tangible and relatable. They help students see how the concepts are applied in clinical practice.

7. **Contextual information:** Concept maps can include contextual information such as references, definitions or additional notes. This supplementary information provides further clarity and depth to the concepts and helps students grasp the nuances and intricacies of the topic.

It is important to note that concept mapping can be adapted and customized based on the specific educational goals and context of the clinical teaching. Providing clear instructions, guidance and examples is essential to ensure students understand the purpose and expectations of the concept mapping exercise. Additionally, fostering a supportive and collaborative learning environment encourages students to actively engage in the process and share their concept maps for discussion and feedback.

TYPE OF CONCEPT MAP

There are many different types of concept mapping that can be used in clinical teaching. Some of the most common types include:

1. **Hierarchical concept maps**: Hierarchical concept maps are organized in a top-down fashion, with the most general concepts at the top and the most specific concepts at the bottom. This type of concept map is often used to help students learn about new concepts by providing them with a visual representation of the concept and its relationships to other concepts.
2. **Network concept maps**: Network concept maps are not organized in a hierarchical fashion. Instead, concepts are connected to each other in a web-like structure. This type of concept map is often used to help students organize their knowledge by providing them with a way to visualize the relationships between different concepts.
3. **Flowchart concept maps**: Flowchart concept maps are used to show the steps involved in a process. This type of concept map can be used to help students learn about clinical procedures or to help them develop a plan of care for a patient.
4. **System concept maps**: System concept maps are used to show the relationships between different parts of a system. This type of concept map can be used to help students understand the human body or to help them understand the healthcare system.

The type of concept map that you choose will depend on the purpose of your map and the level of detail that you want to include. For example, if you are teaching a basic concept, you may want to use a hierarchical concept map. If you are teaching a more complex concept, you may want to use a network concept map.

BENEFITS OF CONCEPT MAPPING IN CLINICAL TEACHING

1. **Enhanced understanding and retention:** Concept mapping promotes active learning, allowing students to actively engage with the material and make meaningful connections between concepts. This process enhances their understanding of complex topics and improves retention of information.
2. **Critical thinking and analysis:** Concept mapping requires students to analyse, evaluate and synthesize information to create meaningful connections. It fosters critical thinking skills by encouraging students to consider the relationships between concepts, identify patterns and think critically about the topic.

3. **Knowledge integration:** Concept mapping facilitates the integration of knowledge from various sources, such as textbooks, lectures and clinical experiences. Students can visually represent and organize concepts, allowing them to see the bigger picture and understand how different pieces of information fit together.
4. **Collaboration and communication:** Concept mapping can be done collaboratively, allowing students to work in groups and exchange ideas. This promotes effective communication, teamwork and the ability to articulate and justify their thinking to others. Collaborative concept mapping encourages students to learn from each other and consider different perspectives.
5. **Clinical reasoning and decision-making:** Concept mapping support the development of clinical reasoning skills. Students can use concept maps to analyse patient cases, identify relevant factors and make informed decisions about interventions. This strengthens their ability to think critically and apply theoretical knowledge to real-world scenarios.
6. **Assessment and feedback:** Concept maps can serve as assessment tools to evaluate students' understanding and application of concepts. Instructors can review concept maps to assess the accuracy and depth of students' knowledge, identify misconceptions and provide targeted feedback for improvement.

CHALLENGES OF CONCEPT MAPPING IN CLINICAL TEACHING

1. **Initial familiarization and skill development:** Some students may initially struggle with the concept mapping process, particularly if they are not familiar with this teaching method. They may require guidance and practice to develop effective concept mapping skills.
2. **Time constraints:** Creating concept maps can be time-consuming, especially for complex topics. Limited time in clinical settings may make it challenging for students to allocate sufficient time to create detailed and comprehensive concept maps.
3. **Grading consistency:** Assessing and grading concept maps can be subjective, and ensuring consistency among different instructors can be a challenge. Clear grading rubrics and guidelines can help address this challenge.
4. **Overemphasis on structure:** Students may focus too much on the structure and aesthetics of the concept map rather than the quality and depth of the content. It is essential to emphasize that the connections and relationships between concepts are the most critical aspects.
5. **Misinterpretation of concepts:** Students may misinterpret or misunderstand certain concepts while creating concept maps. Providing clear instructions, examples and opportunities for clarification can help mitigate this challenge.
6. **Limited application to dynamic situations:** Concept mapping may be less suitable for capturing dynamic or rapidly changing situations. Clinical scenarios that involve quick decision-making or evolving patient conditions may not be easily represented in a static concept map.

Despite these challenges, concept mapping can be a valuable tool for clinical teaching. By understanding the challenges and taking steps to address them, you can help your students to use concept mapping to their advantage. Here are some **tips for overcoming the challenges of concept mapping in clinical teaching**:

- **Provide students with clear instructions and examples**: Make sure that students understand the purpose of concept mapping and how to create a concept map. Provide them with clear instructions and examples of concept maps that you have created.
- **Scaffold the activity**: If students are not familiar with concept mapping, you may need to scaffold the activity by providing them with more support. For example, you could provide them with a list of key concepts or help them to organize their information.

- **Make it fun**: Concept mapping can be a fun and engaging activity if you make it interesting for students. You could use different colours, images or symbols to make your concept maps more visually appealing.
- **Provide feedback**: Provide students with feedback on their concept maps. This will help them to improve their skills and understanding of the material.
- **Use concept maps as a formative assessment**: Use concept maps as a formative assessment to track students' progress and identify areas where they need additional support.

QUESTIONING IN CLINICAL TEACHING

Questioning in clinical teaching plays a crucial role in the education and development of healthcare professionals. It is an interactive and dynamic instructional method that encourages active learning, critical thinking and clinical reasoning. By posing thought-provoking questions, clinical educators can engage learners, assess their understanding and guide them towards deeper levels of knowledge and skill acquisition.

Questioning in clinical teaching is particularly important in nursing education, as it plays a vital role in developing the critical thinking and clinical decision-making skills necessary for safe and effective patient care.

DEFINITIONS

- Phillips and Duke (2008) define questioning as 'a process of stimulating thought and discussion through the use of carefully crafted questions'.
- Clarridge (2011) defines questioning as 'a powerful tool for promoting critical thinking, problem solving, and communication skills'.
- Parkinson (2016) defines questioning as 'a key teaching strategy that can be used to promote student learning'.

PURPOSES

Questioning in clinical teaching within the field of nursing serves several important purposes. Here are some key purposes of questioning in clinical teaching in nursing:

1. **Assessing knowledge and understanding**: Questioning allows clinical educators to assess the knowledge and understanding of nursing students. By asking specific questions related to nursing theory, procedures and concepts, educators can determine the level of comprehension and identify any gaps in knowledge. This assessment helps guide further instruction and provides feedback to students for improvement.
2. **Encouraging critical thinking**: Questioning promotes critical thinking skills among nursing students. By posing thought-provoking questions, educators challenge students to analyse and evaluate information, consider different perspectives and develop well-reasoned responses. This process enhances students' ability to think critically and make sound clinical judgements, ultimately improving their problem-solving skills.
3. **Promoting clinical reasoning**: Questioning in clinical teaching stimulates the development of clinical reasoning skills. Nurses must be able to apply theoretical knowledge to real-life patient

situations, and questioning facilitates this process. By presenting case scenarios and asking relevant questions, educators guide students in applying their knowledge, identifying key clinical issues and formulating appropriate nursing interventions.

4. **Enhancing decision-making skills**: Effective decision-making is crucial in nursing practice. Questioning helps nursing students practice making decisions in simulated or real clinical situations. By presenting dilemmas or complex patient scenarios, educators can ask questions that prompt students to consider various factors, weigh the potential outcomes and make informed decisions. This process contributes to the development of students' decision-making skills in clinical settings.
5. **Encouraging reflective practice**: Questioning prompts nursing students to reflect on their experiences and actions in clinical practice. By asking students to evaluate their own performance, educators facilitate self-assessment and reflection. Reflective practice helps students recognize their strengths, identify areas for improvement and develop a sense of accountability and continuous learning in their nursing practice.
6. **Facilitating effective communication**: Questioning in clinical teaching supports the development of effective communication skills in nursing students. By asking questions related to patient assessment, collaboration with the healthcare team or patient education, educators encourage students to communicate effectively and articulate their thoughts clearly. This enhances students' ability to convey information, listen actively and engage in therapeutic communication with patients, families and colleagues.
7. **Promoting evidence-based practice**: Questioning in clinical teaching encourages nursing students to consider evidence-based practice in their decision-making. By asking questions that involve the application of current research or evidence-based guidelines, educators foster a culture of evidence-based practice. This helps students develop skills to critically appraise research findings, incorporate evidence into their nursing practice and provide the best possible care to patients.

TYPES OF CLINICAL QUESTIONING

In clinical teaching in nursing, various types of questioning techniques can be employed to engage students, promote critical thinking and facilitate learning. Here are some common types of questioning used in clinical teaching in nursing:

i. **Closed-ended questions**: These questions typically require a brief or specific response and often have a single correct answer. They are useful for assessing knowledge, comprehension and recall of facts or information. For example, 'What is the normal range for adult blood pressure?'

ii. **Open-ended questions**: These questions prompt students to provide more in-depth and reflective responses. They encourage critical thinking, analysis and exploration of ideas. Open-ended questions are valuable for assessing higher-order thinking skills and encouraging students to think creatively and independently. For example, 'How would you prioritize the nursing interventions for a patient experiencing multiple health issues?'

iii. **Probing questions**: Probing questions are used to delve deeper into students' understanding and reasoning. They encourage students to provide more detailed explanations, elaborate on their responses and explore different perspectives. Probing questions help educators assess students' thought processes and promote critical thinking. For example, 'Can you explain why you chose that particular nursing intervention? What other options did you consider?'

iv. **Hypothetical questions**: Hypothetical questions present students with hypothetical scenarios or future situations to assess their ability to apply knowledge and make informed judgements. These questions encourage students to think hypothetically and consider potential outcomes or responses in different contexts. For example, 'If you encounter a patient with an unknown allergy during medication administration, what steps would you take to ensure patient safety?'

v. **Reflective questions**: Reflective questions prompt students to think about their experiences, actions and feelings related to clinical practice. They encourage self-assessment, critical reflection and identification of areas for improvement. Reflective questions support students in developing a deeper understanding of their own practice and promoting continuous learning. For example, 'Can you reflect on a challenging situation you faced during clinical practice and discuss what you learned from that experience?'

vi. **Socratic questions**: Socratic questioning follows a structured approach inspired by the Socratic method of teaching. It involves a series of thought-provoking questions aimed at guiding students to discover knowledge and solutions through their own reasoning and analysis. Socratic questions encourage students to critically examine assumptions, consider alternatives and develop logical arguments. For example, 'What are the possible causes of this patient's symptoms? How would you rule out each possibility?'

vii. **Factual questions**: These questions are designed to assess a student's knowledge of a particular fact or concept. For example, 'What is the definition of sepsis?'

viii. **Conceptual questions**: These questions are designed to assess a student's understanding of a particular concept. For example, 'What are the signs and symptoms of sepsis?'

ix. **Problem-solving questions**: These questions are designed to assess a student's ability to apply their knowledge to solve a problem. For example, 'What would you do if a patient with sepsis started to show signs of respiratory distress?'

x. **Critical thinking questions**: These questions are designed to assess a student's ability to think critically about a particular issue. For example, 'What are the ethical implications of withholding treatment from a patient with sepsis?'

GUIDELINE OF EFFECTIVE QUESTIONING IN CLINICAL TEACHING

To effectively use clinical questioning in teaching, clinical educators can follow these guidelines:

1. **Prepare in advance**: Before a teaching session, identify the learning objectives and determine the specific topics or concepts you want to address through questioning. This allows you to plan relevant and meaningful questions that align with the desired outcomes.
2. **Use a mix of question types**: Employ a combination of closed-ended and open-ended questions, as well as probing and hypothetical questions. This variety encourages students to engage in critical thinking, problem solving, and application of knowledge.
3. **Start with foundational knowledge**: Begin with questions that assess students' understanding of basic concepts and facts. This helps establish a foundation and ensures that students have the necessary background knowledge to build upon.
4. **Progress to higher-order thinking**: As the session progresses, gradually introduce more complex questions that require analysis, synthesis and evaluation. These questions challenge students to think critically, make connections and apply knowledge to clinical situations.
5. **Be clear and concise**: Frame questions in a clear and concise manner to avoid confusion. Ensure that questions are easily understandable and focused on the specific topic or concept you want to address.
6. **Allow adequate think time**: After asking a question, provide sufficient think time for students to process the question, formulate a response and gather their thoughts. Silence can be uncomfortable

but allowing a few moments of silence encourages reflection and allows students to gather their ideas.

7. **Encourage participation**: Create a supportive and nonjudgemental learning environment that encourages active participation. Encourage all students to contribute by using techniques like random selection or group discussions. This fosters engagement and allows for diverse perspectives to be shared.
8. **Follow up with probing questions**: After receiving an initial response, use probing questions to encourage students to elaborate on their answers, provide more detail or consider alternative perspectives. Probing questions stimulate deeper thinking and promote thorough exploration of concepts.
9. **Provide constructive feedback**: Use questioning as an opportunity to provide timely feedback. Acknowledge correct responses, provide additional information or clarification when needed and guide students towards accurate understanding. Constructive feedback helps students refine their thinking and enhance their learning.
10. **Foster peer-to-peer interaction**: Encourage students to ask questions to their peers and engage in discussions. Peer-to-peer questioning promotes collaborative learning, active engagement and the sharing of different viewpoints.
11. **Reflect on the session**: After the questioning session, reflect on the effectiveness of the questions used. Consider the students' responses, engagement levels and overall learning outcomes. Reflecting on the session helps identify areas for improvement and informs future teaching strategies.

BENEFITS OF QUESTIONING IN CLINICAL TEACHING

i. Promotes active learning and student engagement.
ii. Encourages critical thinking and clinical reasoning skills.
iii. Stimulates reflection and self-assessment.
iv. Fosters deeper understanding and retention of knowledge.
v. Assesses students' comprehension and knowledge gaps.
vi. Promotes evidence-based practice and application of theoretical knowledge.
vii. Enhances communication and interpersonal skills.
viii. Facilitates collaborative learning and peer-to-peer interaction.
ix. Provides formative assessment opportunities for feedback and improvement.
x. Supports the development of problem-solving and decision-making skills.

LIMITATIONS OF QUESTIONING IN CLINICAL TEACHING

i. Time constraints may limit the number and depth of questions that can be asked.
ii. Some students may feel anxious or intimidated by questioning, hindering their participation.
iii. Assessing and grading students solely based on their responses to questions may not provide a comprehensive evaluation of their clinical competence.
iv. In a large class or clinical setting, it may be challenging to give individual attention to each student's responses.
v. Cultural or language barriers may impact students' ability to fully understand and respond to questions.
vi. Educators need to strike a balance between guiding students through questioning and allowing them to explore and discover knowledge on their own.

PROCESS RECORDING

Process recording refers to a systemically written formal report of a therapeutic conversation, occurred between patient and healthcare provider. According to Walker, 'the process recording is a verbatim account of a visit for purpose of bringing out the interplay between nurse and the patient in relation to the common objectives'. In other words, process recording may be defined as 'a written account or verbalism recording of a conversation that occurred between a patient and the professional nurse, when they are working together towards a common therapeutic objective, which is recorded during and immediately following the nurse–patient interaction'.

I. FEATURES OF PROCESS RECORDING

- It is written during and immediately after the therapeutic nurse–patient interaction.
- Process recording also can be used as an excellent clinical teaching method.
- It also has therapeutic purposes, where recorded conversation is used to understand the patient's behaviour and problem in depth.

II. USES OF PROCESS RECORDING

- As a teaching–learning tool.
- As an evaluation tool.
- As a therapeutic tool.

III. PURPOSES OF PROCESS RECORDING

- Assists the nurse gain competency in interpreting and synthesizing raw data under supervision.
- Helps to consciously apply theory to practice.
- Helps the students develop an increased awareness of their habitual, verbal and nonverbal communication pattern.
- Helps the nurse to learn to identify thoughts and feelings in relation to self and others.
- Helps to increase observation skills as there is a conscious process involved in thinking, sorting and classifying the interaction under the various headings.

IV. ADVANTAGES OF PROCESS RECORDING

- It is the most suitable method of teaching to develop competency in interpreting and synthesizing the abstract concepts.
- It also provides opportunities for students to develop the good communication skills through practice of process recording.
- Process recording also helps to develop the keen observation skills and critical thinking.

V. DISADVANTAGES OF PROCESS RECORDING

- The process recording as a method of teaching is very time-consuming.
- It is not a suitable method of clinical teaching for an average IQ student because it is a highly complex process.
- The students with poor communication skills cannot be benefited with this method of clinical teaching.
- Sometimes patients do not offer the cooperation with this complex process of clinical teaching.

FIELD VISIT

Naturalistic philosophy of education believes that direct experience in natural environment with the learning material, object, situation or a phenomenon is one of the best ways of learning. The field visit is one of the methods of teaching, which is strongly recommended in the naturalistic philosophy of education. The research evidence has also proved the field visit as one of the best methods of teaching and learning where students directly encounter with the particulate learning experience in real environment under the supervision of an expert, who may answer his/her questions or clarify the doubts.

The field visit or field trip may be referred to as an educational procedure by which the students undertake a first-hand experience and exploration of material, object, situation or phenomenon in their natural environment.

A field visit entails a visit to a place outside the regular classroom and is designed to meet certain objectives that cannot be achieved by other methods of teaching. It provides a learner an opportunity to come out of formal classroom and obtain direct new experience in a natural environment. The principal features of a field visit are (1) to facilitate learning of an abstract concept, (2) to enhance students' interest and curiosity and (3) to increase social interaction among students and develop social awareness among them.

I. PURPOSES OF FIELD VISIT

- To make learning more meaningful and memorable.
- To provide an opportunity to learn from actual hands-on experiences rather than by simply reading or hearing about something.
- To supplement the regular classroom instructions and establish a connection between reality and literature.
- To give students experiential learning environment.
- Field visit is also useful in developing the concrete skills, such as note taking and public speaking.
- To help the students to appreciate the relevance and importance of what they have learnt in the classroom.
- To provide authentic learning experience by involving five senses in the learning experiences, that is vision, touch, feel, smell and test.

II. ADVANTAGES OF FIELD VISIT

- Field visit is a first-hand source of knowledge and information and supplements and enriches the classroom instructions.

- It integrates the classroom learning with real-life situations, which in turn help the students to develop a sympathetic understanding of problems as well as enable them to recognize the contribution of other organizations in patient care.
- Students develop a better understanding of the natural history of the disease and aetiological factors like housing, sanitation and socioeconomic conditions.
- It helps students to develop keen observation skills to study problems/situations.
- Field trip provides realistic resource material for study, thus arousing interest and motivation among learners.

III. DISADVANTAGES OF FIELD VISIT

- Most field visits are more time-consuming, which necessitates adjustment of other classes' time schedule.
- The field visit has to be planned as per the convenience of the organizations, which are to be visited.
- Students may not have the necessary data or sufficient background information and understanding to obtain the maximum learning benefit from field visits.
- Transportation may prove to be an inconvenience, if it is not readily available with particular department or organization.
- Field visits are more effective for smaller groups; however, large group is very difficult to supervise and control during field visit.
- It is difficult to create the ideal teaching–learning environment in field setting, which affects the outcome of learning.

Some of the topics related to Clinical Teaching–Learning Methods under clinical teaching strategies such as project (refer to page 223), role-play (refer at page 220), simulation (refer to page 207), problem-based learning (refer to page 238) are discussed in this chapter at pages given with these topics.

REVIEW QUESTIONS

LONG-ANSWER QUESTIONS

1. Explain simulation as teaching methods.
2. Discuss the advantages of case/care studies.
3. Explain the demonstration method.
4. Explain the advantages and disadvantages of micro-teaching.
5. Explain the various methods of clinical teaching.
6. Discuss field trips.
7. Explain panel discussions.
8. Discuss the lecturer method.
9. Discuss the project method.
10. Discuss a symposium.
11. Discuss role-plays.
12. Write in detail about nursing rounds as teaching method.
13. Describe principles of using clinical teaching methods.

SHORT-ANSWER QUESTIONS

1. List down the four clinical teaching methods.
2. Discuss briefly the four purposes of laboratory methods.
3. Mention the four limitations in field trip.
4. Discuss in brief any four advantages of lecturer method.
5. Enumerate the advantages of problem-based learning.
6. Mention two differences between seminar and symposium.
7. Mention four clinical teaching methods.

SHORT NOTES

Write short notes on the following:
1. Bedside clinics.
2. Workshop as a method of teaching.

MULTIPLE-CHOICE QUESTIONS (MCQs)

1. An important aim of lecture method of teaching should be to
   - **(a)** Make students memorize
   - **(b)** Tell and explain
   - **(c)** Use audiovisual aids
   - **(d)** Stimulate thinking
2. Demonstration method strives to achieve the following type of objectives
   - **(a)** Cognitive
   - **(b)** Affective
   - **(c)** Psychomotor
   - **(d)** Observation
3. A nurse educator is interested to teach neonatal assessment to nursing students. The best suitable method would be
   - **(a)** Lecture
   - **(b)** Demonstration
   - **(c)** Project
   - **(d)** Bedside clinic
4. The essential principle behind effective group discussion is
   - **(a)** Formulation of educational objectives
   - **(b)** Timely preparation and execution
   - **(c)** Well-defined responsibility of each group member
   - **(d)** Record of proceedings of discussion
5. Group discussion techniques are best suitable for achievement of
   - **(a)** Complex learning outcomes
   - **(b)** Defined discussion
   - **(c)** Conflicting view points
   - **(d)** Independent learning

6. The topic for panel discussion should be
   (a) Current
   (b) Debatable
   (c) Interesting
   (d) All of these
7. Chances of overlapping of content material are minimal in
   (a) Panel discussion
   (b) Seminar
   (c) Symposium
   (d) Group discussion
8. The teaching technique that has the ability to connect with the audience at an emotional level is
   (a) Role-play
   (b) Demonstration
   (c) Seminar
   (d) Panel discussion
9. The skills of problem solving, analysis and synthesis are best developed by
   (a) Lecture method
   (b) Demonstration method
   (c) Project method
   (d) Role-play method
10. Field trip can be made different from a usual picnic by
   (a) Proper planning and arrangement
   (b) Assigning defined responsibilities to group members
   (c) Seeking prior permission
   (d) Defined educational objectives
11. In which of the following techniques, participants are actively engaged in problem solving?
   (a) Panel discussion
   (b) Workshop
   (c) Exhibition
   (d) Seminar
12. In which of the following methods, subject matter is broken down into small frames and arranged sequentially?
   (a) Programmed instruction
   (b) Role-play
   (c) Field trip
   (d) Simulation
13. All are types of program instruction except
   (a) Linear programming
   (b) Branching programming
   (c) Selective programming
   (d) Computer-assisted programming
14. The main aim of micro-teaching is
   (a) Effective teaching
   (b) Developing specific teaching skills
   (c) Seeking feedback
   (d) Teach a small topic

15. The correct sequence of steps of micro-teaching is
- **(a)** Teach → feedback → re-plan → re-teach → re-feedback
- **(b)** Teach → plan → re-plan → re-teach → re-feedback
- **(c)** Teach → feedback → re-teach → re-plan → re-feedback
- **(d)** Teach → feedback → re-plan → re-teach → re-plan

ANSWERS TO THE MULTIPLE-CHOICE QUESTIONS

1. (d), 2. (c), 3. (b), 4. (c), 5. (a), 6. (d), 7. (b), 8. (a), 9. (c), 10. (d), 11. (b), 12. (a), 13. (c), 14. (b), 15. (a)

FURTHER READING

Abdool, M. A., & Bradley, D. (2013). Twelve tips to improve medical teaching rounds. *Medical Teacher, 35*(11), 895–899.

Agnew, P. W., Kellerman, A. S., & Meyer, J. (1996). *Multimedia in the classroom*. Boston, MA: Allyn and Bacon.

Ahmed, M. (2002). What is happening to bedside clinical teaching? *Medical Education*, 36, 1185–1188.

Alberto, P., & Troutman, A. (2003). *Applied behavior analysis for teachers* (6th ed.). Columbus, OH: Prentice-Hall-Merrill.

Alley, C. (1972). *Classroom*. Boston, MA: Allyn and Bacon.

American Association of Colleges of Nursing (AACN). (2008). *The essentials of baccalaureate education for professional nursing practice*. https://www.aacnnursing.org/Education-Resources/AACN-Essentials

American Nurses Association (ANA). (2015). *Nursing: Scope and standards of practice*. https://www.nursingworld.org/practice-policy/nursing-excellence/standards/

Bevis, E. O., & Oermann, M. H. (1999). *Clinical teaching in nursing*. New York, NY: Springer Publishing Company.

Boud, D. (1985). *Reflection: Turning experience into learning*. London: Kogan Page.

Boud, D., & Feletti, G. (1999). *The challenge of problem-based learning* (2nd ed.). London, UK: Kogan Page.

Boudreau, D., & Butts, J. (2014). *Effective communication in nursing: A guide for health professionals*. Jones & Bartlett Learning.

BPP. (2000). *Success in your research and analysis project*. London, UK: BPP.

Cano, F. (2005). Epistemological beliefs and approaches to learning: Their change through secondary school and their influence on academic performance. *British Journal of Educational Psychology, 75*, 203–221.

Chandler, M. (2007). Using journaling to enhance critical thinking in nursing education. *Nurse Education Today, 27*(3), 203–208.

Chang, C. H., & Cho, H. J. (2010). The effects of debate on critical thinking skills of nursing students. *Journal of Nursing Education, 49*(1), 24–29.

Clark, D. (2010). *Bloom's taxonomy of learning domains*. http://www.nwlink.com/;donclark/hrd/bloom.html

Close, A., & Castledine, G. (2005). Clinical nursing rounds, part 4: Teaching rounds for nurses. *British Journal of Nursing, 14*(18), 982–983.

Collis, B., & Jung, I. S. (2003) Uses of information and communication technologies in teacher education. In Robinson, B., & Latchner, C. (Eds.), *Teacher education through open distance learning* (pp. 171–192). London: Routledge Falmen.

Dewey, J. (1910). *How we think*. New York, DC: Heath & Co.

Dewey, J. (1916). *Democracy & education*. New York: The MacMillian Company.

Dolan, B., & Duffy, J. (2018). *Communication and interpersonal skills in nursing* (6th ed.). New York: Elsevier.

Dolowitz, A. (2020). What is team-based learning, and how is it used in nursing? *Indian Journal of Continuing Nursing Education, 21*, 198–205. https://www.ijcne.org/text.asp?2020/21/2/198/309862

Doody, O., & Condon, M. (2012). Increasing student involvement and learning through using debate as an assessment. *Irish Journal of Nursing*, *23*(2), 33–37.
Everett, D. M. (1926). *The meaning of a liberal education*. New York: W. W. Norton & Co.
Farrell, J. P., & Oliveira, T. (1993). *Teachers in developing countries: Improving effectiveness and managing costs*. Washington, DC: World Bank.
Fitzgerald, M., & O'Connor, P. (2008). Using reflective journaling to enhance learning in nursing students. *Nurse Education in Practice*, *8*(1), 34–39.
Garrison, D. R., & Kanuka, H. (2004). Blended learning: Untangling the confusion. In T. S. Roberts (Ed.), *Online teaching: A practical guide* (pp. 95–112). New York, NY: RoutledgeFalmer.
Gee, J. P. (2003). *What video games have to teach us about learning and literacy?* New York: Palgrave Macmillan.
Gheidanzadeh, M., Baghersad, Z., & Abazari, P. (2017). Nursing students' viewpoints toward two methods of clinical conference and clinical nursing round. *Journal of Education and Health Promotion*, *6*, 71.
Gibbons, P. (n.d.). *Scaffolding language, scaffolding learning: Teaching Second Language learning in the Mainstream Classroom*. Portsmouth, USA: Heinemann.
Giddings, L. S., Dyson, L. C., Entwistle, M. J., Macdiarmid, R., Marshall, D. C., & Simpson, S. M. (2000). Three approaches to use of questioning by clinical lecturers: A pilot study. *Nursing Praxis in New Zealand Inc*, *15*(1), 13–22.
Halpern, D. F. (1998). Teaching critical thinking for transfer across domains. *American Psychologist*, *53*, 449–455.
Henderson, V. (2001). *The nature of nursing: Reflections on the work of Virginia Henderson*. New York, NY: Springer Publishing Company.
Hofstetter, F. T. (1995). *Multimedia literacy*. New York: McGraw-Hill.
Information Communication Technology in Education. https://www.researchgate.net/publication/325087961_Information_Communication_Technology_in_Education. Accessed May 26, 2023.
James, W. (1983). *Talks to teachers on psychology and to students on some of life's ideals*. Cambridge, MA: Harvard University Press. (Original work published 1899).
Jonassen, D. H., Peck, K. L., & Wilson, B. G. (1999). *Learning with technology: A constructivist perspective. Upper Saddle River*, NJ: Merrill/Prentice Hall.
Kitaba K. A. (2022). Effectiveness of pre- and post-clinical conferences in improving clinical learning among midwifery students of Jimma University: Pre-experimental study. *Advances in Medical Education and Practice*, *13*, 1171–1178.
Knowles, M. (1975). *Self-directed learning*. Chicago, IL: Follet.
Kourkouta, L., & Papathanasiou, I. V. (2014). Communication in nursing practice. *Mater Sociomed*, *26*(1), 65–67.
Kozier, B., Erb, G., Berman, A., & Snyder, S. (2017). *Fundamentals of nursing: Concepts, process, and practice* (9th ed.). London: Pearson Education.
Lieberman, A. (2004). *Teacher leadership*. San Francisco, CA: Jossey-Bass.
Lindstrom, R. (1994). *The business week guide to multimedia presentations: Create dynamic presentations that inspire*. New York: McGraw-Hill.
Lucas, J. L., Blazek, M. A., & Riley, A. B. (2005). The lack of representation of educational psychology and school psychology in introductory psychology textbooks. *Educational Psychology*, *25*, 347–351.
Markel, S. M. (1969). *Good frames and bad: A grammar of frame writing*. New York: Wiley.
Monroe, P. (1915). *A text-book in the history of education*. New York: Macmillan.
Moormeier, J. (2017). The use of concept maps as an assessment tool in a baccalaureate nursing program. *Journal of Nursing Education*, *56*(1), 45–47.
National Council of State Boards of Nursing (NCSBN). (2016). *Clinical judgment model*. https://www.ncsbn.org/Clinical_Judgment_Model.pdf
Nordlund, C. Y. (2006). *Art experiences in Waldorf education* (PhD Dissertation). St. Louis: University of Missouri-Columbia.
Redman, B. K. (2008). When is patient education unethical? *Nursing Ethics*, *15*(6), 813–820. doi:10.1177/0969733008095389
Pearson, J. (2003). Information and communications technologies and teacher education in Australia. *Technology Pedagogy and Education*, *12*(1), 39–58.

Prensky, M. (2001). *Digital game-based learning*. New York: McGraw-Hill.

Profetto-McGrath, J., Bulmer Smith, K., Day, R. A., & Yonge, O. (2004). The questioning skills of tutors and students in a context based baccalaureate nursing program. *Nurse Education Today, 24*(5), 363–372.

Quality and Safety Education for Nurses (QSEN). (2018). *Competencies*. http://qsen.org/competencies/pre-licensure-ksas/

Salam, A., Siraj, H. H., Mohamad, N., Das, S., & Rabeya, Y. (2011). Bedside teaching in undergraduate medical education: Issues, strategies, and new models for better preparation of new generation doctors. *Iranian Journal of Medical Sciences, 36*(1), 1–6.

Schweer, J. E. (1972). *Creating teaching in clinical nursing*. St. Louis: Mosby.

Seshan, V., Matua, G. A., Raghavan, D., Arulappan, J., Al Hashmi, I., Roach, E. J., ... Prince, E. J. (2021). Case study analysis as an effective teaching strategy: Perceptions of undergraduate nursing students from a Middle Eastern Country. *SAGE Open Nursing, 7*, 23779608211059265. doi:10.1177/23779608211059265

Shin, H., & Park, C. (2017). Effects of concept mapping care plans on critical thinking and clinical reasoning ability of baccalaureate nursing students. *International Journal of Nursing Practice, 23*(4), e12547.

Squires, D. (2006). From content to context: Video games as designed experiences. *Educational Researcher, 35*(8), 19–29.

Tanner, C. A. (2000). *Teaching and learning: A practical guide*. New York, NY: Springer Publishing Company.

Tapscott, D. (1998). *Growing up digital: The rise of the net generation*. New York: McGraw-Hill.

Taylor, J. (2002). *A different kind of teacher: Solving the crisis of American schooling*. Berkeley, CA: Berkeley Hills Books.

Teo, R., & Wong, A. (2000, December 4–7). Does problem based learning create a better student: A reflection? In *Proceedings at the 2nd Asia Pacific Conference on Problem-Based Learning: Education Across Disciplines*. Singapore.

Thorndike, E. L. (1912). *Education: A first book*. New York: MacMillan.

Vadasy, P., Jenkins, J., Antil, L., Wayne, S., & O'Connor, R. (1997). The effectiveness of one-to-one tutoring by community tutors for at-risk beginning readers. *Learning Disability Quarterly, 20*(2), 126–139.

Vaughan, T. (1998). *Multimedia: Making it work* (4th ed.). Berkeley, CA: Osborne/McGraw-Hill.

Vives, J., & Watson, F. (1913). On education: *A translation of the de tradendis disciplinis of Juan Luis Vives*. Cambridge, MA: Cambridge University Press.

West, C., & Graham, L. (2012). Concept mapping: A tool to promote critical thinking skills and clinical decision-making in nursing students. *Journal of Nursing Education, 51*(7), 375–378.

Woolfolk, A. E., Winne, P. H., & Perry, N. E. (2006). *Educational psychology* (3rd Canadian ed.). Toronto, Canada: Pearson.

World Bank. (2002). *Information & communication technology sector strategy paper*. Washington, DC: World Bank.

Yoder-Wise, P. S. (2006). *Fast facts for the classroom nursing instructor: Classroom teaching in a nutshell*. New York: Springer Publishing Company.

Zare, S., & Othman, M. (2015). Debate as a teaching strategy in nursing education: A systematic review. *Nurse Education Today, 35*(12), 1264–1269.

CHAPTER

Educational media

6

LEARNING OBJECTIVES

This chapter is designed to enable the reader to:

- Define audiovisual aids
- Understand the concept, importance, purposes, characteristics, sources and principles of audiovisual aids
- Classify the types of audiovisual aids
- Describe the concept, characteristics, purposes, types and guidelines for preparation and uses, advantages and disadvantages of different graphic audiovisual aids, such as chalkboard, charts, graphs, poster, flashcards, flannel board, bulletin board and cartoons
- Discuss the concept, characteristics, purposes, types and guidelines for preparation and uses, advantages and disadvantages of different three-dimensional audiovisual aids, such as objects/specimens, models, puppets, exhibitions, museum and dioramas
- Explain the concept, characteristics, purposes, types and guidelines for preparation and uses, advantages and disadvantages of different printed audiovisual aids, such as pamphlets and leaflets
- Appraise the concept, characteristics, purposes, types and guidelines for preparation and uses, advantages and disadvantages of different projected audiovisual aids, such as slide projector, overhead projector, opaque projector, filmstrips, television, video cassette recorder player, camera, microscope and LCD projector
- Explore the concept, characteristics, purposes, types and guidelines for preparation and uses, advantages and disadvantages of different audio/audiovisual aids, such as tape recorder, public address system and computer
- Recognize the guidelines for effective use of audiovisual aids

KEY TERMS

INTRODUCTION

The educational media are the objects that help in teaching and learning activities and enhance the delivery of knowledge to the learners. In other words, educational media are learning devices that help the teacher clarify, establish, correlate and coordinate accurate concepts and interpretation to make learning more concrete, effective, interesting, meaningful and vivid. Audiovisual aids, audiovisual materials, audiovisual media, communication technology, educational or instructional media or learning resources are interchangeably used terms. Broadly speaking, however, all of them have the same meaning.

AUDIOVISUAL AIDS

Scientifically, it is believed that during the communicative process, the sensory register of the memory acts as a filter. The working short-term memory functions are limited by both time and capacity. Therefore, it is essential that the information be arranged in useful bits or chunks for effective coding, rehearsal or recording, and audiovisual aids best suit this function. Therefore, audiovisual aids in the classroom can enhance teaching methods and improve student comprehension. Today's technology offers many choices to the educator who wishes to capitalize on the new generation's appetite for multimedia presentations. An efficient lesson plan that incorporates the use of audiovisual aids consistent with curriculum objectives may do miracles in the achievement of purposes of the teaching–learning process.

I. DEFINITIONS OF AUDIOVISUAL AIDS

Audio-visual aids are those sensory objects or images which initiates or stimulate and reinforce learning.

—Burton

Audio-visual aids are those devices by the use of which communication of ideas between persons and group in various teaching and training situation is helped. These are also termed as multi sensory materials.

—Edgar Dale

Audio-visual aids are anything by means of which learning process may be encouraged or carried on through the sense of hearing or sense of sight.

—Good's Dictionary of education

Audio-visual aids are devices which can be used to make the learning experience more concrete, more realistic and more dynamic.

—Kinder S. James

Audio-visual aids are supplementary devices by which the teacher through the utilization of more than one sensory channel is able to clarify, establish and correlate concepts, interpretations and appreciations.

—**Mckown and Roberts**

Audio-visual aids are those aids which help in completing the triangular process of learning i.e. motivation, classification and stimulation.

—**Carter V. Good**

An audio-visual aid is an instructional device in which the message can be heard as well as seen.

II. CONCEPT OF AUDIOVISUAL AIDS

Audiovisual aids are planned teaching aids that appeal to the senses of people and enhance clear understanding and improve quick learning among learners. A Chinese proverb proves the importance of audiovisual aids in the teaching–learning process:

'I hear, I forget'
'I see, I remember'
'I do, I understand'

It is generally believed that the best learning can be achieved through doing things, but good learning can also be achieved through the use of appropriate audiovisual aids. Furthermore, audiovisual aids help in the completion of the triangular process of learning, enhance motivation, stimulation and improve the clarity of understanding in learners as depicted in Fig. 6.1. It can be inferred that the presentation of content with verbal and audiovisual aids motivates and stimulates the learner, reinforces the learning and enhances the clarity of the content.

Research has shown that oral presentations that use visuals are more persuasive, more interesting, more credible, more professional and more effective than presentations without such aids particularly when the presentation is long (about 20 minutes or more); the audiovisual aids can help the audience follow ideas easily and with fewer lapses in attention. In addition, Edwards and Mercer found in their research study that visual perception contributes about 90% to all human learning. Moreover, audiovisual aids:

- Help to maintain a high level of interest in the lesson and to create interest in the group.
- Help to get students to use the language, especially at the beginning stages.
- Help to promote greater student participation.
- Can be used at all levels of learning.
- Supplement and enrich the teachers' own teaching to make the teaching–learning process more concrete.
- Serve an instructional role in itself.
- Make teaching an effective interactive process.

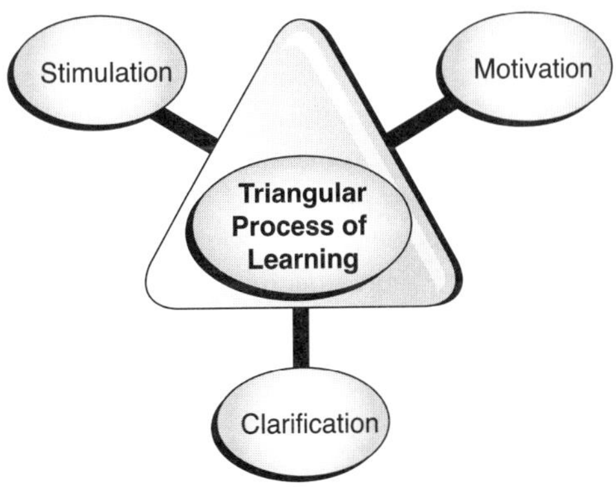

Figure 6.1
Triangular process of learning.

III. IMPORTANCE OF AUDIOVISUAL AIDS

Effective communication can be quite challenging, especially when making a presentation or giving a speech. For communication to be effective, one must keep the attention of the listeners and deliver information in such a way that it is fully understood. Audiovisual aids are one of the most effective ways to get the message across and make it memorable. Joey Papa suggested the following benefits of audiovisual aids (Fig. 6.2):

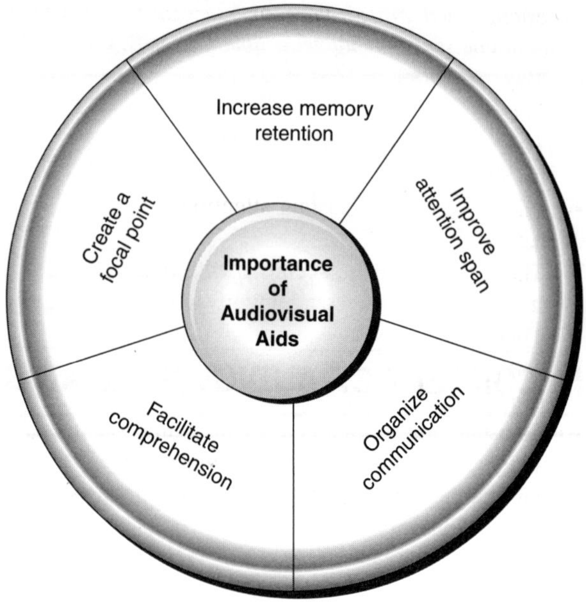

Figure 6.2

Importance of audiovisual aids.

- ***Memory retention:*** The Office of Training and Education of the United States Occupational Safety and Health Administration has reported that psychologists and educators have found the use of audiovisual tools led to retention of information for three days after a meeting or other event. This is six times more than when information is presented by spoken word alone. Visual aids allow the speaker to use verbal and nonverbal communication to solidify the message and provide a point of reference for the mind.
- ***Improved attention span:*** Everyone has a limited attention span. Once this capacity is spent, the mind decreases its ability to retain information and listen effectively. Using audiovisual aids refreshes the mind and engages it in a different way, renewing the attention span. Visual aids keep the mind entertained and therefore sharp and ready to receive information.
- ***Organizing communication:*** Audiovisual aids can be used to organize communication making it easier to remember points made in a presentation. The introduction of a different audiovisual aid for each point of a speech or presentation helps the mind to separate messages into smaller chunks of information. Audiovisual aids also create a point of reference for the mind to quickly refer to when attempting to retrieve information. For example, the use of icons or labels helps trigger messages in the mind.
- ***Comprehension:*** Not everyone understands concepts and information at the same rate. Some people can understand messages quickly while others need help to grasp what is being said. Audiovisual aids are a way of further explanation. If some people are more visual than audio learners, the visual aids may be necessary for comprehension. Audiovisual aids create repetition and the more repetition in communication, the greater the chances are that your audience will understand and remember effectively.
- ***Create a focal point:*** Audiovisual aids help a speaker stay on track. If there is one central visual aid that the speaker can use, then the speaker's thoughts and the audience's attention will stay on course. There is nothing worse than listening to a speaker ramble and lose the audience. Audiovisual aids assist in avoiding such a scenario.

IV. PURPOSES OF AUDIOVISUAL AIDS

Audiovisual aids enhance clarity in communication, provide diversity in the methods of teaching and increase the forcefulness of the subjects being learned or taught. Furthermore, students get direct experience of real-life situations or direct sensory experiences or symbolic experiences through the use of audiovisual aids. Moreover, some essential purposes of the audiovisual aids are as follows:

- They help in effective perceptual and conceptual learning.
- They are helpful in capturing and sustaining the attention of students.
- They are helpful in new learning. New things are interpreted in terms of past experiences.
- Imagery helps preserve and clarify past experiences and provides near realistic experience.
- They increase and sustain attention, concentration and the personal involvement of students in actual learning.
- They create interest, secure attention and motivate students to learn.
- It is easier to understand any given concept through the use of sensory aids.
- They help in saving energy and time of both the teachers and students.
- They give the student an opportunity to touch, feel and see a model, map, picture or specimen and provide a sensory stimulus to enhance learning.
- They provide for purposeful self-activity and student participation.
- They help provide concreteness, realism and lifelikeness in the teaching–learning process.
- Pictures are helpful in studying concrete reality to gain actual meaning.
- They help explicate and increase the meaningfulness of abstract concepts.
- Concrete experience helps combat the tendency to abstractness.
- Visual materials give definite meaning to words.
- They bring remote events of either space or time into the classroom.
- They serve as an open window through which the student can view the world or its entire phenomenon.
- They introduce an opportunity for situational or field type of learning as contrasted with the linear order verbal and written communication.
- It provides direct experience to the student in the clinical setting and observation experience through field trips or such other media.
- They provide, facilitate and advance the process of applying what is learned to realistic performance and life situations.
- They can meet individual demands.
- They are useful for the education of masses.

V. CHARACTERISTICS OF A GOOD AUDIOVISUAL AID

An audiovisual aid must possess the following basic characteristics to be an effective aid for the teaching–learning process:

- ***Meaningful and purposeful:*** An audiovisual aid can be only considered good if it is meaningful and purposeful for the particular teaching–learning process. Very attractive and expensive teaching aids may not have any value until and unless they are meaningful and purposeful for the teacher–taught activity. For example, a tiny tot can be taught the preliminary things with real-life specimens easily rather than with expensive computerized teaching tools.
- ***Motivate the learners:*** A good audiovisual aid must sufficiently motivate the learner so that he can achieve learning swiftly, quickly and promptly. Until and unless an audiovisual aid motivates the learner; it cannot be considered effective in spite of all its other appealing characteristics.
- ***Accurate in every aspect:*** Each audiovisual aid has its peculiar characteristics and must follow some set of rules and principles in preparation and use during the teaching–learning process. Thus, audiovisual aids can only be considered good if they encompass all the essential characteristics and are accurate in all the aspects.

- ***Simple and cheap:*** Along with all the essential characteristics, one of the most essential characteristics of audiovisual aids is their simplicity and cost-effectiveness. The simplicity of an audiovisual aid promotes broader popularity and more adaptability among teachers and learners. In addition, cost-effectiveness of audiovisual aids enhances its acceptability and practicability.
- ***Appropriate size:*** Audiovisual aids used in the teaching–learning process must not be too large or too small. Very large tools create problems of handling and transpiration, while very small tools may not enhance learning because of a poor sense triggering ability due to their small size.
- ***Up to date:*** Science and technology is an ever-progressing field where things are developing and progressing every day and old products are becoming outdated. The field of educational media and technology has also revolutionized to a great extent in the last few years. Therefore, educationists must ensure that audiovisual aids are continuously updated so that a pace can be maintained with other fields. An audiovisual aid can only be considered good if it is up to date with reference to technology and new principles of practice.
- ***Easily portable:*** A good audiovisual tool must have a characteristic of easy portability so that it can be easily handled and transported where required. Easy portability increases the access of audiovisual aids as well as prevents damage and discomfort during handling and transportation.
- ***Customized to the type of educational materials:*** Every tool does not fit all the educational material to be delivered. Therefore, educationists must predetermine which tool will be appropriate for a particular type of teaching content. Appropriately customized and adapted tools promote the teaching–learning process.
- ***Suitable to the mental level of learners:*** While deciding on a tool to be used for teaching a particular group of students, their intellectual ability must be considered so that the objective of the teaching–learning process can be achieved.
- ***Variety:*** A teaching aid may be considered good if it is providing a variety of experiences to the learner so that actual learning can be achieved more swiftly and promptly.

VI. SOURCES OF AUDIOVISUAL AIDS

The development and distribution of audiovisual aids is done by a variety of organizations such as government, premier educational institutions, professional organizations, nongovernment organizations (NGOs), national and international voluntary organizations and commercial industries. Government, premier educational institutions, professional organizations, NGOs, national and international voluntary organizations are generally involved in the preparation and distribution of the audiovisual aids used for mass communication and education. However, for the educational institutions, audiovisual aids are generally supplied by the government, premier educational institutions and commercial companies producing the audiovisual aids. A brief discussion of each of these sources is given below (Fig. 6.3).

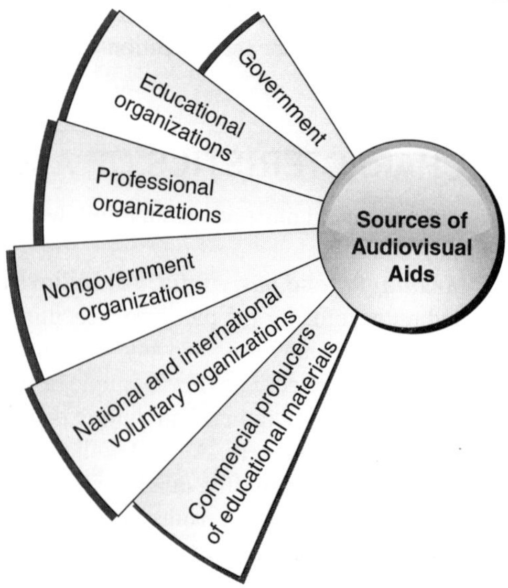

Figure 6.3

Sources of audiovisual aids.

- ***Government:*** The central or state government has two main departments: department of communication, broadcasting and mass media and the department of education, regularly involved in the development and distribution of audiovisual aids for different purposes. The department of communication, broadcasting and mass media is generally planning, preparing and disseminating the audiovisual aids required for mass communication rather than educational institutional media. On the other hand, the department of education has its focus on planning, preparing, developing and disseminating the educational material and media to educational institutions. The experts in these departments make use of latest research and technology developments for designing and disseminating educational aids to the different departments and educational institutions.

- ***Educational organizations:*** Some premier educational institutions have experts involved in regular research and development for generating new empirical evidences for the effectiveness of different teaching tools. These institutions are given the responsibility to use the latest innovations in the development of teaching aids and distribute them to the educational institutions as required.
- ***Professional organizations:*** Some professional organizations involved in using the latest technology towards the development of the most technocratic audiovisual aids may be a source of supply of audiovisual aids. These institutions are involved in the research and development of the most suitable audiovisual aids using technology that meets the latest requirements of educational institutions.
- ***NGOs:*** Some NGOs are also acting as a good source of developing and supplying the educational media. However, these NGOs are usually involved in developing and distributing the educational media to organizations engaged in providing mass education but they may also be a source of educational media for educational institutions.
- ***National and international voluntary organizations:*** Some national and international voluntary organizations provide funds to the educational institutions for direct purchase of the audiovisual aids or voluntary organizations themselves may supply the audiovisual aids to these educational institutions to promote the teaching–learning process. Therefore, educational institutions in need of audiovisual aids may contact these national and international voluntary organizations such as the World Health Organization and World Bank.
- ***Commercial producers of educational materials:*** Commercial producers of educational media are the most largely accessed source of audiovisual aids. There are a lot of national and international commercial companies involved in producing and supplying educational media. Generally, these commercial producers contact the educational institutions themselves or may advertise for commercial promotion of the products. These commercial companies may be contacted to demonstrate their products and may later be asked to provide quotations for buying products. Government educational institutions may receive educational media from different sources; however, private educational institutions primarily depend on commercial suppliers for buying audiovisual aids for the teaching–learning process.

VII. PRINCIPLES FOR USING AUDIOVISUAL AIDS

The following principles must be kept in mind for the effective use of audiovisual aids.

- ***Principle of selection:*** Selection of an audiovisual aid must be based on the basic characteristics of a learner, teacher, educational material, educational institution and the philosophy and objectives of the teaching–learning process. The basic characteristics of a learner that should be considered are age, class, mental ability and interest. For selecting a teaching tool, it must be ensured that teachers have the knowledge, ability and attitude to use a specific audiovisual aid. Furthermore, educational media must be selected according to the type of educational content delivered, resources and readiness of the educational institution. Moreover, educational media must be the best substitute for the real-life experience.

- ***Principle of preparation:*** To promote the efficient use of audiovisual aids, sound preparation is required in special reference to infrastructure, training of teachers and money for the preparation and maintenance of audiovisual aids. Primarily, self-made, cost-effective, locally available and teacher–taught friendly audiovisual aids must be used.
- ***Principle of physical control:*** For the efficient use and durability of audiovisual aids, it is necessary to have an appropriate control of the physical environment, for example a proper place for storage, appropriate environmental temperature and proper cleanliness. An appropriate physical control for audiovisual aids in the classroom and institution promotes the working, durability and hindrance-free use of the audiovisual aids.
- ***Principle of proper presentation:*** The presentation of the teaching aid is the operation stage. The teachers must carefully ensure that the audiovisual aid is in a good working condition. They should acquaint themselves with all the operating systems so that aids can be handled without any undue discomfort. Furthermore, teaching aids must be presented in a manner that every student can visualize them with the greatest comfort and it should catch the attention of students and ultimately enhance learning in the learners.
- ***Principle of response:*** Teachers must ensure that students respond to the stimulus provided by the audiovisual aids so that they can judge the effectiveness of the audiovisual aid in promoting learning in students. In the absence of students' response, teachers will not be able to evaluate the effectiveness of the teaching aids in the achievement of educational objectives.
- ***Principle of evaluation:*** Evaluation is one of the most essential principles because it conveys the efficacy of a particular teaching aid. The teachers can modify their plans of audiovisual aids used in light of the results of evaluation of a particular audiovisual aid. Evaluation of audiovisual aids should be made a regular and continuous process so that timely action can be taken and educational objectives can be achieved without any undue inconvenience and delay.
- ***Other miscellaneous principles:*** Some additional miscellaneous principles for the use of audiovisual aids are as follows:
  - Audiovisual materials should be utilized as an integral part of the educational programme.
  - Educational aids should be central to the teaching–learning process, under special direction and leadership in educational objectives.
  - An advisory committee must be consulted in the selection and utilization of audiovisual materials for different group of students.
  - Educational aids and educational materials must be mutually flexible so that they can be adapted based on the needs.
  - Ethical and legal aspects should be considered in the production and the utilization of educational communication media.

VIII. TYPES OF AUDIOVISUAL AIDS

Edgar Dale's cone of experience is the most fundamental explanation to understand the types of audiovisual aids (Fig. 6.4). A basic classification of the types of different audiovisual aids is given below. Furthermore, a comprehensive description of selected types of audiovisual aids with guidelines for effective use is presented in a later section (Table 6.1).

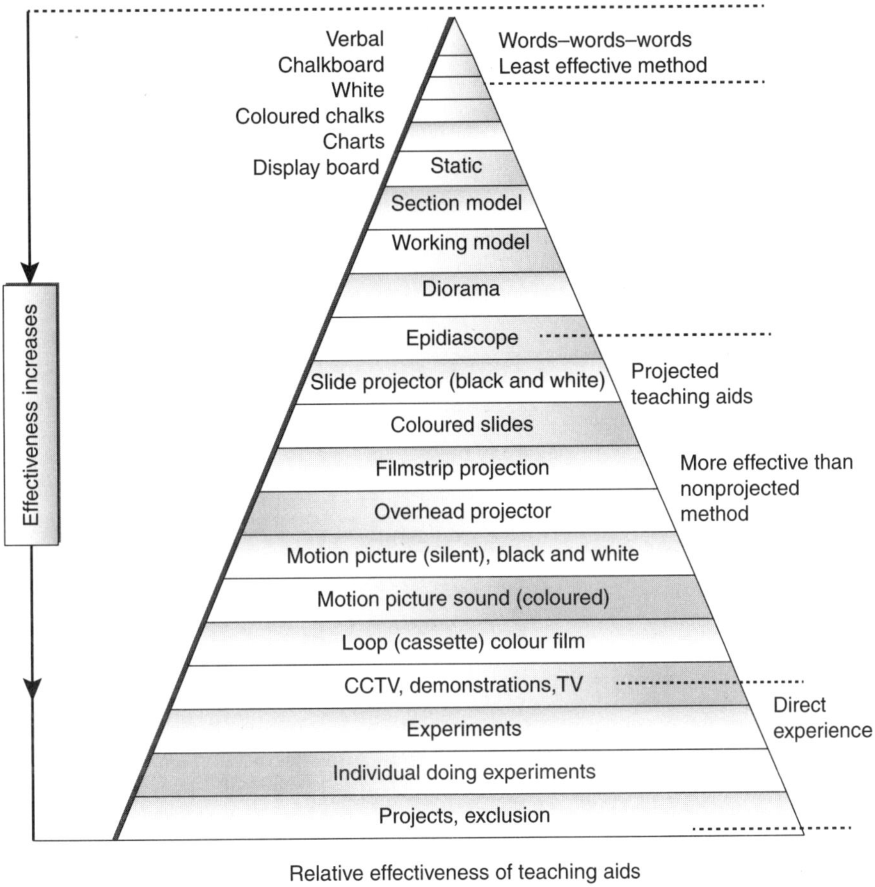

Figure 6.4

Edgar Dale's cone of experience in audiovisual aids.

Table 6.1 Comprehensive Description of Selected Types of Audiovisual Aids

Types of Audiovisual Aids	Standard Size	Essential Characteristics	Basic Guidelines for Preparation and Use
Graphic Audiovisual Aids			
1. Charts	90 × 60 cm or 70 × 50 cm	One chart should display information about one area Should display specific information Can be carefully stored and preserved for use in future	Size of letters for caption, labels should be 2–3 cm Every detail depicted should be visible Display material should be contrasted Should not contain too many details Should be neat and tidy
2. Graphs	Various sizes based on purpose	Principle of simplicity must be kept in mind Give bird's eye view of entire information Attractive to the eye Facilitate comparison of data relating to different periods of time	Must have a title and index Proportion between width and height must be balanced Selection of scale must be appropriate Footnotes should be included wherever needed Neatness and cleanliness must be ensured

Continued

Table 6.1 Comprehensive Description of Selected Types of Audiovisual Aids—cont'd

Types of Audiovisual Aids	Standard Size	Essential Characteristics	Basic Guidelines for Preparation and Use
3. Flash cards	10″ × 12″	Made out of cardboard Simple and understandable 10–12 cards can be used for one talk Message written should be brief	Height of writing should be 5 cm Size of group should not be more than 30 students Arrange in proper sequence Do not cover content with hands while displaying Should be held at chest level against body, not in air
4. Posters	22″ × 28″	Minimal use of words (4–5) Presented idea must be simple and understandable Must be attractive Language should be easy and simple	Use bold illustrations Avoid fancy lettering Attractive and pleasing colours should be used
Display Audiovisual Aids			
1. Chalkboard	5 m × 6 m	Surface should be rough and dull Mounted on appropriate height	Write letters and drawings in large size Writing should be in straight rows Extreme lower corners should not be used Do not use abbreviations Coloured chalks can be used to enhance attraction Avoid spelling mistakes
2. Bulletin board	Size depends on purpose	Framed soft board, straw board or cork board Dark blazer cloth to work as a back drop Height should be 1 m above the ground	Words should catch attention Sort out relevant material Title of the topic must be fixed at the top Should be kept little above the eye level Place bulletin board near the door Board must have neat, ordered and attractive appearance Change the content on the board regularly Overcrowding of the contents must be avoided
3. Flannel board	1.5 m × 1.5 m	A piece of rigid material covered with cotton flannel, wool, suede cloth and paper The cut-outs are provided with rough surface at the back by pasting pieces of sandpaper	Content should be organized around the central theme. Material should be displayed attractively Must be neat and orderly Avoid overcrowding on the board Displayed material should be of sufficient size Remove the material as soon as its purpose is over
Three-Dimensional Aids			
1. Specimen	–	Boxes should be covered with cellophane paper Should be mounted in shallow boxes in an artistic way Label each object or specimen	Plan teaching with certain simple and direct observation of objects and specimen Clarify and emphasize important structural details Provide review and practice to make learning permanent

Table 6.1 Comprehensive Description of Selected Types of Audiovisual Aids—cont'd

Types of Audiovisual Aids	Standard Size	Essential Characteristics	Basic Guidelines for Preparation and Use
2. Model	–	Three-dimensional Simplifies reality Explains the various processes of objects and machine	Must be of adequate size Relevant appearance closely resembling the actual organ/object Material and colours must be of good quality and appropriate in appearance to illustrate originality Must be used for a small group of students so that presentation and visibility can be enhanced Ideal models may have written labels for promotion of self-explanation
3. Puppets	–	Educational cum entertaining aid Easy to carry and operate Material used should be cost-effective and easily available	Age, background and taste of the audience should be considered while writing the puppet play Puppet plays should be short to maintain the interest of audience Size of the puppets should be appropriate Puppeteer should blend his art with dramatization to produce the desired effect Local language should be used while narrating the story

A. Comprehensive Classification Based on the Mode of Presentation

I. Auditory Aids		
– Radio – Phonograms – Gramophone	– Tape and disc recordings – Megaphone – Language laboratories	– Mike (public address system) – Microphone – Tape recorder
II. Nonprojected/Unprojected Visual Aids: Included Both Graphical and Display Aids		
– Models – Flannel boards – Cartoons and comics – Flash cards	– Pictures – Graphs – Maps – Illustrations	– Charts – Chalkboards – Photographs – Posters and printed media
III. Projected Visual Aids		
– Epidiascope – Film projector	– Slide projector – Opaque projector	– Overhead projector – LCD (liquid crystal display)
IV. Audiovisual Aids		
– Television, VCR/VCD	– Video and camera	– Sound-motion pictures
V. Activity Aid		
– Field trips – Exhibition	– Model making – Demonstration	– Collection of material – Computer-assisted instructions – Programmed instructions

VI. Traditional Media		
– Puppets	– Dramas	– Folk songs and folk dance

B. Microscopic Divisional Classification Based on the Mode of Presentation

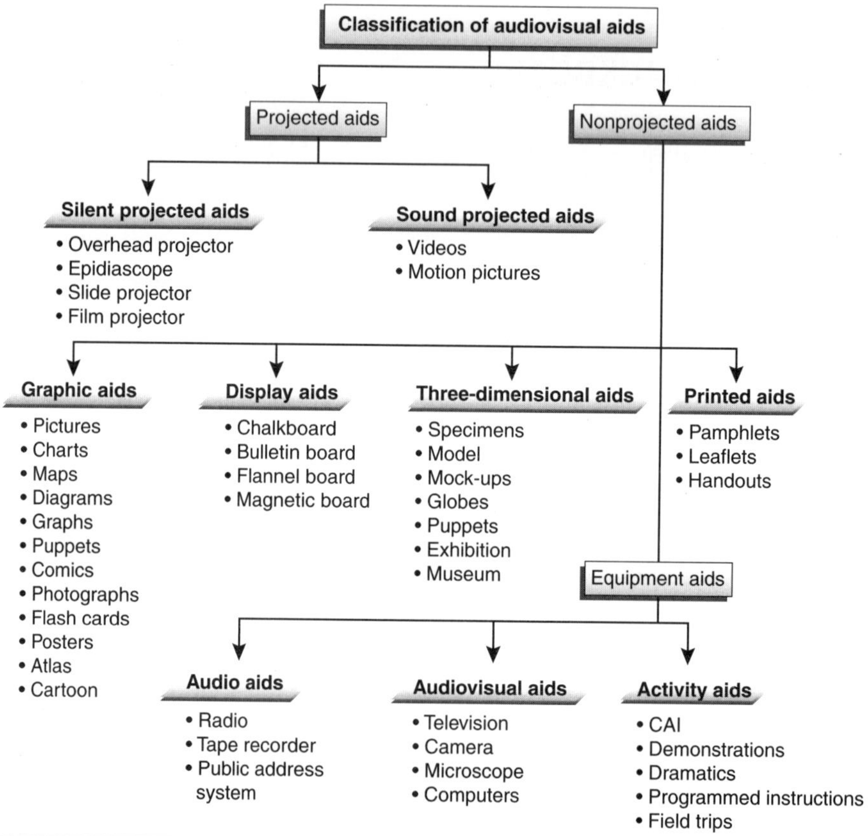

C. Types of Audiovisual Aids Based on the Size of Media

Big Media	Little Media
Computer	Radio, filmstrips
VCR/VCD	Graphic, audio cassettes
Television	And other visuals

GRAPHICAL TEACHING AIDS

The word *graphics* is derived from the Greek word *graphikos* that means visual presentations on some surface, such as a wall, canvas, computer screen, paper or stone to brand, inform, illustrate or entertain. Graphics can be functional or artistic. The latter can be a recorded version, such as a photograph, or an interpretation by a scientist to highlight the essential features, or an artist, in which case the distinction with imaginary graphics may become blurred.

The use of graphic aids in the classroom has become an important teaching strategy in education. As educators learn more about how to reach all types of learners, the use of graphic aids assists in differentiating instructions, giving students greater access to content and helping students achieve greater comprehension of new information. There are multiple graphic aids that can be used in today's classroom and motivate students to learn. The most commonly used graphical teaching aids include chalkboard, chart, graphs, posters, flash cards, flannel board, bulletin board and cartoons, which are discussed below.

I. CHALKBOARD/BLACKBOARD

A blackboard is any dark-coloured, flat, smooth surface on which one can write or draw with a chalk (Fig. 6.5). It is one of the oldest and simplest visual aids. A chalkboard is also known as a *blackboard* that is a dark-coloured writing surface especially black or green in colour used for classroom teaching by writing or drawing illustrations using sticks of chalks. Originally, chalkboards were prepared using smooth, thin sheets of slate or stone of black or dark grey colour. However, in the new era, green-coloured blackboards are becoming more popular because of their better compatibility viewers' vision.

The chalkboard formerly known as the *blackboard* is not a material in itself but a vehicle for a variety of visual materials. In our country, blackboards are mostly black; however, the black colour has given way to either yellow or olive green in the United States and the United Kingdom. The use of colour in the United States for the so-called blackboard has given rise to a new term – the chalkboard. It is documented that the use of chalkboard in American education was found as early as 1801. The origin of the term *blackboard* has been traced to years 1815–1825, while the term *chalkboard* was coined during the years 1935–1940.

It is so much a part of the learning environment that it has become a symbol of education itself. It does not provide ready-made materials; the teacher makes his own meaning as he uses it. It is not only a universally available media of visual instruction but also one of the most valuable devices. A chalkboard is generally installed facing the class which is either built into the wall or fixed or framed on the wall with a ledge to keep the chalk stick and duster.

A. BASIC CHARACTERISTICS OF A CHALKBOARD

The recommended size of chalkboard is 5 × 6 m. For effective use of the chalkboard, the following characteristics should be considered:

- Surface should be rough enough to hold the chalk particles used for writing on the board.
- Surface should be dull enough to eliminate the glare that hampers the visibility of the writing board.

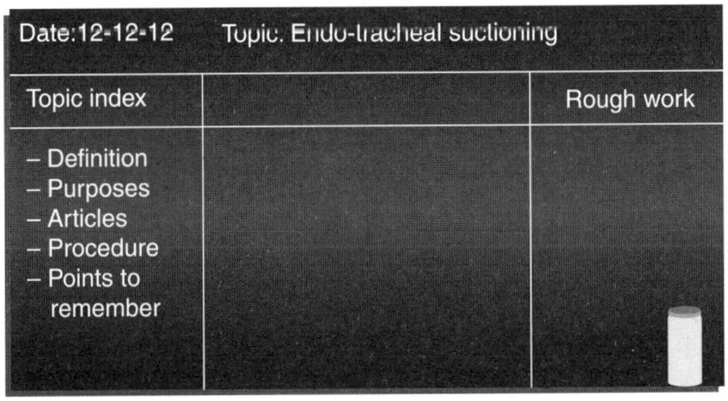

Figure 6.5

Chalkboard/blackboard.

- Surface should be such that chalk can be easily removed with a cloth or foam duster.
- Surface should be mounted on appropriate height within the reach of the teacher and visibility of students.

B. PURPOSES OF A CHALKBOARD

The main purposes of the blackboard are as follows:

- It makes group instruction more concrete and understandable.
- It can set standards of neatness, accuracy and speed, if used properly.
- It can restore the attention of the group.
- It helps in avoiding many vague statements that can be clarified by drawing sketches, outlines, diagrams, directions and summaries.
- It initiates aural and visual sensations and helps in learning.
- It can be a means of motivation and interest.
- It can be used for recording the progress and status.
- It provides many educational opportunities in all curricular and cocurricular activities. The teacher can present facts, principles, processes, procedures, assign individual responsibilities, write questions, problems, sources and references, summaries, outlines, directions, practice individual drills or creative work, make graphic demonstrations, screen for still pictures, projections, symbolic representations and review the total lesson and announcements.
- It can be used to state questions, cite examples of work desired, pose problems and list sources for study.
- It helps in illustrating forms of charting and providing opportunity for nursing students to practice charting.
- It helps in clarifying abstract statements at the exposition stage and providing a summary containing the salient features at recapitulation stage.
- It provides a lot of scope for creative and decorative work.
- It helps in starting afresh by erasing writings and drawings.

C. TYPES OF CHALKBOARD

Blackboards can be fixed or portable and can be made of wood, slate, glass, magnetic materials or sun mica. The main types of boards are as follows:

- ***Ordinary chalkboard held by an easel:*** A portable and adjustable blackboard put on a wooden easel can be taken out of the classroom while taking the class in open, useful for teaching art subjects in a small class.
- ***Roller type chalkboard with mat surface:*** This type of chalkboard is very common in secondary, modern and infant schools. It is made of a thick canvas wrapped on a roller.
- ***Magnetic board:*** These boards are made up of polyvinyl chloride (PVC) materials/sun mica. Small magnets are used to hold suitable objects fixed whenever they are put on this vertical surface. The teachers can make three-dimensional demonstrations with objects on a vertical surface.
- ***Black ceramic unbreakable board:*** These are framed with aluminium or wooden frames as per requirement and chalk is used as writing material.
- ***Black or green glass chalkboard:*** It is the same as the black ceramic unbreakable board but the boards are black/green in colour and made up of glass.
- ***Lobby stand board:*** A lightweight board where the alphabets/figures are interchangeable and mainly used in lobbies. It is easy to carry and has a stand height of 6 feet.

- ***Exhibition board:*** It is easily foldable and expandable and both sides are useable. It is available in 2 panel, 3 panel and 4 panel where pamphlets and papers can be fixed with pushpins.
- ***Double-side stand board:*** In this type of board, one side is whiteboard that is used for marker writing. The other side is blackboard and is used for chalk-piece writing. It is easily moveable and fixed on a wheel stand.
- ***Reception board:*** It is generally used at the reception counters in the corporate sector, hotels, restaurants, etc. Golden letters are fixed and usually framed by golden-coloured aluminium material.
- ***Tariff board:*** It is used at reception counters as a welcome to delegates, at weddings or at hotels to show price lists.
- ***Paging board:*** These are widely used as welcome boards for contacting people at airports and railway stations.
- ***Pressing graph perforated board:*** These perforated boards are commonly used in schools, colleges, corporate offices, hospitals and hotels to display essential information. The boards have either a vertical or horizontal display and have perforations where plastic or metallic alphabets and/or numbers are deployed. The usual size of these letters or numbers used for display on these boards range between ¾ and 1½ inches.
- ***Write and wipe off whiteboard:*** A whiteboard (also known by the terms marker board, dry-erase board, dry-wipe board, pen-board and the misnomer grease board) is a name for any glossy, usually white surface for nonpermanent markings. Whiteboards are analogous to chalkboards, allowing rapid marking and erasing of markings on their surface.
- ***Information notice board:*** Notice boards and pin boards fit nicely into any office environment where they are suitable and are used for posting notices, timetables and other information relating to company news and events. Notices are attached to the boards by pins so that they can be easily posted and removed. Notice boards and pin boards are also ideal for meetings and conferences for the same reason that it is quick and easy to display information and images. Notice boards can be used, for instance, for qualitative research purposes such as focus groups and workshops where images can be arranged quickly for brainstorming and image testing.

D. GUIDELINES FOR PREPARING AND USING A CHALKBOARD

- A blackboard is generally prepared with a piece of plywood about 30 × 40 inch size and painted with blackboard paint.
- To carry from one place to another, it is made in two pieces and hinged in the middle.
- When writing on a blackboard, the teacher should stand on the side and not in front.
- The teacher should not turn his back to the audience for a long time.
- The teacher should write the letters and drawings in a large size.
- The teacher should avoid spelling mistakes.
- Writing should be in straight rows.
- The extreme lower corner of the blackboard should not be used as all members cannot see it.
- The teacher should avoid filling the board with words or figures.
- If the teacher has to write many things or make complicated drawings, he/she should write or draw in advance to save time.
- Abbreviations should not be used.
- Coloured chalks should be used to enhance attraction and clarity in understanding.
- The board should not be cleaned with hands; proper eraser should be used in an up and down motion.
- Before leaving the class, the teacher should make sure the blackboard is clean.

ADVANTAGES OF A CHALKBOARD

- It is simple to use with little practice.
- It is economical and reusable.
- It is easily available and can be used any time.
- It can be used in a wide variety of ways, for simple outlines, drawings, summary of main points, etc.
- It encourages active doing and seeing on the part of the audience.
- It is a natural supplement to all aids and mistakes can be quickly erased.
- It can be easily used for giving lesson notes to students.

LIMITATIONS OF A CHALKBOARD

- It cannot preserve written material.
- It cannot be used for a large audience.
- It requires imagination, initiation, practice and preparation.
- It interrupts communication.
- It becomes smooth and full of glare when used constantly.
- It makes students heavily dependent on the teacher.
- It makes the teacher paced.
- It makes the lesson a dull routine.
- It makes the chalk powder spread, which can be inhaled by the teacher and students.

II. CHART

A chart is a combination of pictorial, graphic and numerical materials, which presents a clear visual summary (Fig. 6.6). It is a diagnostic representation of facts and ideas. The main function of the chart is always to show relationships such as comparisons, relative amounts, developments, processes, classification and organization. Edgar Dale defines charts as, 'a visual symbol summarizing, comparing, contrasting or performing other helpful services in explaining subject-matter'.

A. BASIC CHARACTERISTICS OF A CHART

- Size of the chart could vary based on the type and purpose. However, the standard size of a chart is considered 90 × 60 cm or 70 × 50 cm.
- Charts can be carefully stored and preserved for use in future.
- They have an educational value.
- Usually the charts are teacher made, but students can make it during their presentation as a visual aid.
- Charts display specific information.
- They are easy to carry and store.

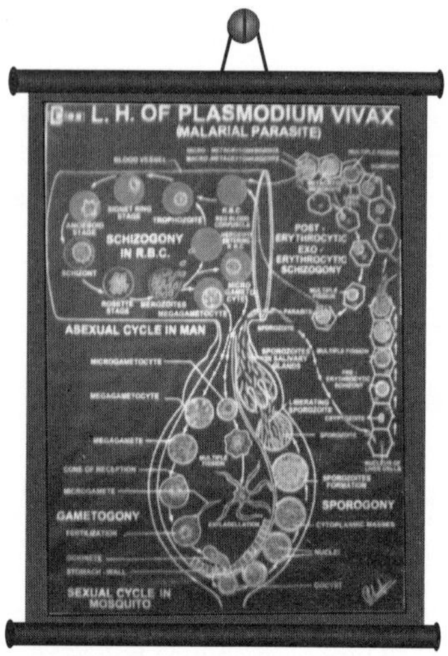

Figure 6.6

Chart.

B. PURPOSES OF CHART

Charts are essential educational aids generally used to:

- Present specific facts, figures and their relationships.
- Symbolically present the educational content.

- Illustrate continuity in a process of certain phenomenon.
- Present abstract ideas in visual forms.
- Present structural developments and organizational structures.
- Help in stimulating the thinking process through illustrative presentations.
- Provide students with motivation for learning.
- Show relationships between facts, figures and statistics.
- Summarize the large information so that comprehension of information may be obtained.

C. TYPES OF CHARTS

The main types of charts used for communication and educational purposes are as follows:

- ***Flowchart:*** Diagrams are used to show organizational elements/administrative/functional relationship boxes connected with lines to show the levels of lines of authority (Fig. 6.7). In this chart, lines, rectangles, circles or other graphic presentations are connected by lines showing the direction of flow.
- ***Flip chart:*** A set of charts related to specific topics that have been tagged together and hung on a supporting stand (Fig. 6.8). The individual charts carry a series of related materials or messages in a sequence. The salient features of specific topics are generally presented through these charts.
- ***Timetable chart:*** These are used to show the schedule of an activity or schedule of an individual. For example, timetable of a class and tour chart. It provides a chronological framework within which events and developments may be recorded. They develop a time sense in students and help them comprehend and visualize the pageant of time and relationships.
- ***Cause and effect chart:*** This kind of chart shows the arrangement of facts and ideas for expressing the relationship between rights and responsibilities, or between a complex of conditions and change or conflict.
- ***Chain chart:*** The arrangement of facts and ideas for expressing transitions or cycles.
- ***Evolution chart:*** Facts and ideas for expressing changes in specific items from the starting data and its projections in the future.
- ***Striptease chart:*** Strip chart has some peculiar characteristics such as (1) it enables speakers to present the information step by step; (2) it increases the interest and imagination of the audience; (3) the information on the chart is covered with thin paper strips applied either by wax, tape or sticky substance or pins; (4) as the speaker wishes to visually reinforce a point with words or symbols, he removes the appropriate strip or paper; and (5) it produces interest and it increases learning and aids recall.

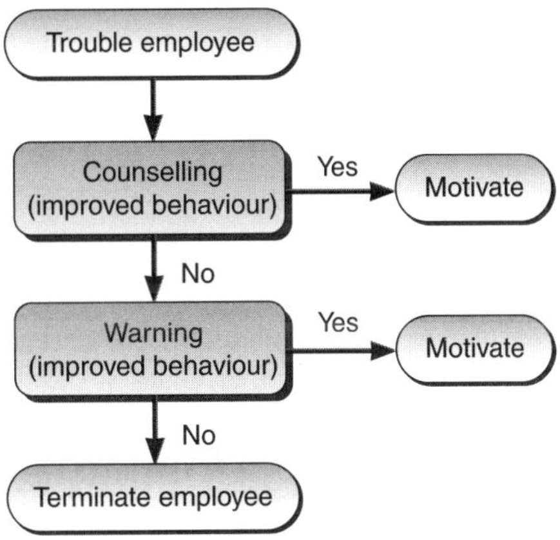
Trouble employee
Counselling
(improved behaviour)
Yes
Motivate
No
Warning
(improved behaviour)
Yes
Motivate
No
Terminate employee

Figure 6.7

Flowchart.

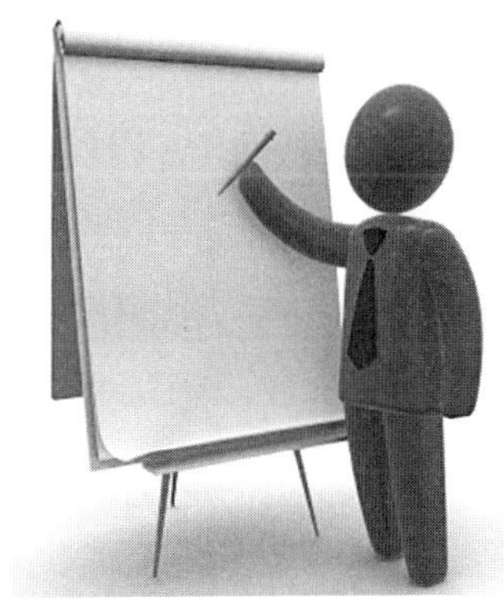

Figure 6.8

Flip chart.

- ***Pull chart:*** It consists of written messages hidden by strips of thick paper. The message can be shown to the viewer, one after another by pulling out the concealing strips.
- ***Tabulation chart:*** It shows the schedule of an activity or of an individual, for example the timetable of a class. These are very valuable aids in the teaching situation where the breakdown of a fact or a statement is to be listed. Also, it is a useful aid for showing points of comparison, distinction and contrasts between two or more things. While making tabulation charts, a few points must be kept in mind. The chart should be 50 × 75 cm or more in size and captioned in bold letters. The vertical columns should be filled with short phrases rather than complete sentences.
- ***Job chart:*** A job chart includes the major responsibilities of the category of personnel for ready reference.
- ***Tree chart:*** Tree charts include the growth and development of specific phenomenon or organizations in a continuous growing process depicted in the form of a tree.
- ***Overlay chart:*** These charts consist of illustrated sheets that can be placed one over another conveniently and in succession. The drawing or illustration on each sheet forms a part of the whole picture. It enables the viewers to see not only the different parts but also see them against the total perspective when one is placed over the other. When the final overlay is placed, the ultimate product is exposed to view.

D. GUIDELINES FOR PREPARING AND USING CHARTS

- The chart should be of standard size (90 × 60 cm or 70 × 50 cm).
- The size of letters for captions and labels should be 2–3 cm and the line thickness should be 2–3 mm.
- Every detail depicted should be visible to everyone in the class.
- Display material should be contrasted with a background.
- Flat pictures and other material should be enlarged before placing on the chart.
- One chart should display information about one specific area in a subject.
- It should not contain too many details.
- It should be neat and tidy.
- The chart should be strong enough to stand for other rough use.

ADVANTAGES OF A CHART

- Charts are helpful in summarizing large information on a single paper so that comprehension and understanding of content can be prompted.
- Illustrative properties of charts catch the attention of students and motivate them for learning.
- The symbolic presentation of information increases quick learning in the learners.

LIMITATIONS OF A CHART

- If the selection of material for preparing charts is not good, they will not last long.
- It takes up a teacher's time if she has to prepare the chart.
- Charts only emphasize on the key points. This leaves the students in doubt if the clarification is not clear.
- Charts lose their charm if they contain too much written matter.
- Poor use of colour combination, improper spacing and margins create confusion in the minds of the students.

III. GRAPHS

Graphs are illustrations to present numerical and statistical data using dots, lines, shapes, colours and pictures. Graphical presentation is a visual art based on the use of visual symbolic and visual-abstract forms. They depict numerical, quantitative relationship or statistical data represented in the form of visual symbols. The common types of graphs are bar graph, line graph, pictorial graphs, histograms, pie graph and cumulative frequency graph.

A. BASIC CHARACTERISTICS OF GRAPHS

The following basic characteristics must be kept in mind while constructing a diagram or graph.

- They must have a title and index.
- The proportion between width and height should be balanced.
- The selection of scale must be appropriate.
- Footnotes may be included wherever needed.
- Principle of simplicity must be kept in mind.
- Neatness and cleanliness in the construction of graphs must be ensured.

B. PURPOSES OF GRAPHS

The main purposes of using graphs in the teaching–learning process are as follows:

- Graphs are one of the most convincing and appealing ways in which statistical results may be presented.
- They give a bird's eye view of the entire information.
- The are attractive to the eye.
- They have a great memorizing effect on the learners.
- They facilitate comparison of data relating to different periods of time.

C. TYPES OF GRAPHS

The most commonly used graphs in the teaching–learning process are bar graphs, pie graphs, histograms, frequency polygons, line graphs, cumulative frequency curves and pictorial graphs.

- ***Bar graphs:*** It is a convenient graphical device that is particularly useful for displaying nominal or ordinal data. It is an easy method adopted for visual comparison of the magnitude of different frequencies. The length of the bars drawn vertically or horizontally indicates the frequency of a character. The bar charts are called *vertical bar charts* (or column charts) if the bars are placed vertically. When the bars are placed horizontally, they are called *horizontal bar charts*. There are three types of bar diagrams: simple, multiple and proportional bar diagrams (Fig. 6.9). The following points to be kept in mind while making a bar diagram:
    - The width of bars should be uniform throughout the diagram.
    - The gap between one bar and another should be uniform throughout.
    - Bars may be vertical or horizontal.
- ***Line graphs:*** It shows the relationships and trends of an event occurring over a period of time. A single line shows the relation and variation in the quantity (Fig. 6.10). The concepts are represented with the help of lines drawn either horizontally or vertically.
- ***Pie/sector graph:*** It is another useful graphical teaching aid for presenting discrete data of qualitative characteristics such as age group, gender and occupational group in a population (Fig. 6.11). The whole area of the circle represents the entire data under consideration.

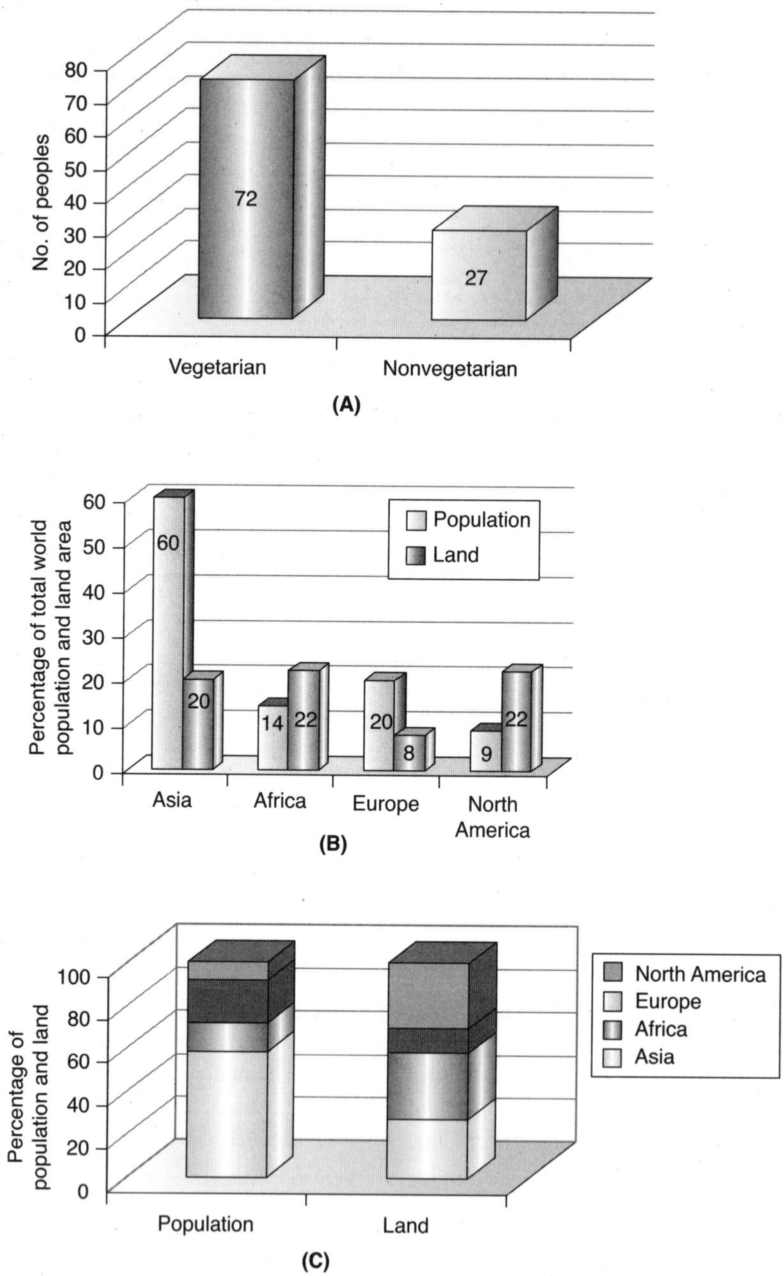

Figure 6.9

Different types of bar graphs: (A) simple bar graph, (B) multiple bar graph and (C) proportional bar graph.

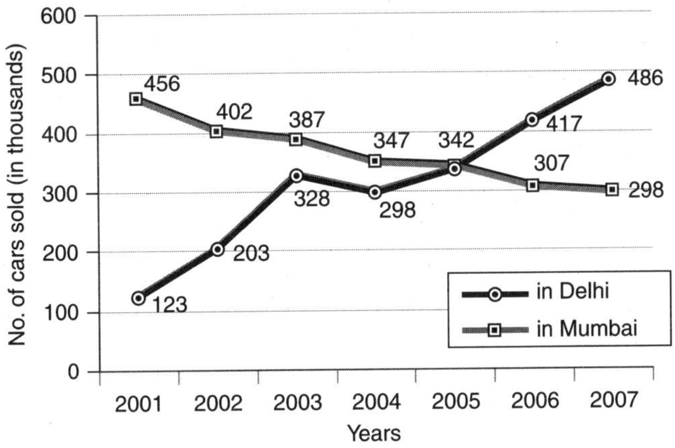

Figure 6.10

Line graph showing car sale in two cities during 2001–2007.

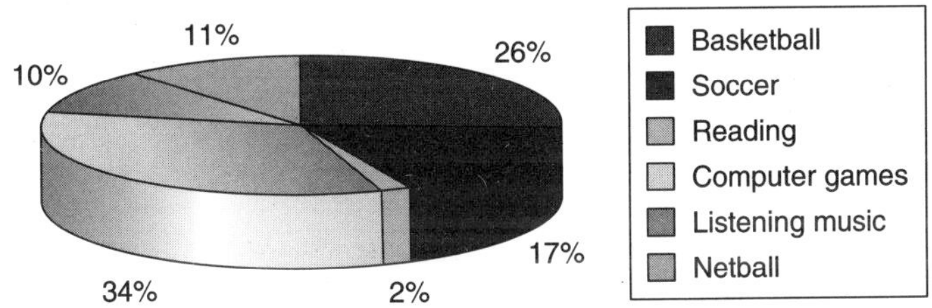

Figure 6.11

Pie diagram showing leisure activities in urban children.

- ***Pictorial graphs:*** This method is used to impress the frequency of the occurrence of events such as attacks, deaths, number operations, admissions, accidents and discharge in a population to the common man (Fig. 6.12).

LIMITATIONS OF GRAPHS

- Sometime may be quite confusing to a lay man.
- Generally presents only quantitative aspect of data.
- Can be used for presenting only one thing or smaller information at one time.
- Can present only approximate values.

IV. POSTERS

S.L. Ahluwalia says 'a poster is a pictorial device designed to attract attention and communicate a story, a fact, an idea, or an image rapidly and clearly'. In other words, a poster is a 'placard, usually pictorial or decorative, utilizing an emotional appeal to convey a message aimed at reinforcing an attitude or

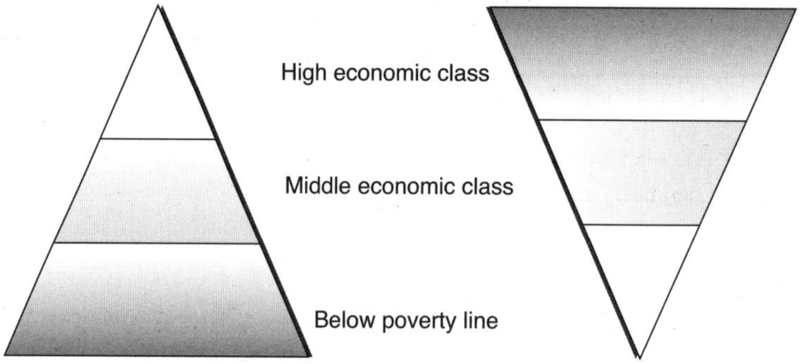

Figure 6.12

Pictorial graph showing proportion of people with economic class: (A) developing countries and (B) developed countries.

urging a course of action'. Posters are generally used for conveying a specific message, teaching a particular thing, giving a general idea, etc. Posters exert great influence on the observer (Fig. 6.13).

The poster can be further defined as a graphic representation of some strong emotional appeal that is carried through a combination of graphic aids like pictures, cartoons lettering and other visual arts on a placard.

Posters are the graphic aids with short quick and typical messages with attention capturing paintings.

A. CHARACTERISTICS OF A GOOD POSTER

- A poster is any piece of printed paper designed to be attached to a wall or a vertical surface, and is typically good substitute for a first-hand experience.
- The ideal size of a poster must be 28 × 22 inches; however the size may vary based on the purpose of poster. For example, conference posters are generally large in size.
- Very effective visual aids vary from a simple printed card to a complicated and artistic design.
- There must be minimal use of words, that is only four to five words.
- The idea or feeling being presented must be original and clearly understandable.
- The layout of the poster must be simple so that it does not distract the student from the main content of learning.
- There must be appropriate use of colours and fonts:
  Use bold illustrations
  Avoid fancy lettering style
  Proper use of colour
- The poster must be as attractive as possible so that students can be motivated for learning.

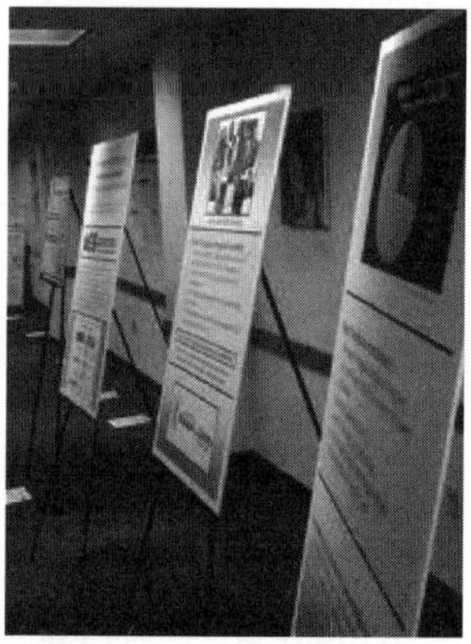

Figure 6.13

Posters.

B. PURPOSES OF A POSTER

Posters are used to:

- Present a single idea or subject forcefully.
- Communicate a more general idea.
- Publicize important school and community events and projects.

- Thrust the message leading to action for the classroom and community.
- Add atmosphere to the classroom.
- Capture attention by some attractive feature and thus convey the message attractively and quickly.
- Motivate the learners in the class.
- Leave a strong lasting impression on the learner's mind.
- Satisfy the viewer emotionally and aesthetically and to create atmospheric effect.

C. GUIDELINES FOR PREPARING AND USING A POSTER

- Promote one point at a time.
- Support local demonstrations and exhibits.
- It should be planned for specified people on a specified topic and a theme should be provided.
- It should have instant appeal.
- It should tell the message in a single glance.
- It should be attractive enough and pleasing colours should be used.
- For headings, bold letters (20 × 30 inch) should be used.
- The language should be easy and simple.
- The most suitable words should be decided upon to provide a title or a slogan.
- A few layouts should be sketched and the best one should be decided on.
- All needed material should be gathered to prepare the poster.
- Smudge marks should be erased and finishing touches added.
- The poster must be displayed at a place with good provision of light and where a large number of people can see it.

ADVANTAGES OF A POSTER

- Because of its impressive presentation, a poster captivates the eye, regardless of the message and is capable of being comprehended.
- A poster is a simple and dynamic medium of presenting a message in a compact form.
- A poster tells the story vividly with the desired effect.

LIMITATIONS OF A POSTER

- A poster conveys a single theme and does not always give enough information.
- The lettering if not attractive and accurate makes the poster illegible.
- Smudge marks make the posters unattractive and futile.

V. FLASH CARDS

Flash cards are used for the presentation of an idea in the form of posters, pictures, words and sentences (Fig. 6.14). A single card or a whole series may be flashed in front of the class. In other words, flash cards are a set of pictured paper cards of varying sizes that are flashed one by one in a logical sequence. Flash cards can be self-made or commercially prepared and are made up of a chart or drawing paper or plain paper using colours or ink on them for drawings.

They aim to develop the power of observation, identification, quick comprehension and retention. Flash cards are small, compact cards, approximately 10 × 12 inches that are flashed before a group. Each card contains important highlights of the topic in the form of words, diagram, photograph and illustrations.

A. BASIC CHARACTERISTICS OF FLASH CARDS

- Flash cards are small, compact cards of varying size approximately 10 × 12 inches in size.
- They are made out of cardboards or any other thick material.
- They are the simplest of all aids to present topic highlights in the form of words, diagrams, photographs and illustration.

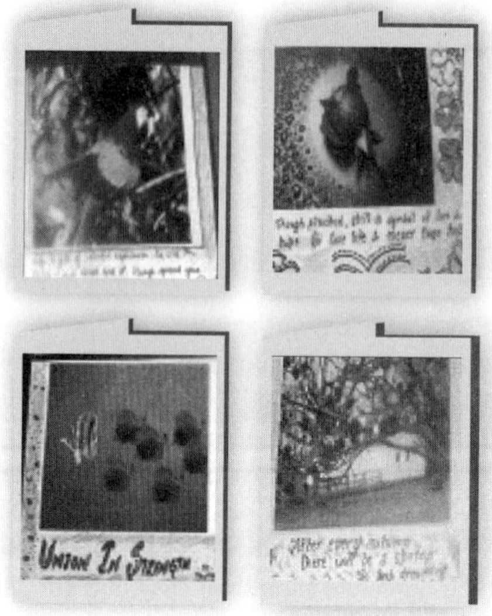

Figure 6.14

Flash cards.

B. PURPOSES OF FLASH CARDS

Flash cards are generally used for the following purposes:

- The pictorial contents presented in a series are easily recognized by the group.
- They are flashed before the class one by one to bring home an idea.
- Communication of new ideas requires repetitive study methods, drill-work and review of the discussion that can be achieved through flash cards.
- They provide students with a systematic approach to drill.
- They are helpful to teach recognition by sight.
- They are easy to carry.

C. GUIDELINES FOR PREPARING AND USING FLASH CARDS

- The messages can be brief, simple line drawings or photographs, cartoons and the content is written in a few lines at the back of each card.
- They are commonly 10 × 12 inches in size.
- Ideally 10–12 cards can be used for one talk. The number of cards should not be less than 3 and more than 20.
- Preparing a picture for each idea which will give visual impact to the idea.
- The height of writing on the flash card is to be approximately 5 cm for better visualization.
- Selection of a topic and the content to be displayed should be planned.
- Illustrations and words should be simple and should give a brief introduction about the lesson to students.
- The size of the group should not be more than 30 students.
- Arrange the cards in proper sequence.
- Significant points should be pointed out and care should be taken not to cover them with hands.
- Look at the card while the concept is explained from the card.
- Be enthusiastic while explaining the matter.
- Flash the card in front of the class by holding it high with both your hands so that all the students can see it. Hold the cards at the chest level where people can see clearly; hold against the body and not in the air.
- Review the lesson by selectively using flash cards.
- Involve the audience in a discussion.

ADVANTAGES OF FLASH CARDS

- They help in the development of cognitive abilities and recognition and recall of students.
- They help to introduce and present topic as well as review the topic.
- They can be used to apply information already gained by students to new situations.
- They can be used for drill and practice in the elementary class.
- They emphasize important points.
- They are very cost-effective because they can be prepared on simple papers.
- They are easy to make, require only hard papers and pens.
- They can work as a useful supplementary aid and can be effectively used with other materials.

LIMITATIONS OF FLASH CARDS

- If used for a prolonged period, they become boring for students.
- The students cannot get a complete view of the concept, as the points are flashed one by one.
- They need to be carefully stored and prevented from bending.
- They are ineffective for large groups.
- They are time-consuming and cannot include the whole topic of presentation. Only a part of a topic can be presented through flash cards.

VI. FLANNEL BOARD

The flannel board or felt board is a piece of rigid material covered with cotton flannel, wool, suede cloth or paper (Fig. 6.15). A piece of rough flannel or khadi fixed over a wooden board provides an excellent background for displaying cut-out pictures, graphs, drawing and other illustrations. The cut-out pictures and other illustrations are provided with a rough surface at the back by pasting pieces of sand paper, felt or rough cloth. They adhere at once when put on the flannel. It is a very cheap medium, easy to transport and promotes thought and criticism.

A. PREPARING FLANNEL BOARD

The following articles and steps are required for preparing the flannel board:

Articles Required

- A piece of plywood, cardboard or poster board
- A piece of flannel large enough to cover the board
- A pair of scissors
- Duct tape (or a staple gun or upholstery tacks if using a plywood)
- Felt squares to make shapes and other cut-outs

Preparation Procedure

- Wrap the piece of flannel around the board you have chosen.
- Secure all edges around the back side with the duct tape, staples or tacks.

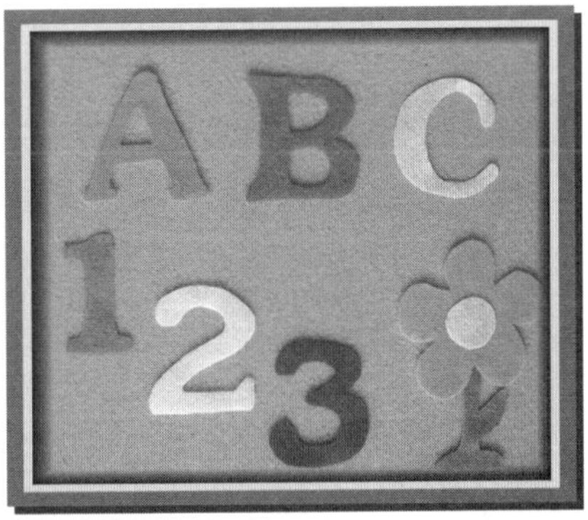

Figure 6.15

Flannel boards.

- The items to be displayed should also be pasted with the same flannel on back side which keeps it adherent to the board without visible support.

B. PURPOSES OF A FLANNEL BOARD

The purposes of using flannel boards are given below:

- They can be used throughout the discussion whenever the needed item can be placed and explained on (if the purpose is served, the item has to be removed).
- They help improve the visual artefact of the written content or illustrations to a large group of learners.
- They also facilitate the illustrative presentation of written content for easy understanding.
- Their use facilitate the auditory, visual and kinaesthetic learning.
  - ***Auditory:*** The learners can hear the content displayed on the board read by someone.
  - ***Visual:*** The learners can visualize the displayed content on the flannel board.
  - ***Kinaesthetic:*** They also can display pieces of information on the board.
- They are generally used as a bridge between the books and in story time programmes.
- They add variety to the storyline.
- They help communicate the idea in an effective manner.
- They describe the way of doing a particular item.
- They motivate the learner.
- They add variety to classroom activity.
- They intensify the impressions and vitalize the instructions.
- They provide information.
- They supplement and correlate information, so saves time.

C. GUIDELINES FOR USING A FLANNEL BOARD

- The contents of the board should be organized around the central theme.
- Appearance must be neat and orderly.
- The material should be displayed in an attractive manner.
- Avoid overcrowding on the board.
- It should be clearly seen by the group members.
- The displayed pictures should be sufficiently large in size.
- Remove the picture as soon as their purpose is over.

ADVANTAGES OF A FLANNEL BOARD

- Makes concepts easy to understand.
- Effectively used for small groups.
- Saves time during the presentation.
- Keeps students well motivated.

LIMITATIONS OF A FLANNEL BOARD

- Cannot be used for large groups.
- Needs more preparatory time.

VII. BULLETIN BOARD

A bulletin board is a display board that shows the visual learning material on a specific subject. It is a soft board that holds pins or tags. It is a simple device placed either indoors or outdoors. Items like photographs, publications, posters, newspaper cut-outs are generally displayed (Fig. 6.16).

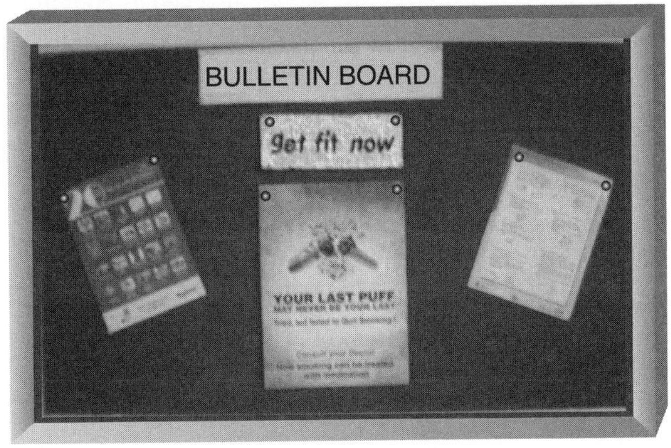

Figure 6.16

Bulletin board.

A bulletin board also known as a *pin board* or a *notice board* is a place where people can display public messages, for example to advertise things, to buy or sell, announce events or provide information. Dormitory corridors, well-trafficked hallways, lobbies and freestanding kiosks often have cork boards attached to facilitate the posting of notices. At some universities, lamp posts, bollards, trees and walls often become impromptu posting sites in areas where official boards are sparse in number.

The items that can be displayed on the bulletin boards are photographs, CD covers, book jackets, news stories, sketches, newspaper and magazine clippings, drawings, cartoons, specimens, real objects, posters, poems, greeting cards, thoughts and even jokes.

A. BASIC CHARACTERISTICS OF BULLETIN BOARDS

- They can be framed soft boards or straw boards or cork boards.
- Their size depends on the purpose.
- Dark blazer cloth works as a back drop.
- The height should be 1 m above the ground.

B. PURPOSES OF BULLETIN BOARDS

Bulletin boards are used for the following purposes:
- Communication of ideas
- Giving correct initial impression
- Broaden the sensory experience
- Intensify impressions
- Vitalize instructions
- Add variety to classroom activity
- Provide information
- Supplement and correlate instructions
- Save time
- Help students learn how to communicate ideas visually
- Facilitate class study of single copy material
- Encourage participation
- Provide a review

C. TYPES OF BULLETIN BOARDS

- Felt board
- Magnetic board
- Fixed type
- Movable type
- Folded type

D. GUIDELINES FOR PREPARING AND USING BULLETIN BOARDS

- ***Thumbnail sketches:*** Make several and then select one.
- Procurement of material on a given subject.
- Sorting out relevant material.
- ***Decide on a theme:*** Words should catch attention of viewers.
- Use of attention-directing devices.
- Should be displayed in an aesthetic manner and the area should be well lighted.
- Should be kept a little above eye level.
- Place the bulletin board near the doorway.
- The content of a bulletin board should be organized around a central theme.
- Title of the topic must be fixed at the top and the material placed should be appropriately dated and revised from time to time.
- The material should be organized properly by dividing the board, overcrowding of content must be avoided.
- The board must have a neat, ordered and attractive appearance.
- Give due thoughts to eye catching leads.
- Make special reference during course of study.
- Students can be asked to collect display material.
- The content on the board should be changed regularly.
- There should be a separate board for posting routine notices of the institution.
- A bulletin board committee is responsible for editing the board from time to time.
- Do not leave the board for long after the teaching purpose is over.
- Take down displays from the board, return the borrowed items and file useful material.

ADVANTAGES OF BULLETIN BOARDS

- Display can be effectively used as a follow-up of chalkboard work.
- Adds colour and liveliness in communicating the message to the audience.
- Good supplement for other teaching aids.
- Introduces a new topic to a large number of people.
- Explains important events, reports and special activities.

LIMITATIONS OF BULLETIN BOARDS

- Not effective for illiterate groups.
- Takes a lot of time for preplanning and preparation.
- Cannot be used for an all-inclusive teaching.
- Has to be used as a supplementary aid to other teaching aids.

- Collection of relevant materials for certain topics may sometimes be difficult.

VIII. CARTOONS

A cartoon is a humourous caricature which gives a subtle message. In a cartoon, the features of objects and people are exaggerated along with their general symbols. In short, a cartoon is a figurative and subtle graphic aid. It is a metaphoric representation of reality and makes learning more interesting and effective, as it creates a strong appeal to the emotions. A cartoon is an interpretative illustration which uses symbols to portray an opinion, a scene or a situation (Fig. 6.17).

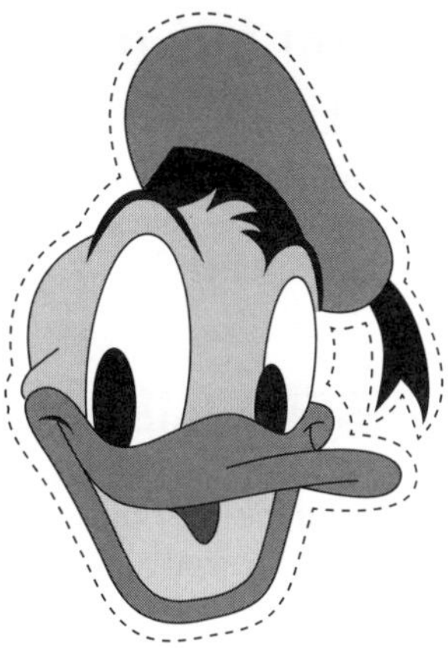

Figure 6.17

Cartoon.

Cartoons are a novel way of using pictures or symbols for presenting a message or a point of view concerning a personality, news, situation or an event. They are more attention-drawing and provide a lot of imagination, particularly on current happenings, in a small space. They are blended with humour and satire.

A. BASIC CHARACTERISTICS OF CARTOONS

- Cartoons should be of appropriate size so that everyone can see them and understand the message appropriately.
- Cartoons must be drawn according to the age and educational level of the learners to ensure their appropriateness for the target group.
- The symbols used in cartoons must be clear and understandable.
- Use of text must be minimal and should be meaningful.
- Cartoons should be self-explanatory and instructive.
- Cartoons should be funny, interesting and humourous.

B. PURPOSES OF CARTOONS

The main purposes of cartoons in the teaching–learning process are as follows:
- They are primarily designed for capturing the attention of the targeted group.
- They are successful tools for student motivation and the promotion of learning.
- They create humour and fantasy among the learners so educational stress can be minimized.
- A single cartoon can easily present multiple ideas and concepts.
- They trigger innovative thinking in the learners.
- They can present educational content in an interesting manner.

ADVANTAGES OF CARTOONS

- Cartoons are humourous caricatures so they capture the attention of the learners and prevent boredom among them.
- They are quite successful in motivating the learning, and messages can be easily understood by the learners.
- They can easily present multiple ideas and concepts to the learners.

LIMITATIONS OF CARTOONS

- A skilled specialist is required to prepare educational cartoons.
- Many educational topics can be presented only through cartoons.
- Cartoons as educational aids may sometimes distract the students from the main learning purpose and objectives.

THREE-DIMENSIONAL AUDIOVISUAL AIDS

Three-dimensional aids are considered good substitutes of real objectives. A variety of three-dimensional audiovisual aids are also known as *realia.* They are used to substitute the real objectives so that students can get the experience of real objectives in their natural setting. Sometimes it is not possible to provide a real object experience. In these cases, the three-dimensional aids could be the best option to be used as a teaching tool. For example, a teacher can use a model of the heart to teach about the heart's anatomy when real body dissection is not possible. On the other hand, sometimes real-life objectives could be too large or expensive to bring into the classroom, then the three-dimensional audiovisual objectives may be a good alternative. Three-dimensional objects stimulate the imagination, thinking and abstraction in the students by offering first-hand experiences about real-life situations. Some of the main three-dimensional audiovisual aids, that is objects and specimens, models, puppets, exhibitions, museums and dioramas, are discussed below.

I. OBJECTS AND SPECIMENS

A collection of real things for instructional use refers to objects. A specimen is a sample of the real object or material. Objects and specimens should be mounted in shallow boxes in an artistic way and the boxes should be covered with cellophane paper (Fig. 6.18). Also each object or specimen should be labelled using self-adhesive paper.

While using the specimen and objects as teaching aids, a teacher must keep the following points in mind:

- Planning of the object or specimen display should be such that a simple and direct visualization of the object or specimen is possible by all the learners with a great level of ease.
- The display of object or specimen must be supplemented with an active question–answer session, so that the teacher can be sure that students have clearly understood the object or specimen under observation.
- The teacher must provide details of the structure of an object or specimen under display and offer clarification when and where needed.
- The teacher must ensure feedback and further practice so that students can learn the object or specimen thoroughly under observation.

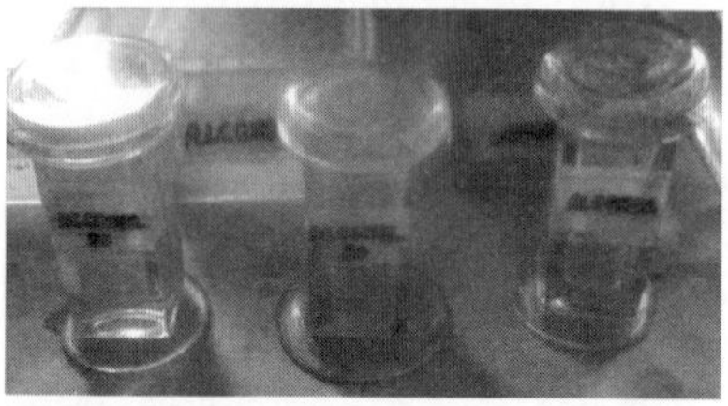

Figure 6.18

Specimen.

A. SOURCES OF OBJECTS AND SPECIMENS

- Local markets.
- Manufacturers and factories.
- Discarded material from houses.

- Specimens found in nature can be collected by students from field trips and nature hunts.
- Plaster casts can be purchased.
- Wild flowers, leaves, shells, stones, butterflies, moths and insects can also be procured.

ADVANTAGES OF OBJECTS AND SPECIMENS

- Collection of objects and specimens by students requires interaction with others leading to the development of social skills and values.
- When students collect and display objects and specimens, they derive satisfaction of contributing something worthwhile to the school and the teacher.
- The student's power of observation and first-hand experience is enhanced by the collection of objects and specimens.
- Student's personal collection of objects and specimens can be a good source of doing investigatory projects.
- Collection of objects and specimens becomes an interesting educational pursuit of the teacher and the students alike.
- They arouse some interest in students for learning.
- They involve all the five senses in the process of learning.
- They heighten the reality in the classroom.

II. MODELS

A model is a recognizable representation of a real thing three dimensionally, that is height, width and depth is felt as reality. In other words, a model is a life size miniature or over size or original size whether workable or not, whether it differs or not from original size of an object to be studied, which is very useful in teaching (Fig. 6.19).

Further, a model means imitation, replica and copy of the real-life object. However, if the model is larger or smaller than the real thing, the students should be given a clear idea of its actual size. In some cases, models are oversimplified, such models should be used with great caution.

A. PURPOSES OF MODELS

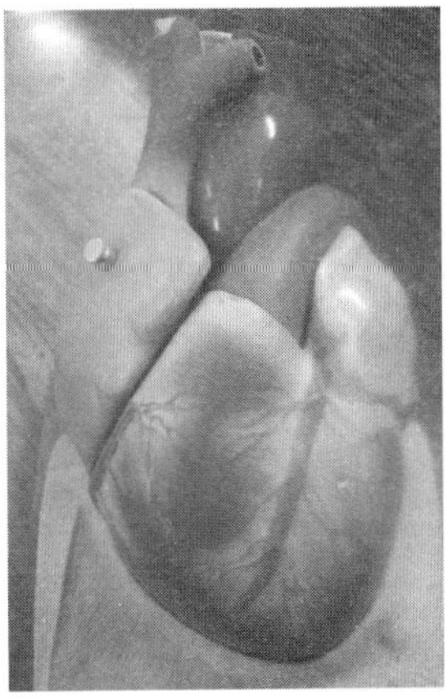

Figure 6.19

Model.

Models are useful and necessary because:

- The real thing may not be available in that season or may be far away from the institute.
- The real thing may be too big to be brought to the institute.
- The real thing may be too dangerous to be felt or handled by the students.
- The real thing may be too expensive.
- The real thing may be too small to be seen at all or seen properly.

Other core purposes of models used as teaching aids are as follows:

- Models simplify reality.
- Models help in clarifying the abstract concept of knowledge.
- They also facilitate visualization and learning of the large objects. It is generally not possible to visualize at one snapshot.
- Models also offer a clear and correct concept of invariably large real objects such as a dam, bridge and mountain.

- Furthermore, functional models also help in understanding the real working of various objects, instruments and machines.
- Promotes creative interest in students.

B. TYPES OF MODELS

- ***Solid models:*** They are a replica of an original thing made with suitable materials, such as clay, plaster of Paris, wood and iron, to show the external parts of thing. For example, a globe, clay model of a human or animal.
- ***Cutaway and X-ray models:*** They are the replicas of the original things to show their internal parts. They show how something looks from inside. There are many situations particularly in technical subjects and in the study of hygiene where it is necessary to see the interior of an organ or a machine to understand how it works. Cross-sectional models are difficult to make in the classroom or institutions as they require expertise to construct them. For example, a cross-sectional model of the human body.
- ***Working models:*** These models are either actual working things or miniature replicas for illustration of an operation. In some lessons, working models that show how things function or operate in a simple way are very helpful. In many cases, they are used in place of real articles because they are easier to understand. For example, a motor, a generator or a model showing blood flow in the body.
- ***Sand models:*** Sand models are made by using sand, clay and saw dust. For example, a tribal village or a forest area.
- ***Scale models:*** In some study situations, we need a correct representation of things through exactness of a scale. Small-scale models of the Damodar valley and other projects help students as well as others form a good idea of big enterprises. Further, a scale is one measurement that represents another value of measurement. For example, architects may use a scale of ¼ inch = 1 foot for construction drawings. At this scale, a building of 100 feet on each side could be represented as a 25-inch square.
- ***Simplified models:*** There are, however, many learning situations in which models that show the external form of an object roughly are required. The animals, birds and fish which children of primary schools make out of clay, sand or straw have great educational value.

C. ESSENTIAL QUALITIES OF A MODEL

A model must have the following qualities:
- Usefulness
- Accuracy
- Simplicity
- Utility
- Solidity
- Ingenuity

ADVANTAGES OF MODELS

- Models heighten the reality of things and make learning direct and meaningful as they are three-dimensional.
- Models illustrate the application side of certain principles and laws.

- Models explain complex and intricate operations in a simplified way and thus make comprehension easier.
- Models are long lasting and ultimately work out to be cheaper teaching aids.
- Still models are easy to make with the help of discarded materials like empty boxes, pins, clips, nails and clay.
- Models should be reasonable in size and convenient to handle.
- Models involve the use of all the five senses and make learning effective.

LIMITATIONS OF MODELS

- They require expertise to make.
- They are time-consuming.
- Some models may be very expensive.

III. PUPPETS

One of the old and popular arts in Indian villages is puppetry. Puppetry is an education cum entertaining aid where puppets are manipulated by the performer (Fig. 6.20). In writing or selecting a puppet play, the age, background and tastes of students should be taken into consideration. A short puppet play is always preferable.

A puppet is a manipulative doll dressed as a character and the performer is a person termed as a puppeteer. A good puppeteer has to blend his art with dramatization to produce the desired effect. It is used as an effective teaching aid for languages and social sciences.

D. TYPES OF PUPPETS

- ***String or marionette puppets:*** Marionettes consist of puppets with hinged body parts which are controlled by nine strings producing the required movements in the puppet. These puppets are mainly manipulated by professional puppeteers.
- ***Stick puppets:*** Stick puppets are painted cut-outs attached by sticks. The actions of these puppets are manipulated by the teacher and students by hiding behind a screen so that only the puppets are visible to the audience or the class.
- ***Shadow puppets:*** Shadow puppets are silhouettes of cardboard that produce shadows on a white screen. The motion of these silhouettes is manipulated by the teacher and students.
- ***Finger of hand puppets:*** Hand puppets are round balls painted as heads with overflowing, colourful costumes. They are worn on fingers which operate their movements. They are operated from below the stage.

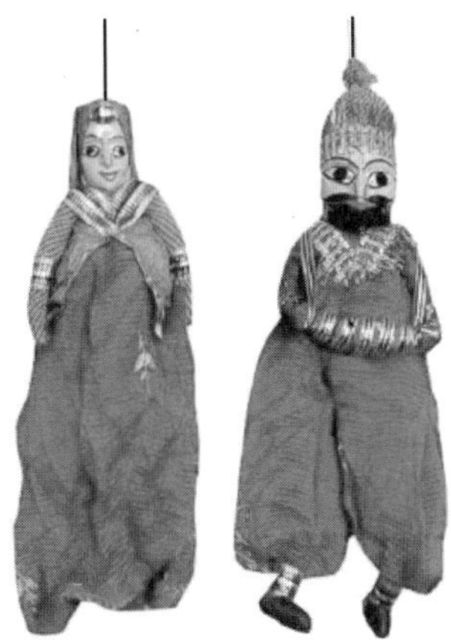

Figure 6.20

Puppets.

ADVANTAGES OF PUPPETS

- They create interest.
- They give knowledge in a brief period.
- They are an effective method in teaching.

- They motivate students.
- They are easy to carry and operate.

LIMITATIONS OF PUPPETS

- They need group cooperation and coordination.
- They require skills in preparation and supply.
- Skills are needed for presentation.

IV. EXHIBITIONS

Many times in the school, a department of the school or class puts up their work for showing it to the people outside the school, such a show is called an *exhibition* (Fig. 6.21). The pieces of work done by the students for an exhibition are called *exhibits*.

A. BASIC CHARACTERISTICS OF AN EXHIBITION

- The exhibition should have a central theme with a few subthemes to focus attention to a particular concept.
- The exhibits should be clean and labelled properly.
- The concepts of contrast in colour and size should be used for laying out the exhibitions.
- The exhibits should be so placed so most visitors can see them.
- The place and exhibits should be well lighted.
- Both motion and sound should be utilized to capture the attention and interest of the visitors.
- The exhibition should have some exhibits with operative mechanism such as switches and handles to be operated by the visitors to observe some happenings.
- The exhibition should include a lot of demonstrations as they involve the students and the visitors deeply.
- The exhibition should be able to relate various subject areas to provide integrated learning.

ADVANTAGES OF AN EXHIBITIONS

- Exhibitions inspire students to learn by doing things themselves and get a sense of involvement.
- Exhibitions give students a sense of accomplishment and achievement.
- Exhibitions develop social skills of communication, cooperation and coordination.
- Exhibitions foster better school community relations and make community members conscious about the school.
- Exhibitions couple information with pleasure.
- Exhibitions foster creativity in students.

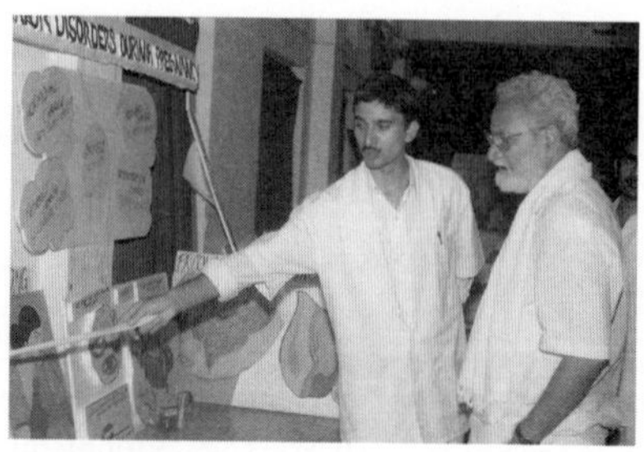

Figure 6.21

Exhibition.

LIMITATIONS OF AN EXHIBITIONS

- Exhibitions require thorough preparation.
- They are time-consuming.
- They require a large amount of funds or budget.

V. MUSEUMS

A museum is a building that displays a collection of historical relics, antiques, curiosities, works of arts, works of science, literature and other artefacts of general interest. Museums can be useful both for public education and specific classroom instructions.

A. SETTING UP A SCHOOL MUSEUM

- Schools should have enough space.
- Take the help of students, collect old and new objects and articles.
- Accept donations from various organizations who donate articles.
- Students can be guided to prepare exhibits for museum.
- All the collected and prepared articles should be displayed and labelled.
- A detailed report book should be maintained giving a brief description of each museum pieces.
- The museum rooms should be well lighted.
- It should be clean and well maintained for use.

VI. DIORAMAS

A diorama is a three-dimensional arrangement of related objects, models and cut-outs to illustrate a central theme or concept. The objects and models are generally placed in a big box or showcased with a glass covering and the background is printed with a shade or a scene, for example a harvest scene and a planting scene.

ADVANTAGES OF DIORAMAS

- They provide a good opportunity to learn.
- They give the appearance of actual things which cannot be brought to the classroom.
- They are interesting and enhance creativity.
- Live things can also be shown in dioramas, for example an aquarium.
- They provide an opportunity for the students to carry out a creative activity.

LIMITATIONS OF DIORAMAS

- Sometimes they are not a cost-effective method.
- They need expatriation for preparation.
- They may require a large budget.
- They may sometimes misguide the student if is not a replica of the actual thing.

PRINTED EDUCATIONAL AIDS

Printed educational aids have been used since a long time and are found essentially important in the classroom as well as mass education. However, rapid development in science and technology has revolutionized the use of educational aids in the teaching–learning process. Today, we have so many advanced educational aids which are far advanced in technology and usefulness than conventional educational aids. However, conventional educational aids still have their importance in the teaching–learning process. Some important printed educational aids are pamphlets, handouts, handbills and leaflets. However, this chapter presents the most commonly used printed educational aids, that is pamphlets and leaflets.

I. PAMPHLETS

Pamphlets are a type of nonprojected audiovisual aids. A pamphlet is a paper that can be folded into two or three or five, and the matter can be printed either on a single or on both sides. In other words, a pamphlet is an unbounded booklet without a hard cover or binding. It may consist of a single sheet of paper that is printed on both sides and folded in half, in thirds, or in fourth, or it may consist of a few pages that are folded in half or stapled at the crease to make a single book. A pamphlet gives a chance to explain to the people who do not have time to stay and discuss the content of information. A pamphlet must be self-explanatory (Fig. 6.22).

A. PURPOSES OF PAMPHLETS

Pamphlets are used for the following purposes:

- To mobilize people to support a cause.
- To advertise a meeting or a specific event.
- To popularize a slogan or a message.
- Furthermore, pamphlets are used for the following purposes:
  - Explain an issue to the community.
  - Inform people of their rights.
  - Win support for a campaign you are running.
  - Win support for any organization's point of view.

B. PREPARING PAMPHLETS

To prepare a good pamphlet, the following things must be followed:

- Discuss the purpose, the message, the target people and content.
- Discuss the quantity and quality of pamphlets.
- If printing is done on both sides of a pamphlet, each side should have an interesting *bold* headline to get peoples' attention.
- Each side should also carry the organization's logo or name.
- Keep the language simple by avoiding long and complicated sentences.
- The best pamphlets are short and simple.
- All facts should be correct.

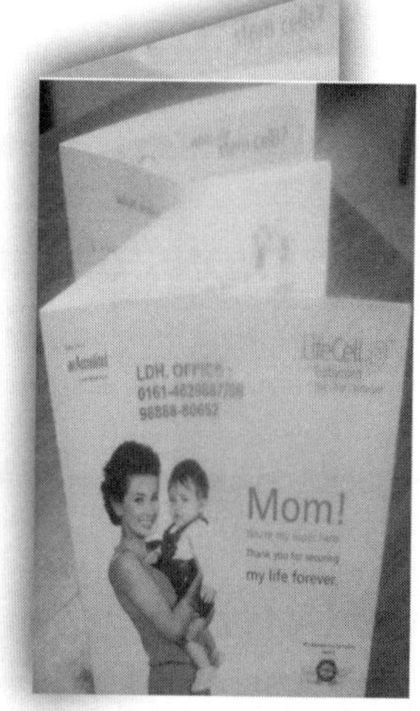

Figure 6.22
Pamphlet.

STEPS FOR PREPARING PAMPHLETS

- Initially, the purpose and nature of the pamphlets and the target group must be determined. The target group may be a general person, professionals such as doctors and nurses.
- The second priority should be to define the dimensions of the pamphlet. The best and most used size is with the dimensions of 8.5 × 11 inches^2.

- Some people, however, choose a larger, smaller and more expensive pamphlet sizes if the budget can handle it.
- Design the pamphlet by writing the content and identifying the images to be included in the pamphlet.
- Give the pamphlet for proof printing and then check for any mistake, ensure modification, if required.
- Finally print out the needed pamphlets and distribute them according to the best method.
  - Think carefully about the target group before you plan for distribution because different sectors of people gather in different places, for example outside the school gates, factory gates, public places.
  - The best way of distributing is door to door where a team drops the pamphlets off at each house in the target area or with newspapers.

C. STYLES FOR ORGANIZING A PAMPHLET

- ***Tutorial style:*** This is the first and the most basic style of pamphlets. It gives information on a particular subject or explains how something is done.
- ***Frequently asked question style:*** This is a very effective technique to get an answer to any question fast.
- ***Testimonial style:*** This is a storytelling mode. A story is narrated about the pamphlet issue. The concepts are introduced one by one historically. This makes the learning process easier for most learners.

ADVANTAGES OF PAMPHLETS

- They are the best method of dissemination of information or a message to larger group of people.
- They save time and recourses in dissemination of information to a large group of people.

LIMITATIONS OF PAMPHLETS

- The main disadvantage of pamphlets is that they can waste a lot of money and time if printed pamphlets are not distributed properly.
- Only literate and educated people can be benefited with this educational aid. Furthermore, because of more written content, they capture less attention.
- They do not ensure that the targeted group has surely paid attention and time to read the pamphlet.

II. LEAFLETS

Leaflets are printed educational aids of a single sheet paper folded to make a full page of printed matter on a single side. A leaflet is commonly referred to as any piece of printed information, which includes fact sheets, guides, small booklets, brochures and usually distributed for a campaign to disseminate the information or message to a large population (Fig. 6.23). Leaflets are printed educational media used to propagate a message to a mass population in a short time.

A. TYPES OF LEAFLETS

- ***Persuasive leaflets:*** Persuasive leaflets are used to spread a message and convince people through the reason and logic printed in the leaflets.

- ***Informative leaflets:*** These leaflets are used to present the facts that are already known to the people in a target group, and therefore attract and satisfy their curiosity.
- ***Directive leaflets:*** As the name suggests, these leaflets are used to offer special instructions and directions to the people in a target group which is useful for directing and controlling their activities.

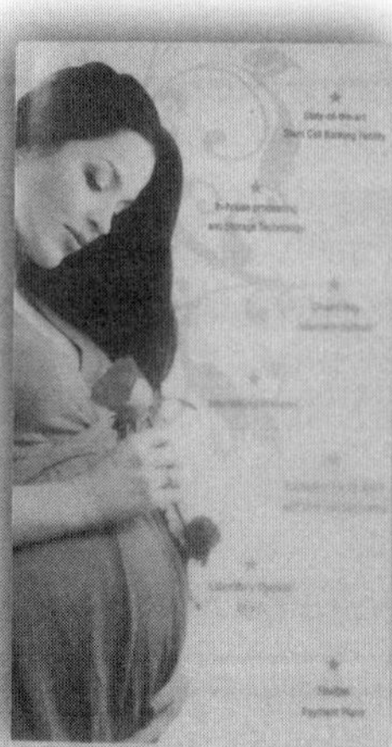

Figure 6.23

Leaflets.

B. GUIDELINES FOR PREPARING LEAFLETS

- A leaflet must be organized under the following headings:
  - ***Heading:*** Leaflet heading is the part which is most prominently responsible for catching the attention of people and is therefore considered as the most important part of the leaflet. The heading must be precise, focused on the main theme and written in eye-catching words and colours.
  - ***Subheadings:*** Leaflet subheadings are essential when the main heading is not successful in covering the theme of the main text. Further, subheadings may be required if stress is required on a specific point or used to introduce a new paragraph in text so that a gap between the main heading and text can be obtained.
  - ***Text:*** The text in leaflets must be as brief as possible and should begin with impressive and interesting sentences to capture the attention of readers. Creditable and verifiable facts must be presented so that readers can believe in the content and can make use of those facts.
  - ***Pictures:*** To make the leaflet more eye catching, the pictures are mixed in the text so that it becomes more easily understandable, interesting and meaningful.
- Good colour combinations and background must be used in organizing the leaflet so that the leaflet could be more attractive and amazing.
- The size of the leaflet must be customized so that it is easy to carry and read.
- The written words must be large enough so that everyone including the elderly people with diminished eyesight may read the content.
- Leaflets must be a good mixture of text, illustrations and pictures so that they become more interesting for the readers.

ADVANTAGES OF LEAFLETS

- Leaflets are a good combination of written words, illustrations and pictures so they are more widely accepted.
- They should have facts to enjoy a high level of credibility and prestige in readers.
- They are considered a permanent source of message which cannot be alerted until and unless the leaflet is tampered with.
- A wide range of people may be targeted to spread the message through leaflets.
- A very personal question can also be answered through leaflets which can be read in private, for example questions and answers related to safe sexual practices.

LIMITATIONS OF LEAFLETS

- Illiterate people can be targeted through leaflets to spread a message. They remain deprived of the message if leaflets are used as an education aid for them.

- Planning, printing and designing the leaflets require a lot of time, effort, men and money.
- Expert, skilled professional manpower is required for planning and designing leaflets.
- Distribution of leaflet is not an easy task, it requires a strong coordination, efforts, time and money.

PROJECTED AUDIOVISUAL AIDS

The use of projected audiovisual aids is not a very recent phenomenon; however, rapid contribution of science and technology in the development of newer projecting audiovisual aids has revolutionized the field of audiovisual aids. Today, there is an availability of the most technologically advanced projecting educational aids such as liquid crystal display (LCD) projectors, which are the most widely media nowadays in educational purposes. The other projected audiovisual media that have been popular in the educational fraternity are overhead projectors (OHPs), slide projectors, opaque projectors (epidiascope), television, VCR/VCD, cameras and microscopes. Some valuable projected audiovisual aids are discussed below, namely slide projector, OHP, opaque projector, filmstrip, television, video cassette recorder (VCR)/DVD player, camera, microscope and LCD player.

I. SLIDE PROJECTOR

A slide projector is a projecting audiovisual device, where small sized (about 2 × 2 inches) transparent pictorial or diagrammatic slides are arranged in a proper sequence for presentation on a large screen. Slide projectors were the most popularly used audiovisual aids in health sciences where teachers used them during lectures to show still pictures using slides prepared from photographs, pictures or a special diagram (Fig. 6.24).

A slide is a small piece of transparent material on which a single pictorial image or scene or graphic image has been photographed or reproduced. Slides are a form of projected media that are easy to prepare. They are still pictures on a positive film which you can process and mount individually yourself or send to a film laboratory. The standard size of the slides is 2 × 2 inches and any 35 mm camera will make satisfactory slides.

The preparation of slides requires imagination and creative ability and they may be prepared from diagrams, pictures and photographs generally captured during life experiences or certain learning experiences, such as a picture of a patient with a rare clinical presentation, a specific finding of a pathological laboratory test and so on. At the time of presentation, slides must be presented in a sequence of topics so that they may be used appropriately and efficiently during presentation.

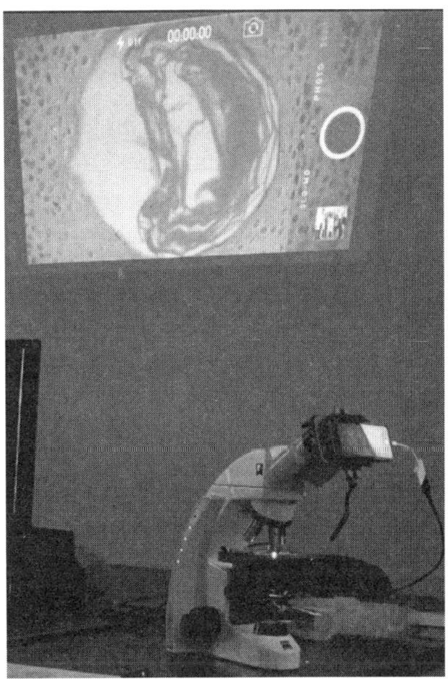

Figure 6.24

Slide projector. *Source: Stoff, BK, Streicher JL, Kini, SP. Innovative dermatopathology teaching in a resource-limited environment.* J Am Acad Dermatol, *74(5);2016. ISSN: 0190-9622.*

A. TYPES OF SLIDES

- ***Photographic slides:*** The ideal size is 2 × 2 inches to 3 × 4 inches. Photographic slides could be black and white or coloured.
- ***Handmade slides:*** Slides used in slide projectors may be handmade using an acetate sheet, cellophane, etched glass, plain glass or a lumarith.

ADVANTAGES OF A SLIDE PROJECTOR

- Requires only filming, processing and mounting by self or laboratory.
- Results in colourful and realistic reproduction of original subject.
- Preparation with any 35 mm camera for most uses.
- Easy to revise and update.
- Easily handled, stored and rearranged for various uses.
- Can be combined with taped narration or can be controlled for time during a discussion.
- May be adapted to group or individual use.

LIMITATIONS OF A SLIDE PROJECTOR

- Only diagrams, pictures, photographs and abbreviated text can be presented. It can be used to present the written descriptive text.
- Slide preparation requires a lot of predevelopmental work such as collecting or taking a snapshot of the pictures or photographs.
- This method requires a significant amount of imaginative and creative skills.

II. OVERHEAD PROJECTOR

The OHP is mostly used in all audiovisual aids. It projects transparencies with brilliant screen images suitable for use in a lighted room. The teacher can write or draw diagrams on the transparency while he teaches; these are projected simultaneously on the screen by the OHP (Fig. 6.25).

A. PURPOSES OF AN OVERHEAD PROJECTOR

- To develop concepts and sequences in a subject matter area.
- To make marginal notes on transparencies for the teacher's use that can carry without exposing them to the class.
- To test student performances while other classmates observe.
- To show relationships by means of transparent overlays in contrasting colours.
- To give the illusion of motion in the transparency.

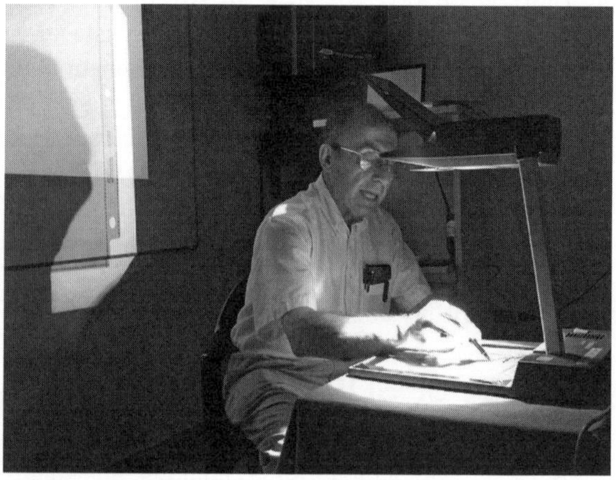

Figure 6.25

Overhead projector. *Source: Dreskin SC. Dr. Henry N. Claman.* Ann Allerg Asthma Immunol, *121(5);2018. ISSN: 1081-1206.*

B. OVERHEAD PROJECTOR TRANSPARENCIES

- Transparencies are a popular instructional medium. They are simple and easy to prepare and easy to operate with the OHP which is lightweight.

- A 10 × 10 inch sheet with printed, written or drawn material is placed on the platform of the projector and a large image is projected on the screen.
- The projector is used from rear to the front of the room with the teacher standing or sitting beside the projector, facing the student.

GUIDELINES FOR MAKING EFFECTIVE TRANSPARENCIES

- Have one main idea on each transparency.
- Include only related figures and diagrams.
- Ensure that all transparencies are as simple as possible and as easy to read.
- Avoid too much information on any single transparency.
- Use a simple letter style in writing.
- Do not use all capital letters.
- Do not overcrowd the transparency with written content.
- Use diagrams in proportion to its lettering.
- Keep the message clear and simple.
- Emphasize the key messages.
- Use colour and words with discretion.
- Colour can enhance a visual but can also reduce the effectiveness of the message. Do not overuse the colours in texts of a transparency.
- Be sure what the transparency says is immediately evident in the transparency in the form of an illustration to enhance understanding.

C. POINTS TO REMEMBER DURING AN OVERHEAD PROJECTOR PRESENTATION

- Keep the screen above the participants heads (Fig. 6.26).
- Keep the screen in full view of the participants.
- The presenter must make sure that he is not blocking anyone's view when presenting.
- Darken the room appropriately by blocking out sunshine and dimming nearby light.
- Turn the screen off between slides if you are going to talk for more than 2 minutes.
- Talk to the audience, not to the screen.
- Switch off the bulb of the OHP when not in use to save electricity but the fan must keep running to keep the OHP cool.
- Do not move the OHP when it is in use; it may increase the chances of losing the lamp of the OHP.

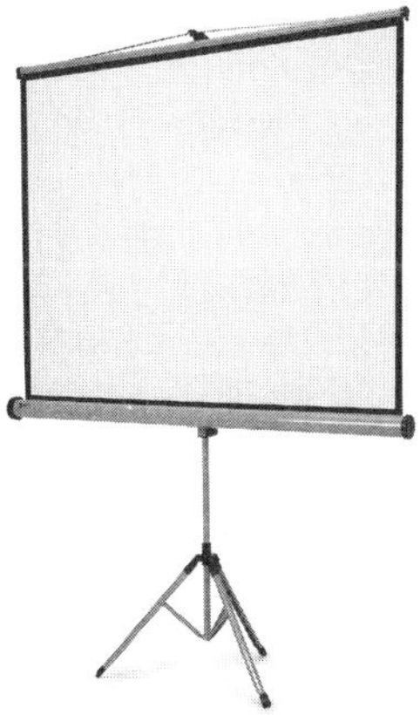

Figure 6.26

Projector screen.

ADVANTAGES OF AN OVERHEAD PROJECTOR

- Permits the teacher to stand in front of the class while using the projector, thus enabling her to point out features appearing on the screen by pointing to the materials at the projector itself and at the same time, to observe the students' reactions to her discussion.
- Gains the students' attention.
- Permits face-to-face interaction with the students.
- Can be used in daylight with a slight darkening of the room.
- Can present information in systemic developmental sequences.

- Requires limited planning and can be prepared in a variety of inexpensive methods.
- Use of an OHP can be quite cheap and transparencies can be used repeatedly.
- Easily available.
- Easy to operate and handle.

LIMITATIONS OF AN OVERHEAD PROJECTOR

- Cannot be used in situations of power supply interruptions.
- Requires careful handling as OHP bulbs are very sensitive to power fluctuations and jerky movements.
- Preparing transparencies is a time-consuming process and requires good handwriting abilities.

III. OPAQUE PROJECTOR

Opaque projector is also commonly known as *epidiascope*. It can present images or printed matter or small opaque objects on a screen. Opaque projector is the only projector on which you can project a variety of materials like book pages, objects, coins, postcards or any other similar flat material that is nontransparent. The opaque projector will project and simultaneously enlarge all kinds of written or pictorial matter directly from the originals in any sequence derived by the teacher (Fig. 6.27).

It works on the principle of horizontal straight line projection with a lamp; plane mirror placed at a 45 degree angle over the projector reflects the light so that it passes through the projection lens forming a magnified image on the screen. This large size projector requires a dark room with a fixed place because it is not easily movable due to its heavy weight and size.

ADVANTAGES OF AN OPAQUE PROJECTOR

- Stimulates attention and arouses interest.
- Can project a wide range of materials like stamps, coins and specimens when one copy is available.
- Can be used for enlarging drawings, pictures and maps.
- Does not require any written or typed materials, handwritten material can be used.
- Helps students retain knowledge for a longer period of time.
- Can be used to review instructional problems.
- Can be used to test knowledge and ability.
- Simple operation.

LIMITATIONS OF AN OPAQUE PROJECTOR

- Costly equipment, requires careful handling.
- Very large and heavy object, cannot be moved easily to other classrooms or place.
- Needs a dark room for projection.

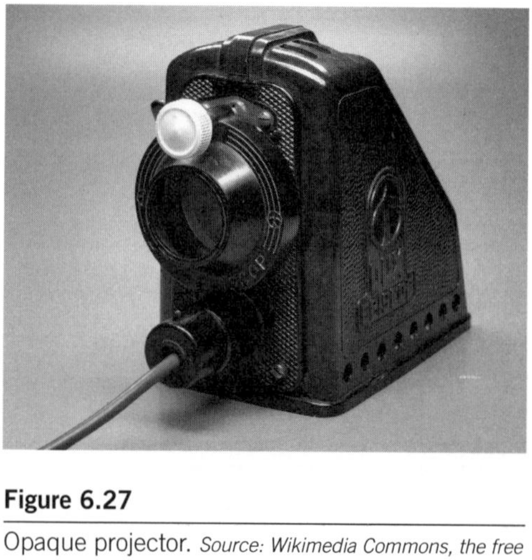

Figure 6.27

Opaque projector. *Source: Wikimedia Commons, the free media repository.*

IV. FILMSTRIPS

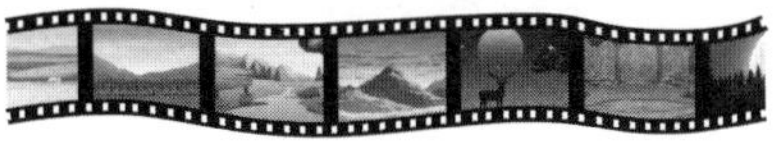

Figure 6.28

Filmstrip.

A filmstrip is a continuous strip of film consisting of individual frames or pictures arranged in a sequence usually with a specific title (Fig. 6.28). In other words, filmstrips are a sequence of transparent still pictures with individual frames on a 35 mm film. A tape-recorded narration can be synchronized with a film strip. Each strip contains between 12 and 18 or more pictures. It is a fixed sequence of related stills on a roll of a 35 mm or an 8 mm film.

Filmstrips are basically used to present a process in a logical consistency and continuity with still pictures so that the whole filmstrip makes a complete presentation. Filmstrips are used to stimulate emotions, build attitudes and point out problems. Filmstrips have been very commonly used for presenting the still pictures in a sequence and continuity along with verbal or audiotape explanation to demonstrate common nursing procedures such as bed bath, back care, crutch walking, intravenous cannulation and nasogastric tube insertion.

A. TYPES OF FILMSTRIPS

- ***Discussion filmstrip:*** It is a continuous strip of film consisting of individual frames arranged in a sequence usually with explanatory titles.
- ***Sound slide film:*** It is similar to a filmstrip but instead of explanatory titles or spoken discussion, the recorded explanation is audible and is synchronized with the pictures.

B. GUIDELINES FOR USING FILMSTRIPS

- Select the filmstrips carefully to meet the needs of the topic to be taught and preview them before actual presentation.
- An appropriate and efficient congruence must be established between the filmstrip and the topic of study. Before starting the presentation of the filmstrip, it must be appropriately introduced so that the audience is adequately charged to receive the important message.
- The specific details and important points on the filmstrip must be focused by the presenter using a pointer.
- A part of the filmstrip may be shown again if the content needs to be stressed on or needs more specific study.

ADVANTAGES OF FILMSTRIPS

- Filmstrips are compact, easy to handle and always in proper sequence.
- They can be supplemented with a recorded audiotape or verbal explanation.
- They are inexpensive when quantity reproduction is required.
- They are useful for group or individual study as the projection rate is controlled by the instructor or user.
- They are projected with a simple, lightweight equipment.

LIMITATIONS OF FILMSTRIPS

- Preparing the slides is a cumbersome job and requires a lot of effort.
- If the filmstrip is not supplemented with an audiotape, the verbal explanation becomes difficult to understand, especially to the new learners.

V. TELEVISION

Television (TV) is a telecommunication medium for transmitting and receiving moving images that can be monochrome (black and white) or coloured with accompanying sound. Television is a very commonly and widely used medium for sharing and disseminating information between large groups. It is also very popular and widely viewed by different strata of the society because of its specific feature, the combination of audio and visual technology. Televisions have wide variety of uses such as entertainment, sharing information and may also be very effective for educational purposes because of their easy and wide accessibility (Fig. 6.29).

The educational use of television was first reported at the State University of Iowa, the United States, in 1932. Later, the popularity of television steeply grew, and by 1972, it had become a popular medium for educational instructions. India reportedly started the use of TV in 1959, and in the 1990s, the popularity and use of TV grew steeply. Today, TV in India covers more than 70 million homes giving a viewing population more than 400 million individuals through more than 100 channels.

A. EDUCATIONAL USES OF TELEVISION

The instructional television may have the following principal educational uses:

- Television could be *interactive* (allowing the viewers to interact with the instructor or other students live) or *passive* (airing prerecorded programmes) to share educational material for general students that are broadcasted at a particular time so that everyone who is interested may view them.
- Television can be used in a classroom setting where either a telecasted or prerecorded programme may be displayed for students to supplement traditional learning.
- Television may be used for teaching students social, cultural, political and religious affairs of the country by exposing them with the general basic television programmes.
- Television may be used for behaviour modification through showing specific therapeutic programmes.
- Television may also be used for educational entertainment so that students can feel fresh to carry out the next traditional educational activity.

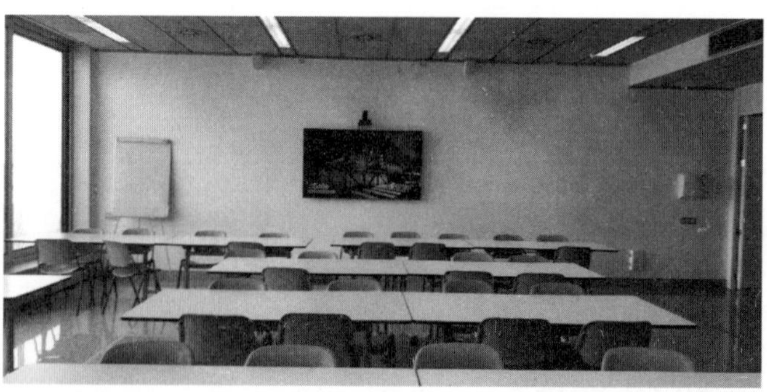

Figure 6.29

Television. *Source: Iriondo I., Korres O., Paños-Castro J., et al. Digital transformation in higher education: A qualitative evaluative study of a hybrid virtual format using a smart classroom system.* Heliyon, *9(6);2023. ISSN: 2405-8440.*

ADVANTAGES OF TELEVISION

Television is a visually stimulating medium and is of interest to children. Therefore, it can be used to assist reluctant learners by creating interest and removing pressure that can accompany traditional learning techniques. The main advantages of using television in education are as follows:

- A cost-effective educational media, which is easily available everywhere and large proportion of students may be covered by a single teacher in interactive television programmes.
- A multiple sensory stimulating educational media (sight and sound), which makes learning a recreational and leisure activity by providing real experiences in a stimulating way to learn faster and quicker.
- Television ensures uniformity in learning experience because it offers same basic ideas, information techniques to everyone viewing the educational programme.
- Television provides quicker and long-lasting visual and sound impression because it improves concentration by eliminating the possibilities of environmental distraction.
- Television stimulates and reinforces learning by repetitive presentation of ideas, information and beliefs to the learner that brings permanent change in the behaviour of an individual.
- Revision and repetition of the same educational programme is possible to telecast, which may be used to reinforce knowledge to achieve long-lasting learning.
- Real-life impossible experiences are achieved in the classroom through television because the naturally impossible things such as forests, wild animals and snakes may be brought to the classroom electronically through television.
- Media for mass education: Television is considered as a good education aid for teaching a large group because of television's universal availability.

LIMITATIONS OF TELEVISION

- Television educational instructions are generally a one-way process; therefore doubts of the students cannot be clarified.
- It is not a student-centric approach, where instructions are prepared and are not flexible to be moulded according to the situation of a particular group of students in a classroom.
- Underprivileged group of students in schools where television is not available remain deprived of these educational programmes.
- School schedules have to be customized according to the telecast schedule of television educational programmes.

VI. VIDEO CASSETTE RECORDER/VIDEO COMPACT DISC PLAYER

The VCR is an electromechanical educational medium which constitutes an electronic machine, prerecorded video cassettes and the television screen for display (Fig. 6.30). This educational medium is considered as a useful teaching aid because preplanned tailor-made teaching programmes may be prepared and used as and when required for multiple times with audio as well as video stimulation for the learners. Gradually

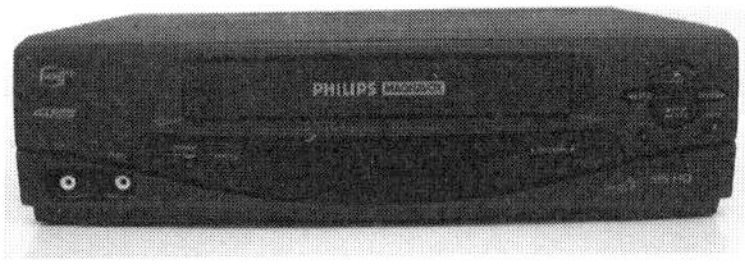

Figure 6.30

Video cassette recorder. *Source: Wikipedia: User:VHSVideos2006.*

with the development of science and technology, the conventional VCR has been replaced by more sophisticated electronic advanced video compact disc (VCD) players because of their handiness and cost factors.

A. EDUCATIONAL USES OF VCR/VCD PLAYER

The VCR and the VCD player are considered as potential educational media for learning a wide range of motor, intellectual, cognitive, and interpersonal and affective skills. These audiovisual educational media have certain specific qualities to bring visual and auditory stimulus, which finally leads to a permanent memory impact and learning. They are used for a wide range of educational purposes ranging from simple classroom content delivery to facilitating distance education.

ADVANTAGES OF VCR/VCD PLAYER

- Easy to access and use for educational purposes.
- Multiple use and repetition of the same content several times is possible.
- They can be used in daylight in the classroom without any special preparation.
- Recording and playing content does not require any special skills and techniques.
- Combines the advantages of both the motion pictures and a tape recorder.

LIMITATIONS OF VCR/VCD PLAYER

- Older playback equipments are bulky and large to transport to different situations.
- Power supply is mandatory to run these equipments; without power supply they do not have any use.
- Recorded content cannot be edited in basic equipments.
- Good quality video recording is a time-consuming and cumbersome task.

VII. CAMERA

Camera is an electromechanical device capable of recording and storing still or movable images (Fig. 6.31). The camera is the most commonly used device in medical and nursing education. The use of camera has further increased with the availability of more advanced assistive education media such as slide projectors, film projectors and LCD projectors, where images taken from real clinical practice are used to educate students using the abovementioned assistive educational devices. The emergence of the digital camera has significantly influenced the use of camera in medical and nursing education because the user may obtain any image and can instantly use the image for teaching.

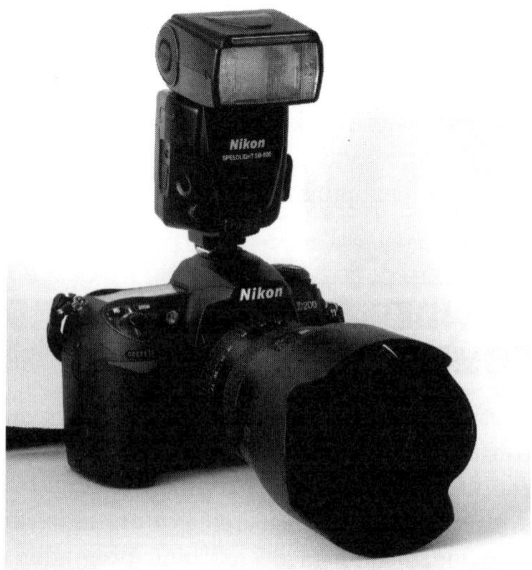

Figure 6.31

Camera. *Source: Wikimedia Commons, the free media repository.*

A. EDUCATIONAL USES OF CAMERA

The camera is very widely and significantly used in education; some of the most essential uses of a camera in education are as follows:

- Cameras can improve the teaching presentation by making it more illustrative by adding the images obtained through the camera.
- Some of the images of the patients' rarer clinical issues may be obtained and published to educate other people in the profession.
- Pursuing regular photography and making use of relevant images for teaching purpose.
- Assisting students in special education and autistic applications.
- Providing close-up, macro or micro views of objects, plants or animals.
- Enhancing slideshows or presentations by incorporating current relevant pictures from own scenario.
- Encouraging effort through immediate recognition of achievement.
- Recording student progress (including difficult-to-record evidence for process outcomes).
- Analysing physical education activities through photography.
- Recording sequences of events in science experiments (e.g. lifecycles, motion).

B. SOME REAL-WORLD EXAMPLES OF CAMERA USE IN EDUCATION

- Using camera for obtaining images of an advanced nursing procedure to disseminate knowledge to people sitting at remote places through telenursing.
- A nurse may monitor the progress of bedsore heeling in a diabetic patient by taking images at different intervals and the same may also be used for teaching the nursing students about the process of bedsore wound healing in a diabetic patient.
- A surgeon may take a few images of a rarer surgical procedure and may use these for publication, presentation in a conference and teaching students.

VIII. MICROSCOPE

The word *microscope* is derived from the Greek word *mikrós* meaning 'small' and 'to look' or 'see'. It is an instrument used to see objects that are too small for the naked eye (Fig. 6.32). The microscope is a device used for visualization of objects or living things such as tissue samples, microorganisms and micro-objects, which cannot be seen by naked eyes. In health sciences, a microscope is the most commonly used teaching device for preclinical and paraclinical subjects such as anatomy, physiology, biochemistry, microbiology, pathology and genetics. The initial microscope used for diagnostic and teaching purposes was the optical microscope where light was used to image the sample. Other advanced microscopes used for medical diagnostic tests and teaching are transmission electron microscope, scanning electron microscope and scanning probe microscope.

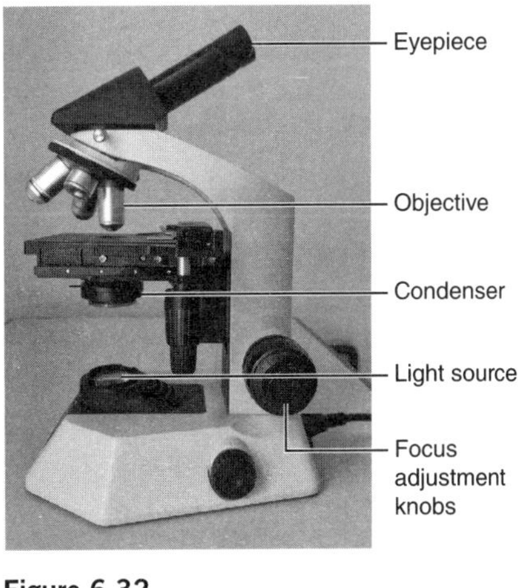

Figure 6.32

Microscope. *Source: Anuthama K., Prasad H. Atlas of Oral Histology, 3rd ed. Elsevier, 2023.*

A. USES OF MICROSCOPE IN NURSING AND MEDICAL EDUCATION

- The microscope has played a significant role in nursing and medical education; microscope is used for teaching anatomy, physiology, microbiology and pathology to medical and nursing students.

- Microscopes are used in diagnostic laboratories to carry out tests, ranging from the simple blood test to the complex histopathological or genetic test, where students can be practically taught through showing live slides of the disease diagnostic tests. This live practical experience helps them comprehend the theory more conveniently and easily.
- Today, microscopes are used to produce and develop pictures of diagnostic findings, which could be used for teaching in classrooms.

IX. LCD PROJECTOR

An LCD projector is a type of video projector for displaying video, images or computer data on a screen or other flat surfaces (Fig. 6.33). The LCD projector was invented by the New York inventor, Gene Dolgoff, in 1984. LCD projectors are increasingly being used in meetings, training sessions, classroom education and visual entertainment. They appeal to all the sensory organs and the impact is always greater than simple speech.

B. TYPES OF LCD PROJECTORS

According to their size and portability, LCD projectors are classified into the following three categories:

- Ultralight portable projectors
- Conference room projectors
- Fixed installation projectors

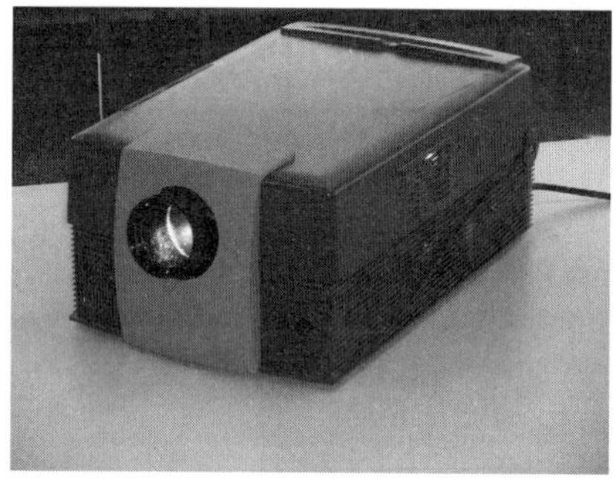

Figure 6.33

LCD projector. *Source: Wikimedia Commons, the free media repository.*

C. GUIDELINES FOR USING LCD PROJECTORS

The following guidelines must be followed while using the LCD projector for educational purposes:

- ***Projection surface:*** White projecting, the surface should be a neutral colour and best suited for natural colour tones.
- ***Setting up the system:*** The following steps must be followed to set up the LCD projection system:
  - The LCD projector must be placed 5–15 feet away from the projection screen, either with a permanently fixed ceiling or placed on a stable surface.
  - Computer/laptop cable should be connected at the back of LCD projector on a video pot and computer/laptop and projector should be effectively connected (Fig. 6.34).
  - The power cable of the projector should be connected to the three-way electrical port which is grounded.
  - Then the lens cap of the projector should be removed.

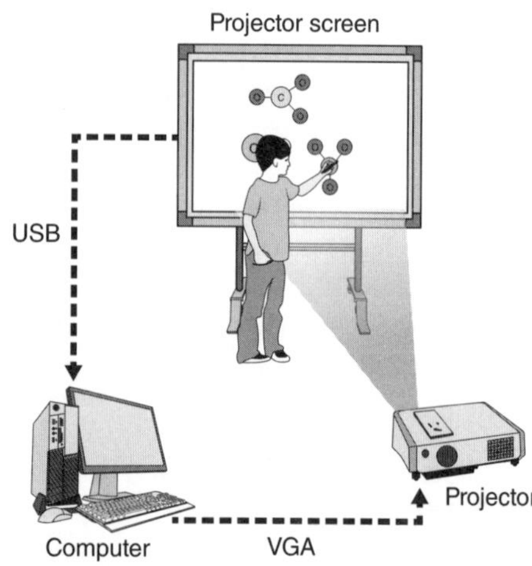

Figure 6.34

Connecting LCD projector with computer.

  - The projector should be switched on by pressing the power button on the top of projector which will lead to a flash of light followed by the projection of image.
  - The computer/laptop should then be started. Then the teacher should right click on the desktop screen and proceed to the graphical properties and graphical output. There, the teacher should click on the Notebook + Monitor option to have content display on the projection screen and computer/laptop screen both or the same may be done through the keyboard function key and F3 key.
  - The content to be projected should be clearly projected on the projection screen. If projection is not clear then the focus of projection should be fixed using the rings on the lens.
  - Further, projection may be adjusted by manipulating the foot of the projector on the bottom at the front and back.
- ***Shutting down the LCD projector:***
  - To shut off the LCD projector, the power button should be pressed; a message may appear to check if you actually want to turn off the projector, the power button should be pressed again and finally the projector will turn off.
  - The teacher should wait for the projector fan to turn off before the projector is unplugged from the electrical port. Also, it must be ensured that the flashing light is off before the projector is unplugged.
- ***Warning lights:*** In addition to the power button light, there are two additional warning light buttons, which are lamp warning light and temperature warning light.
  - The blinking of lamp warning light notifies the need of the lamp to be changed.
  - The blinking of orange colour temperature status light notifies the need to change the air filter, and the red colour temperature status light notifies the increased temperature of the projector and the need to turn off the lamp and allow the running fan to cool the warm lamp.
- ***Additional audio and video devices:***
  - The projector has several other additional ports to connect VCR, DVD and cameras, which can further improve the utility of the LCD projector in education.

D. GUIDELINES FOR POWERPOINT PRESENTATIONS

PowerPoint presentations are the most popular audiovisual aid in the present educational community because they are believed to be more interesting and visually attractive. A PowerPoint presentation is preferred because of its flexibility in both preparation and presentation. The following guidelines must be followed for the preparation and presentation of PowerPoint presentations:

- Use the horizontal/landscape format for slides.
- Limit the information on each slide to a single topic or idea.
- Use action words and short phrases rather than sentences.
- Pictures, drawings and illustrations make the presentation interesting but as a general rule keep the slides simple and clear.
- Keep the slide simple and clear without overburdening the slides with special effects and irrelevant pictures. Irrelevant images and effects may distract the audience.
- Maintain consistency in use of colour throughout the slides and avoid overuse of multiple colours and graphics.
- Use dark-coloured text on a light background and vice versa, for example using white or yellow text on a black background slide.
- Use of bullets instead of numbers is always considered good; only use the numbers to show sequence or rank of presented content.

- Do not overboard the slide with text; try to keep enough open space around the written text on slide.
- Use the 6 × 6 rule that is 6 lines of text and 6 words per line.
- Ensure the text on the slide is readable. It is recommended to use a minimum of 36 points for the slide title and 24 points for the body text.
- Ensure the use of standard styles of written text such as Arial fonts, which are easily readable.
- Avoid using only uppercase text (CAPITAL), rather, use upper and lower case text, which is more legible.
- Use contrasting colours to present and highlight specific points but avoid small red text, which is generally not visible.
- Significant points in text may be presented using bold, italic and large size fonts to ensure emphasis.
- To make the presentation more interactive, limit the written content and use simple illustrations.
- Do not use multiple animations and transition effects on a single slide. Limit to one or two animations or transition effects per slide.
- Try developing visual aids that are visually pleasing as well as clear.
- It is generally considered good to limit the number of slides to the number of minutes the presenter has in hand.

ADVANTAGES OF LCD PROJECTORS

- It is a technologically advanced audiovisual aid that can be used for presentation of still slides as well as videos. Slide show and video can be clubbed together and customized in a single presentation.
- It is considered very interesting and visually attractive for the audience.
- Back and forth movement of presenting content can be easily carried out for reinforcing or recapitalizing the whole presentation.

LIMITATIONS OF LCD PROJECTORS

- It is quite an expensive electronic gadget that is not easy to afford.
- Teachers and faculty require technical skills of computer and PowerPoint presentation while using LCD projector.
- In case of power failure or technological failure, it may cause a lot of problems, which are very difficult to manage at the last minute.

AUDIO EDUCATIONAL AIDS

Audio educational aids are popularly known as *auditory aids* and are considered significantly important educational aids because of their access, cost-effectiveness and easy operability. Audio educational aids are very popular in language-learning strategies. The common educational aids that come under this category are radios, tape recorders and gramophones, and most commonly used is tape recorder, which is discussed below.

I. AUDIOTAPES AND COMPACT DISCS

Audiotapes and compact discs (CDs) play an important role in the educational field. Now audiotapes has become obsolete, therefore, CD has been discussed in detail. Compact Disc Read Only Memory

(CD-ROM) is a technology, where a range of data types, including text, graphics, audio and photographs, can all be stored digitally. This technology can then be accessed using conventional personal computers. In the past, learning meant face-to face lectures, reading handouts or printed books, taking notes, answering questions and completing assignments. In traditional method of education, learning and teaching are impossible without books, chalkboards and teachers. Education and training today have a new meaning. Education and training are now completely different concepts. Computers are an integral part of every classroom. Teachers use DVDs, CD-ROMs, and videos to demonstrate how things work. Students can interact with their subject matter using these web-based tools and CD-ROMs. CD-ROMs are commonly used for teaching–learning processes, where learning material in the form of recorded videos, PPTs, photographs, world files and learning software may be stored, which can be used by learners at their convenience.

DEFINITIONS

- Audiotape is a magnetic tape used for recording the sound or verbal instructions of teaching–learning purposes.
- CD, a moulded plastic disc containing digital data that is scanned by a laser beam for the reproduction of recorded sound and other information.
- CD, a multimedia storage media disc, stores a variety of data types including text, graphics, animations, photographs and video digitally, and can be retrieved by CD-player or computers.

TYPES BASED ON FORMAT OF MEDIA

- Originally developed to store and play sound recordings.
- Later adapted for storage of data (CD-ROM).
- Further derivatives are detailed below:
  - i. CD-R (once audio and data storage)
  - ii. CD-RW (rewritable media)
  - iii. VCD (video compact disc)
  - iv. SVCD (super video compact disc)
  - v. Photo CD
  - vi. Enhanced music CD

ADVANTAGES OF COMPACT DISCS IN EDUCATION

- This is a beneficial resource for all students and all subjects.
- It may fulfil some of an instructor's duties and provide support to students without the personal involvement of an instructor.
- It plays a significant part in computer-assisted learning.
- CDs can be used as instructors.
- CDs can be used as an audio-visual learning tool.
- It facilitates quick and inexpensive search for data in different forms.
- It encourages development of concepts, influences various strategies and promotes interconnectedness.
- Animations, graphics, audios and videos can spark interest in learners. Also, background music or sounds can increase reading enjoyment.
- These devices are used to store and reproduce data in the teaching–learning process.

- Students have some control over the pace and order of their learning.
- It is effective with at-risk or special learners.

DISADVANTAGES OF COMPACT DISCS IN EDUCATION

- Students often work individually, with limited contact with instructors or other students.
- It has copyright issues and cannot be duplicated without permission.
- Not effective in development of motor and interpersonal skills domains.
- CDs teach at the lowest levels of knowledge and understanding.
- Memory-holding capacity of CD-ROM is less and we cannot rewrite the data into the CD-ROM.
- The data inside this CDs may get corrupted easily and hence cannot be reused or read.
- The CDs are not completely secured and the data information inside them can be stolen and can be replicated or even someone can make illegal copies of your information and misuse them.

II. RADIO

Radio has been used in education over the past more than a century and it has been used in many ways. Its main uses in education include school broadcasting, adult learning, literacy and informal general education. Radio is an efficient system for delivering education to larger audiences. It acts as a 'community telephone' by facilitating information exchange at the community level. Radio has a crucial role in education as it is the only medium for formal and informal education.

DEFINITION

- Radio is a scientific device that functions as an effective auditory instrument for communication.
- Radio is an efficient audio aid technology capable of assisting teachers in the classroom by offering important information and learning experiences to a large number of learners.

TYPES OF RADIO BROADCASTS

There are two types of radio broadcasts: general broadcast and educational broadcast.

a. ***General broadcast:*** It broadcasts general information about activities and incidents, integrating knowledge about the globe, society and life.
b. ***Educational broadcast:*** Educational broadcasts that are expressly produced and transmitted to help the purpose of education and the classroom in the form of radio lessons, lectures and so on.

ADVANTAGES OF RADIO IN EDUCATION

- **Simple accessibility:** Radio is much more accessible than other media. Low-cost transistors are easily accessible to even the most economically poor. Therefore, it can be used to educate all stratas of the society.
- **Broad coverage:** We can now cover large areas of our territory using radio broadcasts, which are available all over the subcontinent. Radio can reach remote rural audiences quickly and effectively, extending learning at a distance.
- **Cost-effective:** Radio technology has a low operating cost and capital investment. Radio broadcasts are easy to set up and require less manufacturing area than other forms of electronic media.

- **Easy reception:** Listening to radio broadcasts while doing manual work is easy for learners. Distance learners can listen from anywhere and at any time to the programmes they choose.
- **Effective thought promotion:** Because hearing is usually always accompanied by simultaneous information processing, radio taps into the learner's cognitive process. Through the use of music and the technique of pauses, radio may spark listeners' imaginations.
- **Supportive and motivative technologies**: Broadcasting is a great way to make education more interesting and enjoyable if used creatively. Music and other sound effects can help stimulate the motivation and feeling of listeners.
- **Easier production**: Radio programming is much simpler than a TV or video production. For such production, there is no need for complex machinery or advanced instruments. Producing such a programme requires less manpower than producing a television/video programme.
- **Effective reality building: A powerful 'audio' version puts a scene into clear focus while also successfully establishing 'movement'**. Listeners can share the experience of watching a live broadcast, even though they are 100 miles away. The broadcast can allow listeners to experience a scene from the past that occurred, for example 100 years ago.
- **Possibility of learner enrichment:** The most common purpose of technology in learning is learner enrichment. This function is simple and inexpensive to implement using radio.
- **Direct instruction**: This method has been used. However, this requires extensive and systematic radio usage. Such programmes are based on syllabus and broadcast for specific target groups.

DISADVANTAGES OF RADIO IN EDUCATION

- The radio is not an adaptable medium. Radio is not an interactive medium that allows for conversation, dialogue or face-to-face interaction between listeners and speakers. Without motivation, guidance and supervision, learning becomes a one-way process of information transfer.
- A learner's doubts and questions cannot be addressed immediately. The learner cannot receive immediate feedback and there is no feedback regarding the content's quality.
- It might not be the best medium for all kinds of subject content. Radio is not able to teach certain subjects, such as those that require demonstrations or visual illustrations.
- For educational programming, there is a shortage of qualified personnel. Radio programming requires someone who is both creative and skilled in production. It is hard to find someone with this experience.
- Educational radio programmes are not given enough and adequate broadcast time-chunk. This is a problem for learners, who must make themselves available during the scheduled broadcast times regardless of any other engagements.
- Most academics in developing world must devise programmes that cater to a diverse range of audiences (e.g. the jobless, school dropouts and illiterates). A radio programme of common utility/appeal is harder to create more diverse audience.

If special efforts are not made to reassure learners, their attention span will be limited.

III. TAPE RECORDER

A tape recorder is a portable electronic gadget used to record, reproduce, erase and rerecord sound on a magnetic tape. This device can be used without any problem by anybody by operating the press buttons attached to the recorder, namely, stop, play, wind, rewind, record, pause and eject (Fig. 6.35).

DEFINITIONS

- A tape recorder is a device that records and plays back sound using magnetism.
- An audio tape recorder, often termed as a tape deck, tape player, tape machine or generally a tape recorder, is an audio recording and reproducing system that captures and plays back recordings on magnetic tape.
- Tape recorder, a recording system that makes use of electromagnetic phenomena to record and reproduce sound waves.

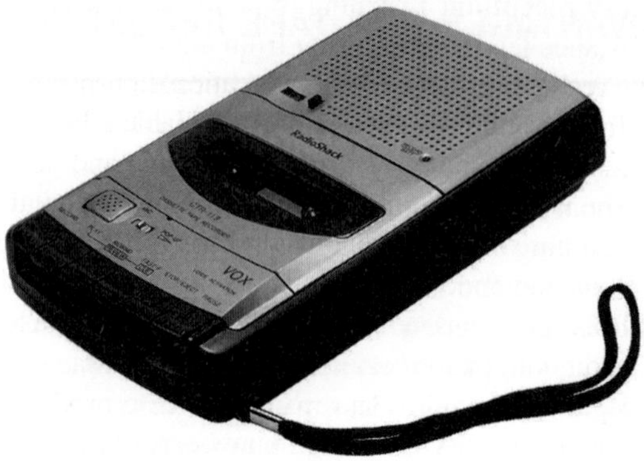

Figure 6.35

Tape recorder. *Source: Wikimedia Commons, the free media repository.*

A tape recorder is a portable electronic gadget to record, reproduce, erase and rerecord sound.

USING OF A TAPE RECORDER IN TEACHING

A record player can be used in the following ways in the actual classroom situation:

- Supplementing a lesson with tape recorder to provide additional information or content.
- Can be used as an appreciation lesson in music or literature class.
- Can be used for students to acquire singing ability, deliver a speech properly and recite a poem in the right way.
- Can be used for reviewing a lesson already presented.
- A tape recorder can be used for physical exercises, yoga or meditation accompanied with relevant music.
- It could be used for recording interviews, talks, discussions of various experts, which could be later used for teaching purposes.

GUIDELINES FOR USING A TAPE RECORDER IN TEACHING

The following guidelines must be followed for using the tape recorder for educational purposes:

- The teacher must be familiar or practice the basic functioning of the tape recorder before using it in the classroom setting.
- Proper functioning of the tape and recorded cassette must be ensured by the teacher before final use in the classroom.
- The teacher must prepare, customize and practice the tape-recorded lesson before use in the actual classroom.
- The teacher must prepare tape-recorded material and catalogue it properly.
- The teacher may use prerecorded programmes in a tape recorder from previously recorded actual lessons, radio educational programmes, television programmes, etc.
- The teacher must maintain a tape recorder cassette library on particular subjects, which could be used later by the teacher or other faculty members.

ADVANTAGES OF A TAPE RECORDER

Tape recorder when used for educational purposes has the following advantages:

- Tape recorders are commonly available educational aids that are economical, as recording tapes can be used multiple times and erasing and rerecording is also possible.
- The tape recorder is the most commonly available electronic gadget; therefore, most people are familiar with its use and functioning.
- A valuable recording can be recoded, stored and used multiple times whenever required.
- In language learning, a tape recorder is very useful because spoken conversation can be recorded and replayed for correcting the individual.
- Hearing of one's own recorded voice provides a positive psychic stimulation; therefore, by using the tape recorder, children may be actively involved in the learning programme.
- Recorded cassettes of interviews or discussion can become an evidence of facts having high legal value and may be used in case of disputes.

DISADVANTAGES OF TAPE RECORDER

- The recorded lecture lacks a visual representation, which is essential in the teaching and learning process.
- The system does not take into account individual variances.
- Communication is generally one-way from the speaker to the audience, not the other way around.
- Tape recorders are sometimes employed to replace the teacher, which should not be done because the teacher is intended to guide the students throughout the programme.
- The effectiveness of employing a tape recorder is dependent on the learners' listening abilities, which is beyond the teacher's control because it is impossible to determine whether or not the learners are truly listening.
- It is ineffective in large classrooms since the audio may not cover all learners.
- Some schools may not be able to afford the tape recorder machine and all required accessories.
- There is no personal contact with speaker.
- It does not provide a practical or laboratory experience.

IV. PUBLIC ADDRESS SYSTEMS

A public address system is an electronic amplification system made up of the tape recorder, amplifier and loudspeaker to distribute the sound to a large group of people. For example, loudspeakers used for speeches for a large group of people, DJ playing prerecorded music (Fig. 6.36). Small public address systems are commonly used in schools and colleges in the auditorium and examination halls. They may also be used in playgrounds for making announcements and address a large group of students.

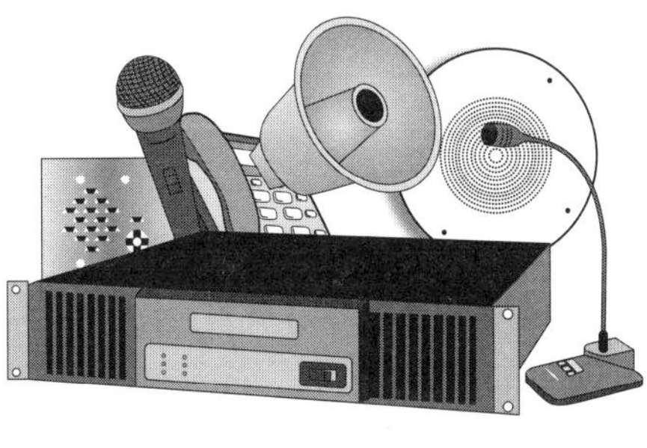

Figure 6.36

Public address systems.

TYPES OF PUBLIC ADDRESS SYSTEMS

- ***Small public address systems:*** The simplest public address system consists of a microphone, a modestly powered mixer amplifier and one or more loudspeakers. Simple public address systems of this type often provide 50–200 watts of power and are often used in small venues such as school auditoriums, churches and small bars. A sound source such as a CD player or a radio may be connected to a public address system so that music or sound can be played through the system.
- ***Large public address systems:*** Some public address systems have speakers that cover an entire campus of a college or an industrial site, or an entire outdoor complex (e.g. an athletic stadium). More often than not, this public address system is used as a voice alarm system that makes announcements during emergencies to evacuate the occupants in a building.

ELECTRONIC EDUCATIONAL MEDIA

I. COMPUTER

A computer is a programmable machine designed to sequentially and automatically carry out a sequence of arithmetic or logical operations. The particular sequence of operations can be changed readily, allowing the computer to solve more than one kind of problem. A computer is an electronic machine that can work under the control of stored programmes, automatically accepting data to produce the desired results (Fig. 6.37). Conventionally, a computer comprises two basic components: hardware and software.

Computers are extremely fast, information processing machines. They take a given input, process it and deliver a certain output. The developments in microelectronics and transistors have gone so far that computers are classified in terms of different generations. The first computer ENIAC (Electronics Numerical Integrator and Calculator) was invented in 1946. From that point, we have moved into the age of the fifth generation of supercomputer (based on artificial intelligence). In our lives today, however, fourth generation personal computers are predominantly used. At present, we have the most sophisticated, handy and modern cost-effective computers that have become an essential part of the education system. Computers have become an integral part of each discipline of human operation including the education system because of its specific qualities and characteristics like speed, accuracy, diligence, versatility, vast memory for storage and automation. Unfortunately, the computer has no brain.

IMPORTANCE OF A COMPUTER IN EDUCATION

Educational uses of the computer are concerned with more effective learning with the help of the computer. In fact, the computer should be regarded as an add-on rather than a replacing device. It is a technological tool that deserves to be used at the right time, to the right extent and in the right way to improve what has been learnt using other media and source material. The decision of when, how and how much computers should be used for learning should ideally be left to the teacher. The educational applicability of the

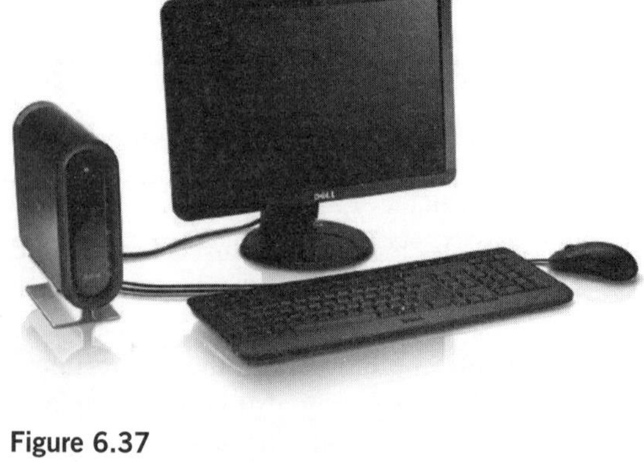

Figure 6.37

Computer. *Source: Shiland BJ. Medical Assistant: Nervous System, Law and Ethics, Psychology and Therapeutic Procedures—Module G. Elsevier, 2050.*

computer covers almost all subjects ranging from mathematics (the most structured) to music (one of the least structured). The essential uses of computers in education as an educational aid are as follows:

- Computers facilitate active learning in students as they learn through working with computers.
- Computers help in improving the recall ability of learners because of visual impressions.
- They also offer fresh innovative instructional stimuli so that undivided attention of the learner may be ensured.
- They also enhance interactive learning through constant, systematic and desired feedback.
- The interactive computer system can make the learners more autonomous and help them assume greater responsibility for their learning by providing individual adaptive instructions supported by graphics, synthesized speech and modelling software.
- The educational uses of the computer have special significance in distance education because of economic reasons. The computer enables a large number of students in distance education to develop new skills at a much lower cost than is possible through the formal learning system. In distance education, the computer can function as a surrogate for the human tutor even though it lacks the latter's intelligence and flexibility.

ADVANTAGES OF A COMPUTER

Certain essential capabilities and qualities that make computers highly suitable for use in education and training are as follows:

- Computers help to work in a fast and accurate way.
- They are reliable.
- They save time because they perform operations at a high speed.
- They help in doing repetitive work.
- Ideas can be understood quickly and easily through a presentation.
- Photographs or images can be transferred to computers with the help of a scanner or a digital camera.
- They are used as a voice recognition system.
- They store huge amounts of information in formats such as text, sound, picture and film.
- They take up very little space, usually that of one table; you can also have just a *notebook*-type computer on your palm.
- They are portable. One can work on a *notebook* or *laptop* computer even while making a trip.
- They are highly interactive and also enable communication from one place to another.
- They are user-friendly and easy to operate.

DISADVANTAGES OF A COMPUTER

- Computer is not a very cost-effective tool to be used in all educational settings. Everyone cannot afford a computer for educational purposes.
- Health and safety is crucial to the effective operation of a computer. Stress is widely accepted as a common and possibly the most dangerous aspect of using a computer.
- Computer use is also associated with physical problems such as musculoskeletal problems, eye strain and electromagnetic radiation risk of foetus in pregnant women.

II. WEB-BASED VIDEO CONFERENCING

In recent years, video conferencing is becoming more popular in education. This technology is rapidly expanding and allows people to connect instantly via audio and visual. It also makes it easier to share documents and files online. Direct video streaming has been used by many educators for live teaching and sharing of experiences with students.

Web conferencing is generally a term that refers to a variety of online collaborative services like webcasts, webinars, and meetings. You can make it possible using IP or TCP connections via the internet. In the past, internet was used to send texts through web conferencing tools. Later it became capable of sending audios and can now send high definition videos. Different types of web conference tools are available today for different formats.

DEFINITION

- Video conferencing is defined as an online technology that allows users in different locations to hold face-to-face meetings without having to move to a single location together.
- Web conferencing is a phrase that is used to describe a variety of approaches that permit two or more individuals in different places to communicate in real time through the internet.

TYPES OF WEB CONFERENCING

Web conferencing is typically grouped into three types based on their forms, such as meetings, presentations and collaborations. However, these three forms may be employed in a variety of ways to expand the varieties of web conferencing. Web conferencing has therefore been categorized into distinct forms based on their intended application. This chapter has briefly presented the various types of web conferencing, such as webinars, webcasts, web-meetings, online collaboration and online presentation as detailed below:

- **Webinars:** Webinars are actually seminars that are conducted online. Webinars allow presenters to share information with participants, and participants can ask or answer questions about that topic under discussion. This online conferencing option allows for minimal interactivity between speakers and audiences.
- **Webcast:** This is a web conference, which is another type of broadcast that can be made on TV. However, they are distinct in that the broadcast can be done using web instead of TV. Although webcast is possible to broadcast to large numbers of people at once, there are very few or no interactions between participants and the presenter in this form of web conferencing.
- **Web-meeting:** This category includes virtual meetings via the internet. This allows participants to interact with each other. Information can flow both forward and backward, that is the information can flow from the host to the audience or vice versa. Web meetings allow participants to initiate the conversation and others can respond to the original presenter. There are many web conferencing software options available, such as '*ezTalks*' cloud meeting and Zoom meetings, which allow hosts and audiences to send documents, images and videos in real time, rather than uploading prerecorded conversations.
- **Web-based collaboration:** These web conferencing types are very useful and can be used for a variety of purposes. It can be used for audio conferences if text messages are not shared. But live videos can be added to make it even more effective. The web-based collaboration format allows you to instantly view and edit files, documents or papers. A web-based collaboration allows participants to do more than simply communicate with each other via the internet. They can collaborate to edit and exchange any document. Online collaboration tools allow participants to exchange the information and data they have gathered in an interactive fashion. Web collaboration allows for all modifications to be made immediately without any need for special software. This allows people from different areas to come together and work on documents or files to complete the project.

- **Online Presentations:** Online presentations can be made via web conferencing. Online presentations can also be done using web-based chats, streaming audios/videos and slide presentation. To view these presentations, participants must log-in to the conference website. Participants can interact with the presenter via web-based chat or their smartphone.

ADVANTAGES OF WEB-BASED VIDEO CONFERENCING IN EDUCATION

- Allows multiple institutes to effortlessly communicate and interact (boost global collaboration).
- Connects with experts.
- Facilitates virtual field trips.
- Helps students prepare for the world of work.
- Improves the convenience and ease of studying outside of the classroom.
- Allows users to record information for future reference.
- Makes scheduling of parent–teacher meetings convenient.
- Increases engagement.
- Saves valuable time.
- No time constraint.
- Increases productivity of the employees.
- Self-paced learning is rampant.

DISADVANTAGES OF WEB-BASED VIDEO CONFERENCING IN EDUCATION

- Removes the element of human interaction.
- It is more expensive to purchase and install video conferencing equipment.
- Bound to experience technical problems.
- Limits the number users who can engage simultaneously.

III. E-LEARNING

E-learning is often referred to as the intentional use of networked communication and information technology in teaching or learning. E-learning can also be described using a number of terms. These include online learning, virtual learning, distributed learning, networked learning and web-based learning. The term 'e-learning' encompasses much more than online, virtual, distributed, networked and web-based learning. The letter 'e' stands for electronic and it could include all educational activities that are performed online or offline by individuals or groups. They can also be done synchronously or asynchronously using standalone or networked computers or other electronic devices.

DEFINITIONS

- A learning system based on formalized teaching but with the help of electronic resources is known as e-learning.
- E-learning is the learning facilitated and supported by Information Communication Technologies to enable people to learn anytime and anywhere.
- E-learning can also be termed as a network-enabled transfer of skills and knowledge through which the delivery of education is made to a large number of recipients at the same or different times.

- Experts in education and educational technology define e-learning as 'the delivery of training and education via networked interactivity and a range of other knowledge collection and distribution technologies'.

TYPES OF E-LEARNING

Educational experts have classified e-learning into many kinds and paradigms based on factors such as learning style, delivery mode and educational technologies employed. The following are the several forms of e-learning that are now in use:

1. ***Computer-Managed Learning (CML):*** CML environments allow instructors to set learning goals and assess performance of the learner. Instructors can create learning objectives and assess students' achievement in CML environments. Many activities may be performed by computer-managed education systems. These include the generation of tests, analysis of test results and keeping records about learners' progress. The system's ranking parameters allow students to tailor the learning process to their own preferences. CML systems can also be used by institutions for the storage and retrieval of classroom information, training content and curriculum information.
2. ***Computer-Assisted Instruction (CAI):*** It is also known as computer-assisted learning and is a type of e-learning in which computers are used with traditional teaching methods. This method combines a variety of tasks, including drill-and-practice, lesson and simulation exercises. These assignments can be used instead of or in addition to typical teacher-directed instruction. The main advantage of CAI is interaction, which helps learners to become more active participants in the learning process.
3. ***Synchronous Online Learning:*** Students can participate in group activities simultaneously online, wherever they may be, using synchronous online learning. Online chat and video conferencing facilitate this real-time interaction, allowing students and instructors to communicate with one another without delay. This community-oriented e-learning model is the fastest growing type of e-learning.
4. ***Asynchronous Online Learning:*** Asynchronous e-learning is a different type of online learning than synchronous. It allows students to study at their own pace and in different places, with no need for real-time communication. Students are able to be more flexible with their schedules through this self-paced learning method. Email, blogs, e-books, discussion boards, CDs and DVDs are all used to asynchronously e-learning tools.
5. ***Fixed E-Learning:*** Fixed e-learning ensures that the content utilized in the course of learning is not changed after it has been developed. It ensures that all learners get the same content. Instructors typically determine the course content. This means that it cannot be altered to accommodate student learning needs or preferences.
6. ***Adaptive E-Learning:*** Learning materials can be adapted and modified to meet the individual needs of learners in adaptive e-learning. Educational approaches can be more student-centred and personalized by taking into account parameters such as student performance, goals and abilities.
7. ***Linear E-Learning:*** E-learning can also have a classification based on the type of communication used. Linear e-learning allows information to be passed from sender and receiver. The sender decides when, how and at what pace the information will be received. No feedback is provided by the receiver to the sender. The classic example of linear learning is instruction delivered via television, radio and newspapers.
8. ***Interactive E-Learning:*** Interactive e-learning is a two-way method of communication that allows for both the sender and receiver to communicate. This is opposed to previous linear e-learning. The sender can be the recipient in this scenario and vice versa. Instant messaging as well as discussion boards and forums are examples of today's technologies. Instructors and students may readily communicate and alter learning and teaching techniques as needed.

9. ***Individual E-Learning:*** Individual E-learning allows learners to study the material in their own time and is designed for students to achieve learning goals individually. This is similar to traditional classroom learning.
10. ***Collaborative E-Learning:*** The collaborative approach to e-learning is more modern and efficient than individual e-learning. Collaborative e-learning is a method where two or more individuals participate in the learning process as part of a group. Collaborative e-learning is based upon the notion that knowledge is most effective when it is shared in a group environment where people can learn from each other and use their strengths and weaknesses to help each other.

ADVANTAGES OF E-LEARNING

- Students may work at their own speed using self-paced learning modules.
- Students may be able to choose educational content that fit their level of knowledge and awareness.
- Coursework can be scheduled without interfering with work or family obligations.
- Off-campus students' travel time and expenditures are reduced.
- Students may study whenever and wherever they choose as long as they have a computer and an internet connection.
- It is simple to participate in discussion at any time, or to communicate with peers and teachers remotely in chat rooms.
- It encourages more interaction between learners and teachers than traditional lecture method.
- It may suit students with different learning preferences and allow for learning through a number of tasks.
- Develops internet and computer abilities that will benefit students for the rest of their lives and professions.
- Completing online or computer-based courses builds confidence and inspires learners to accept responsibility.
- Learners can test themselves and focus on acquiring new abilities.

DISADVANTAGES OF E-LEARNING

- Learners who lack self-discipline or poor organizational skills may fall behind.
- Learners may feel alone in the absence of a teacher and peers.
- When students have a question, the teacher or professor may not be available.
- Accessing course materials may be difficult due to poor internet connections or ageing of computer.
- Students may become lost or confused about coursework and time limits if there are no timetables like in a typical classroom.
- Managing computer data and online learning tools might be difficult for students with basic computer abilities.

IV. SMART CLASSROOM

Technology-enabled education is transforming classrooms and paving the way for smart education. Smart classroom is a revolutionary concept. They integrate advanced hardware and new software technology to enhance teaching and maintain control over students' learning. Smart classrooms or digital classrooms are able to foster creativity. Interactive environments can help you bring in more innovative ideas and queries and provide more solutions.

Although the process of creating a smart classroom has been slow, it is becoming more and more complex. An interactive whiteboard is a step up from the traditional chalkboard-based classroom. It replaces the traditional concept of teaching with the most advanced 'digital ink technology'. It helps the children remain focused on the classroom teaching and entertains them.

It could be as simple as a way to add audio and video components to a lesson. This is something that many educational institutions are doing now. It could also involve performing virtual reality-based nursing and medical procedures.

DEFINITIONS

- Smart classroom is technology-enhanced classrooms that foster opportunities for teaching and learning by integrating learning technology, such as computers, specialized software, audience response technology, assistive listening devices, networking and audio/visual capabilities.
- A smart classroom is one that is digitally enabled and offers a wide range of teaching and learning approaches via the use of technologies.
- A smart classroom provides the students and teachers with virtual interactive sessions, access to adaptive and collaborative learning, performance-based assessments and developing students' abilities and performances.
- A smart classroom is an Edtech-enhanced classroom that fosters education by increasing access to digital teaching and learning techniques for both instructors and learners by integrating the most recent technological breakthroughs with education.

FEATURES OF SMART CLASSROOM

The main features of smart classroom are as listed below (Fig. 6.38):

- Adaptation of digitally smart equipment.
- Facility of quick internet search.
- Sensing and inferring data.
- Monitoring and analysing students' performance.
- Collaborative learning.
- Self-organization of learning communities.
- Self-assessment tools.
- Monitoring and feedback of students' skills.
- Digital cloud big data handling.

TYPES OR LEVELS OF SMART CLASSROOM

Smart classrooms are outfitted with cutting-edge technology to improve learning and teaching. Here are some examples of smart classrooms depending on their equipment:

I. **Basic/Level-1:**

Minimally includes:

- Computer
- Projector (either ceiling or desktop) with connections for audio/video/data
- Screen

II. **Teaching Station/Level-2:**

Minimally includes:

- Computer
- Projector

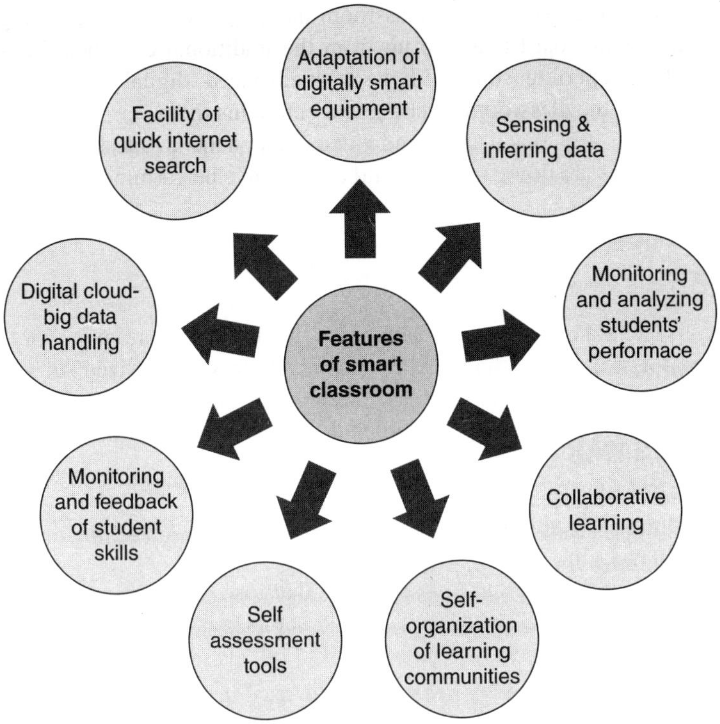

Figure 6.38

Features of smart classroom.

- Screen
- DVD/VCR combination player and/or Blu-Ray player
- Teacher station

III. Technology-Enabled Teaching Room/Level-3:

Minimally includes:

- Connections for a user-supplied computer
- Projector
- Screen
- Connections for a portable VCR/DVD or document camera
- Ceiling speakers

IV. Dedicated Smart Classroom/Level-4:

Teacher's podium which includes:

- Computer
- Dual monitors
- An interactive pen display
- Projector
- Screen
- Wireless mouse
- A DVD/VCR combination player and/or Blu-Ray player
- Ceiling speakers
- Connections for a user-provided laptop computer
- Document camera

- Wide-angle webcam
- USB wireless microphone
- Basic lecture capture

V. Advanced Smart Classroom/Level-5:

All aspects of a Level 4 smart classroom with the addition of the following:

- Room audio reinforcement
- May have multiple projectors/screens
- Interactive whiteboard

VI. R-Portable Cart:

- Computer
- Projector
- Portable teacher station

ADVANTAGES OF SMART CLASSROOM

1. It provides students with access to an online resource database.
2. Smart classrooms improve students' and instructors' learning and teaching opportunities.
3. It is available at all times for their educational process.
4. It facilitates interactive sessions between students and professors in the classroom.
5. It enables students and instructors to keep in touch and share information for improved learning results.
6. Environmentally friendly technology instruments are used in smart classrooms.
7. Smart classes have easy accessibility to everything, which allows for more time to be spent on more beneficial activities.
8. It gives chances for academics to study and practice, as well as the available resources for improved learning results.
9. It improves teamwork and general engagement in the learning process.
10. A well-equipped and physically appealing classroom encourages learners to think critically and behave logically.
11. It enables instructors to give lectures more efficiently, resulting in improved learning experience for students.
12. It is a perfect option for students with different IQs.
13. Smart classes employ electronic tools which are easy to use and maintain.
14. It provides flexibility in teaching and learning.
15. It helps teachers to instruct remote and local students simultaneously.
16. It provides a facility to update the content.
17. It improves students' academic achievement, consequently increasing their mental and physical growth.

DISADVANTAGES OF SMART CLASSROOM

1. The expenses of infrastructure, ongoing software updates, maintenance and teacher training are issues for smart classrooms.
2. Electronic devices are prone to technical malfunctions.
3. Distractions are common when studying on a personal computer or smartphone with an internet connection; students can explore other websites, social networking applications and so on.
4. A lack of qualified instructor is more of a hindrance than a reward.

5. It is tough to create presentations, movies and programmes.
6. Devices such as laptops, digital boards and so on are delicate and difficult to use.
7. Extremely reliant on electricity.
8. Requires network access such as local-area network (LAN), wide-area network (WAN), internet and so on.

TELECOMMUNICATION/DISTANCE EDUCATION

Telecommunication or distance education is a structured learning where the instructor and learners are separated by time and place, is the rapid-growing form of international and domestic education and is currently the most popular. The once unique form of education that utilized nontraditional delivery systems was now an important part of mainstream education.

Technology has made it possible to offer courses in a wide range of media to students from different locations. This allows them to meet the growing educational needs of the population. Many times, technology has allowed distance education programmes to offer specialized courses to students from remote locations. The interactivity between teacher and student is increasing. Even though the implementation of distance education can vary from country to country greatly, most programmes use technology that is either already in place or being looked at for cost-effectiveness. This is especially true for those who cannot afford traditional education because they are physically and financially limited.

DEFINITION

- Distance education is defined as instruction between a teacher and student when they are separated by physical distance, and communication is accomplished by one or more technological media.
- Distance education is defined as institution-based formal education where the learning group is separated, and where interactive telecommunications systems are used to connect learners, resources and instructors.
- Distance education is a structured and planned activity that includes selecting, didactically preparing and presenting instructional materials, as well as supervising and supporting student learning. It is accomplished by using at least one acceptable technical medium to bridge the physical gap between learners and instructors.
- Distance education is defined as the practice of using correspondence, either written or virtual, to learn.

CHARACTERISTICS OF DISTANCE EDUCATION

Keegan (1986) lists seven key features that he believes are required for any meaningful definition:

- the separation of instructor and student
- the dominance of an educational institute
- the application of technological media
- the availability of two-way communication
- the lack of group learning, with learners taught mostly as individuals
- enrolment in the most industrialized kind of learning
- the privatization of education (learning that happens outside of the group)

TYPES OF DISTANCE EDUCATION

Distance education types are classified depending on delivery techniques, pacing models and delivery methods.

1. **Based on Delivery Methods**
   The delivery method refers to the general way that distance education courses or classes are actually delivered. There are currently two main delivery methods. However, it is possible to cross-over.
   i. **Cable TV:** Education is delivered through cable TV, which is also popularly known as educational television programmes.
   ii. **Satellite broadcasting:** EduSat is the first satellite of India designed and launched by ISRO specifically to serve the educational sector. EduSat was created primarily for the purposes of providing connectivity to school, college and higher levels of education and also to support nonformal education including developmental communication.
   iii. **Video conferencing:** In the present era, video conferencing is commonly used for distance learning for smooth teacher-taught interaction and teaching–learning process. Furthermore, it also helps in keeping close in touch with the experts, enhances communication with peer group and facilitates enhancing personalized learning experience. The commonly used online platforms for video conferencing are Zoom, Google Meet, Microsoft Teams, ezTalks cloud meeting, Yammer, Evernote, Prezi, Skype, Cisco WebEx, office 365, etc.
   iv. **Telephone:** Mobile phone has become very popular for educational media use during the pandemic-19 and thereafter. There are several mobile-based educational programmes or apps developed to be used for every level of students including professional students.
   v. **Correspondence:** While online delivery is the preferred method of delivery, correspondence courses are more traditional and can be sent by mail.
2. **Based on Pacing Models**
   A pace model describes how distance learning can be controlled. This is how quickly courses can be completed, and how quickly students are able to move. The two most important models for pacing are:
   i. **Paced:** Paced distance learning is an approach that allows the school, college or university to control the pace of the students' progress so that they all complete the work at the same time. This will often mean that students will have a clear start/end date and modules for each course. The deadlines for assignments will be the same as those for exams.
   ii. **Self-paced:** The self-paced model of distance learning allows learners to choose how fast they want to progress. This means that the pace at which students' complete lessons or courses will depend on how long they have been available to study and their level of ability.
3. **Based on Modes of Delivery**
   The mode of delivery is the method by which distance education content is delivered to students and how they engage with it. These are the main modes:
   i. **Synchronous:** Synchronous learning refers to distance education where teachers and students interact from different places at the same time. This is an emerging trend in e-learning. Technology like Skype, Google Hangouts or Microsoft Teams facilitates it. Synchronous learning is essentially live or in real time. It is similar to in-person education but the learners are geographically distant. Students might be required to take part in mandatory learning activities, which could include group chats, virtual classroom sessions and many more at a set time.
   ii. **Asynchronous:** Asynchronous learning refers to distance learning that takes place outside of live sessions. This type of learning involves more self-study. Students can complete tasks

at different times and have access to learning materials on an on-demand basis. It is possible to stream audio and video files and download documents.

iii. **Mixed:** Mixed delivery is a mix of synchronous and nonsynchronous learning. One example is that a course could be based on an asynchronous work. However, the learning group would need to meet up for live sessions every other week to share their ideas. It could also be that students work primarily independently but must have one-on-one sessions with the teacher occasionally.

ADVANTAGES OF DISTANT EDUCATION

- It can accommodate students with special needs.
- Greater focus on the student and his needs.
- Greater interactivity and dynamism.
- Flexibility of time and space.
- It helps students develop their technical skills.
- It is a wonderful instrument for enhancing the adult population's academic and professional growth.
- It enables students to complete previously postponed courses.
- It has flexible timetables that allow students to organize their time while still respecting family life and professional responsibilities.
- It assumes low cost.
- It provides an opportunity for individualized focus as the tutor observes, monitors and corrects each student.
- There is information feedback so that the teacher knows if the student responds to the method and reaches the objectives initially set.

DISADVANTAGES OF DISTANT EDUCATION

- Difficulty staying motivated.
- Absence of physical interaction.
- Difficulty staying in contact with instructors.
- Difficulty interacting with peers.
- Difficulty completing all courses for a degree/Difficult to choose a quality educational programme.
- It does not help in developing oral skills and social interactions.
- It has technical difficulties.
- Employer's reluctance to accept distance mode of training.

MOBILE-BASED EDUCATIONAL TECHNOLOGY

Mobile learning (m-learning) is an important part of the professional and educational training of specialists. Mobile technologies are rapidly evolving and can be integrated into the education process to increase the quality of education. Many educational institutions around the globe are using mobile technology to access multimedia learning web resources (audio, video, maps, images) and to quickly access to resources, dictionaries and learning sites.

DEFINITIONS

- Mobile education is an extension of mobile learning, including the full range of opportunities mobile technologies and systems offer for improving learning, teaching, assessment and educational administration and management.
- Mobile learning, also known as m-learning, is a new way to access learning content using mobile devices.
- It is the point of intersection, where mobile computing goes through e-learning to provide a learning experience anytime and anywhere.
- Mobile learning is 'any sort of learning that happens when the learner is not at a fixed, predetermined location, or learning that happens when the learner takes advantage of the learning opportunities offered by mobile technologies'.

BASIC REQUIREMENTS FOR MOBILE-BASED EDUCATION

The minimum criteria for mobile technology that enable learning outside of the classroom. These technologies should be as follows:

- *Highly mobile:* The technology is accessible anytime he or she needs to study.
- *Individual:* The technology may be tailored to an individual learner's talents, expertise and learning preferences, and it is intended to promote personal learning rather than typical office work.
- *Unobtrusive:* The student can collect experiences and retrieve knowledge without the technology being distracting or intrusive on the scenario.
- *Accessible:* The student may utilize the technology from any location to communicate with teachers, professionals and classmates.
- *Adaptable:* The technology may be tailored to the learning situation as well as the learner's increasing abilities and knowledge.
- *Persistent:* The learner may utilize technology to handle learning throughout a lifespan so that the learner's own collection of information and knowledge is always available, regardless of technological changes.
- *Useful:* The technology is appropriate for daily purposes such as communication, entertainment, employment and education.
- *Simple to use:* Individuals with no prior knowledge with the technology may quickly understand and operate it.

ADVANTAGES OF MOBILE-BASED EDUCATION

Mobile devices for education offer several advantages, such as:

- Learners have continual access to the most up-to-date books, audio books, videos and digital learning experiences from across the globe, and they may learn whenever and wherever they prefer.
- Assignments and projects, integrating text, photos, audios and videos may be made on a mobile device and aggregated by the student in an online portfolio.
- Learners (and instructors) may communicate with one another at any time and from any location to discuss and share their learning.
- By using mobile devices to introduce concepts and administer examinations, teachers may spend less time in front of a class delivering and evaluating knowledge, allowing for more interaction with students and exploring.

- Information and comments may be readily delivered directly to students, instructors, mentors, parents and so on and will be recognized and followed up on promptly.
- Mobile devices may be used by online planning systems to manage and send notifications regarding classes, seminars, activities and vacations.
- Test papers may be properly and safely assessed, collated, pooled and marked when students are ready, rather than at predetermined intervals throughout the year.
- Mobile education can be less expensive than traditional methods, allowing for better use of space and employee time and saving money, such as on photocopy, printing, shipping, books and staff travelling.
- Mobile technologies make it simpler for instructors to give more diversified learning opportunities and formative evaluation for students with varying skills and learning styles.
- Mobile-linked devices can enable learners to access information quickly and easily, whether inside or outside of the classroom.
- It reduces need for students to carry around heavy textbooks.
- A student can access the same educational materials from everywhere and anytime.
- Students can modify educational content without causing physical copies to become damaged.

DISADVANTAGES OF MOBILE-BASED EDUCATION

1. Using mobile learning creates a lot of distraction.
2. Many students misuse the device for different purposes.
3. It requires good internet connection or electricity.
4. It requires training of new technology personnel and their applications.
5. Lack of mobile technology compatibility with students and teachers.
6. Extended screen time can lead to various physical and mental problems.
7. It has lack of physical interaction.
8. It has a copyright or content security problem.
9. It has a risk of sudden obsolescence.

GUIDELINES FOR EFFECTIVE USE OF AUDIOVISUAL AIDS

The key to using graphics and visual aids effectively requires using them so that they make the maximum impact (Table 6.1). The principles of using audiovisual aids are as follows:

- Begin the presentation with no aids, as presenters want their audience to be listening to them, not looking at props, specimens or other visual aids.
- Present the aid at the appropriate point in the presentation and then remove it immediately.
- Present the aid, give audience a few seconds to comprehend it and then comment on the aid.
- Use a pointer, such as a laser pointer, to focus the audience on the part of the graphic that is being discussed by the presenter.
- Be sure to speak slowly and deliberately as the presenter; explain or use a graphic to avoid confusing the audience.
- In addition, remember to talk to the audience maintaining eye contact with them, not only to the visual aid.
- When using slides, tell the audience what they will see, show them the slide, give them time to digest what they are seeing, then comment on the slide.
- Turn off the projector lamp between slides.

- Do not begin talking about another topic while a slide, depicting a past topic, is still showing.
- Remember people cannot see and listen at the same time.
- Use colour to influence mood and emotion.
- The colours for type, illustrations and backgrounds influence the way they are perceived. Here is a basic guide to using colour in presentations:

Red: excitement, alert	*Purple:* dignity, sophistication
Green: growth	*Yellow:* confidence, warmth, wisdom
Blue: truth, justice	*White:* professionalism, new, innocence
Black: authority, strength	*Orange:* action, optimism
Brown: friendliness, warmth	*Grey:* integrity, maturity

- **Text size:** Projected text should be large enough to be read by all viewers (even the people at the end of the room). Ideally, the following text size must be followed:
  - ***Headline text:*** 36–44 points
  - ***Subtext:*** 34–36 points
  - ***Second-level text:*** 24–28 points
  - 28–24 points is a minimum for most situations.
- **Font style:** Regarding the font style, the following guidelines must be followed:
  - Use simple bold running styles of written text content.
  - Use only standardized font styles, such as Arial font, which are easily readable.
  - Do not use only capital text, they are difficult to read; use both upper and lower case text.
- **Images**
  - Use images to supplement text content, which improves understanding.
  - Use images for emphasizing the specific points of the presentation.
  - Do not use an image or illustration to fill the space.
  - Do not use irrelevant pictures or images with text. Those will rather distract the learner.
- **Animation:** It is good to use animation in presentations but keep the animations simple and effective.
- **Other miscellaneous principles**
  - The instructional programme should be organized and administered such that the audiovisual material functions as an integral part of the educational programme.
  - The audiovisual education programme should be organized and administered in such a way that the programme is centralized with a specialized direction and leadership.
  - The audiovisual education programme should be flexible. In addition to those education communication media which are available through purchase, rental or loan, opportunities should be provided which encourage the teacher to personalize their instruction through the preparation of their own instructional materials where feasible.
  - An advisory committee should be appointed to assist in the selection and coordination of audiovisual materials.
  - Audiovisual materials should be available as and when they are needed if they are to be utilized effectively as an integral part of the curriculum.
    - They eliminate frequent duplication of materials.
    - Pooling of equipment makes for more frequent and better use of equipment.
    - They are readily available and accessible to the entire instructional staff.
    - They provide for space for adequate preparation or production of audiovisual materials.
  - Provision should be made for helping the instructors to acquire skills in the use of audiovisual materials.

  - Budget appropriation should be made regularly for the audiovisual education programme.
  - Evaluation of the audiovisual education programme should be made at regular intervals. Evaluation of the function and the use of each audiovisual aid should be done continuously.
  - Legal aspects should be considered in the production and the utilization of educational communication media.
- **Additional presenter tips:** A presenter may follow the following tips to make presentation more successful:
  - Arrive early for the presentation so that the presenter can feel psychologically comfortable and ready.
  - Check out the equipment, lights and set-up so that the presentation may proceed smoothly later.
  - Get oriented to rooms, lighting and audiovisual aid for effective operation during needs.
  - Brush up on giving your presentation to feel comfortable.
  - Give yourself time to feel prepared and confident before the presentation.

REVIEW QUESTIONS

LONG-ANSWER QUESTIONS

1. Discuss audiovisual aids.
2. Explain the importance of audiovisual aids in teaching nursing and describe the principles in use for any two educational aids.
3. Discuss audiovisual aids and their use in teaching. Explain with suitable examples.
4. Discuss audiovisual aids in nursing education.
5. Discuss blackboard/chalkboard.
6. Define audiovisual aids and write the importance of using audiovisual aids in nursing education.
7. Discuss bulletin board and its principles.
8. List the various audiovisual aids and discuss how a blackboard is a simple and effective visual aid used for teaching.
9. Differentiate between blackboard and bulletin board.
10. Discuss educational communication media.
11. Discuss the effective use of overhead projector.
12. Discuss the role of a teacher in using teaching aids effectively.
13. Enumerate the criteria for the selection of audiovisual aids.
14. Discuss flash cards.
15. Discuss the importance of a blackboard.
16. List the purposes of audiovisual aids in nursing education and elaborate the advantages of computer as a teaching aid.
17. List the types of audiovisual aids and write about three-dimensional aids used in nursing education.
18. Discuss posters.
19. Write about projected teaching aids.
20. Discuss puppets.
21. Discuss slide projectors.
22. Write about tape recorders.
23. Explain the uses of a flannel board.
24. Discuss the types, advantages and disadvantages of blackboards.

25. Discuss the principles in use in audiovisual aids.
26. Discuss the role of audiovisual aids in teaching.
27. Discuss the various types of audiovisual aids.
28. Discuss graphic audiovisual aids.
29. Enumerate sources of audiovisual aids.
30. Explain the principles to be followed for the effective use of audiovisual aids.
31. Explain different types of chart.

SHORT-ANSWER QUESTIONS

1. Discuss briefly four characteristics of good audiovisual aids.
2. Mention four types of blackboard.
3. List down the projected audiovisual aids.
4. Classify instructional aids.

MULTIPLE-CHOICE QUESTIONS (MCQs)

1. Leaflet is made up of
   (a) Full page
   (b) Two pages
   (c) Half page
   (d) Five pages
2. How many folds do pamphlets contain?
   (a) 2–5
   (b) 2–6
   (c) 2–7
   (d) 2–8
3. Full page, single side printed material is called
   (a) Leaflet
   (b) Handout
   (c) Pamphlet
   (d) Flash card
4. A paper that is both sides printed with threefold is known as
   (a) Leaflet
   (b) Pamphlet
   (c) Handout
   (d) Flash card
5. What is the appropriate size of flash card?
   (a) 10″ × 10″
   (b) 10″ × 12″
   (c) 12″ × 14″
   (d) 12″ × 12″
6. Flash card can be used for group of
   (a) 40
   (b) 20

(c) 35
(d) 45

7. Ideally how many flash cards can be used for one health talk/one session?
   (a) 01–02
   (b) 10–12
   (c) 20–25
   (d) 25–30
8. Appropriate size of letter for making posters
   (a) 10″ × 20″
   (b) 15″ × 25″
   (c) 22″ × 28″
   (d) 5″ × 15″
9. Percentile, quartile deviation can be drawn on
   (a) Cumulative frequency
   (b) Ogive
   (c) Histogram
   (d) Frequency polygon
10. Angle of pie graph is
   (a) 90 degrees
   (b) 180 degrees
   (c) 360 degrees
   (d) None of these
11. Graphical presentation of data can be drawn for
   (a) Qualitative data
   (b) Quantitative data
   (c) Raw data
   (d) Abstract data
12. Which one of the following is not a type of map?
   (a) Relief maps
   (b) Historical maps
   (c) Distribution maps
   (d) Overlay maps
13. To show the complication of disease, you will use
   (a) Job chart
   (b) Flow chart
   (c) Tree chart
   (d) Pie chart
14. To show family history of patient, you will use
   (a) Tabulation
   (b) Genealogy chart
   (c) Flow chart
   (d) Tree chart
15. Which one of the following is one-way communication aid?
   (a) Television
   (b) Radio
   (c) Both (a) and (b)
   (d) None of these

ANSWERS OF THE MULTIPLE-CHOICE QUESTIONS

1. (a), 2. (a), 3. (b), 4. (b), 5. (b), 6. (b), 7. (b), 8. (a), 9. (c), 10. (c), 11. (b), 12. (c), 13. (b), 14. (d), 15. (c)

FURTHER READING

Alexander, M., Lenahan, P., & Pavlov, A. (2005). *The future of cinemeducation*. Abingdon, UK: Radcliffe Publishing.

Amory, A. (2001). Building an educational adventure game: Theory, design, and lessons. *Journal of Interactive Learning Research, 12*(2–3), 249–263.

Anglin, G. J., Vaez, H., & Cunningham, K. L. (2004). *Visual representations and learning: The role of static and animated graphics*. Mahwah, NJ: Lawrence Erlbaum Associates Publishers.

Atkinson, R. K. (2005). *Multimedia learning of mathematics*. New York: Cambridge University Press.

Barron, A. E. (2004). *Auditory instruction*. Mahwah, NJ: Lawrence Erlbaum Associates Publishers.

Belliveau, P. P., & Perla, R. J. (2007). Antibiogram-derived radial decision trees: Innovative visual educational tools for discussing empirical antibiotic selections. *Pharmacy Education, 7*(1), 43–51.

Betrancourt, M. (2005). *The animation and interactivity principles in multimedia learning*. New York: Cambridge University Press.

Block, G., Miller, M., Harnack, L., Kayman, S., Mandel, S., & Cristofar, S. (2000). An interactive CD-ROM for nutrition screening and counselling. *American Journal of Public Health, 90*(5), 781–785.

Bouman, M. (2004). *Entertainment-education television drama in the Netherlands*. Mahwah, NJ: Lawrence Erlbaum Associates Publishers.

Brett, R. P. (2003). Allocation of support levels to hearing-impaired children: Moving away from using audiometric descriptors. *Deafness & Education International, 5*(3), 167–181.

Burn, A., & Durran, J. (2006). *Digital anatomies: Analysis as production in media education*. Mahwah, NJ: Lawrence Erlbaum Associates Publishers.

Carey, M., Schofield, P., Jefford, M., Krishnasamy, M., & Aranda, S. (2007). The development of audio-visual materials to prepare patients for medical procedures: An oncology application. *European Journal of Cancer Care, 16*(5), 417–423.

Casarotti, M., Filipponi, L., Pieti, L., & Sartori, R. (2002). Educational interaction in distance learning: Analysis of a one-way video and two-way audio system. *Psychnology Journal, 1*(1), 28–38.

Chang, C. K. (2004). Constructing a streaming video-based learning forum for collaborative learning. *Journal of Educational Multimedia and Hypermedia, 13*(3), 245–263.

Clark, R. C. (2005). *Multimedia learning in e-courses*. New York: Cambridge University Press.

Clark, R. E., & Feldon, D. F. (2005). *Five common but questionable principles of multimedia learning*. New York: Cambridge University Press.

Clarke, J. O. (1975). Improving teaching techniques through the use of A-V materials. *Journal Pendidikan*, U.K.M., No. *14*, 7–59.

Claudet, J. (2002). Integrating school leadership knowledge and practice using multimedia technology: Linking national standards, assessment, and professional development. *Journal of Personnel Evaluation in Education, 16*(1), 29–43.

Claudet, J. (2002). Issues and directions in technology-integrated personnel assessment and professional development. *Journal of Personnel Evaluation in Education, 16*(1), 7–10.

Cobb, S., & Fraser, D. S. (2005). *Multimedia learning in virtual reality*. New York: Cambridge University Press.

Copley, J. (2007). Audio and video podcasts of lectures for campus-based students: Production and evaluation of student use. *Innovations in Education and Teaching International, 44*(4), 387–399.

Creighton-Zollar, A. (2006). *Communicating across preferences: A comparative family systems example*. New York: Haworth Press.

Croker, S. (2003). Review of secrets of the mind CD ROMs. *Psychology Learning & Teaching, 3*(1), 69–70.

Curran, V. R. (2006). Tele-education. *Journal of Telemedicine and Telecare, 12*(2), 57–63. doi:10.1258/135763306776084400

Damore-Petingola, S., Lightfoot, N., Vaillancourt, C., Mayer, C., Steggles, S., & Gauthier-Frohlick, D. (2002). Hear how I feel: Evaluation of a video depicting the experiences of adolescents and young adults with a parent diagnosed with cancer. *Journal of Psychosocial Oncology*, *20*(4), 57–69.

Davies, D. K., Stock, S. E., & Wehmeyer, M. L. (2002). Enhancing independent task performance for individuals with mental retardation through use of a handheld self-directed visual and audio prompting system. *Education & Training in Mental Retardation & Developmental Disabilities*, *37*(2), 209–218.

Dewald, B. W. A. (2000). Turning part-time students' feedback into video programs. *Education & Training*, *42*(1), 33–39.

Different types of distance learning_elearning_eztalks_video conferencing, webinar, online meeting, screensharing tips and reviews [Internet]. ezTalks. [cited 2021Nov21]. https://eztalks.com/elearning/different-types-of-distance-learning.html

Dillon, A., & Jobst, J. (2005). *Multimedia learning with hypermedia*. New York: Cambridge University Press.

Douglas, G. (2001). ICT, education, and visual impairment. *British Journal of Educational Technology*, *32*(3), 353–364.

Dowaliby, F., & Lang, H. G. (1999). Adjunct aids in instructional prose: A multimedia study with deaf college students. *Journal of Deaf Studies and Deaf Education*, *4*(4), 270–282.

Elbon, S., Nsubuga, P., Knowles, J., Bobrow, E., Parvanta, I., Timmer, A., & van der Haar, F. (2006). Micronutrient action plan instructional tool (MAPit): A training tool to support public health professionals' efforts to eliminate micronutrient malnutrition. *Innovations in Education and Teaching International*, *43*(4), 353–368.

Endri, E. (2021). The effect of visual communication on children's reading interest. *Library Philosophy and Practice (e-journal)*. 6440. https://digitalcommons.unl.edu/libphilprac/6440

Eschenbrenner, B., & Fui-Hoon, Nah. (2007). Mobile technology in education: uses and benefits. *International Journal of Mobile Learning and Organisation*, *1*(2), 159–183. doi:10.1504/ijmlo.2007.012676

Finlayson, R., Schneider, J., Wan, M., Irons, R., & Sealy, J. (1999). Sexual addiction portrayed in cinema. *Sexual Addiction & Compulsivity*, *6*(2), 151–159.

Fleming, M. (1982). Changing conceptions in research on pictures. *Communication & Cognition*, *15*(1), 53–60.

Fletcher, J. D., & Tobias, S. (2005). *The multimedia principle*. New York: Cambridge University Press.

Franks, F. L., & Glass, R. (1985). Microslide Cassette Programs for low vision students. *Education of the Visually Handicapped*, *17*(1), 11–16.

Galvez Diaz, V., & Waldegg, G. (2004). Science and scientific knowledge in educational television. *Ensenanza de las Ciencias Revista de Investigacion y Experiencias Didacticas*, *2*(1), 147–158.

Goodman, S. (2005). *The practice and principles of teaching critical literacy at the educational video center*. Malden, MA: Blackwell Publishing.

Gouzouasis, P. (1994). Multimedia constructions of children: An exploratory study. *Journal of Computing in Childhood Education*, *5*(3–4), 273–284.

Graff, M. (2003). Assessing learning from hypertext: An individual differences perspective. *Journal of Interactive Learning Research*, *14*(4), 425–438.

Graves, D., Ray, R., & Thompson, D. (1986). Audiovisual training materials to support mainstreaming. *Pointer*, *31*(1), 29–33.

Hayes, M. T., & Petrie, G. M. (2006). We're from the generation that was raised on television: A qualitative exploration of media imagery in elementary preservice teachers video production. *International Journal of Qualitative Studies in Education*, *19*(4), 499–517.

Hegarty, M. (2005). *Multimedia learning about physical systems*. New York: Cambridge University Press.

Hernandez-Ramos, P. (2007). Aim, shoot, ready! Future teachers learn to 'do' video. *British Journal of Educational Technology*, *38*(1), 33–41.

Higgins, J. A., & Dermer, S. (2001). The use of film in marriage and family counselor education. *Counselor Education and Supervision*, *40*(3), 182–192.

Hizal, A. (1983). *Uzaktan Ogretim Surecleri ve Yazili Gerecler (Distance Teaching Process and Print Materials)*. Ankara, Turkey: Ankara Universitesi Egitim Fakultesi Yayinlari.

Iqbal, H., Parra, R., Ramirez-Mendoza, R. A., & Zavala-Yoe, R. (2020). Smart educational tools and learning management systems: Supportive framework. *International Journal on Interactive Design and Manufacturing, 14*, 1179–1193.

Jeste, D. V., Dunn, L. B., Folsom, D. P., & Zisook, D. (2008). Multimedia educational aids for improving consumer knowledge about illness management and treatment decisions: A review of randomized controlled trials. *Journal of Psychiatric Research, 42*(1), 1–21.

Jewell, J., Hupp, S., & Luttrell, G. (2004). The effectiveness of fatal vision goggles: Disentangling experiential versus onlooker effects. *Journal of Alcohol and Drug Education, 48*(3), 63–84.

Johnson, L. (2006). Lights...camera...educate: A tool to engage and enthuse students in medical education. *PsycCRITIQUES, 51*(9), 2006.

Jonassen, D. H., Lee, C. B., Yang, C. C., & Laffey, J. (2005). *The collaboration principle in multimedia learning*. New York: Cambridge University Press.

Jones, L., & McNamara, O. (2004). The possibilities and constraints of multimedia as a basis for critical reflection. *Cambridge Journal of Education, 34*(3), 279–296.

Keegan, D. (1986). *The foundations of distance education*. London: Croom Helm.

King, J. (2002). Using DVD feature films in the EFL classroom. *Computer Assisted Language Learning, 15*(5), 509–523.

Kirkpatrick, H. A. (2005). *Technological considerations*. Abingdon, UK: Radcliffe Publishing.

Kompolt, P. (1984). Function and tasks of film in education. *Jednotna Skola, 36*(3), 243–253.

Konrad, J. L., & Yoder, J. D. (2000). Adding feminist therapy to videotape demonstrations. *Teaching of Psychology, 27*(1), 57–58.

Kozma, R., & Russell, J. (2005). *Multimedia learning of chemistry*. New York: Cambridge University Press.

Krupinski, E. A., Lopez, A. M., Lyman, T., Barker, G., & Weinstein, R. S. (2004). Continuing education via telemedicine: Analysis of reasons for attending or not attending. *Telemedicine Journal and e-Health, 10*(3), 403–409.

Lajoie, S. P., & Nakamura, C. (2005). *Multimedia learning of cognitive skills*. New York: Cambridge University Press.

Lan, W. Y., & Morgan, J. (2003). Videotaping as a means of self-monitoring to improve theater students' performance. *Journal of Experimental Education, 71*(4), 371–381.

Lancioni, G. E., O'Reilly, M. F., Singh, N. N., Sigafoos, J., Oliva, D., Baccani, S., ... Stasolla, F. (2004). Technological aids to promote basic developmental achievements by children with multiple disabilities: Evaluation of two cases. *Cognitive Processing, 5*(4), 232–238.

Lemaire, E. D., & Greene, G. (2003). A comparison between three electronic media and in-person learning for continuing education in physical rehabilitation. *Journal of Telemedicine and Telecare, 9*(1), 17–22.

Lepard, D. H. (2002). Using peers and technology to strengthen leadership. *Journal of Personnel Evaluation in Education, 16*(1), 11–28.

Lowe, R. K. (2005). *Multimedia learning of meteorology*. New York: Cambridge University Press.

Mayer, R. E. (2005). *Introduction to multimedia learning*. New York: Cambridge University Press.

Mayer, R. E. (2005). *Principles for managing essential processing in multimedia learning: Segmenting, pretraining, and modality principles*. New York: Cambridge University Press.

Mayer, R. E. (2005). *Principles of multimedia learning based on social cues: Personalization, voice, and image principles*. New York: Cambridge University Press.

Mehdipour, Y., & Zerehkaf, H. (2013). Mobile learning for education: Benefits and challenges. *International Journal of Computational Engineering Research, 3*(6), 93–101.

Metha, A. A. (2003). *Learning in high dimensional spaces: Applications, theory, and algorithms. Dissertation Abstracts International: Section B: The Sciences and Engineering*. Washington DC: University of Washington.

Moore, M. G., & Anderson, W. G. (2003). *Handbook of distance education*. Mahwah, NJ: L. Erlbaum Associates.

Moreno, R. (2005). *Multimedia learning with animated pedagogical agents*. New York: Cambridge University Press.

Moss, J., Deppeler, J., Astley, L., & Pattison, K. (2007). Student researchers in the middle: Using visual images to make sense of inclusive education. *Journal of Research in Special Educational Needs, 7*(1), 46–54.

Ofiesh, N. S., Rice, C. J., Long, E. M., Merchant, D. C., & Gajar, A. H. (2002). Service delivery for postsecondary students with disabilities: A survey of assistive technology use across disabilities. *College Student Journal, 36*(1), 94–108.

Olivero, F., John, P., & Sutherland, R. (2004). Seeing is believing: Using videopapers to transform teachers' professional knowledge and practice. *Cambridge Journal of Education, 34*(2), 179–191.

Parish, S. J., Weber, C. M., Steiner-Grossman, P., Milan, F. B., Burton, W. B., & Marantz, P. R. (2006). Teaching clinical skills through videotape review: A randomized trial of group versus individual reviews. *Teaching and Learning in Medicine, 18*(2), 92–98.

Parra-Medina, D., Wilcox, S., Thompson-Robinson, M., Sargent, R., & Will, J. C. (2004). A replicable process for redesigning ethnically relevant educational materials. *Journal of Women's Health, 13*(5), 579–588.

Pearson, S., & Ralph, S. (2007). The identity of SENCos: Insights through images. *Journal of Research in Special Educational Needs, 7*(1), 36–45.

Peraya, D. (1984). Audiovisual pedagogy: Myths and actual trends. *Revue Belge de Psychologie et de Pedagogie, 46*(185–186), 19–32.

Plass, J. L., & Jones, L. C. (2005). *Multimedia learning in second language acquisition*. New York: Cambridge University Press.

Prosser, J., & Loxley, A. (2007). Enhancing the contribution of visual methods to inclusive education. *Journal of Research in Special Educational Needs, 7*(1), 55–68.

Puzanov, B. P. (1983). Use of graph-projector at the history lessons in the school for mentally retarded children. *Defektologiya, 2*, 44–47.

Ramirez, A. (2000). *Assessing the cognitive fit of hypertext-based learning aids for advanced learning in complex and ill-structured domains. Dissertation Abstracts International Section A: Humanities and Social Sciences.* Washington DC: University of Washington.

Reinking, D. (2005). *Multimedia learning of reading*. New York: Cambridge University Press.

Rieber, L. P. (2005). *Multimedia learning in games, simulations, and microworlds*. New York: Cambridge University Press.

Robertson, M., & Collins, A. (2003). The video role model as an enterprise teaching aid. *Education & Training, 45*(6), 331–340.

Rouet, J. F., & Potelle, H. (2005). *Navigational principles in multimedia learning*. New York: Cambridge University Press.

Roy, M., & Chi, M. T. H. (2005). *The self-explanation principle in multimedia learning*. New York: Cambridge University Press.

Saykılı, A. (2018). Distance education: Definitions, generations, key concepts and future directions. *International Journal of Contemporary Educational Research, 5*(1), 2–17.

Schnotz, W., & Rasch, T. (2005). Enabling, facilitating, and inhibiting effects of animations in multimedia learning: Why reduction of cognitive load can have negative results on learning. *Educational Technology Research and Development, 53*(3), 47–58.

Shapiro, A. M. (2005). *The site map principle in multimedia learning*. New York: Cambridge University Press.

Sharma, V. (1988). Educational technology and multi-media language learning: A psychological consideration. *Psycho-Lingua, 18*(1), 1–10.

Shephard, K. (2003). Questioning, promoting and evaluating the use of streaming video to support student learning. *British Journal of Educational Technology, 34*(3), 295–308.

Sivakumar, R. (2014). 3G-Mobile technology in education. *Cognitive Discourses International Multidisciplinary Journal, 2*, 50–54.

Skouge, J. R., Rao, K., & Boisvert, P. C. (2007). Promoting early literacy for diverse learners using audio and video technology. *Early Childhood Education Journal, 35*(1), 5–11.

Sloan, D., Stratford, J., & Gregor, P. (2006). Using multimedia to enhance the accessibility of the learning environment for disabled students: Reflections from the skills for access project. *ALT-J Research in Learning Technology, 14*(1), 39–54.

Sweller, J. (2005). *Implications of cognitive load theory for multimedia learning*. New York: Cambridge University Press.

Sweller, J. (2005). *The redundancy principle in multimedia learning*. New York: Cambridge University Press.

Team, S. P. (2014). *Pros & cons of distance learning* [Internet]. Scholarship Positions 2021 2022 [cited 2021 Nov 21]. https://scholarship-positions.com/pros-cons-distance-learning/2014/07/25/

Thierry, K. L., Goh, C. L., Pipe, M. E., & Murray, J. (2005). Source recall enhances children's discrimination of seen and heard events. *Journal of Experimental Psychology Applied, 11*(1), 33–44.

Thompson, D. E., Brooks, K., & Lizarraga, E. S. (2003). Perceived transfer of learning: From the distance education classroom to the workplace. *Assessment & Evaluation in Higher Education, 28*(5), 539–547.

Wiley, J., & Ash, I. K. (2005). *Multimedia learning of history*. New York: Cambridge University Press.

Wilksch, S. M., Tiggemann, M., & Wade, T. D. (2006). Impact of interactive school-based media literacy lessons for reducing internalization of media ideals in young adolescent girls and boys. *International Journal of Eating Disorders, 39*(5), 385–393.

Williams, C., Griffin, K. W., Macaulay, A. P., West, T. L., & Gronewold, E. (2005). Efficacy of a drug prevention CD-ROM intervention for adolescents. *Substance Use & Misuse, 40*(6), 869–878.

Zabel, B. (2007). *Using technology and music to motivate science students*. Thousand Oaks, CA: Corwin Press.

Zahn, D. K. (1972). *A study to evaluate the effectiveness of audio-tutorial slide/tape instruction versus the flowcharted method of self-instruction in machine calculation*. Graduate Student Theses, Dissertations, & Professional Papers, 9799. https://scholarworks.umt.edu/etd/9799

Zeedyk, M. S., & Wallace, L. (2003). Tackling children's road safety through edutainment: An evaluation of effectiveness. *Health Education Research, 18*(4), 493–505.

CHAPTER

Assessment and evaluation

7

LEARNING OBJECTIVES

This chapter is designed to enable the reader to:

- Understand the concept of measurement, assessment and evaluation
- Describe the meaning, purposes, scope and types of assessment
- Describe principles for selection of assessment methods and guidelines for development of assessment test
- Illustrate barriers to evaluation
- Classify the assessment tools and techniques
- Discuss the concept, purposes, features, principles, advantages and disadvantages of different assessment techniques, such as essay type questions, short answer questions, multiple-choice questions, observation checklist, rating scale, videotapes, written assignments, practical examination, oral examination, simulation-based assessment, clinical portfolios and clinical logs
- Demonstrate the skills in conducting the objective structured clinical examination
- Explain the concept, purposes, features, principles, advantages and disadvantages of different attitude measurement scales such as Likert scale and semantic differential scale
- Appraise assessment tests for higher learning such as interpretative questions, hot spot questions, drag and drop questions and ordered response questions.

KEY TERMS

INTRODUCTION

Assessment is part of the everyday activities of nursing professionals. People also regularly check out our life progress by evaluating our achievements in life. Assessment is the most important but often neglected part of nursing education as well as nursing care provided by nurses through the nursing process approach. Assessment is the only way by which a teacher can know how successful his teaching was and what areas in teaching need improvement. Similarly, a student can know his learning difficulties and also at what position he stands in the crowd of students. Assessment is also necessary to determine to what extent the curriculum objectives have been achieved and the need for improvement.

CONCEPTS OF MEASUREMENT, ASSESSMENT AND EVALUATION

Evaluation, measurement and assessment are three different terms that are certainly connected and interchangeably used. However, it is essential to consider them distinct as well as interconnected ideas and processes.

Measurement refers to the process by which the physical specifications (length, height, weight) of an object are determined. Measurement is the process of assigning a number to an attribute (or phenomenon) according to a rule or set of rules. The term can also be used to refer to the result obtained after performing the process. Measurement is a collection of quantitative data. Measurement is made by comparing a quantity with a standard unit. As this comparison cannot be perfect, measurements are subjected to error.

Educational settings may involve the measurement of attitude, IQ, etc. For measurement, we require standardized tools and a person who is skilled in administering those tools. For example, we require a thermometer to measure temperature, a BP instrument to measure blood pressure, a pulse oximeter to measure oxygen saturation and so on. We will also require a physician or nurse to administer these tools to gather data. The end result of measurement is the collection of data. Measurement is the application of a standard scale or measuring device to an object, event or condition, according to practices accepted by those who are skilled in the use of the device or scale.

Now let us see what *assessment* means. Students frequently hear from a teacher that they will have an assessment test on so and so date. The idea of assessment should now be clear in your mind; it is simply a test that is conducted to test the progress of the student against some predetermined learning objectives. Remember, all tests are assessments but all assessments are not tests. Sometimes, a teacher may require some tools for the assessment, for example basic life support skill assessment checklist to assess the Basic Life Support (BLS) skills of undergraduate nursing students. Assessment is the specified condition by which the behaviour laid down in an objective may be ascertained. Such specifications are usually in the form of written descriptions. So, assessment is the process of documenting, usually in measurable terms, knowledge, skills, attitude and beliefs.

Evaluation is perhaps the most frequently used and the least attended term. It is not simply administering the test, checking answer sheets and announcing marks to the students. What remains in the heart of evaluation is the 'value or quality judgement'. Without using these two core words, evaluation cannot be explained. Evaluation is the most powerful tool in the hands of the teacher to enhance learning. Evaluation is a process that starts with the specification of the criteria or objectives for evaluation; preparing and administering the test (reliable and valid) based on the prespecified criteria; gathering data and facts, and making a judgement whether the objectives are achieved or not; making judgements about the quality, appropriateness, worthiness, validity and goodness of this achievement; and if the criteria or objectives are not achieved, searching for reasons behind this failure, generating solutions to overcome the barriers leading to failure. Evaluation is the process of systematically assessing the design, implementation and impact of programmes, policies or projects.

For example, I often tell my students if they wanted to determine the temperature of the classroom, they would need to get a thermometer and take several readings at different spots and perhaps average the readings. That is simple measuring. The average temperature tells us nothing about whether or not it is appropriate for learning. To do that, students would have to be polled in some reliable and valid way. That polling process is what evaluation is all about. An average classroom temperature of 75°F is simply information. It is the context of the temperature for a particular purpose that provides the criteria for evaluation. A temperature of 75°F may not be very good for some students, while for others, it is ideal for learning.

MEANING OF EVALUATION

Evaluation is the process of determining to what extent the educational objectives are being realized.

—Ralph Tyler

Evaluation is the process of determining the extent to which objectives are being achieved, the effectiveness of the learning experiences provided in the classroom and how well the goals of education have been accomplished.

—NCERT

Evaluation is the assessment of merits and or worth.

—Scriven

Evaluation is a value judgment on an observation, 'performance test' or indeed any data whether directly measured or inferred.

—International Dictionary of Education

Evaluation is a systematic examination of educational and social progress.

—Conbach et al.

Educational evaluation is a process of estimating and appraising the degree and dimensions of student's achievement. Further, it is also a process of estimating and appraising the proficiency level of the particular educational practice, which is being conducted. It is a way of appraising the application of educational theory in practice.

—K. Sudha Rao

Evaluation in education is a systematic process which enables the extent to which the student has attained the educational objectives to be measured. Evaluation always includes measurements (quantitative or qualitative) plus a value judgment.

—J.J. Gulbert

Evaluation involves assessing the strengths and weaknesses of programs, policies, personnel, products, and organizations to improve their effectiveness.

—American Evaluation Association

Continuous evaluation is evaluating patient needs and their progress and determining how well their healthcare needs are being met. Evaluation is a means of helping an individual or a group to become self-directing; it assists in the establishment of goals which, in turn, serve as a criterion for judging desirable changes. A complete evaluation programme for a teacher of nursing would encompass the evaluation of the following:

- Educational objectives
- Teaching and learning procedures
- Student's progress outcome

PURPOSES OF EVALUATION

Evaluation serves distinct purposes for students, teachers, curriculum and society. The teacher should have a complete programme of evaluation, which should be considered an integral, continuous part of teaching as it enables the teacher to accomplish essential purposes. Imagine what will happen if individuals are provided with nursing degrees without proper and objective evaluation? It will ultimately lead to a compromised and poor quality nursing care because incompetent candidates may obtain nursing degrees or licenses in the absence of an efficient evaluation system, which may be disastrous for the profession in long term. Evaluation serves the following distinct purposes for students, teachers, curriculum and society:

- To provide short-term goals to the students to work towards the achievement of educational objectives.
- To clarify the intended learning outcome.
- To determine the level of knowledge and understanding in students.
- To diagnose the strengths and weaknesses of students.
- To encourage student learning by measuring their achievement and informing them about their success.
- To provide information to students for overcoming learning difficulties and selecting future learning experiences.
- To estimate the effectiveness of the instructional media used and the usefulness of instructional materials.
- To help students acquire the attitude and skills of self-evaluation.
- To assess the nonscholastic domains of the student's personality (interests, attitudes and values).
- To provide feedback to the students about their strengths and weaknesses requiring their special attention.
- To assess the student's progress throughout the year.
- To determine whether a particular student is competent enough to be advanced to the next class.
- To ascertain if the teaching strategies are effective and if there is a need to change the teaching strategies.
- To improve curriculum in light of recent advances.
- To satisfy the university requirements for a curriculum.
- To recommend the names of students eligible for a degree to the university.
- To report the student's progress to parents.
- To prevent the society from quacks and incompetent professionals by blocking them from getting degrees/diplomas.
- Evaluation is carried out for general and educational research.

SCOPE OF EVALUATION

There is a broad and wide scope of assessment and evaluation as discussed below (Fig. 7.1):

- **Selection of students:** Selection of students in the institute is the first and foremost scope of assessment because the right students in the right educational programmes are essential for the ultimate growth and development of a country. This can be ensured through the means of assessment for student selection.
- **Feedback to students:** Feedback is necessary for efficient remedial measures in time. Therefore, assessments have a wide scope to offer timely feedback to students so that they can improve and the educational objectives may be achieved.
- **Feedback to teachers:** Assessment does offer feedback to teachers about the student's progress so they can plan and implement corrective measures to support the students in achieving the educational objectives.
- **Incentive to learning:** Students feel an incentive to learning when they are assessed and feedback is given to them. They get a feeling of incentive that reduces boredom in the routine, monotonous teaching–learning process.
- **Motivation of learning activities:** The teaching–learning activities do not remain interesting without timely assessment and evaluation. Therefore, scheduled assessment processes are required for motivating students.
- **Certification of competence:** Student assessment is one of the principle prerequisite to certify the competence or knowledge in a particulate aspect of curriculum.
- **Decision for success or failure:** Assessment offers the ability to decide about the ultimate success or failure of students in the achievement of preplanned educational objectives.

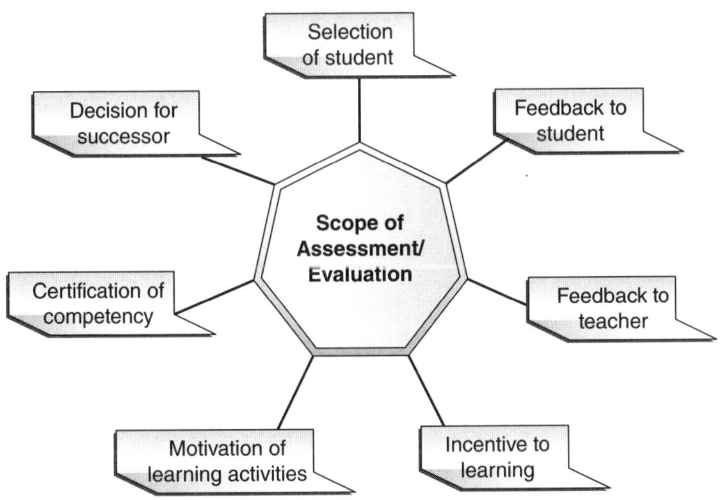

Figure 7.1

Scope of the assessment/evaluation.

TYPES OF EVALUATION

- The description of the types of assessment or evaluation may be seen in Box 7.1. Furthermore, the basic classification of assessment tools and techniques is also given in Box 7.2.

PRINCIPLES FOR SELECTION OF EVALUATION METHODS

Each assessment technique and method has unique features; however, the selection of an assessment technique and method requires careful consideration of the criteria as shown in Fig. 7.2 so that the assessment process can be efficient. Assessment is considered the most tedious task, therefore, the selection of an appropriate technique and method is an essential responsibility of an evaluator. These

BOX 7.1 DESCRIPTION OF TYPES OF ASSESSMENT/EVALUATION

Parameters	Formative Assessment	Summative Assessment
Meaning	It is an ongoing assessment of the student's achievement while the instructional course/ programme is in progress.	It is the final assessment of the student's achievement at the end of a unit/course/programme.
Purposes	To monitor the progress of students and provide feedback for improvement while instructions are in progress.	To finally assign the grades or pass/fail status in a particular educational module or programme.
Frequency	Carried out quite frequently ranging from daily to weekly while instructions are in progress.	Carried out monthly, biannually, annually or at the end of a semester course/progress.
Content focus	Detailed focus on content.	General and broad content scope.
Methods	Methods of formative assessment include classroom questioning, daily assignments, regular formal/informal observation, class tests and internal assessments.	Methods of summative assessment include project evaluation, term examination and final external examination.

BOX 7.2 CLASSIFICATION OF ASSESSMENT TOOLS AND TECHNIQUES

Assessment of Knowledge	Assessment of Skills	Assessment of Attitude
• Essay type questions ◦ Extended response essay ◦ Restricted response essay	• Observation checklist • Rating scale • Anecdotal records	• Likert attitude scale • Semantic differential scale
• *Short answer questions* ◦ Fill in the blank type ◦ Statement completion ◦ Labelling a diagram ◦ Short answer in 5–10 words	• Cumulative records • Written clinical assignments • Critical incident record • Practical examination • Viva voce (oral examination)	
• *Objective type of questions* ◦ Multiple-choice questions ◦ Multiple-response questions ◦ True and false questions ◦ Matching type question	• Objective Structured Clinical Examination (OSCE) • Objective Structured Practical Examination (OSPE)	

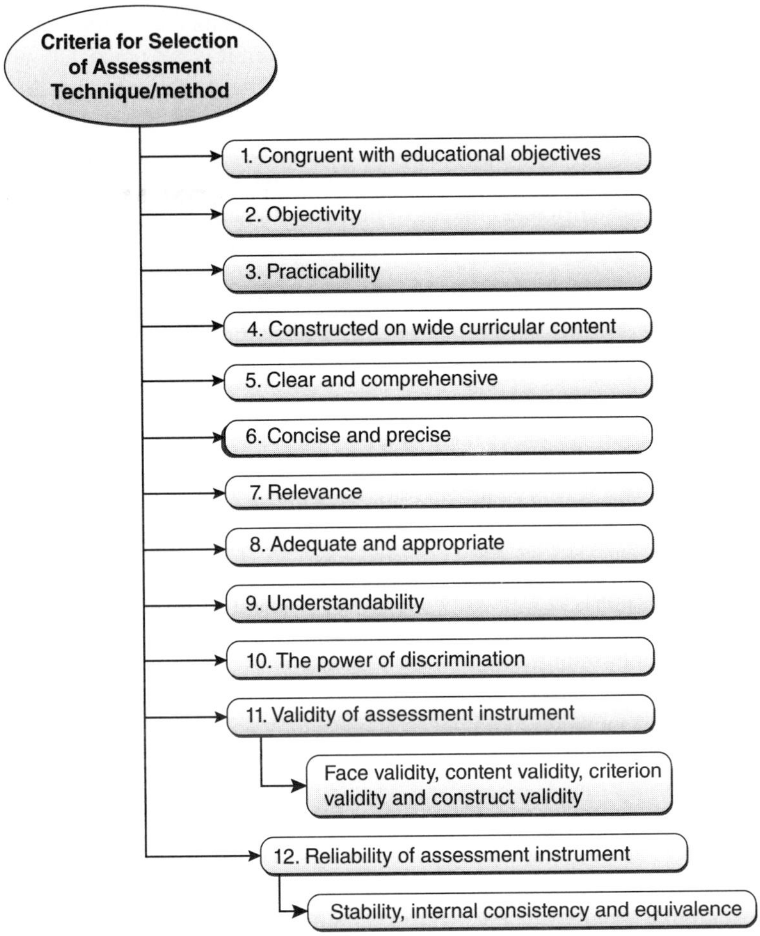

Figure 7.2

Criteria for the selection of assessment technique/method.

principles or criteria described below are also known as *qualities of good assessment tools, techniques and methods*:

- **Congruent with educational objectives:** The assessment techniques and methods must be directly related to the educational objectives so that planned educational objectives can be met. Therefore, evaluators generally base their evaluation techniques and methods on the respective educational objective of a particular curriculum.
- **Objectivity of assessment techniques and methods:** Objectivity is the extent to which independent and competent examiners agree on what constitutes a good answer for each of the elements of a measuring instrument. A good tool used for assessment must be objective so that the evaluator's subjective bias may be avoided. For example, multiple-choice questions (MCQs), short answer questions (SAQs) and objective structured clinical examination (OSCE) are more objective methods of evaluation where there is a minimal risk of subjective bias of the evaluator. However, essay type questions or informal observation in practical examinations may have a high risk of subjective bias and may not be considered an objective means of evaluation.

- **Practicability of measuring techniques and methods:** Evaluators sometimes develop complex methods and tools of evaluation in overenthusiasm. However, it is not practically possible to implement such complex tools and methods of evaluation. For example, a set of MCQs may not be practical to assess clinical skills of nursing students. An evaluator may require an observational rating scale or checklist to appropriately measure their clinical skills.
- **Evaluation tools constructed on wide curricular content:** A good evaluation tool must be constructed from the wide curricular content so that essential and vital areas may not be neglected and the evaluator is assured that the learner is competent in all the essential curricular areas and domains.
- **Clear and comprehensive:** The constructed evaluation tools must be clear to promote understanding in students and they should be comprehensive so that unnecessary time is not wasted in learning and comprehension is easy.
- **Concise and precise:** An evaluation instrument must be as concise as possible and precise so that the face and contract validity of the evaluation tools may be ensured. Furthermore, a concise and precise evaluation tool makes the evaluation process more easy and convenient.
- **Relevance:** The measuring tool must be relevant in reference to the curricular content to be evaluated, the domain of learning to be evaluated and the learner's age and ability to answer the constructed items.
- **Adequate and appropriate:** An evaluation tool must be adequate enough to cover all the essential aspects of the content to be evaluated and it must be appropriate for the evaluation of the domain of learning and the student's ability.
- **Understandability:** An evaluation tool must be easily understandable by the respondent; the understandability of an evaluation tool may be enhanced by using simple and familiar language, avoiding ambiguity in the written content of the items and clear presentation.
- **The power of discrimination:** The basic and essential function of each evaluation tool and technique is to efficiently discriminate in the particular domain of learning among students. Before the selection of an evaluation tool, it must be ensured that it has the ability and strength to discriminate between students with poor and good knowledge. The power of discrimination in an evaluation tool signifies that the students with good knowledge will be able to score more marks as compared to poor students.
- **Validity of assessment instrument:** Validity of an evaluation technique and method is the extent to which the particular evaluation tool and technique measures what it is intended to measure. The validity of an evaluation tool is the most primary and essential characteristic of evaluation tools and techniques because if a tool is not valid then it will not measure what it is supposed to measure. For example, a valid evaluation tool developed to assess the ECG interpretation skills of nursing students must include only the items related to the different clinical ECG situations rather than simple ECG knowledge-related questions. Generally, the validity of an evaluation tool is ensured by seeking the opinions and suggestions from experts of the respective fields. Furthermore, developing standardized evaluation tools may require the statistical measure to establish the validity of the respective evaluation tool. Validity of an evaluation tool may be affected by unclear directions to attempt the questions in a test or examination, difficult professional jargons used to construct the questions, ambiguous terms and sentences, use of unfamiliar language for respondents/students and inexperienced and unqualified persons preparing the questions. Basically, the validity of an assessment tool is classified into the following four categories:
    - ***Face validity:*** Face validity involves the overall look of an instrument regarding its appropriateness to measure a particular aspect of knowledge and skill or to affect the domain of learning.

Though face validity is not considered a very important and essential type of validity for an instrument, it may be taken in consideration to assess the other aspects of validity of an evaluation instrument. In simple words, this aspect of validity refers to the face value or the outlook of an instrument. For example, for a questionnaire constructed to assess the knowledge of nursing regarding 'endotracheal suctioning', an expert of the respective field or evaluator may judge the face value of this instrument (whether it looks good or not), but it provides no guarantee about the appropriateness and completeness of an evaluation instrument with regard to its content, construction and measurement score.

- ***Content validity:*** It is concerned with the scope of coverage of the content area to be measured. It is often applied in tests of knowledge measurement. It is a case expert judgement about the adequacy, appropriateness and completeness of the content area included in the evaluation instrument to measure a particular phenomenon. Judgement of the content viability may be subjective and based on the previous researcher's and expert's opinion about the adequacy, appropriateness and completeness of the content of the instrument. Generally, this viability is ensured through the judgements of experts about the content.
- ***Criterion validity:*** This type of validity is a relationship between the measurements of the instrument with some other external criteria. The instrument is valid if its measurements strongly respond to the score of some other valid criterion. The problems with criterion-related validity is finding a reliable and valid external criterion. Mostly, we are to rely on a less than perfect criterion because the rating found by empirical and supervisory methods may be computed mathematically that can correlate the score of the instrument with the score of criterion variable. The range of coefficient ≥ 0.70 is desirable. Criterion-related validity may be differentiated by predictive validity and concurrent validity.
  - *Predictive validity:* It is the degree of forecasting judgement; for example, some personality tests and academic futures of students can be a predictive behaviour pattern. It is the differentiation between the performances on some future criterion and instruments ability. An instrument may have predictive validity when its score significantly correlates with some future criteria.
  - *Concurrent validity:* It is the degree of the measures in the present time. It relates to the present specific behaviour and characteristics, hence the difference between the predictive and concurrent validity refers to the timing pattern of obtaining the measurements of a criterion.
- ***Construct validity:*** Construct validity is a key criterion for assessing the quality of an evaluation instrument. It has most often been addressed in terms of measurement issues. The key construct validity questions with regard to measurements are as follows: What is this instrument really measuring? Does it adequately measure the abstract concept of interest? Construct validity gives more importance to testing the relationship predicted on theoretical measurements. The evaluator can make predictions in relation to other such type of constructs. One such method of construct validation is known as *group technique*.

- **Reliability of the assessment instrument:** Reliability is the degree of consistency and accuracy with which an instrument measures the attribute it is designed to measure. Further, reliability is defined as the ability of an instrument to create reproducible results. Therefore, reliability is concerned with consistency of the measurement tools. A tool can only be considered reliable if it measures an attribute with similar results on repeated use. There are several ways to measure the reliability of research tools, which depends on several factors such as nature of the instrument as well as aspects of reliability the evaluator wants to measure. The main aspects of reliability that are considered important in evaluation are stability, internal consistency and equivalence.

- ***Stability:*** The stability aspect of reliability means that the research instrument provides the same results when it is administered consecutively two or more times. Stability is estimated to make sure that the research instrument is consistent in providing similar results with repeated administrations. It is also known as *test-retest reliability*. To assess test-retest reliability, the test is administered twice at two different points in time. It is used to assess the consistency of a test across different times. This type of reliability assumes that there will be no change in the quality or construct being measured. Test-retest reliability is best used for things that are stable over time, such as intelligence. Generally, reliability will be higher when little time has passed between tests. The test-retest method is a relatively easy and straightforward approach to establish reliability. It is used for questionnaires, observation checklists and observation rating scales. It can be statistically calculated by using Karl Pearson's correlation coefficient formula.
- ***Internal consistency:*** Internal consistency is also called *homogeneity*. It ensures that all the subparts of a research instrument are measuring the same characteristics. An evaluation tool can only be considered internally consistent if all the subparts of the tool are measuring the same characteristics. One of the most primitive approaches of assessing the internal consistency is the split half technique. However, to overcome its drawback as an estimation tool of different correlation coefficient results with different combination of split half (odd–even or first half–second half, etc.). This method is replaced by formulas that compensate this deficiency such as Cronbach's alpha and Kunder–Richardson formula-20.
- ***Equivalence:*** This aspect of reliability is estimated when an evaluator is testing the reliability of a tool, which is used by two different observers to observe a single task performed by the learner independently or two presumably parallel instruments are administered to the individual at about the same time. For example, a rating scale is developed to assess wound dressing skills among nursing students. This rating scale may be administered to observe the clinical skills of nursing students for wound dressing by two different observers simultaneously but independently. This is also known as *interrater reliability* or *interobserver reliability*, which is estimated by the administration of tools to observe single events simultaneously and independently by two or more trained observers.

BARRIERS TO EVALUATION

Evaluation is an integral part of nursing education and it is entirely different from other education programmes. There are various barriers that interfere with the accuracy of evaluation in nursing educational assessments which are described below:

- **Personal barriers:** These are the obstacles to evaluation which are associated with the teacher and student dimensions.
  - *Teacher related barriers:* Lack of academic and clinical skills, personal biases, poor communication skills, personality traits, heavy work load and time constraints, poor planning of educational assessment, resistance to learn novel methods of evaluation, lack of collaboration with professionals in the clinical areas.
  - *Student related barriers:* Lack of motivation, lack of achievement and inherent skills, lack of interest according to subjects and teachers, etc.
- **Organizational barriers:** These are the obstacles to evaluation which are associated with the institutional dimensions such as lack of cooperation and support, insufficient resources, large student intake and mismatch between teacher and student ratio, lack of clinical and academic facilities, limited patients in the clinical areas and negative attitude towards profession.

Curriculum-related barriers: These are the obstacles to evaluation which are associated with the nursing curriculum dimensions, such as problems and biases related to evaluation methods (halo effect, horn effect, central tendency errors, generosity errors, etc.). Inappropriate evaluation system such as inconsistency, uncertainty in the evaluation criteria, distrust and subjective ranking methods, ambiguous internal and external consensus in evaluation methods, unsystematic evaluation, etc., may be key barriers.

GUIDELINES TO DEVELOP ASSESSMENT

A right assessment tool to measure right skills is essential. However, development of a good assessment is a tedious work and it has some of the prerequisites such as (1) prior understanding about purpose of assessment and (2) establishing a link between expected learning objectives, teaching methods and assessment. Further, assessment development requires precise language, a good exercise of revision and effectively aligned with learning objectives and instructional methods.

Development of assessment involves planning for assessment, design of assessment and quick check on quality and accuracy of assessment. It is important to ensure that assessment is valid, reliable, flexible and fair. The general principles to develop an assessment are that the assessment must:

- Measure all instructional objectives.
- Cover all the learning domains.
- Use appropriate test items.
- Make test valid and reliable.
- Use test to improve learning

The steps of developing assessment are illustrated in Fig. 7.3.

GUIDELINES FOR DEVELOPMENT OF GOOD ASSESSMENT

Five important guidelines for development of a good assessment includes:

i) ***Understanding about purpose and functions of assessment:*** It is essential to understand the clear purpose and functions of assessment for the development of a good assessment. An assessment has the 'triple function' of assessment (Fig. 7.4), that is assessing what learner knows before (diagnostic assessment), during (formative assessment and after the formal learning exercises (summative assessment).

ii) ***Know the required levels of assessment based-on taxonomy of learning objectives:*** Assessment must be intended to measure predetermined learning objectives or outcomes covering all the domains of learning (cognitive, affective and psychomotor) and levels of learning objectives. For example, as per Bloom's taxonomy of learning objectives, the cognitive domain has six levels from lower to height order of thinking skills, such as remembering → understanding → applying → analysing → evaluating → and creating.

iii) ***Using right tools and techniques to assess right set of knowledge, skills and attitude:*** The various tools and techniques are available for the assessment, but it is important to choose the right to tool or technique to assess particular set of domain and levels of learning. The different methods of assessment with the details about what can assessed using the particular method and what are their advantages and disadvantages have been given in Box 7.3.

iv) Choose balanced combination of open and closed ended methods of assessment: The closed ended questions or select response type of questions such as MCQs, true/false, matching, binary and checklist type questions are only good to assess recall and recognition of facts but not good for assessment of deeper understanding and reasoning as well as psychometric skills. On the other hand, open-ended or construct response type questions, such as essay, short-answer, cloze/fill-in-the-blank and sentence completion type questions help to assess the higher-order of thinking, deductive and inductive reasoning, creative thinking and organization skills. Therefore, it is

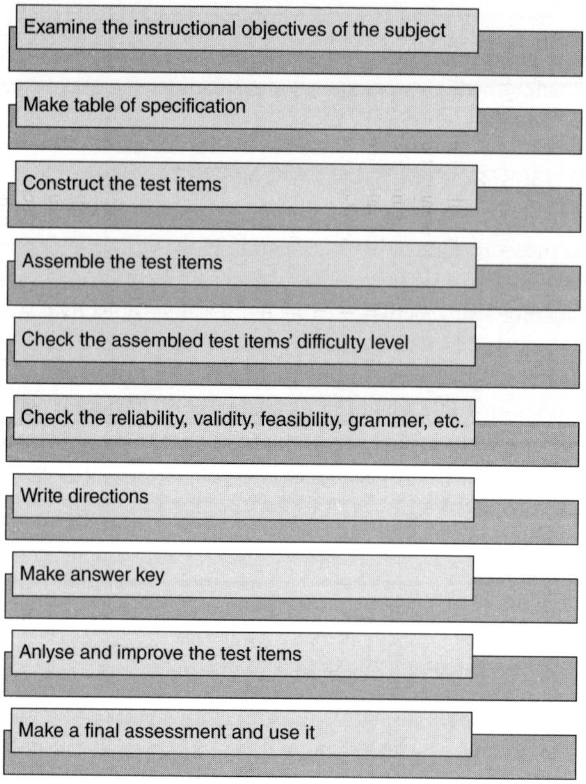

Figure 7.3

The steps of developing assessment.

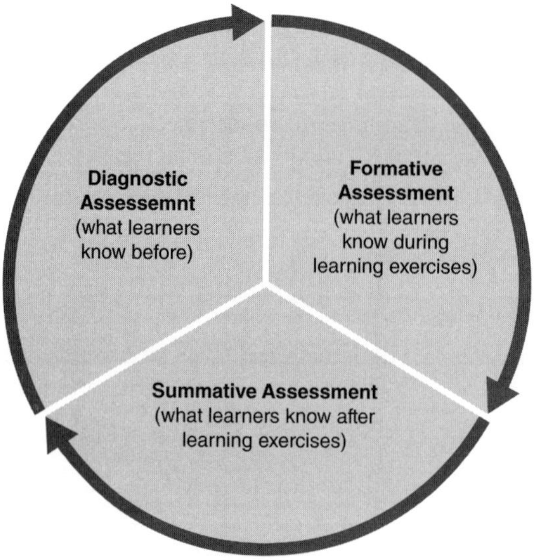

Figure 7.4

The triple function of assessment.

BOX 7.3 COMMON TYPES OF ASSESSMENTS AND THEIR ADVANTAGES AND DISADVANTAGES

Assessment Method	What Can Be Assessed	Advantages	Disadvantages
Multiple-choice questions (MCQs)	- Facts - Understanding of ideas - Application of principles	- Fast and reliable evaluation - Assesses large number topics broadly - Possible to declare of exam results quickly	- Not possible to assess procedural or conceptual knowledge - It is difficult to prepare good quality MCQs - Difficult to assess higher level of thinking, though not impossible - Not possible to assess skills of inductive reasoning, creativity and organization
Essays	- Understanding of ideas - Ability to think critically - Ability to formulate an argument, support it with ideas and evidences - Formulate a conclusion based on ideas and evidences	- Assesses higher-order thinking - Assesses procedural or conceptual knowledge - Allows students to express their knowledge in a less constrained, more open format than a closed test (such as MCQs, short answer and fill in the blank)	- Needs evaluation scoring rubrics - More difficult to ensure validity of scoring - It takes too long time to evaluate and grade each question - Potential subjectivity, lack of validity and reliability without well-designed rubric for evaluation, students with poor writing skills remain in disadvantage in spite of knowing the subject well.
Project	- Reveals depth of knowledge - Assesses skills of creativity and organization of content - Assesses skills of writing and documentation	- Mainly assesses procedural and conceptual knowledge – what students can do and metaunderstanding of ideas - Assesses higher-order thinking	- Time consuming to evaluate - Needs well-designed scoring rubric - Potential subjectivity, lack of validity and reliability without well-designed rubric for evaluation
Portfolio	- Reveals depth of knowledge - Assesses skills of creativity and organization of content - Assesses skills of writing and documentation - Multiple levels of assessment (from knowledge of facts to analysis and evaluation of information to self-reflection	- Encourages learners to display knowledge and understanding in multiple formats - Mainly assesses procedural and conceptual knowledge – what students can do and metaunderstanding of ideas - Assesses higher-order thinking	- Time consuming to evaluate - Needs well-designed scoring rubric - Potential subjectivity, lack of validity and reliability without well-designed rubric for evaluation

Source: Adapted from Commonwealth of Learning & Asian Development Bank, 2008.

important to have a good combination and balance of selected assessment methods to ensure holistic 360-degree assessment of the student.

v) Right set of questions for the assessment: It is important to develop the right set of questions for the development of the most effective assessment tool. Some of the key guidelines related to develop the right set of questions have been presented below:

- Provide instructions that are brief and clear, such as:
  - How to provide answer, diagram required, number of question attempted.
  - The scoring system of various items.
  - If an answer sheet is provided, instructions on how to use it.
- Begin with the easiest question in each division to gain confidence.
- Making assessments cumulative allows learners to integrate the information.
- Calculate how much students usually will require to complete a test using the following suggestions:
  - Each true/false item has a time limit of 30 seconds.
  - Each multiple-choice item has a time limit of 60 seconds.
  - Each short answer item has a time limit of 120 seconds.
  - Each essay question should take 10–15 minutes to complete.
  - Allow students should take 5–10 minutes to review their work.
- Choose questions that at least 50%–70% of students can answer properly or that are of average complexity.
- Longer exams are regarded more reliable than shorter exams.
- Be careful that many test banks and/or review books with question items rarely measure higher learning levels.
- Specific guidelines to develop good MCQs:
  - Ensure that the stem of the question is precise, unambiguous and clear to understand.
  - The stem should provide additional information to support higher-level questions (e.g. an emphasis on analysis, synthesis or assessment), but it should remain succinct.
  - Keep the answers succinct, with no unnecessary information. The student should never be able to determine the correct response just by looking at it.
  - Do not provide 'All of the above' or 'None of the above'. These alternatives incentivize students who do not know the answers.
  - Ensure that the length, style and content of all answers – both the right and wrong answers – are consistent. Do not allow the learners to get the correct answer simply because it differs from the incorrect ones.
  - Select reasonable distractors by providing additional information.
  - Observe the language chosen. Avoid errors in syntax, spelling and mechanics that may make it difficult for students to comprehend the responses.
  - Do not use categorical words – always, never. There is no such thing as 'always', 'never', or any other term. This is a red flag.
  - Do not use double negatives.
  - Common student misconceptions should be dispelled by distractions. It is essential to know how to distinguish between high, medium and low-level performers. Each question should be considered an independent entity. Do not relate or connect questions.

ASSESSMENT OF KNOWLEDGE

Cognitive domain of learning or knowledge is fundament to any field of learning including nursing. Assessment of knowledge is an inseparable part of evaluation process, which can be carried out by various methods and techniques, which include select response type of questions and construct response type of questions. The commonly used select response type of questions includes MCQs, true/false, matching and binary type questions. On the other hand, common routine in practice construct response type of questions are essay, short-answer, cloze/fill-in-the-blank and sentence completion type of questions.

The most commonly used methods and techniques for assessment of knowledge such as essay type of question, SAQs and MCQs have been presented in detail in this chapter.

ESSAY TYPE QUESTIONS

Educators choose essay questions over other forms of assessment because essay items challenge students to create a response rather than to simply select a response. Some educators use them because essays have the potential to reveal students' abilities to reason, create, analyse, synthesize and evaluate. In short, essay items are used for the advantages they offer. Despite the advantages associated with essay questions, there are numerous disadvantages also. However, essay type questions are the most frequently used method of evaluation in most Indian universities, colleges and schools.

> *Essay questions are defined as a test item which requires a response composed by the examinee, usually in the form of one or more sentences, of a nature that no single response or pattern of responses can be listed as correct, and the accuracy and quality of which can be judged subjectively only by one skilled or informed in the subject.*
>
> **—John M. Stalnaker**

> *An essay type test presents one or more questions or other tasks that require extended written responses from the persons being tested.*
>
> **—Robert L.E. and David A.F.**

> *Essay type questions are a test containing questions requiring the students to respond in writing. It emphasizes recall rather than recognition of the correct alternative.*
>
> **—Gilert Sax**

Based on Stalnaker's definition, an essay question should meet the following criteria:

- They should require examinees to *compose* rather than select their response.
- They should elicit student responses that must consist of many interlined sentences.
- They should allow different or original responses or a pattern of responses.
- They should require subjective judgement by a competent specialist to judge the accuracy and quality of responses.
- They should provide students with an indication of the types of thinking and content to use in responding to the essay question.

Essay questions are different from these other constructed response items because they require more systematic and in-depth thinking. An effective essay question will align with each of the four criteria given in Stalnaker's definition and provide students with an indication of the types of thinking and content to use in responding to the essay type questions.

I. FEATURES OF ESSAY TYPE QUESTIONS

- Questions are used both as formative and summative assessments.
- They require a great deal of thought and planning.

- Students prepare their own answers.
- They evaluate knowledge areas alone.
- Student's handwriting, spelling, neatness, organization and way of expressing ideas may be considered while scoring the items.
- No single answer can be considered thorough or correct.
- The examinee is permitted freedom of response.
- Answers vary in their degree of equality or corrections.

II. PURPOSES OF ESSAY TYPE QUESTIONS

Essay type questions are subjected to criticism by educationists but are still used in university exams across the globe. One might wonder if there are so many loopholes, why they are consistently being used for evaluation in nursing. This is because essay type questions serve distinct purposes which cannot be accomplished by any other type of questions. These purposes are discussed below:

- ***Students get a chance to express own views:*** It provides students with an opportunity to express their views on particular phenomena.
- ***To assess factual recall of knowledge:*** Sometimes teachers might be interested in knowing how well students can recall the facts they have learned. This purpose can be fulfilled by having essay type questions in the test paper.
- ***Analysis and explanation of relationships:*** When the teacher is interested in knowing how well the students can explain the relationship between two or more concepts, essay type questions are used because no other form of question can serve this purpose.
- ***Assessment of non-content-related attributes of students:*** Creativity, writing style, organization, neatness and cleanliness are some other attributes that can be more appropriately assessed through essay type of questions.

III. PRINCIPLES FOR CONSTRUCTION OF ESSAY TYPE QUESTIONS

The following guidelines must be followed for the construction of essay type questions:

- The learning objective supposed to be evaluated by an essay type question should be clearly defined in simple words.
- If a learning objective can be evaluated by any other type of question, the use of essay type question should be avoided.
- It is always better to use several short essay type questions instead of a long one.
- The question and the task in a problem situation should be clearly defined by ensuring the following:
  - Clearly define the question so that students understand what to write.
  - Delimit the scope of the question so that students do not feel that they need to write infinite number of pages.
  - Clearly develop the problem or problem situation so that students can be focused.
- The approximate time and word limit for each essay type question should be specified.
- The distribution of marks for different segments of a particular question and organization, neatness and expressive language should be explained.
- The use of complex and ambiguous words should be avoided.
- Questions that are too broad in scope and allow for blunders should be avoided.
- Words like differentiate and compare should be used at the beginning of the question to restrict the scope of the question.

- Simple unambiguous language well understood by all students should be used.
- A reasonable question should be presented to students, so that they do not feel that it is outside their ability and scope to answer.
- Questions can be written in declarative as well as interrogative statements.
- The relative point value and the approximate time limit should be specified in clear directions.
- The criteria for grading should be stated so that students know what to include in the answer.
- The use of optional questions which may confuse the students and make evaluation difficult should be avoided.
- The essay question should be improved through preview and review.

Preview: Before administration the evaluator must

- Predict student responses.
- Write a model answer.
- Ask a knowledgeable colleague to critically review the essay question, the model answer and the intended learning outcome for alignment.

Review: After the administration of essay type questions, the evaluator must

- Review student responses to the essay question.

ADVANTAGES OF ESSAY TYPE QUESTIONS

- Assess higher-order or critical-thinking skills in learners.
- Evaluate student thinking and reasoning.
- Provide an opportunity to assess the problem-solving and decision-making abilities in learners.
- Help evaluate thinking, recall, analysis and synthesis of facts.
- Provide an opportunity for creative expression and organization of facts.
- Are relatively easy to construct but require a good knowledge of essay type question contraction among evaluators.
- Provide very limited scope of guessing answers.

DISADVANTAGES OF ESSAY TYPE QUESTIONS

- These questions lead to vague answers if the wording of questions is ambiguous and difficult to understand.
- They assess a limited sample of the range of content from the entire curriculum.
- It is difficult and time consuming to grade the answers.
- Evaluation is subjective; different teachers may mark the same answer differently.
- There is a scope of a lot of subjective biasness.
- These questions provide practice in poor or unpolished writing.
- They have a limited range of application.

SHORT ANSWER QUESTIONS

SAQs are very similar to objective items as a clearly defined answer is required in both. However, in SAQs, the answer has to be generated and supplied by the learner rather than chosen from a number of options provided. SAQs are sometimes called *objective questions* because they can be marked with a very high degree of reliability if suitably designed. Strictly speaking, however, they are not truly objective as the marker may sometimes have to exercise a certain amount of subjective judgement in deciding whether an answer is satisfactory. The evaluator may, for example, have to decide whether a wrongly spelt word, a partly correct answer or a perfectly good answer that the question setter did not anticipate is acceptable, and may also have to decide whether an explanation or description is satisfactory. Obviously, the subjective judgement involved tends to increase with the length and complexity of the required answer, while the degree of 'objectivity' shows a corresponding fall.

I. PURPOSES OF SAQs

- Useful to assess the recall ability of students (lower cognitive domain).
- Used to assess students in a classroom while a lecture is in progress.
- Useful in formative assessment.
- May be used in summative evaluation to supplement other forms of questions.

II. PRINCIPLES FOR CONSTRUCTION OF SAQs

The following guidelines must be followed for the construction of essay type questions:

- The learning objective which is supposed to be evaluated by the short answer type question should be clearly defined in simple words.
- The overall purpose and content of the item should be determined.
- SAQs should be written using the following guidelines:
  - The item should be expressed in such a way that only a single, brief answer is possible.
  - The item should be expressed in a clear, simple language, making it as concise as possible while avoiding looseness or ambiguity.
  - The item should be expressed in a positive form wherever possible as it has been found that positively phrased test items tend to measure more important learning outcomes than negatively phrased items.
  - One should try to avoid providing clues to the required answer unwittingly.
  - Where a numerical answer has to be supplied, the degree of precision expected and (if appropriate) the units to express it should be indicated. For example, how many milligrams of Lasix a nurse will administer to a patient with renal failure in a day?
  - Precise, simple and unambiguous language should be used.
  - Action-oriented verbs should be used.
  - Each question should deal with important content area of a unit.
  - Long complex sentences should be avoided and the questions should be kept as simple as possible.
  - Phrases like 'write briefly on, short notes on' should be avoided.
  - Space should be provided for answers below each question as per the requirement of the question being asked.
  - Specific problems for questions that will have distinct specific answers should be chosen.
  - Fill-in-the-blank type questions should use statements that omit only one or two key words (answer) at the end of sentence.
- While finalizing the layout of questions, it must be ensured that:
  - The item is presented in such a way that the learners are in no doubt as to what they are expected to do and how they are required to indicate their response.
  - The wattage for each question and criteria for marking is mentioned clearly.
- Items to be evaluated by the subject experts panel: An expert must ensure the availability of the following information before finalizing the evaluation of each short answer item:

- Is the item relevant to the course/module/syllabus to which it relates?
- Is the item style appropriate to the topic being covered and the specific educational skills or outcomes being assessed?
- Does the item present the learners with a clearly defined task?
- Is the item logically and structurally sound?
- Is the item stated in a simple and clear language?
- Is the item free from extraneous clues?
- Is the stated difficulty of the item likely to prove accurate?
- Is this stated difficulty appropriate?

III. TYPES OF SAQs

FILL-IN-THE-BLANK TYPE

Example: **Q.1:** A patient is diagnosed with brain tumour. The nurse's assessment reveals that the patient has difficulty in interpreting visual stimuli. Based on these findings, the nurse suspects injury in the....................lobe of the brain.
Answer: Occipital

STATEMENT COMPLETION

Example: **Q.1:** A 45-year-old patient is admitted with excruciating paroxysmal facial pain. He reports that the episodes occur most often after feeling cold draft and drinking cold beverages. Based on these findings, the nurse determines that the patient is most likely suffering from....................................
Answer: Trigeminal neuralgia

LABELLING A DIAGRAM

Example: **Q.1:** An elderly patient fell and fractured the neck of his femur. Identify the area where the fracture occurred.

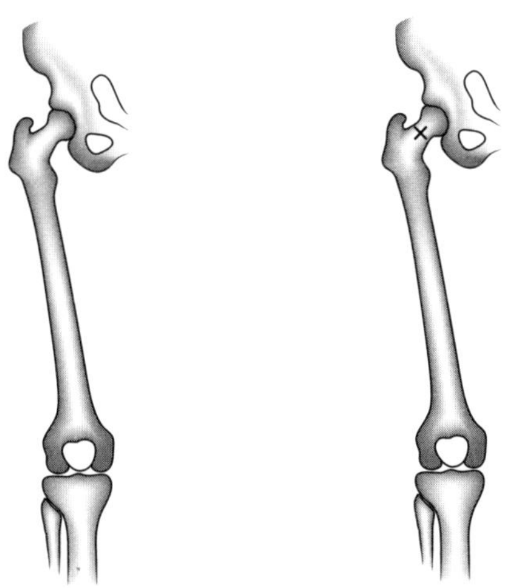

SHORT ANSWER IN 5–10 WORDS

Example: **Q.1:** Mention the five commonly occurring signs and symptoms of hypothyroidism.

1. ______________________ **4.** ______________________
2. ______________________ **5.** ______________________
3. ______________________

ADVANTAGES OF SAQs

- Provide the opportunity to cover a much wider content of the syllabus to evaluate the students.
- Can be administered to a large group of students for a short formative assessment.
- Useful to assess the recall of information without any assistance or cues or alternatives.
- Provide less scope for guesswork.
- Require less stationary as compared to essay type questions.
- Less scope of subjectivity as compared to essay type questions when judging answers.
- Easy to administer and mark the tests; ensure more objective scoring.

DISADVANTAGES OF SAQs

- They are not particularly well suited for testing some types of higher cognitive and noncognitive outcomes, especially if these are of a multifaceted or complex nature, or involve the assessment of 'life skills'.
- They can lead to cheating within a group of students if the examination hall is not spacious enough.
- They can lead to difficulties in scoring if not worded carefully.
- They provide no scope to assess the writing ability, expression, organization of answer, etc.

MULTIPLE-CHOICE QUESTIONS

MCQs are the form of assessment where respondents are asked to select the best possible answer (or answers) out of choices from a list. Although E.L. Thorndike developed an early multiple-choice test, Frederick J. Kelly was the first to use such items as part of a large-scale assessment. MCQs are a special type of questions that are widely used in various entrance exams where thousands of students attempt the exams. These are standardized tests with high reliability and validity. A typical MCQ begins with a *stem* which may be an incomplete statement, picture or a graph, which is followed by 4–5 *alternatives* or choices. All the wrong answers or alternatives are known as *distractors.* The correct answer/answers are known as the key (Fig. 7.5). Clear instructions are provided at the beginning of the questionnaire about the selection of the answer (e.g. choose one response that is correct; choose all responses that are correct) or instructions are provided within the questionnaire whenever necessary. Scoring in MCQs is easier as compared to essay type and short answer type questions but the other side of the coin is that it is equally difficult to construct good quality MCQs and there is a high chance of cheating and guesswork practices.

I. STRUCTURE AND CHARACTERISTICS OF MCQs

- MCQs consist of a stem and a set of options. The *stem* is the beginning part of the item that presents the item as a problem to be solved, a question asked to the respondent or an incomplete statement to be completed and any other relevant information.

Q.1: Which artery is most commonly used to assess the pulse rate in a two-year-old child? } **Question Stem**

a) Radial artery
b) Femoral artery } Distracters
c) Pedal artery
d) Apical artery } Answer

(a–d: Alternatives)

Figure 7.5

Basic structure of multiple-choice questions.

- The stem follows by 4–5 options. The options are possible answers that the examiner can choose from with the correct answer called the *key* and the incorrect answers called *distractors.* Generally, only one answer can be keyed as correct. However, when more than one answer is keyed as correct, then these questions are named as *multiple-response questions* (Box 7.4).
- Usually, a correct answer earns a set number of points towards the total marks and an incorrect answer earns nothing. However, tests may also award a partial credit for unanswered questions or penalize students for incorrect answers to discourage guessing.
- Markings of the answers made by the teacher are objective as there is no scope of subjectivity.
- Answers can be checked by computers or by any other person supplied with the answer key.

II. GUIDELINES TO CONSTRUCT GOOD MCQs

The following basic rules must be observed for writing good MCQs:

A. GENERAL TIPS

- Design each item to measure an important learning objective or learning outcome.
- Before writing a question, think about what it is that you want to test. Lecture notes, textbook readings, assigned problems and other course materials can be an inspiration to write items.

BOX 7.4 EXAMPLES OF MULTIPLE-CHOICE AND MULTIPLE-RESPONSE QUESTIONS

Multiple-Choice Question

Q: A patient is admitted to the hospital with a diagnosis of chronic bronchitis. He has a 10-year history of emphysema. The nurse should place him on which of the following positions?

A. Side-lying
B. Supine
C. High-Fowler's
D. Semi-Fowler's

Answer: C

Multiple-Response Question

Q: The nurse is assessing a 2-year-old patient diagnosed with bacterial meningitis. Which of the following signs and symptoms of meningeal irritation is the nurse likely to observe?

Select all that apply:

A. Generalized seizures
B. Nuchal rigidity
C. Positive Brudzinski's sign
D. Positive Kernig's sign
E. Babinski reflex
F. Photophobia

Answer: B, C, D, F

- Control the difficulty of the item either by varying the problem in the stem or by changing the alternatives.
- Make certain that each item is independent of the other items in the test.
- Make sure that each item is grammatically accurate to avoid ambiguity in understanding.
- Keep the question stem and alternatives as short as possible. Use few words. Avoid repeating words from the question stem in the alternatives.
- Make sure to have a sufficient number of easy and more challenging questions so that the poor, fair, good and excellent students are effectively judged and separated.
- Try to make the first few MCQs relatively quick and easy, to help calm students down so they can focus on the more challenging questions to come.
- Avoid the temptation to test many things in one question. If possible, try to write more than one MCQ rather than test multiple concepts in one question.
- Ask more than one question when a fair amount of information must be provided as it takes time for students to carefully read and understand the information you provide in a test. For example, you could give them a table of results, a graph or a scenario and then ask two or three different MCQs about it.
- Do not try to write the entire test in one day; it takes time, creativity and thought to write good MCQs.
    - After constructing the MCQ test, a try-out may be planned on nearly similar subjects and an item analysis must be carried out before preparation of a final draft of the test.

B. CONSTRUCTION OF THE STEM

- Present a single, clearly formulated problem in the stem of the item/question.
- Phrase the question stem as clearly and concisely as possible, avoiding complex language.
- State the stem of the item in a positive form, wherever possible.
- Emphasize negative wording whenever it is used in the stem of an item; for example, which of the following is **NOT** an appropriate method of back massage?
- Avoid verbal clues, which might enable students to select the correct answer or to eliminate an incorrect alternative. Similarity of wording in both the stem and the correct answer is one of the more obvious clues.

C. CONSTRUCTION OF ALTERNATIVES

- Make certain that the intended answer is correct or clearly the best.
- Make all alternatives grammatically consistent with the stem of the item and parallel in form.
- Avoid the use of the alternative ‘all of the above’ and use ‘none of the above’ with great caution.
- Do not include alternatives such as ‘both (A) and (D)’ or ‘all but (C)’, as these complicate the structure of the question and tend to confuse students and/or slow them down.
- Vary the position of the correct answer in a random manner.
- Vary the relative length of the correct answer to eliminate length as a clue.
- There is no set rule about the number of options you should include in MCQs. The greater the number of options, the smaller the mathematical chance of correct guesswork. Therefore, generally 4–5 alternatives are used.
- Make the distracters plausible and attractive to the uninformed, by:
    - Using common misconceptions or common errors of students as distracters.
    - Using good sounding words (e.g. accurate, important, etc.) in the distracters, as well as in the correct answers.

- Making the distracters similar to the correct answer in both length and complexity of wording.
- Stating the alternatives in the language of the student.
- Construct the destructors as close as possible to the correct answer to make most effective destructors.

D. ADVANTAGES OF MCQs

- Easy to use and administer.
- Can cover a large content area of syllabus.
- Easy to check answers.
- High reliability and validity.
- No scope of subjective biasness.
- Allow more adequate sampling of content.
- Tend to more effectively structure the problem to be addressed.
- Questions can be used more efficiently and reliably than just supplying items.
- Different response alternatives can provide diagnostic feedback about the planned questions (item analysis is possible).
- Questions can be constructed to address various levels of cognitive complexities.

E. DISADVANTAGES OF MCQs

- Not useful to test the highest level of cognitive domain.
- Difficult to construct good MCQs.
- Provide an opportunity to guess the answer if the question is not properly constructed.
- More suitable format for cheating in students if the invigilator is not highly keen in observing students.
- A time-consuming process to construct good questions.
- Can lead the instructor to favour simple recall of facts.
- High degree of dependence on student's readings and instructor's writing ability.
- Measuring synthesis and evaluation can be difficult.
- Inappropriate for measuring the outcomes that require skilled performance.

ITEM ANALYSIS

It is important that a newly constructed MCQ test must be valid and reliable, which depends on characteristics of each question item included in the test. The value and suitability of each constructed question item are evaluated through a specific method named as *'item analysis'* so that eventually the final draft of test is functional and useful. The item analysis is one of the important phases of test construction (see Box 7.5).

Item analysis is referred to as a specific method of systemically examining the effectiveness of each item created for the test that includes three main characteristics, which are evaluating the item difficulty, discrimination index and effectiveness of destructors.

PURPOSES OF ITEM ANALYSIS

The item analysis serves the following main purposes:

- Item analysis provides information about (1) difficulty level of each item in test, (2) discriminating power of each item in test and (3) effectiveness of each destructor used in an item.

BOX 7.5 PHASES OF AN MCQ TEST CONSTRUCTION

1. Preparing a draft of items.
2. Tryout of test in similar setting.
3. Item analysis
4. Final draft of test

- It is helpful in construction of a functional, useful and a more effective test.
- It helps in accepting the good items and revises or rejects the poor items to construct the most suitable test for the target group.

COMPONENTS OF ITEM ANALYSIS

The main characteristics of the item analysis are the item difficulty, discrimination index and effectiveness of destructors.

(a) ***Item difficulty:*** It is a proportion of students who are with the correct answer for a particular test item.

$$\text{Item Difficulty} = \frac{\text{No. of students with correct answer}}{\text{Total No. of students}}$$

For example, MCQ No. 03 is answered correctly by 45 students out of 80 students. The item difficulty (p-value) for this MCQ item will be 45/80 = 0.56. The ideal range of item difficulty is 0.26–0.75; the items with p-value in this range should be considered with appropriate difficulty. However, an item with p-value above the 0.76 is considered very easy and a p-value below 0.25 is considered very difficult. Therefore, those items need to be revised or discarded.

(b) ***Discrimination index:*** It is a difference between the proportion of the upper group who are with the correct answer and the proportion of the lower group who are with the correct answer.

Discrimination Index = DU – DL

$$\text{DU} = \frac{\text{No. of students in the upper 25\% with correct answer}}{\text{Total no. of students in upper 25\%}}$$

$$\text{DL} = \frac{\text{No. of students in the lower 25\% with correct answer}}{\text{Total no. of students in lower 25\%}}$$

For example, in a question item, 15 students are with correct answer in upper 25% students (20 students) and the same question item is answered correctly by 5 students among lower 25% students (20 students). In this case, DU = 15/20 = 0.75 and DL = 5/20 = 0.25. Thus, the discrimination index will be 0.75 – 0.25 = 0.50. The discrimination index ranges between –1.0 and 1.0. The discrimination index score between –1.0 and –0.50 can discriminate but the item is questionable and this must be discarded. Furthermore, the discrimination index score between –0.55 and 0.45 is considered as nondiscriminatory and thus it must be revised, while score of discrimination index between 0.45 and 1.0 is considered as discriminating score for the particular item and this item must be included in the test.

(c) ***Effectiveness of destructors:*** It is very important in the MCQ test that the destructors created are very effective. The effectiveness of a particular destructor can be evaluated by the total number of students who have chosen a destructor in a particular item in a tryout test. A destructor chosen by less than 5% student is considered as inappropriate and must be revised.

ASSESSMENT OF SKILLS

Clinical evaluation of nursing students has higher importance because nursing is a skill-oriented discipline. Assessment of clinical skills and competencies is a tedious work and require multiple approaches to ensure that finally clinical practice-ready nurse graduates enter the health industry, who are capable to provide safe and quality care.

George Miller proposed a theoretical model to assess clinical skills or competence in 1990. Miller claimed that traditional assessment methods were too focused on testing students' knowledge and not on real-life situations. Miller's model, also known as the Miller pyramid, helped to shift away the traditional theoretical knowledge-based assessments towards clinical performance-based examinations.

Miller's pyramid of assessment offers a framework for assessing clinical competence. Clinical teachers can use it to match learning outcomes (clinical competencies), with expectations of what the learner should do at each level.

Miller's pyramid model splits clinical competence development into four hierarchical processes. Knowledge (knows) is at the bottom of the pyramid, followed by competence (knows how), performance (shows how) and action (does).

Knowledge is represented by the bottom or first two levels. The first level of knowledge, the 'Knows', refers to principles, concepts and facts that students are able to recall and explain. Written exams and traditional MCQs test this knowledge. The second level of 'Knows how' refers to the ability of the students to apply these principles, concepts and facts to solve problems. This level is called 'application of knowledge'. It is assessed through essays, clinical problem-solving exercises and extended MCQs. The third level, 'Shows', requires students to perform/demonstrate a procedure in a simulation setting. The third tier of this pyramid is 'clinical skills competency'. It is evaluated through standardized patient exercises and simulations, as well as clinical exams. The final tier is the 'Does' level. This refers generally to what learners do in real life, usually in the context of medical education. The top of the pyramid is 'clinical performance'. This can be evaluated through direct observation in real clinical settings (Fig. 7.6).

Each method has its strengths and weaknesses. When deciding which method to use, it is important to remember the ABCs.

- Assess at the appropriate level in Miller's pyramid and Bloom's taxonomy.
- Be aware of the strengths of each method as well as the factors that may affect validity in the setting you are working in.
- Consider how different methods can be combined in an overall assessment programme to harness the strengths and mitigate their individual weaknesses.

This section of chapter presented commonly used methods and techniques of clinical assessment, that is observation checklist, rating scales, violates assessment, written assignments, oral examination, simulation-based assessment, OSCE, self-evaluation, clinical portfolio and clinical logs.

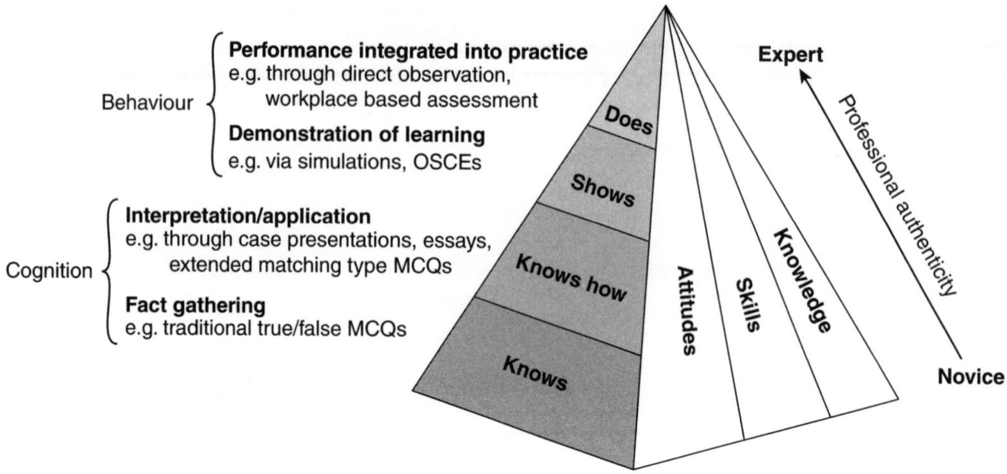

Figure 7.6

Miller's prism or pyramid of clinical competencies. *Source: Based on work by Miller GE. The Assessment of Clinical Skills/Competence/Performance; Academic Medicine, 1990, 65(9), 63–67. Adapted by Drs. R. Mehay & R. Burns, UK (Jan 2009).*

OBSERVATION CHECKLIST

An observation checklist is the most commonly used instrument for performance evaluation. A checklist enables the observer to note only whether a trait is present or not. It consists of a listing of steps, activities or behaviours the observer records when an incident occurs. The observer has to judge whether a certain behaviour has taken place.

Observation checklist is simply a list of the performer's behaviours associated with particular nursing interventions within a space for the assessor to check or tick off whether or not that particular behaviour occurred (Box 7.6).

DEFINITIONS OF CHECKLIST

A checklist is a simple instrument consisting prepared list of expected items of performance or attributes, which are checked by an evaluator for their presence or absence.

Checklists are constructed by breaking a performance and the quality of a product, which specifies the presence or absence of an attribute or trait which is then 'checked' by the rater/observer.

CHARACTERISTICS OF A CHECKLIST

- Observe one respondent at one time.
- Clearly specifies the characteristics of the behaviour to be observed.
- Use only carefully prepared checklists to avoid more complex traits.
- The observer should be trained how to observe, what to observe and how to record the observed behaviour.
- Use checklists only when you are interested in calculating a particular characteristic.

BOX 7.6 CHECKLIST FOR EVALUATION OF STUDENT'S PERFORMANCE DURING INTRADERMAL INJECTION

Steps	Place for (√) Tick Mark		
	Yes	No	Remarks
1. Wash hands			
2. Collect all articles			
3. Check the medication order with medication card			
4. Load the syringe with the required amount of medicine			
5. Identify the patient by name and other details			
6. Explain the procedure to the patient			
7. Select the site and clean the area with a sprit swab			
8. Stretch the patient's skin tightly with the thumb and finger			
9. Insert the needle at 5–15 degree angle, advance about 3 mm through the epidermis layer			
10. Inject contents watching for a bleb			
11. Do not massage the area			
12. Mark with a pen around the wheel and note the date, time, sight and medication			
13. Wash hands and replace the articles			

**Each step carries one mark* *Total marks obtained:* ....

Signature of examiner: .... Date: ....

CONSTRUCTION OF A CHECKLIST

While constructing or preparing checklists, the following points should be kept in mind:

- Express each item in a clear and simple language.
- An intensive survey of the literature should be made to determine the type of checklist to be used in a particular assessment/evaluation.
- The list of items in the checklist may be continuous or divided into groups of related items.
- These lists of the items are formulated on the basis of the judgement of experts and each item is evaluated with respect to the number of favourable and unfavourable responses.
- Avoid negative statements whenever possible.
- Avoid lifting statements verbatim from the text.
- Ensure that each item has a clear response: *yes* or *no*, or *true* or *false*.
- Review the items independently.
- Checklists must have the quality of completeness and comprehensiveness.

A. ADVANTAGES OF CHECKLISTS

- Checklists allow interindividual comparisons.
- They provide a simple method to record observations.
- They are adaptable to subject matter areas.
- Checklists are useful in evaluating learning activities expected to be performed.
- They are helpful in evaluating procedure work.
- Properly prepared checklists allow the observer to constrain the direct attention.

- Checklists have objectivity to evaluate characteristics.
- Useful for evaluating the processes that can be subdivided into a series of actions.
- Decreases the chances of errors in observation.

B. DISADVANTAGES OF CHECKLISTS

- Checklists do not indicate quality of performance so the usefulness of checklists is limited.
- Only a limited component of overall clinical performance can be evaluated.
- Only the presence or absence of an attribute, behaviour or performance parameter may be assessed. However, the degree of accuracy of performance can be assessed.
- It has limited use in qualitative observations.
- Checklists are not easy to prepare.

RATING SCALE

Rating is the term used to express opinion or judgement regarding some performance of a person, object, situation and character. The rating scale involves qualitative description of a limited number of aspects of a thing or traits of a person. When we use rating scales, we judge an object in absolute terms against some specified criteria, that is we judge properties of objects without reference to other similar objects.

I. DEFINITIONS OF A RATING SCALE

Rating scale refers to a scale with a set of opinion, which describes varying degree of the dimensions of an attitude or a phenomenon being observed.

Rating scale is a device by which judgements may be qualified or a opinion concerning a trait can be systematized.

—Suresh K. Sharma

A rating scale is a tool in which one person simply checks off another person's level of performance. It could be a 3-point (Fig. 7.7), 5-point (Fig. 7.8) or 7-point rating scale. Rating scales measure how much or how well something happened, where generally quantitative and qualitative terms are used

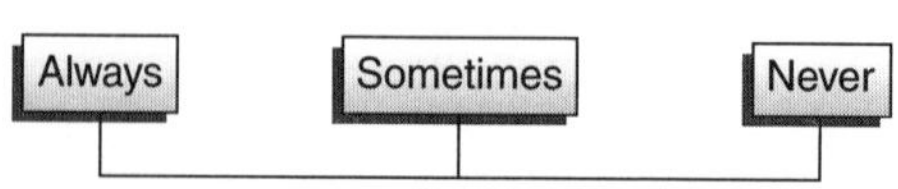

Figure 7.7

Three-point rating scale.

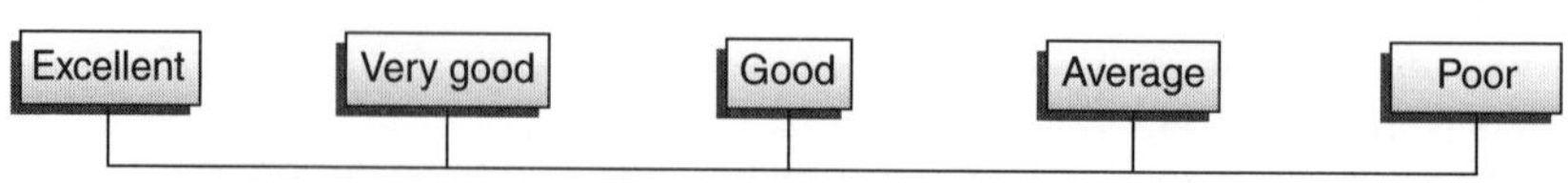

Figure 7.8

Five-point rating scale.

BOX 7.7 COMMON CONTENT OF APPRAISAL IN RATING SCALE

Quantity of Work	Volume of Work	Quality of Work	Dependability
Reliability	Initiative	Judgement	Neatness
Accuracy of work knowledge	Cooperative	Ability to work	Willingness

to judge the performance. A wide variety of attributes may be assessed by using rating scales; details may be perused from Box 7.7.

Q. How frequently do you discuss with your clinical instructor the difficulties encountered during clinical posting?

Q. The overall performance of the student in a mouth care procedure.

II. TYPES OF RATING SCALES

(a) ***Graphic rating scale:*** In this scale, the performance is printed horizontally at various points from lowest to highest. It includes the numerical points on the scale. It is anchored by two extremes presented to the respondents for the evaluation of a concept or object. For example: How satisfied are you with the lecture delivered by Professor X?

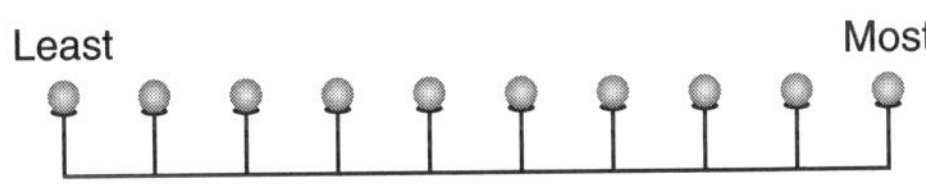

Graphic rating scale.

(b) ***Descriptive rating scale:*** This type of rating scale does not use numbers but divides the assessment into a series of verbal phrases to indicate the level of performance.

For example: Q. Judge the level of performance of the nursing personnel in a medical ICU.

	Level of Clinical Performance			
Nursing Personnel in a Ward	**Very Active**	**Active**	**Moderately Active**	**Passive**
1. *Amandeep*				
2. *Jasveen*				
3. *Tara*				
4. *Kirandeep*				

(c) ***Numerical rating scale:*** It divides the evaluation criteria into a fixed number of points and defines only numbers except at the extremes. In these scales, each statement is generally assigned a numerical score ranging from 1 to 10 or even more. For example: Pain assessment numerical scale.

(d) ***Comparative rating scale:*** In this type of rating scale, the rater makes a judgement about a person's attributes by comparing to another similar person(s). For example, Mr Ram's decision-making abilities closely resemble that of Mr Shyam and Mr Gopal. In this type of rating scale, the rater must have prior knowledge about the selected attributes of the people with whom the subjects are supposed to be compared.

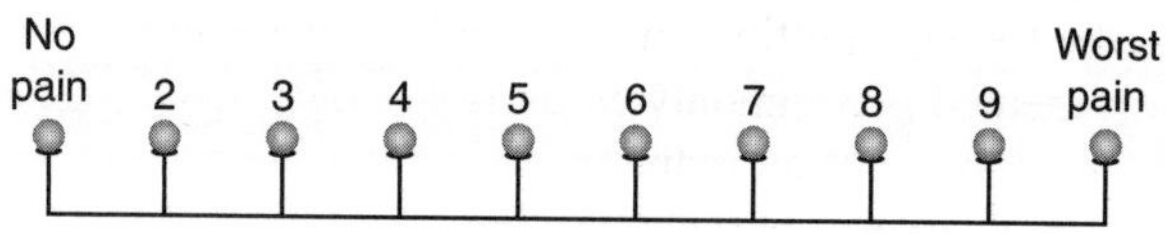

Numerical rating scale.

III. CHARACTERISTICS OF A RATING SCALE

- Rating scales are value judgements of the attributes of one person by another person.
- These scales are most commonly used tools to carry out structured observations.
- They are generally developed to make quantitative judgements about qualitative attributes.
- They provide more flexibility to judge the level of performance or the presence of attributes among subjects.
- Guilford (1954) identified that a rating scale must have the following basic characteristics that must be taken care of while constructing a rating scale.
  - *Clarity:* The rating scale must be constructed using short, concise statements in simple and unambiguous language.
  - *Relevance:* The statement designed in a rating scale should be relevant to the phenomenon and should be exactly in accordance with the variables under study.
  - *Variety:* While developing the rating scale, monotony of the statements must be avoided and variety in different statements must be ensured.
  - *Objectivity:* The statement formed in a rating scale must be objective in nature so that it is convenient for the rater to judge the attributes or performances of the subjects under study.
  - *Uniqueness:* Each statement constructed in a rating scale must be unique in itself so that the attributes can be judged appropriately.

IV. ADVANTAGES OF A RATING SCALE

- Rating scales are easy to administer and score the measured attributes.
- They have a wide range of application in nursing educational evaluation.
- Graphic rating scale is more easy to make and less time-consuming.
- Rating scales can be easily used for a large group.
- They are also used for quantitative methods.
- They may also be used for the assessment of interests, attitudes and personal characteristics.
- They are used to evaluate performance, skills and product outcomes.
- Rating scales are adaptable and flexible assessment instruments.

V. DISADVANTAGES OF RATING SCALES

- It is difficult or dangerous to fix up rating about many aspects of an individual.
- Misuse can result in a decrease in objectivity.
- There are chances of subjective evaluation thus the scales may become unscientific and unreliable.

VIDEOTAPE-BASED ASSESSMENT

Videotape-based assessment is a powerful method used to evaluate and analyse an individual's performance, skill or behaviour in nursing education. By recording relevant activities or interactions on video, assessors can review the footage multiple times, providing a unique opportunity for objective observation and analysis. This method is commonly employed in nursing educational, professional and clinical settings to assess various aspects of an individual's competence and provide valuable feedback for improvement. Videotape-based assessment may be defined as:

- Dowrick and Dove (1980) defined videotape-based assessment as 'the use of videotape to record and analyze behaviour for the purpose of making decisions about intervention'.
- Gersten et al. (1995) defined videotape-based assessment as 'a procedure in which student's behaviour is videotaped in a natural setting and then analysed by a trained observer'.
- O'Neill et al. (1997) defined videotape-based assessment as 'a method of collecting data on student's behaviour that involves recording the student's behaviour on videotape and then coding the behaviour using a standardized coding system'.

Videotape-based assessment can be used to assess a variety of behaviours, including social skills, academic skills and emotional regulation. It can also be used to assess the effectiveness of interventions and performance.

PURPOSES OF VIDEOTAPE-BASED ASSESSMENT

- Objective observation and analysis of an individual's performance or behaviour.
- Identification of strengths, weaknesses and areas for improvement.
- Facilitation of constructive feedback and evaluation.
- Support for training and professional development.
- Enhancement of self-reflection and self-awareness.
- Promotion of skill refinement and technique development.
- Identification of specific areas for targeted intervention or support.
- Documentation and evidence of performance for assessment or evaluation purposes.
- Comparison of performances over time to track progress and growth.
- Research and analysis of specific interactions or learning behaviours.
- Development of teaching or coaching strategies based on observed performance.
- Calibration and standardization of assessment criteria.
- Quality assurance in educational, professional or clinical settings.
- Identification and analysis of effective teaching or intervention techniques.
- Enhancing objectivity and reducing biases in assessment processes.

GUIDELINE TO CONDUCT VIDEOTAPE-BASED ASSESSMENT

The following guidelines may be used for conducting videotape-based assessment effectively, which provides valuable insights and feedback to support individual development and growth.

- ***Determine the purpose:*** Clearly define the purpose and objective of the assessment. Identify what specific skills, behaviours or interactions will be observed and evaluated through the videotape-based assessment.
- ***Obtain consent:*** Ensure that all participants involved in the recording and assessment process provide informed consent. Explain the purpose, process and potential uses of the video footage and address any concerns or questions.
- ***Select appropriate recording equipment:*** Choose suitable recording equipment, such as video cameras or digital devices, based on the context and requirements of the assessment. Ensure the equipment is properly set up, tested and functioning correctly before starting the recording.

- ***Establish clear guidelines:*** Develop specific guidelines or criteria for the assessment. Clearly define the behaviours or skills that will be observed, evaluated and rated during the assessment. This will provide a structured framework for the analysis of the video footage.
- ***Conduct the recording:*** Record the relevant activities, interactions or performances using the chosen recording equipment. Ensure that the camera angle, lighting and audio are optimal to capture the necessary details for accurate assessment.
- ***Securely store and protect the footage:*** Safeguard the recorded video footage to maintain confidentiality and privacy. Follow appropriate data protection protocols and ensure that only authorized individuals have access to the recordings.
- ***Multiple viewings and analysis:*** Review the recorded footage multiple times to conduct a thorough analysis. Pay attention to specific behaviours, actions or skills outlined in the assessment guidelines. Take notes and document observations during the viewing process.
- ***Assess and evaluate:*** Evaluate the performance or behaviours based on the established assessment criteria. Consider both strengths and areas for improvement. Use the video footage as evidence to support evaluations and provide constructive feedback.
- ***Provide feedback:*** Schedule a feedback session with the individual being assessed. Use the recorded footage as a visual reference to discuss specific observations, strengths, weaknesses and areas for improvement. Offer constructive feedback, suggestions and guidance to support their development.
- ***Reflect and enhance:*** Encourage individuals to reflect on their performance and the feedback provided. Help them identify strategies and actions to enhance their skills, behaviours or interactions based on the assessment results.
- ***Consider ethical and legal obligations:*** Ensure compliance with ethical and legal obligations related to data privacy, confidentiality and consent. Obtain necessary permissions for using video recordings for assessment purposes and follow relevant policies and guidelines.
- ***Continuous improvement:*** Use the insights gained from the videotape-based assessment to inform ongoing training, professional development or intervention strategies. Continuously monitor progress and reassess as needed to track improvement and growth.

By following these guidelines, one can effectively conduct a videotape-based assessment, providing valuable insights and feedback to support individual development and growth.

ADVANTAGES OF VIDEOTAPE-BASED ASSESSMENT

- ***Enhanced objectivity:*** Videotape-based assessment allows for objective observation and analysis of performance or behaviour, reducing the influence of biases that can occur during real-time assessments.
- ***Multiple viewings:*** Video recordings can be reviewed multiple times, enabling assessors to closely analyse and capture details that may have been missed during live assessments. This leads to more accurate evaluations and assessments.
- ***Constructive feedback:*** Video footage provides a visual reference for providing specific and targeted feedback. It allows assessors to illustrate strengths and areas for improvement, enhancing the effectiveness of feedback sessions.
- ***Self-reflection:*** Individuals being assessed can review their own performances, promoting self-reflection and self-awareness. They can observe their behaviours objectively, identify areas for improvement and take ownership of their professional growth.
- ***Training and professional development:*** Videotape-based assessment supports training and professional development by providing opportunities for individuals to learn from their own performances, refine their skills and develop strategies for improvement.

- ***Standardization:*** Video recordings offer a standardized assessment method, ensuring consistent evaluation across different assessors and settings. This promotes fairness and reliability in the assessment process.
- ***Documentation and research:*** Video footage serves as a documented record of performances, interactions or behaviours. It can be utilized for research purposes, analysis of teaching techniques or evidence-based practices.

DISADVANTAGES OF VIDEOTAPE-BASED ASSESSMENT

- ***Limited context:*** Video recordings may not capture the full context or environment in which the performance or behaviour occurred. Factors such as physical presence, nonverbal cues and situational dynamics may be missed or distorted.
- ***Observer bias:*** Even though video recordings can reduce biases, the interpretation of the footage can still be influenced by observer bias. Different assessors may perceive and evaluate the same footage differently.
- ***Selective editing:*** The act of editing or selecting specific segments of the video footage for assessment purposes may introduce bias or omit important contextual information.
- ***Privacy and consent:*** Obtaining consent and ensuring privacy can be challenging when recording and storing video footage. Ethical considerations should be carefully addressed to protect the rights and confidentiality of the individuals involved.
- ***Technical challenges:*** Technical issues such as poor video quality, audio disruptions or difficulties in recording certain activities may impact the effectiveness and reliability of the assessment.
- ***Time-consuming:*** Reviewing and analysing video footage can be time-consuming, especially when conducting detailed observations and assessments. This may limit the scalability and efficiency of the assessment process.
- ***Subjectivity in assessment criteria:*** While video recordings provide a visual reference, the assessment criteria and guidelines used for evaluation can still be subjective and vary among assessors, impacting the reliability of the assessments.

By recognizing these benefits and limitations, practitioners can make informed decisions and effectively utilize videotape-based assessment as a valuable tool for evaluation, feedback and professional development.

WRITTEN ASSIGNMENT-BASED ASSESSMENT

Progress notes, nursing care plans, process recording and projects are used as written assignments-based assessment. These assessment method plays a vital role in nursing education, allowing students to demonstrate their understanding of nursing concepts, apply theoretical knowledge to real-world scenarios and develop essential skills required for professional nursing practice. Written assignment-based assessment in nursing refers to the evaluation and assessment of nursing students' knowledge, critical thinking and communication skills through written tasks specific to the field of nursing. Written assignment-based assessment may be defined as:

- John T.E. Richardson defines written assignment-based assessment as 'a method of evaluating student learning that involves the completion of written assignments, such as essays, reports, and research papers etc'.
- David Boud defines written assignment-based assessment as 'a process of gathering evidence of student learning through the completion of written tasks'.

- Rebecca Black defines written assignment-based assessment as 'a form of assessment that requires students to produce a piece of written work, such as an essay, report, or research paper'.

It is important to note that there is no single, universally accepted definition of this type of assessment. However, all of the definitions cited above emphasize the importance of using written assignments to assess student learning.

PURPOSES OF WRITTEN ASSIGNMENT-BASED ASSESSMENT

- Assess understanding of nursing concepts and theories.
- Evaluate critical thinking skills in nursing practice.
- Assess ability to apply theoretical knowledge to clinical scenarios.
- Evaluate communication skills, both written and professional.
- Assess knowledge and application of evidence-based practice in nursing.
- Evaluate problem-solving skills in nursing care planning and decision-making.
- Assess understanding and application of ethical principles in nursing practice.
- Promote integration of theory and practice in nursing education.
- Encourage continuous learning and professional development.
- Provide feedback and guidance for improvement in nursing competencies.
- Prepare students for real-world nursing challenges and patient care scenarios.

GUIDELINES TO CONDUCT WRITTEN ASSIGNMENT-BASED ASSESSMENT IN NURSING

1. ***Clearly define learning outcomes:*** Clearly define the learning outcomes and objectives that the written assignments aim to assess. Ensure alignment with the nursing curriculum and programme goals.
2. ***Provide clear instructions:*** Provide clear and detailed instructions for each written assignment, including formatting requirements, word limits and specific guidelines related to the assignment topic or scenario.
3. ***Incorporate realistic scenarios:*** Develop written assignments that reflect real-world nursing scenarios and challenges. This helps students apply theoretical knowledge to practical situations, promoting critical thinking and problem-solving skills.
4. ***Use rubrics or grading criteria:*** Develop rubrics or grading criteria to ensure consistency and transparency in the assessment process. Clearly outline the criteria for evaluation, including content, critical thinking, organization, communication and adherence to professional standards.
5. ***Encourage evidence-based practice:*** Encourage students to incorporate evidence-based practice in their written assignments. Provide guidance on how to locate, critically appraise and integrate relevant research and evidence into their work.
6. ***Promote professional writing skills:*** Emphasize the importance of professional writing skills in nursing. Provide resources or workshops on effective communication, proper documentation and professional writing style. Consider incorporating elements such as nursing terminology, accurate referencing and appropriate citation.
7. ***Allow sufficient time for completion:*** Ensure students have sufficient time to complete the written assignments. Consider the complexity of the assignment and the workload of the students to determine appropriate timelines and deadlines.

8. ***Offer feedback and evaluation:*** Provide timely and constructive feedback on the written assignments. Highlight strengths and areas for improvement and offer suggestions for further development. Use the feedback as a learning opportunity to enhance students' understanding and application of nursing concepts.
9. ***Maintain academic integrity:*** Promote academic integrity by clearly communicating expectations regarding plagiarism and proper citation of sources. Encourage students to cite their references accurately and consistently adhere to ethical standards in their written work.
10. ***Supportive resources and assistance:*** Provide students with access to supportive resources, such as reference materials, databases, writing centres or writing mentors, to help them develop their writing skills and meet the requirements of the written assignments.
11. ***Ensure confidentiality and privacy:*** Safeguard students' confidentiality and privacy by handling their written assignments securely. Protect sensitive information and ensure compliance with data protection regulations.
12. ***Reflect and improve:*** Reflect on the effectiveness of the written assignment-based assessment process. Collect feedback from students and assessors to identify areas for improvement. Make necessary adjustments to enhance the assessment process and ensure its alignment with desired learning outcomes.

ADVANTAGES OF WRITTEN ASSIGNMENT-BASED ASSESSMENT IN NURSING

- ***Critical thinking skills:*** Assignments encourage students to think critically and analyse information in a structured manner. By researching, organizing thoughts and presenting ideas in writing, students develop their critical thinking skills, which are crucial for nursing practice.
- ***Communication skills:*** Writing assignments improve students' written communication skills, which are essential for effective documentation and professional communication in nursing. Clear and concise writing helps nurses convey information accurately, ensuring patient safety and effective collaboration with the healthcare team.
- ***Knowledge application:*** Assignments provide an opportunity for students to apply theoretical knowledge to real-life scenarios. By researching and writing about specific nursing topics, students can demonstrate their understanding and apply theoretical concepts to practical situations, enhancing their ability to transfer knowledge to clinical practice.
- ***Self-reflection:*** Written assignments often require students to reflect on their learning experiences, clinical practice or ethical dilemmas. Engaging in reflective writing promotes self-awareness, personal growth and the development of empathy, which are important qualities for nursing professionals.
- ***Time management and organization:*** Completing a written assignment requires students to manage their time effectively, plan their work and meet deadlines. These skills are transferable to nursing practice, where nurses must prioritize tasks, manage their time efficiently and handle multiple responsibilities simultaneously.

CHALLENGES OF WRITTEN ASSIGNMENT-BASED ASSESSMENT IN NURSING

- ***Subjectivity:*** Grading written assignments can be subjective, as interpretation and evaluation of content may vary among different faculty members. Students may feel that their work is not fairly assessed, especially if grading criteria are not clearly defined.
- ***Limited assessment of clinical skills:*** While written assignments assess theoretical knowledge and critical thinking, they may not adequately evaluate students' clinical skills, such as physical assessment, technical procedures or hands-on interventions. Practical assessments and simulations

are needed to complement written assignments for a comprehensive evaluation of nursing competencies.

- ***Time-intensive:*** Creating, reviewing and grading written assignments can be time-consuming for both faculty members and students. It may pose challenges for faculty who have limited time to provide prompt feedback, and students may find it challenging to balance assignment workload with clinical placements and other responsibilities.
- ***Plagiarism and academic integrity:*** Written assignments can be susceptible to plagiarism, especially in the digital age where information is readily available online. Ensuring academic integrity and promoting original work can be a challenge for educators, requiring the implementation of plagiarism detection tools and educational interventions to emphasize ethical writing practices.
- **Language barriers and writing skills**: Nursing programmes often consist of diverse student populations, including international students who may face language barriers or have different levels of proficiency in academic writing. It is essential to provide support and resources to enhance writing skills and ensure that language proficiency does not hinder students' ability to demonstrate their knowledge effectively.

Overall, while written assignment-based assessment in nursing offers various benefits, it is important to balance its use with other forms of assessment to ensure a comprehensive evaluation of nursing competencies. Integrating practical assessments, simulations, and clinical evaluations alongside written assignments can provide a more robust evaluation of students' knowledge and skills in nursing.

PRACTICAL EXAMINATION

Practical examination is concerned with the assessment of practical performance skills and practice competency acquired by a student during the course of a particular programme. The nursing profession has used practical examination since long to assess the ability of nurses to perform specific expected practical tasks or practice competencies. Generally, in addition to assessment of cognitive domain of learning through theory examination, a practical profession like nursing also imposes a demand to assess the psychomotor and affect domain through practical examination. Traditionally, practical examinations are conducted in practice laboratories or real-life practice areas such as patients admitted in a hospital ward. The successful completion of a nursing programme requires a nursing student to pass the practical examination of a particular subject independently over and above the theoretical assessment. Practical examination is considered the most essential part of the overall assessment process in nursing because it is believed that merely theoretical knowledge of a nurse does not make them a qualified, competent nurse. Therefore, nurses must be assessed for their practical skills through practical examinations.

I. PURPOSES OF PRACTICAL EXAMINATIONS

Traditionally, practical examinations are used in nursing for the following purposes:

- To assess the practical skills and practice competencies of nursing students.
- To assess the development in practice domain of students by observing their reactions to real-life or simulated situations.
- To assess the student's problem-solving skills.
- To assess the recording and reporting skills of nursing students.
- To assess how well the students are successful in transforming their theoretical knowledge in practice.

- To assess multiple performance tasks such as assessment, planning, implementation, communication and evaluation.

II. GUIDELINES FOR CONDUCTING PRACTICAL EXAMINATIONS

The following guidelines may be followed for conducting the practical examinations:

A. PLANNING PHASE OF PRACTICAL EXAMINATION

- Consider the learning experience and learning objectives before planning the practical examination.
- Decide the appropriate place for the practical examination. Preliminary practical examinations must be conducted on simulators in a nursing laboratory. However, the final practical must be conducted on real-life situations. For example, patients admitted in the respective ward of a hospital or a field area for community health nursing.
- Preferably, plan to conduct the practical examination in a familiar place for students so that they can be psychologically comfortable.
- The selected area for practical examination must have an adequate supply to carry out the expected nursing procedures and the area should be well planned to accommodate the nursing students and examiners.
- The ward nurse managers or clinical area in-charges must be informed well in advance so that they are well prepared to support in the conduction of the practical examination.
- The overall evaluation criteria must be planned and students must be informed about the evaluation criteria so that they can prepare accordingly.

B. CONDUCTING PHASE OF PRACTICAL EXAMINATION

- Students and examiners must reach the place of examination as scheduled well in advance so that necessary changes may be adapted comfortably without any undue discomfort.
- Students must be called in a group and they must be conveyed with all the rules and regulations of the examination and examination stations or the patients may be randomly assigned through the lottery method to avoid subjective bias.
- Students must be assigned with routine nursing procedures performed by them regularly to make them psychologically comfortable with the practical situation.
- Generally, students feel nervous and anxious during practical examinations so a stress-free atmosphere must be offered to students so they can perform better without undue stress and pressure.
- Practical examinations must proceed using the steps of the nursing process such as assessment, planning, implementation and evaluation. For example, a student may initially assess the assigned patient, then plan and implement the care for priority needs and finally evaluate the effect of implemented care.
- Each student must be given sufficient time to perform the nursing procedure and accomplish the practical examination. Each examiner should not examine more than 20 students in a day (INC, 1986).
- Any sort of undue discomfort to the patients during practical examination must be avoided.
- On completion of the practical examination, the marks obtained by students must be compiled and sent to the examining body, that is university or nursing board in a sealed envelope under confidentiality.

C. ADVANTAGES OF PRACTICAL EXAMINATIONS

- Practical examination provides an opportunity to assess the skills and competency acquired by the students.
- Practical examination offers an opportunity to the examiners for assessing the use of compartmentalized knowledge in an integrated manner by a student while providing holistic nursing care to the assigned patient.
- An examiner also gets an opportunity to assess the communication and interpersonal skills of the students along with their clinical competence in performing the nursing procedures.

D. DISADVANTAGES OF PRACTICAL EXAMINATIONS

- Practical examination is not considered a standardized assessment practice when students are assessed while working with patients.
- It is not considered an objective method of assessment because there are higher chances of subjectivity and personal bias.
- It is a time-consuming process when an examiner assesses the complete practices and procedures of a student.
- It cannot be considered a feasible method for assessing a large group of students.
- Sometimes it is considered as unethical to expose patients for examining students.
- The emergencies and complex ward routines may be considered as disturbance factors to the smooth conduction of the practical examination.

ORAL EXAMINATION

Viva voce is a Latin phrase literally meaning *with living voice* but is most often translated as *by word of mouth*. Furthermore, viva voce is also termed as an *oral examination* which consists of a dialogue between the examiner and a student where the examiner asks question and the student replies. The examiner may ask short open questions, MCQs or a series of other type of questions not necessarily related to each other.

In nursing, viva voce is generally used to supplement the practical examination where two examiners, that is internal and external, ask several questions related to a particular subject matter. The viva voce might form a part of the validated assessment for a course, assessed by an oral examination. In these situations, the viva voce is a useful tool that assists in authenticating that the student has got enough knowledge in the subject matter.

I. PURPOSES OF VIVA VOCE

There are a variety of circumstances which might require the use of a viva voce and provision for these is contained in the academic and organizational regulations. There are several legitimate reasons for asking a student to attend a viva voce examination, all of which may have a different impact on the student. The main purposes of viva voce are mentioned below:

- To assess student's ability to communicate with another person.
- To supplement the information obtained through other evaluation techniques.
- To use stimulation methods like role play and telephone conversation.
- To identify and analyse the student's presence of mind.

- To evaluate the student's spontaneity and mannerism.
- To acquire soundness of knowledge through various forms of question.
- To diagnose the student's limitation and weakness and take remedial action.

II. PRINCIPLES TO CONDUCT VIVA VOCE

- The viva should not be limited to a single topic but should cover a range of different issues to avoid the results of the viva being skewed by selecting a topic which the candidate can answer exceptionally well or about which he/she knows nothing of. All questions should be strictly relevant to the purpose of the viva.
- Do not use long preambles to questions. Examiners should talk as little as possible during the viva.
- The chair of the examiners must remain in charge of the session and must deal appropriately with any problem candidate or difficult situation.
- When the last question is being asked, allow the student to complete his/her answer and end the session formally.
- Viva voce examinations should not normally exceed 30 minutes.
- Candidates should be examined individually.
- Candidates should be given adequate notice of the possibility of being called to attend a viva, and this should normally not be less than 24 hours.

A. ADVANTAGES OF A VIVA VOCE

- Provides direct contact with the candidates to assess their communication, presentation skills and overall impression.
- Provides opportunity to mitigate circumstances into accounts.
- Provides flexibility in moving the candidates from strong to weak points.
- Makes students formulate replies without cues, and the reaction is observed for a specific stimulus.
- Facilitates simultaneous assessment by two or more examiners.
- Provides an opportunity for the examiner to get feedback on the performance of the students and the university.

B. DISADVANTAGES OF A VIVA VOCE

- Lacks standardization, objectivity and reproducibility of the result.
- Permits favouritism and cannot be used for future references.
- Suffers from undue influence of irrelevant factors.
- Costly in terms of professional time.

SIMULATION-BASED ASSESSMENT

Simulation-based assessment in nursing is an innovative approach that provides an immersive and realistic learning and assessment environment for nursing students to practice and demonstrate their skills and competencies. This method involves recreating real-life patient scenarios using high-fidelity mannequins, computer programs, or standardized patients, allowing students to engage in hands-on experiences that closely mimic clinical practice. Simulation-based assessments have gained popularity in nursing education due to their ability to bridge the gap between theoretical knowledge and practical application. Simulation-based assessment may be defined as follows:

- David Gaba defines simulation-based assessment as 'the use of simulated environments to assess the knowledge, skills, and attitudes of learners'.
- Mark S. Allen defines simulation-based assessment as 'a method of evaluating student learning that involves the use of simulated environments to assess the learner's ability to apply knowledge and skills in a realistic setting'.
- Michael I. Cohen defines simulation-based assessment as 'a form of assessment that uses simulated environments to assess the learner's ability to perform tasks or solve problems'.

PURPOSES SIMULATION-BASED ASSESSMENT

- Provide a realistic and controlled environment for nursing students to practice and apply their clinical skills.
- Assess students' competency in performing nursing procedures, critical thinking, decision-making and problem-solving.
- Evaluate students' ability to communicate effectively, collaborate with healthcare teams and demonstrate professional behaviour.
- Identify strengths and areas for improvement in students' clinical performance and skills.
- Enhance students' confidence and competence in managing complex patient scenarios.
- Bridge the gap between theory and practice by allowing students to apply their knowledge in a realistic setting.
- Promote the development of clinical reasoning skills and the ability to prioritize patient care.
- Assess students' ability to adapt to unexpected situations, handle emergencies and manage patient safety.
- Foster the development of interprofessional collaboration and teamwork skills.
- Provide a safe and supportive environment for students to make mistakes, learn from them and receive constructive feedback.
- Prepare students for real-world clinical practice by simulating various healthcare settings and scenarios.
- Increase students' understanding of ethical considerations, cultural sensitivity and patient-centred care.
- Encourage self-reflection and self-assessment among nursing students.
- Validate the effectiveness of nursing education programmes and curriculum by measuring students' performance in simulated clinical situations.

GUIDELINES TO CONDUCT SIMULATION-BASED ASSESSMENT IN NURSING

Simulation-based assessments in nursing can provide valuable opportunities for students to develop and demonstrate their clinical skills in a controlled and realistic environment. Here are some guidelines to conduct simulation-based assessments in nursing:

- ***Define objectives:*** Clearly identify the learning objectives and outcomes desired to be achieved through the simulation. These objectives should align with the specific skills and competencies need to be assessed.

- ***Design realistic scenarios:*** Develop realistic scenarios that reflect the clinical situations nursing students are likely to encounter in their practice. Consider using case studies, standardized patients or high-fidelity mannequins to create lifelike scenarios.
- ***Set up the simulation environment:*** Create a simulated healthcare environment that closely resembles an actual clinical setting. Ensure that the simulation room is well-equipped with necessary medical equipment, supplies and resources.
- ***Provide prebriefing:*** Before the simulation, provide students with a prebriefing session to explain the objectives, expectations and guidelines for the assessment. This session should also include a review of relevant theory and concepts.
- ***Establish clear guidelines:*** Clearly communicate the guidelines and rules for the simulation to the students. Discuss the expected behaviour, ethical considerations and safety precautions. Emphasize the importance of professional conduct, communication and teamwork.
- ***Facilitate the simulation:*** During the simulation, play the role of a facilitator or instructor. Guide the students, provide support and feedback and ensure that the simulation progresses smoothly. You may also consider involving other healthcare professionals or faculty members as additional facilitators.
- ***Encourage reflection:*** After the simulation, allow time for debriefing and reflection. Encourage students to discuss their actions, decisions and thought processes during the simulation. Facilitate a constructive discussion to help students recognize strengths, areas for improvement and lessons learned.
- ***Provide feedback:*** Offer timely and constructive feedback to students based on their performance during the simulation. Highlight their strengths and provide specific recommendations for improvement. Feedback should focus on both technical skills and nontechnical skills, such as communication and critical thinking.
- ***Assess performance:*** Develop a standardized assessment rubric or checklist to evaluate student performance during the simulation. Assess both the technical and nontechnical aspects of their skills. Use objective criteria to ensure fairness and consistency in the assessment process.
- ***Follow ethical guidelines:*** Adhere to ethical guidelines and ensure that students' confidentiality is maintained during the simulation. Obtain necessary consents and permissions when using standardized patients or recording simulation sessions for assessment purposes.
- ***Evaluate the effectiveness:*** Continuously evaluate the effectiveness of your simulation-based assessments. Collect feedback from students and faculty to identify areas of improvement. Make necessary adjustments to enhance the learning experience and assessment process.

Remember, simulation-based assessments are intended to be a safe and controlled learning and assessment environment. Emphasize the importance of learning and improvement rather than focusing solely on grades or outcomes.

ADVANTAGES OF SIMULATION-BASED ASSESSMENT IN NURSING

- ***Realistic practice:*** Simulation-based assessments provide a realistic practice environment that closely mimics real-life clinical scenarios, allowing students to apply their theoretical knowledge and develop practical skills.
- ***Safe learning environment:*** Simulations offer a safe space for students to make mistakes, learn from them and build confidence without compromising patient safety.
- ***Standardized assessment:*** Simulation-based assessments allow for standardized evaluation criteria, ensuring fairness and consistency in assessing students' performance.

- ***Immediate feedback:*** Students receive immediate feedback on their performance during debriefing sessions, enabling them to reflect on their actions, identify areas for improvement and make adjustments in real time.
- ***Enhanced critical thinking:*** Simulation-based assessments promote critical thinking skills by requiring students to make decisions, prioritize care and manage complex patient situations in a time-sensitive and dynamic environment.
- ***Teamwork and communication:*** Simulations provide opportunities for students to practice interprofessional collaboration, teamwork and effective communication skills, which are essential in healthcare settings.
- ***Experiential learning:*** Through simulations, students can experience a wide range of patient conditions and scenarios, allowing them to develop skills, build clinical judgement and gain confidence in managing various situations.

LIMITATIONS OF SIMULATION-BASED ASSESSMENT IN NURSING

- ***Cost and resource intensive:*** Developing and maintaining a simulation centre, acquiring high-fidelity mannequins and implementing simulation-based assessments can be expensive and require significant resources.
- ***Time constraints:*** Conducting simulation-based assessments can be time-consuming, requiring dedicated sessions for each student or small group, which may pose challenges in terms of scheduling and logistics.
- ***Limited reproducibility:*** It may be challenging to reproduce identical simulation scenarios for multiple groups of students, which can impact the comparability of assessment outcomes.
- ***Instructor dependency:*** The quality and consistency of simulation-based assessments heavily rely on the facilitator's expertise and ability to provide accurate feedback and guidance to students.
- ***Generalization challenges:*** Students may excel in simulation environments but struggle to translate their skills and knowledge to actual clinical practice due to the contextual differences between simulations and real-world patient care settings.

OBJECTIVE STRUCTURED CLINICAL EXAMINATION

OSCE is a modern type of examination often used in health sciences (e.g. medicine, dentistry nursing, pharmacy and physiotherapy) to assess clinical skill performance and competence in skills, such as communication, clinical examination, medical and nursing procedures/prescription, exercise prescription, joint mobilization/manipulation techniques and interpretation of results.

I. DEFINITIONS OF OSCE

Objective Structured Clinical Examination (OSCE) is a form of performance-based testing used to measure candidates' clinical competence. During an OSCE, candidates are observed and evaluated as they go through a series of stations in which they interview, examine and treat standardized patients who present with some type of medical problem.

The OSCE is an approach to the assessment of clinical competence in which the components of competence are assessed in a planned or structured way with attention being paid to the objectivity of the examination.

—Harden

OSCE is an assessment tool in which the components of clinical competence such as history taking, physical examination, simple procedures, interpretation of lab results, patient management problems, communication, attitude etc. are tested using agreed check lists and rotating the student round a number of stations some of which have observers with checklists.

—N. Ananthakrishnan

II. USES OF OSCE

OSCE can be used for undergraduate as well as postgraduate nursing students to assess their clinical competencies. Generally, ranges of basic and advanced clinical practice skills are assessed by using a 10-station OSCE session which comprises practice stations such as physical examination stations, history-taking stations, stations that cover communication skills and stations to perform nursing procedures followed by response stations to ask related MCQs or SAQs. Generally, the following range of practical skills are typically assessed in nursing using OSCE:

- Interpersonal and communication skills
- History-taking skills
- Physical examination of specific body systems
- Mental health assessment
- Clinical decision-making, including the formation of differential diagnosis
- Clinical problem-solving skills
- Interpretation of clinical findings and investigations
- Management of a clinical situation, including treatment and referral
- Patient education
- Health promotion
- Acting safely and appropriately in an urgent clinical situation
- Basic and advanced nursing care procedure practices

III. ORGANIZING THE OSCE

- The OSCE examination consists of about 10–15 stations, each of which requires about 4–5 minutes. The number of stations and time spent on each station may vary based on needs of evaluation.
- All stations should be capable of being completed in the same time.
- The students are rotated through all stations and have to move to the next station at the signal.
- As the stations are generally independent, students can start at any procedure stations and complete the cycle.
- Thus, using 15 stations of 4 minutes each, 15 students can complete the examination within 1 hour.
- Each station is designed to test a component of clinical competence.
- At some stations, called the *procedure stations* (Fig. 7.9), students are given tasks to perform on patients or simulators (some of the essential examples of procedure stations that may be used for first year B.Sc. Nursing students are given in Box 7.8). At all such stations there are observers with agreed upon checklists or rating scales to score the student's performance (Box 7.9).
- At other stations called *response stations* (Fig. 7.10), students respond to questions of the objective type or interpret data or record their findings of the previous procedure stations. An example of a mode OSCE is depicted in Box 7.10.

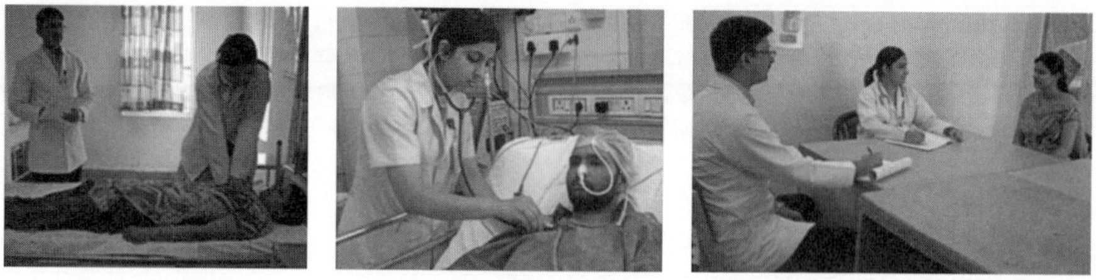

BLS skill station | Chest examination station | History taking station

Figure 7.9

Examples of a procedure station.

BOX 7.8 EXAMPLES OF THE PROCEDURE STATION FOR FIRST YEAR B.SC. NURSING STUDENTS

- Brief history taking
- Chest assessment
- Identifying nursing needs
- Identification and uses of different gadgets
- Oral medication
- Back care
- Intramuscular injection and such nursing procedures

BOX 7.9 PROCEDURE STATION CHECKLIST

Procedure: Oral Medications	Please Tick (√) Mark	
Steps to Be Followed	**Yes**	**No**
1. Wash hands		
2. Recall safety measures, locate the drug, read the label on the bottle and see that it is the right medicine and shake the bottle		
3. Collect medicine into the container		
4. Measure liquids accurately with a minim glass and read the lower level of the meniscus		
5. Pour liquid from the opposite side of the label, wipe the mouth of the bottle and recap the bottle		
6. Take the tablet/capsule in a spoon or medicine cup		
7. Identify the patient with the patient chart		
8. Explain the procedure		
9. Place patient's towel under the chin		
10. Position the patient comfortably in the upright sitting position		
11. Administer each drug separately followed by water		
12. Record the drug administering details of dose, route, date, time, signature and omissions		
13. Clean and replace the articles		

**Each step carries one mark*

Signature of examiner: .... Date: ....

RESPONSE STATION-1

Interpret the following ABG report.

$pH = 7.27$

$PaCO_2 = 49$

$HCO_3 = 24$

$PaCO_2 = 92$

Name this condition: ....

RESPONSE STATION-2

Patient-G had prescription of 1200 mL fluid for 12 hours. How many drops per minute nurse will administrator through macro drip set?

a) 27

b) 30

c) 32

d) 40

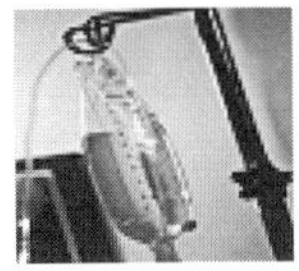

Figure 7.10

Examples of response stations for OSCE.I

BOX 7.10 EXAMPLE OF A MODEL OSCE FOR CRITICAL CARE NURSING STUDENTS

Procedure Station-1

Assess the patient X; identify the three priority nursing needs:

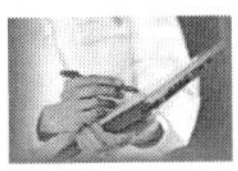

i. ....

ii. ....

iii. ....

Procedure Station-2

Conduct chest assessment of patient A and identify two abnormal respiratory findings:

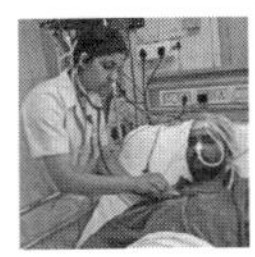

i. ....

ii. ....

Procedure Station-3

Carryout ET suctioning of patient Y and record the procedure:

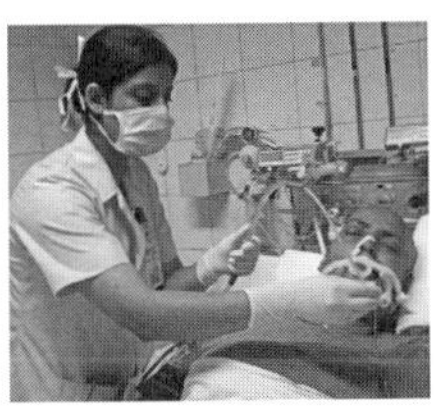

Procedure Station-4

Change 'PEEP' from 10 to 5 of patient Z, who is on ventilator:

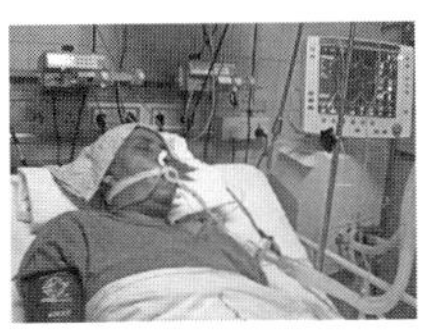

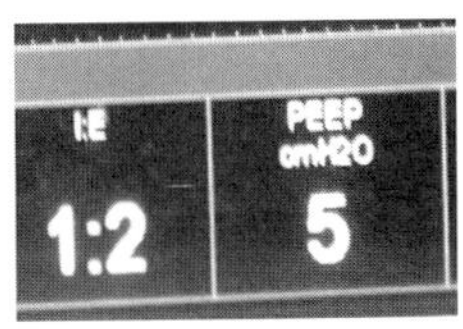

Response Station-5

Interpret this ABG report:

pH = 7.27

$PaCO^2 = 49$

$HCO^3 = 24$

$PaCO^2 = 92$

Name this condition: ....

Response Station-6

Patient G had a prescription of 1200 mL fluid for 12 hours. How many drops per min nurse will the administrator through macro drip set?

a) 27

b) 30

c) 32

d) 40

BOX 7.10 EXAMPLE OF A MODEL OSCE FOR CRITICAL CARE NURSING STUDENTS—cont'd

Procedure Station-7

Mention indications, dose and any four nursing consideration of this medicine:

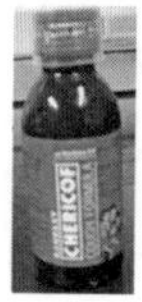

i. Indication: ....
ii. Dose: ....
iii. Three essential nursing considerations:
....
....

Response Station-8

Interpret the following ECG strip:

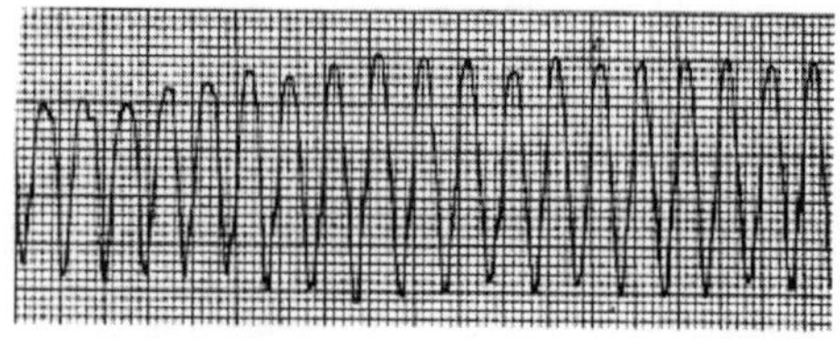

Name the condition: ....

IV. SIMULATED VERSUS REAL-LIFE OSCE STATIONS

This is one of the controversial issues; however, most of the clinicians support real-life OSCE station for procedures. A study conducted on the preference and efficacy of simulation versus real-life OSCE station revealed that students preferred and felt comfortable in simulated stations. But candidates who performed better over simulators were not found to be confident real-life practitioners. However, simulators and real-life OSCE stations have their unique positive aspects as discussed below (Fig. 7.11):

The positive aspects of simulated OSCE stations are as follows:

- They are controlled and safe.
- Feedback from modern sophisticated simulators can be obtained.
- Simulators are readily available when required.
- Simulated stations can be tailored to the level of skill to be assessed.

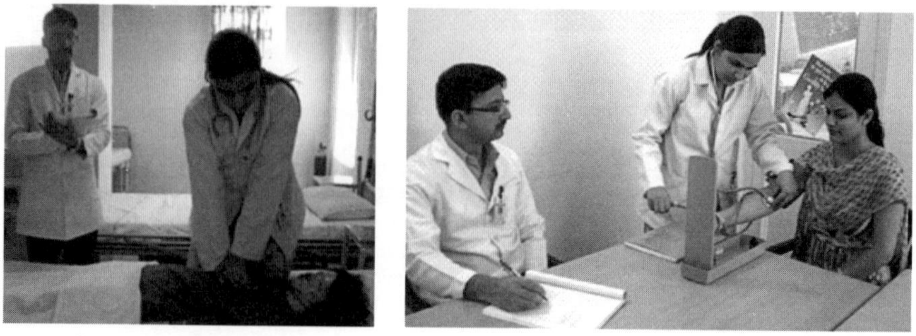

Simulated OSCE station | Real life OSCE station

Figure 7.11

Simulated versus real-life situation for an OSCE station.

- Scenarios that are distressing to real patients can be simulated.
- In simulated stations, the patient variable in examination is uniform across trainees.

The positive aspects of real-life OSCE stations are as follows:

- Real-life stations provide actual competence of a person on performance because idealized 'textbook' scenarios may not mimic real-life situations.
- They allow assessment of complex skills which may not be possible at simulated stations.
- Real-life situations may be more cost-effective.

V. PROBLEMS OF USING OSCE IN THE INDIAN SCENARIO

The main reasons OSCE has not become a routine assessment method for clinical examination of nursing students either for formative or summative evaluation in India are as follows:

- Lack of feasibility due to time constrains.
- Shortage of training for use of OSCE.
- Shortage of observers/examiners.
- Lack of interest in examiners.
- Lack of enforced guidelines for practical examination by universities (number of students examined and format of evaluation used).

A. ADVANTAGES OF OSCE

- More valid than the traditional approach to clinical examinations.
- Examiners can decide in advance what is to be tested and can then design the examination to test these competencies.
- Examiners can have better control on the content and complexities.
- Emphasis can be moved away from testing factual knowledge to testing a wide range of skills including advanced clinical skills.
- More reliable because variables of the examiner and the patient are removed to a large extent.
- The use of checklists by examiners and the use of MCQs results in a more objective examination.
- More practical because it can be used with a large numbers of students.

B. DISADVANTAGES OF OSCE

- Students' knowledge and skills are tested in compartments and they are not tested on their ability to look at the patient as a whole.
- Demanding for both examiners and patients.
- Examiners are required to pay close attention to students repeating the same task on a number of occasions.
- The time involved in setting up the examination is greater than for the traditional examination.
- Maintaining uniform difficulty levels is not always possible.

SELF-EVALUATION

It is well said that 'no one knows better than self' and self-evaluation has gained more importance recently and been utilized more frequent in the field of education including nursing education. Self-evaluation is the process of systematically observing, analysing and improving one's own actions or results. Self-evaluation can be defined as:

- Self-evaluation is a process of critical evaluation of one's performance, in which explicit criteria are being used to scrutinize and appraise work against a set of agreed upon standards.
- Self-evaluation is defined as the evaluation or judgement of 'the worth' of one's performance and the identification of one's strengths and weaknesses with a view to improving one's learning outcomes.
- Self-evaluation is a procedure to systematically observe, analyse and value own professional action and its results in order to stabilize or improve it.
- Self-evaluation is defined as learners judging the quality of their work, based on evidence and certain criteria, for the purpose of improvement.

PURPOSES OF SELF-EVALUATION

- Objectively reflect on and critically evaluate their own progress and skill development.
- Identify gaps in their understanding and capabilities.
- Discern how to improve their performance.
- Learn independently and think critically.

STEPS OF SELF-EVALUATION

There are seven steps of self-evaluation, which are detailed below and also illustrated in Fig. 7.12.

1. ***Set measurable goals:*** The first step in self-evaluation is to set and clarify effective goals, against which one can assess their performance.
2. ***Providing criteria:*** Generation of specific criteria is essential to generate internal feedback or setting the standard against which one can assess themselves.
3. ***Giving opportunities:*** Preparation of multiple opportunities to assess own performances help to close the gap between current performance and the desired performance.
4. ***Record information about changes:*** The next step is to continue collecting information that will help to see the progress.
5. ***Interpret the data:*** Interpretation of data is to ensure the accuracy and relevancy of data according to the set objectives.
6. ***Draw actionable conclusions and using results as feedback:*** In this a reasonable conclusion is made according to the interpretation of the findings. In this step, students use the results as feedback.

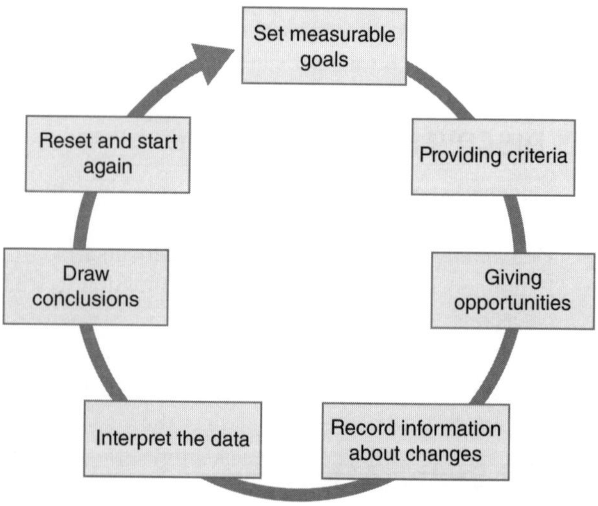

Figure 7.12

Steps of self-evaluation.

7. ***Reset and start again:*** If the goals have not been met to a great extent, then it is essential to reconsider the goals and organize subsequent learning activities.

The following are some of the questions used in the self-evaluation tool.

- 'What have I learned this week?'
- 'What do I need to do to further my personal development?'
- 'What specific areas do I need to consider for future learning?'

ADVANTAGES OF SELF-EVALUATION

- This method is a very simple but very effective means of allowing students time to reflect on their learning and development.
- It offers students how to write a detailed analysis of their performance, identifying their strengths and weaknesses in various areas.
- It allows learners to think about, reflect on, and jot down their issues and constraints.
- Students have the opportunity to forecast their primary goals for the future year and consider career opportunities.
- It aids in setting future goals and considering professional development and training needs.
- There is no peer pressure when students evaluate themselves.
- It encourages learners to take a more active role in their own education.
- It assists students in developing their analytical abilities.

DISADVANTAGES OF SELF-EVALUATION

- Self-evaluation is subjective, as learners may be untruthful or even exaggerate their own performance.
- It takes a lot of time for learners.
- It is possible that students are unfamiliar with the assessment standards.

CLINICAL PORTFOLIO

The term 'portfolio evaluation' has a lot of different connotations. A portfolio is a collection of student work that showcases a student's accomplishments, progress and efforts in a variety of areas. In simple words, a clinical portfolio is a record of clinical activities that represents the students learning activities according to the areas set in the curriculum. A portfolio assessment might be a collection of student-selected work experiences or papers linked to the outcome being evaluated. It can help students achieve academic objectives such as achieving predetermined clinical competencies. Clinical portfolio can be defined as:

- The South African Qualifications Authority defines a portfolio as the 'collection of different types of evidence relating to the work being assessed. It can include a variety of work samples' (SAQA, 2001).
- 'A clinical portfolio is a private collection of evidence that demonstrates the continuing acquisition of skills, knowledge, understanding and achievement in clinical areas. It is both retrospective and prospective, as well as reflecting the current stage of development and activity of the individual' (Norman, 2008).
- 'A portfolio provides evidence of a person's competence and reflective thinking, and illustrates critical analysis skills and self-directed learning' (Scholes et al., 2004).

STEPS IN CLINICAL PORTFOLIO

1. Determine and decide the purpose of the portfolio and setting the learning outcomes.
2. Setting the contents of portfolio according to the prescribed curriculum.
3. Selction of the grading or assessment criteria according to the desired objectives and content of portfolio.
4. Selection of outcomes of perfomance standards upon which evaluation can be made (e.g. examples of a high, medium and low scoring portfolio).
5. Preparation of general detailed instructions regarding the student activities (e.g. how students should collect, select, reflect, format and submit their work).

CONTENT OF CLINICAL PORTFOLIO

- A title page that includes the student's name, position and year of study, as well as the name of the supervisor.
- A contents page outlining the teachers' feedback and evaluation, recording experiences and mentoring, nursing process, educational activities, self-evaluation, etc.

ADVANTAGES OF CLINICAL PORTFOLIO

- It facilitates the student's active participation in the clinical setting, as well as reflection on his or her experiences and skills.
- A portfolio is an excellent way to demonstrate the shift from pedagogy to andragogy in learning styles.
- It enables a learner to accumulate and exhibit evidence of their strengths and proficiency of abilities in order to supplement traditional academic assessment methods.
- It monitors students' progress towards stated learning objectives and performance criteria embedded in the curriculum.
- It serves as a more comprehensive means of assessment throughout the curriculum.
- It facilitates the examination of areas that are difficult to evaluate using conventional approaches, such as emotions, personal characteristics, critical thinking and professionalism.
- It promotes more effective learning through constant reflection and the development of learning strategies.
- It establishes a consistent and longitudinal framework across the curriculum.
- It enables a mentor to assess a learner's abilities based on the contents provided in the portfolio.
- It is used to identify whether a learner is prepared to go to the next stage of learning.
- It can be utilized to determine where an individual's learning is lacking.
- It streamlines the process of maintaining current curriculum vitae.
- It can facilitate a process in which a learner engages in self-reflective, personalized professional growth.
- It can serve as a repository for procedure/clinical experience/encounter data.

DISADVANTAGES OF CLINICAL PORTFOLIO

- Faculty time is needed to create the portfolio assignments and to help learners to complete it. Arrangement of logistics can be difficult.

- Students are expected to retain and compile their own work, which is typically done outside of class. It may be challenging to persuade students to take the portfolio seriously.
- Transferred students may struggle to adhere to programme-portfolio criteria.

CLINICAL LOGS

A clinical log is used as part of a student learning portfolio, to monitor the quantity and quality of student early and longitudinal clinical experience provided in healthcare setting. It is created as a longitudinal self-directed organized record of student learning activities, with reflection on these activities for personal and professional development, and learning activities planned or taken. The clinical log can be defined as:

- The clinical log specifies the types of patients and clinical conditions to be encountered, the skills to be performed, the appropriate clinical settings for these experiences and the expected levels of medical student responsibility.
- The clinical logs are the repository of activities regarding the attainment of professional competencies prescribed in each course's clinical disciplines and learning objectives.

PURPOSES OF CLINICAL LOGS

- To facilitate development of students' reflective skills with recording of increasing level of involvement and confidence over time.
- To cultivate an attitude of critical reflection during the course of learning and to provide feedback on learning progress to students and the institution.

USE OF CLINICAL LOGS FOR CLINICAL EVALUATION

The following criteria outline the optimal use of clinical logs in clinical teaching and evaluation.

1. Make use of all available resources and avoid duplicating previously completed tasks.
2. Keep evaluation structured, succinct and precise.
3. Use an easy-to-read structure.
4. Integrate the logbook into the curriculum, which implies that the curriculum's learning outcomes and the log's learning objectives should be aligned.
5. Serve as a mentor and oversee learning objectives.
6. Make time and space available for the instructions and learning.
7. Establish an easy-to-follow workflow that includes updating log content, printing and storing it, turning it over to trainees, academic staff or mentors, introducing and explaining the log's use, inspecting and collecting them, and reviewing them at the conclusion of the educational period.
8. Communicate with students. The information should include a formal introduction to logs and its contents, a discussion of the clinical log's purpose and a recommendation to view every circumstance as an opportunity to learn.
9. Train supervisors and mentors, which includes repeated instruction on how to utilize the clinical logbook in clinical evaluation and providing recommendations for evaluation on the fly, as well as information regarding the logbook's structure, content and purpose.

ADVANTAGES OF CLINICAL LOGS

- Clinical logs compile a list of learning objectives to ensure that clinical training adheres to uniform educational standards.
- Clinical logs provide a concise assessment of clinical training criteria and their current stage of fulfilment.
- Clinical log records are especially beneficial when clinical training takes place across many sites.
- Clinical logs enable supervisors and trainees to quickly determine which learning objectives remain unachieved and to develop a learning plan.
- Clinical logs assist trainees and clinical teachers in communicating.
- Standardized clinical logs in clinical training can result in an increase in the quantity and quality of procedures performed.
- Log analysis can show training weaknesses and determine whether trainees have met the training's basic criteria.

DISADVANTAGES OF CLINICAL LOG

- It is time-consuming.
- There might be variability in grading the students by different teachers; thus have significant risk of subjectivity.
- It seems difficult to create a clinical log which is simple to use and still yield reliable and valid data.
- Students may fill information dishonestly.

ASSESSMENT OF ATTITUDE

The main intended outcome of nursing education is not only to develop knowledge and skills among budding nurses but also to focus on achieving desired change in their behaviour, which may include developing integrity, honesty, dependability, reliability, confidentiality and ethical professional behaviour. Achieving desired behaviour is more important than merely gaining knowledge and skills. Therefore, it is important to assess the desired changes in attitude and behaviour of nursing student in nursing discipline. There are different methods to measure the change in attitude, and some of the most commonly used methods or attitude-measuring scales such as Likert scale and semantic differential scale have been described in this chapter.

ATTITUDE SCALES

An attitude is a dispositional readiness to respond to certain situations, persons or objects in a consistent manner, which has been learned and has become one's typical mode of response. An attitude has a well-defined object of reference. For example, one's views regarding a class of food or drink, sports and math are attitudes.

A scale is a device designed to assign a numeric score to people to place them on a continuum with respect to attributes being measured, like a scale for measuring attitudes or weight. These rating scales are used to assess the attitudes and feelings of self-concept. The expressions in view of any point are accounted as measurements towards any item, object or concept. It shows a person's positive or negative attitude towards any concept. Measuring the score between two opposite words tells us the attitude, feeling and perception of a person or study subject towards the directions of positive or negative attitude in a scale. Visual scales illustrate visual depiction of any culture; photographs are given to get feelings, belief, opinions about contrast, texture, colour and elements.

I. TYPES OF ATTITUDE SCALES

There are two attitude scales commonly used to assess the attitude of individuals: Likert scale and semantic differential scale.

LIKERT SCALE

Likert scale was named after a psychologist Rensis Likert, who developed it in 1932 as a psychological concept measurement scale. Likert scale is the most commonly used scaling technique. It was developed to measure the attitudes, values and feelings of people. Primarily, the original version of this scale was developed with a five-point scale (strongly agree, agree, uncertain, disagree and strongly disagree) containing a mixture of positive and negative declarative statements regarding measuring variables (Box 7.11). However, one can even observe the Likert scale now with four point (strongly agree, moderately agree, disagree and uncertain) to seven point (very strongly agree, strongly agree, agree, uncertain, disagree, strongly disagree and very strongly disagree) scaling categories.

I. DEFINITIONS OF A LIKERT SCALE

Likert scale is a composite measurement scale used to measure attitude, values and feelings of the people that involve summation of scores on the set of positive and negative declarative statements regarding measuring variables to which respondents are asked to indicate their degree of agreement or disagreement.

Likert scale is a composite measure of attitudes that involve summation of scores on set of items (statements) to which respondents are asked to indicate their degree of agreement or disagreement.

BOX 7.11 EXAMPLE OF THE FIVE-POINT LIKERT SCALE TO ASSESS THE ATTITUDE WITH HIV/AIDS

	Please Tick (√) in Appropriate Column for Each Statement				
Statement	***Strongly Agree***	***Agree***	***Uncertain***	***Disagree***	***Strongly Disagree***
1. Person with multiple sex partners are at high risk of AIDS					
2. You can get AIDS by sharing utensils					
3. You may have HIV by sharing needles with others					
4. Only gay men can get AIDS					
5. One way of getting AIDS is infected blood transfusion					
6. AIDS is a curable disease					

II. USES OF A LIKERT SCALE

- It is basically used to measure the attitudes, values and feelings of the people about a specific concept such as a situation, people, place, object, programme, practice and policy.
- This scale is used to have quantified measurement of the qualitative attributes of people such as feelings, values and attitude.
- It may also be used to assess the opinion of people about a particular abstract concept.
- It spreads out people with various attitudes, emotions and feelings towards a particular concept.

III. CHARACTERISTICS OF A LIKERT SCALE

The main characteristics of a Likert scale are as follows:

- ***Psychological measurement tool:*** Likert scale is basically a psychological measurement tool to assess the attitudes, values and feelings of the people about a specific concept.
- ***Illustrative in nature:*** This scale is generally illustrative in nature, where each statement in the scale is stated in an explicitly graphical way so that a person can make a clear judgement about the degree of agreement or disagreement with the particular item of scale.
- ***Neutral statements:*** The scale must contain neutral statements without incorporation of any bias of the evaluator.
- ***Bipolar scaling method:*** This is composed with an alternative mixture of positive and negative declarative statements, so that the respondent's casual response bias can be eliminated. Positive statements get a high score with agreement and negative statements get a high score with disagreement with the statement.
- ***Measurement of the specific number of scaling categories:*** This scale is originally developed with five scaling categories and later the scales even develop with four, six and seven scaling categories.

IV. SCORING OF THE LIKERT SCALE

Scoring of the Likert scale is done on the basis of the type of statement and the level of the respondents' agreement with the statement.

- For a positive statement, respondents get a higher score if there is agreement with a statement. However, in case of negative statements, respondents get a higher score if there is disagreement with a statement or vice versa as depicted in Box 7.12.

BOX 7.12 SCORING OF STATEMENTS IN LIKERT SCALE

Statement	Strongly Agree	Agree	Uncertain	Disagree	Strongly Disagree
(Positive statement) 1. Person with multiple sex partners are at high risk of AIDS	5	4	3	2	1
(Negative statement) 2. You can get AIDS by sharing utensils	1	2	3	4	5

V. GUIDELINES FOR THE CONSTRUCTION OF LIKERT SCALE

- A five-point or seven-point Likert scale may be designed with appropriate degrees of agreement and disagreement phrases.
- The statements should be brief, concise and precise.
- Each statement should convey only one complete thought. More than one idea should not be included in a single statement; it is better to construct more statements.
- The statement should belong to the attitude variable that is to be measured.
- Care should be taken about language:
  - use simple sentences
  - avoid double negatives
  - avoid: all, always, none or never
  - use with care: only, just, merely
  - avoid words with more than one meaning.
- The statements should cover the entire range of the affective scale of interest.
- Statements should be such that they can be endorsed or rejected (agreed/disagreed).
- Acceptance and rejection should indicate something about the attitude measured.

A. ADVANTAGES OF A LIKERT SCALE

- It is relatively easy to construct this scale.
- Likert scale is considered a more reliable and valid tool to measure psychosocial variables.
- It is easy to administer as the respondents only have to place a tick in the provided spaces against each statement.
- It is less time consuming during construction and administration.

B. DISADVANTAGES OF A LIKERT SCALE

- In a Likert scale, the respondents may feel forced to answer the question against each preplanned item and its categories.
- Feelings of the respondents may not be fully assessed due to researcher's preplanned statements and categories.
- Difficulty in justifying the selection of the number of categories and numerical assignment to these categories.
- Casual approach of respondents in these scales may provide misleading data.

SEMANTIC DIFFERENTIAL SCALE

Semantic differential scale is the most effective and most widely used technique these days. In 1967, Osgood, Suci and Tannenbaum introduced this method for the first time in their book, *The Measurement of Meaning*. Although the original purpose of the scale was not necessarily to measure the assessment of attitude, the procedure was well adopted for attitude assessment.

Semantic differential questions measure people's attitude towards stimulus, words, objects and concepts. This question type consists of a series of contrasting adjective pairs (e.g. good–bad, beneficial–harmful) listed on opposite ends of a bipolar scale. Many studies have shown that semantic differential questions can work effectively with different age groups, cultures and languages. This scale is popular

Experience Working with Patients

Unpleasant	1	2	3	4	5	6	7	Pleasant
Rude	1	2	3	4	5	6	7	Polite
Cold	1	2	3	4	5	6	7	Warm
Callous	1	2	3	4	5	6	7	Considerate
Inhuman	1	2	3	4	5	6	7	Human
Noncommunicative	1	2	3	4	5	6	7	Communicative
Disrespecting	1	2	3	4	5	6	7	Respectful
Insincere	1	2	3	4	5	6	7	Friendly
Unconcern	1	2	3	4	5	6	7	Empathy

Figure 7.13

Example of a semantic differential scale to assess the attitude of student nurses towards patients.

because it is extremely easy to construct and administer and provides reasonably valid and reliable quantitative data. An example of a semantic differential scale to assess the attitude of student nurses towards patients is illustrated in Fig. 7.13.

I. DEFINITION OF A SEMANTIC DIFFERENTIAL SCALE

Semantic differential scale is a type of rating scale designed to measure the connotative meaning of objects, events and concepts. These connotations are used to derive the attitude of the objects, events and concepts.

II. CONSTRUCTING A SEMANTIC DIFFERENTIAL SCALE

For the preparation of semantic differential scale, the following adjective pairs are used (Box 7.13):

- The bipolar adjective pairs can be used for a wide variety of subjects.
- The adjective pairs are selected according to the objectives of the survey.
- The adjective pairs can be grouped into three large categories and each survey question usually includes a few points from each category. These categories are evaluation, potency and activity.
- Often, the attitude scale needs to be constructed for a particular aspect that one wishes to measure and the following steps are used in construction of an attitude scale:
    - Specify the attitude variable that is to be measured.
    - Collect a wide variety of statements.
    - Edit the statements.
    - Sort out the statements into (an imaginary) scale.
    - Calculate the scale value.

A. ADVANTAGES OF A SEMANTIC DIFFERENTIAL SCALE

- A convenient method to assess beliefs, attitudes and values in quantitative form.
- Easy to administer.
- Provides reasonable, valid and reliable quantitative data.

BOX 7.13 ADJECTIVE PAIRS USED FOR CONSTRUCTION OF SEMANTIC DIFFERENTIAL SCALE

Evaluation	Potency	Activity
Good — Bad	Hard — Soft	Active — Passive
Kind — Cruel	Strong — Weak	Fast — Slow
Wise — Foolish	Heavy — Light	Hot — Cold
Beautiful — Ugly	Deep — Shallow	Motivated — Aimless
Happy — Sad	Potent — Impotent	Moving — Still
Sociable — Unsociable	Large — Small	Excitable — Calm
Friendly — Unfriendly	Simple — Complex	Alive — Dead
Willing — Unwilling	Difficult — Easy	Emotional — Unemotional
Honest — Dishonest	Submissive — Assertive	Bright — Dim

B. DISADVANTAGES OF A SEMANTIC DIFFERENTIAL SCALE

- It is difficult to select the relevant concepts that are appropriate for any given investigations.
- It is time consuming, if anyone is not able to find the appropriate adjective pairs.

ASSESSMENT TESTS FOR HIGHER LEARNING

Assessments tests for higher education are crucial in measuring the effectiveness and quality of education. Assessments help and answer various questions about student development, the value of specific courses and the credibility of an institution. The assessment for higher learning is best described 'as a process by which assessment information is used by teachers to adjust their teaching strategies, and by students to adjust their learning strategies'.

METHODS FOR HIGHER LEARNING ASSESSMENT

There are many types of assessment methods for testing higher learning. These include rating scales, extended matching items, critical reading papers, clinical vignettes, modified essay questions (MEQs), extended multiple-response questions, matrix or grid type questions, interpretative questions, hot spot questions, drag and drop (cloze) type questions and ordered response questions. Some of the most commonly used methods and techniques for assessing higher education, that is interpretative questions, hot spot questions, drag and drop questions and ordered response questions are discussed in this section.

INTERPRETATIVE QUESTIONS

An interpretive question has an answer that can be supported with evidence from the text. Interpretative questions may be answered differently by different students, but the evaluator still can consider each different answer correct as long as evidence supports the answer of the question. Interpretative questions can be defined as:

- 'An interpretive question has more than one answer that can be supported with evidence from the text'.

- 'Interpretive questions ask students to make inferences about the meaning of a selection. More than one answer to an interpretive question can be considered correct. However, answers to interpretive questions must be supported by evidence in the selection'.

GUIDELINES TO DEVELOP INTERPRETIVE QUESTIONS

The following guidelines can assist in the development of good interpretive items:
- The opening material should be contextually appropriate.
- This item's effectiveness is contingent upon the introductory information. It should not be overly basic or very complicated.
- The introduction content should be appropriate for the students' curricular experience and reading abilities.
- The introduction should provide unique material. It should not be the same as the ones used in instruction.
- The introduction content should be concise and informative.

ADVANTAGES OF INTERPRETIVE QUESTIONS

- Allows one to test knowledge through the use of media that might be encountered in everyday situations (e.g. charts, pictures, etc.).
- Measure more complex knowledge through the analysis of data.
- Since there are several questions about the same information, it is possible to measure more reasoning skills in greater depth.
- Because it establishes a same structure for all students and evaluates them objectively, the findings are more reliable.

DISADVANTAGES OF INTERPRETIVE QUESTIONS

- Difficult to construct and time consuming.
- The exam items must correspond to the educational goals and objectives.
- Possibly a heavy demand on reading skill and puts poor readers at disadvantage.

HOT SPOT QUESTIONS

Hot spot questions test higher congnitive abilities using image as a medium in which examinees respond by selecting an area or region within the image. A hot spot is a test item type that allows students to click areas on an image. With hot spot questions, candidates are presented with an image and they select an area or 'Hot Spot' on the picture as the answer. For example, identify the area where the nurse should place the stethoscope to auscultate heart sounds heard at the Erb's point (Fig. 7.14).

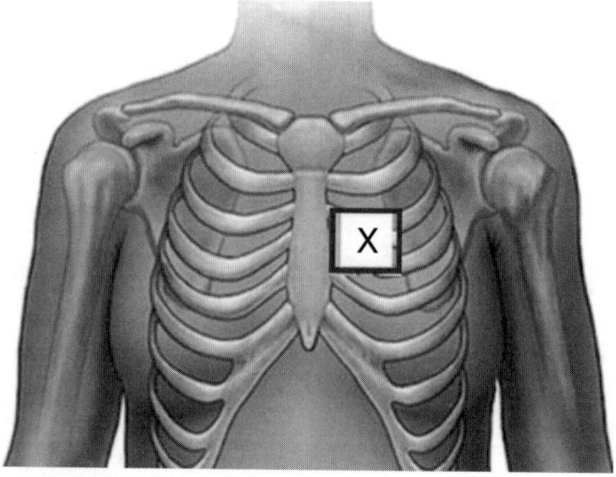

Figure 7.14

Example of hot spot question.

Q. The nurse performs a physical assessment on an adult client. Identify where the nurse places the stethoscope to auscultate the heart sounds heard at Erb's point.

ENHANCED HOT SPOT QUESTIONS

Furthermore, there are more complex host spot questions, which are named as 'Enhanced Hot-Spot Questions'. The enhanced hot spot questions generally present a case-study with details on health history and clinical progress of a patient, where student is asked to highlight the specific section which is related to particular clinical condition.

For example, 'Q. The nurse reviewing the patient's electronic health record to determine the patient's health status. Click to highlight the information in the record that would indicate to the nurse the patient is experiencing stroke'.

Electronic Health Record of Patient

The patient and his spouse were walking with their pet dog around 9.00 am. The spouse states that around 10.00 am during the walk, the patient suddenly started to report headache and dizziness, along with slurred speech, right-sided hemiplegia and confusion developed. The spouse called 108 ambulance and patient arrived in Emergency Room of nearby hospital by 11.00 am. The patient is alert and present with right-sided facial drooping with dysarthria, mild aphasia, no vision changes and right-sided hemiplegia. Vital signs are HR 99, BP 210/116, RR 15, oxygen saturation 98% on room air and temperature 98.8°F. Health history includes hypertension, smoker for last 30 years, hyperlipidemia, diabetes type-2, no head trauma or recent surgery and BMI is 32.

STEPS TO CREATE HOT SPOT ITEMS

The steps of hot spot items include determining the objectives of assessment, formulating the text item, inserting image, providing space to select specific part of image, provide reference and finally provide feedback (Fig. 7.15).

ADVANTAGES OF HOT SPOT QUESTIONS

- When compared to MCQs with single or multiple correct answer item type, a picture can supply more distracters and therefore is more useful for assessing higher learning.
- Faculty use visuals to help solidify key concepts and to ensure that students can correctly identify key components visually and not just in theory.
- Hot spot questions improve retention of knowledge as well as allow a student to demonstrate skills too in an effective manner.
- This item type is excellent when measuring visual content since it reduces the chance of cueing or guessing because participants can click on any portion of the image.

DISADVANTAGES OF HOT SPOT QUESTIONS

- Hot spot questions may be more difficult to develop because of the need to have an illustration as a reference point.
- Hot spot questions are more effective in computer application.

DRAG AND DROP QUESTIONS

Using drag and drop question is a good way to test higher learning. The phrase drag and drop describes the action of selecting an object or section of text, moving it (dragging) and then placing it (dropping) in an alternate area. It includes multiple drag sources and drop targets that require learners to match correctly. It is a type of e-learning and assessment questions in which users can select an object or a section of text and can move it to a desired location and 'drop' it there. In nursing education, drag and drop type of questions may also be used to assess correct sequence of clinical nursing procedure steps.

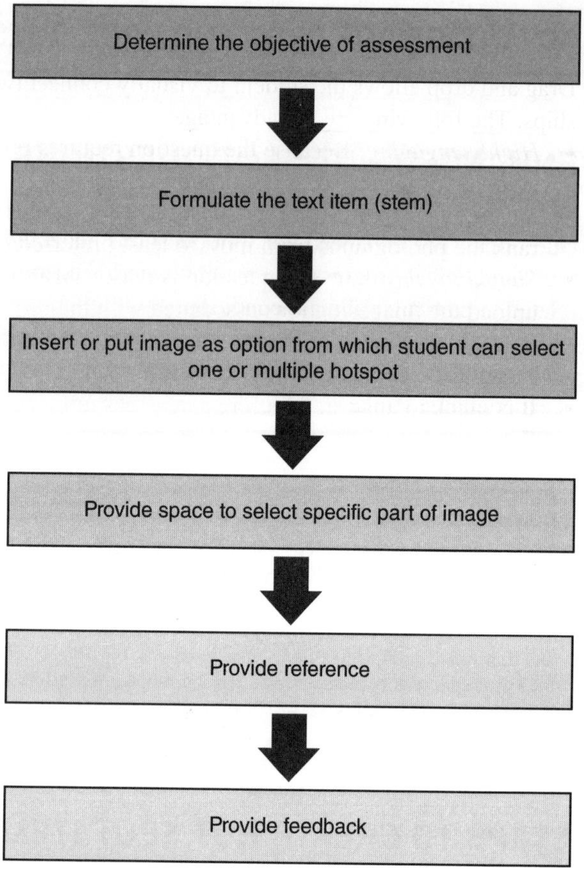

Figure 7.15

Steps to create hot spot items.

TYPES OF DRAG AND DROP QUESTIONS

1. ***Drag and drop into text:*** This question type can be used in various ways and can be a unique alternative to 'fill in the blank' style questions. Where 'fill in the blank' only allows one response that must be typed in by the student, drag and drop into text allows for multiple responses within one question.
2. ***Drag and drop markers:*** The second type of drag and drop question is the drag and drop markers. Drag and drop markers are primarily used for identifying items in an image.
3. ***Drag and drop onto image:*** The third type of drag and drop question is the drag and drop onto image. Images or text labels are dragged and dropped into specifically displayed drop zones on a background image.

WHEN TO USE DRAG AND DROP QUESTIONS

Drag and drop allows the students to visually connect two more objects or steps of a procedure and establish logical connections/relationships. The following are some examples where drag and drop type of questions may be used:

- Group items that are related or have something in common.
- Match an object to another object.
- Arrange elements in the proper order.
- Arrange steps of nursing procedure in the proper order.

ADVANTAGES OF DRAG AND DROP QUESTIONS

Drag and drop allows the student to visually connect two or more objects and establish logical relationships. The following are the advantages.

- *Highly engaging:* Because the question requires responders to physically drag and drop response alternatives into a list, it is extremely enticing.
- *Simple to comprehend:* This question style is quite straightforward. The respondent is required to rank the photographs from most to least preferred/liked.
- *Simple to construct:* The question is reasonably simple to create. The assessor is only required to upload the images/options associated with the response choices in the allocated area.
- It is a good method for testing dates, events, locations and persons.
- It can test recognition of relationships.
- It is quick to answer, therefore can assess more content.
- Easy and fast to score.

DISADVANTAGES OF DRAG AND DROP QUESTIONS

- Difficult to assess student learning beyond the recall level.
- It is time consuming to construct drag and drop type of questions.

ORDER RESPONSE QUESTIONS

An order response question asks respondents to order answer choices by way of preference. This allows assessor to not only understand how respondents feel about each answer option, but it also helps to understand each one's relative popularity. This type of question requires the analysis of many true assertions and then organize them appropriately, either sequentially (which comes first?) or according to their importance.

Order response question is defined as 'a question type that allows respondents to rearrange and rank multiple-choice options in a specific order'.

For example, in the question below:

Q. The nurse prepares to insert a nasogastric tube (NG tube) of an older female patient who has developed an intestinal obstruction. Arrange the following actions in the sequence in which they should be completed by the nurse. All available choices must be addressed.

A. Provide High Fowler's position to patient.
B. Lubricate the tube's tip with a lubricating jelly.
C. As the tube is inserted further, remind the patient to swallow.
D. Estimate the length of the tube starting at the tip of the nose and continuing to the earlobe and xiphoid process.
E. Secure the tube in place.
F. Through the naris, insert the tube. Gently press downward.

- You must be familiar with the procedure for inserting a nasogastric tube in order to answer this question. Assemble the steps in the correct order by mentally visualizing the method.
- You have the correct answer if you ranked the answer choices in this order: A, D, B, F, C, E.

The order response question provides the respondent with a list of items, created by evaluator, which they can rank according to their liking or knowledge. This allows respondents to compare different items to each other by placing them in order of how they score (or rank) at a specific aspect, such as steps of procedure, design, cost, functionality and importance. Often with the most important or preferred item ranked first or on top of the list.

ADVANTAGES OF ORDER RESPONSE QUESTIONS

- It helps to generate advanced respondent insights.
- It is effective in collecting feedback quickly.
- Respondents find it quite easy to answer them.
- It requires less time to answer.
- This type of question has higher response rate.

DISADVANTAGES OF ORDER RESPONSE QUESTIONS

- Calculation and interpretation are difficult. Order response questions are more difficult to analyse and comprehend than other types of questions.
- It compels responders to prioritize/order one item above another.
- It is easier for respondents to guess or answer randomly.

REVIEW QUESTIONS

LONG ANSWER QUESTIONS

1. Describe the advantages and disadvantages of essay type questions.
2. Describe the advantages and disadvantages of practical examinations.
3. Describe the advantages of MCQs.
4. Explain observational checklists.
5. Describe the criteria for the selection of evaluation techniques and devices.
6. Describe OSCE with examples.
7. Describe the types of reliability used for an assessment tool.
8. Describe the disadvantages of MCQs.
9. Explain Likert attitude scale.
10. List the purposes of educational evaluations and explain the qualities of an evaluation tool.
11. Describe the scope of evaluation.
12. Describe the validity of assessment tools.
13. Mention the criteria for the selection of evaluation methods.
14. Discuss the MCQs/items.

SHORT ANSWER QUESTIONS

1. Define evaluation.
2. Mention the parts of a MCQ with an example.
3. Give one example for any type of rating scale.
4. Write any two characteristics of MCQ.
5. List down the characteristics of a Likert scale.
6. Define OSCE.

7. Define summative and formative evaluation.
8. Mention the advantages of essay type questions.
9. Discuss the purposes of short answer questions.
10. Discuss the characteristics of a checklist.

MULTIPLE-CHOICE QUESTIONS (MCQs)

1. What do you mean by term *evaluation*?
   (a) Process of finding out the level of achievement based on predecided criteria
   (b) Measurement of quantity of pupil's attainment in a subject
   (c) By the use of some test check the performance of students
   (d) Testing the quality and quantity of students
2. Evaluation of students' performance is based on which law?
   (a) Law of effect
   (b) Law of motivation
   (c) Leadership law
   (d) Both (a) and (b)
3. Evaluation is a
   (a) Static process
   (b) Continuation process
   (c) Motivational process
   (d) Helpful only for students
4. Evaluation process involves
   (a) Teacher
   (b) Learner
   (c) Question
   (d) Teacher and learner
5. Evaluation process involves the maximum use of
   (a) Motivation
   (b) Learning
   (c) Knowledge
   (d) Insight
6. What do you mean by term *measurement*?
   (a) Quantifying and describing of pupil's achievement
   (b) It is a tool for measuring evaluation
   (c) It shows a measurement as 50 out of 100
   (d) All of these
7. Is measurement a part of evaluation?
   (a) Evaluation includes measurement and a wider process of judgement
   (b) Measurement includes evaluation and a wider process of judgement
   (c) Measurement includes evaluation and a narrow process of judgement
   (d) Evaluation includes measurement and a narrow process of judgement
8. Validity of an instrument varies with
   (a) Influence of extraneous variables
   (b) Difficult levels of items
   (c) Both (a) and (b)
   (d) Expert opinion

9. Validity of a measurement tool means
   (a) The accuracy with which a test measures whatever it is intended to measure
   (b) The inaccuracy is tested in this method to remove error
   (c) It is a degree of consistency of result when measured by particular instrument
   (d) It is a test–retest method
10. Reliability of a measurement tool means
   (a) A test measures whatever it is intended to measure
   (b) Consistency with which test measures a given variable
   (c) Both (a) and (b)
   (d) None of these
11. Which one of the following is the type of validity of a measurement tool?
   (a) Reality, concurrent, parallel, content, predictive validity
   (b) Content, reliability, face, predictive, content validity
   (c) Predictive, face, concurrent, content, construct validity
   (d) Face, construct, concurrent, reliability, content validity
12. What should be the quality of a good measurement tool?
   (a) Validity
   (b) Reliability
   (c) Practicability
   (d) All of these
13. Student evaluation is for what?
   (a) Motivation
   (b) Feedback
   (c) Certification of competence
   (d) All of these
14. Validity is measurement in
   (a) Degree: high, moderate, low
   (b) Levels: level 1, level 2, level 3
   (c) Present or absent
   (d) Consistent or nonconsistent
15. Approaches/methods used for establishing reliability of a measurement tool include
   (a) Mean, median and mode
   (b) Test–retest method and split half method
   (c) Mean, median, mode and range
   (d) Geometrical mean and test–retest method

ANSWERS OF THE MULTIPLE-CHOICE QUESTIONS

1. (a), 2. (d), 3. (b), 4. (d), 5. (a), 6. (a), 7. (a), 8. (c), 9. (a), 10. (b), 11. (c), 12. (d), 13. (d), 14. (c), 15. (b)

FURTHER READING

A guide to creating drag-and-drop quizzes in iSpring QuizMaker [Internet]. (2021). Explore the eLearning world with us. [cited 2021Dec14]. https://www.ispringsolutions.com/blog/how-to-make-drag-and-drop-quiz

Adams, R. J., Doig, B. A., & Rosier, M. J. (1991). *Science learning in Victorian schools: 1990, ACER Monograph No. 41*. Hawthorn, Vic.: Australian Council for Educational Research.

Anupama, K. (2019). Objective Structured practical examination (OSPE) in nursing. *International Journal of Evidence Based Nursing*, 2(2), 12–17.

Black, P., & Wiliam, D. (1998). Assessment and classroom learning. *Assessment in Education*, 5, 7–74.

Bloom, B. S., Hastings, T., & Madaus, G. (1971). *Handbook on formative and summative evaluation of student learning*. New York: McGraw-Hill.

Bowling, A. (2002). *Research methods in health: Investigating health and health services*. Buckingham, UK: Open University Press.

Bridge, P. D., Musial, J., Frank, R., Roe, T., & Sawilowski, S. (2003). Measurement practices: Methods for developing content-valid student examinations. *Medical Teacher*, 25, 414–421.

Brown, G., & Pendlebury, M. (1992). *Assessing active learning part 1: Core materials*. Sheffield, UK: CVCP Universities' Staff Development and Training Unit.

Brown, G., & Pendlebury, M. (1992). *Assessing active learning part 2: Illustrative examples of the core materials*. Sheffield, UK: CVCP Universities' Staff Development and Training Unit.

Brown, S., Rust, C., & Gibbs, G. (1994). *Strategies for diversifying assessment in higher education*. Oxford, UK: Oxford Centre for Staff Development.

Burnard, P. (1988). Self-evaluation methods in nurse education. *Nurse Education Today*, 8(4), 229–233.

Burns, R. (2000). *Introduction to research methods*. London, UK: Sage.

Case, S. M., & Swanson, D. B. (2001). *Constructing written test questions for the basic and clinical sciences* (3rd ed.). Philadelphia, PA: National Board of Examiners.

Crooks, T. J. (1988). The impact of classroom evaluation practices on students. *Review of Educational Research*, 58, 438–481.

Crossley, J., Humphries, G., & Jolly, B. (2002). Assessing health professionals. *Medical Education*, 36, 800–804.

Crow, L. D. (1951). *Introduction to education: Fundamental principles and practices*. New York: American Book Company.

Doig, B. A., Piper, K., Mellor, S., & Masters, G. (1994). *Conceptual understanding in social education, ACER Research Monograph No. 45*. Melbourne, Vic.: Australian Council for Educational Research.

El Idrissi, W. E., Chemsi, G., Kababi, K. E., & Radid, M. (2021). Assessment practices of student's clinical competences in nurse education. *The Open Nursing Journal*, 15(1), 47–54.

Evans, A. W., McKenna, C., & Oliver, M. (2002). Self-assessment in medical practice. *Journal of the Royal Society of Medicine*, 95(10), 511–513.

Gleeson, F. (1997). *AMEE Education Guide No. 9: Assessment of clinical competence using the objective structured long examination record (OSLER)*. Dundee: Association for Medical Education in Europe.

Gronlund, N. E. (1968). *Constructing achievement tests*. Englewood Cliffs, NJ: Prentice Hall Inc.

Gwenna Moss Centre for Teaching and Learning. (2018). *Methods of assessment: An introduction. Teaching and learning*. https://teaching.usask.ca/articles/methods-of-assessment.php. Accessed December 5, 2021.

Haladyna, T. M. (1999). *Developing and validating multiple-choice test items* (2nd ed.). Mahwah, NJ: Lawrence Erlbaum Associates.

Harden, R., & Gleeson, F. (1979). Assessment of clinical competence using an objective structured clinical examination (OSCE). *Medical Education*, 13, 41–54.

Harlen, W., & James, M. (1996). *Creating a positive impact of assessment on learning*. New York: Paper presented at the annual meeting of the American Educational Research Association.

Heidgerhen, L. E. (1994). *Teaching and learning in school of nursing, principles and method* (3rd ed., pp. 629–668). New Delhi: Konark Publish Pvt. Ltd.

Heidgerkan, L. E. (1966). *Teaching and learning in schools of nursing* (3rd ed.). Philadelphia: J B Lippincott Co.

Henrysson, S. (1971). Gathering, analyzing, and using data on test items. In R. L. Thorndike (Ed.), *Educational measurement* (2nd ed., pp. 130–159). Washington, DC: American Council on Education.

Hopkins, C. D., & Antes, R. L. (1990). *Classroom measurement and evaluation*. Itasca, IL: Peacock.

Importance of hot spot questions in teaching and assessment [Internet]. (2019). ExamSoft. [cited 2021Dec14]. https://examsoft.com/resources/importance-of-hot-spot-questions-in-teaching-and-assessment

Izard, J. (1991). *Assessment of learning in the classroom*. Geelong, Vic.: Deakin University.

Izard, J. (1997). *Trial testing and item analysis in test construction*. Paris: International Institute for Educational Planning.

Jeffries, P. R. (2012). Simulation in nursing education: From conceptualization to evaluation. In P. R. Jeffries (Ed.), *Simulation in nursing education: From conceptualization to evaluation* (2nd ed., pp. 1–25). National League for Nursing.

Johnson, L. M., Henderson, J. M., & Bates, A. (2019). Utilizing videotape-based assessment for competency evaluation in nursing education. *Journal of Nursing Education*, 58(10), 594–598. doi:10.3928/01484834-20190919-09

Jones, A. B., & Brown, C. D. (2018). Designing effective assignments for authentic assessment. In K. Miller & L. White (Eds.), *Assessment practices for higher education: Implications for student learning* (pp. 87–105). England: Routledge.

Khan, K. Z., Gaunt, K., Ramachandran, S., & Pushkar, P. (2013). The objective structured clinical examination (osce): Amee guide no. 81. Part II: Organization and administration. *Medical Teacher*, 35, e1447–e1463.

Klenowski, V. (1995). Student self-evaluation processes in student-centred teaching and learning contexts of Australia and England. *Assessment in Education: Principles, Policy & Practice*, 2(2), 145–163.

Lagoo, J. Y., & Joshi, S. B. (2021). Introduction of direct observation of procedural skills (DOPS) as a formative assessment tool during postgraduate training in anaesthesiology: Exploration of perceptions. *Indian Journal of Anaesthesia*, 65(3), 202–209.

Linn, R. L., & Gronlund, N. E. (2000). *Measurement and assessment in teaching* (8th ed.). Upper Saddle River, NJ: Prentice-Hall.

Liu, C. (2012). An introduction to workplace-based assessments. *Gastroenterology and Hepatology from Bed to Bench*, 5(1), 24–28.

Masters, G. N., Lokan, J., Doig, B., Khoo, S. T., Lindsey, J., & Robinson, L. (1990). *Profiles of learning: The basic skills testing program in New South Wales, 1989*. Hawthorn, Vic.: Australian Council for Educational Research.

Mehay, R., & Burns, R. (2009). Miller's pyramid of clinical competence. In R. Mehay (Ed.), *The Essential handbook for GP training and education*. London: Radcliffe Publishing Limited.

Mehrens, W. A., & Lehmann, I. J. (1984). *Measurement and evaluation in education and psychology* (3rd ed.). New York: Holt, Rinehart and Winston.

Miller, G. E. (1990). The assessment of clinical skills/competence/performance. *Academic Medicine*, 65(9), S63–S67.

Mollahadi, M., Khademolhoseini, S. M., Mokhtari-Nouri, J., & Khaghanizadeh, M. (2018). The portfolio as a tool for mentoring in nursing students: A scoping review. *Iranian Journal of Nursing and Midwifery Research*, 23(4), 241–247. doi:10.4103/ijnmr.IJNMR_195_17

Nayar, U., Malik, S. L., & Bijlani, R. L. (1986). Objective structured practical examination: a new concept in assessment of laboratory exercises in preclinical sciences. *Medical Education*, 20(3), 204–209.

Norcini, J. J. (2003). ABC of learning and teaching in medicine. Work based assessment. *BMJ*, 326(7392), 753–755.

Norcini, J., & Burch, V. (2007). Workplace-based assessment as an educational tool: AMEE Guide No. 31. *Medical Teacher*, 29(9-10), 855–871.

Norman, J., Riker, A., & Shellenbarger, T. (2017). Simulation as a tool to improve patient safety: Bridging the gap between theory and practice. *Nursing Clinics of North America*, 52(4), 597–609. doi:10.1016/j.cnur.2017.07.005

Oosterhoff, A. (2003). *Developing and using classroom assessments* (3rd ed.). Upper Saddle River, NJ: Pearson Education.

Osterlind, S. J. (1998). *Constructing test items: Multiple-choice, constructed-response, performance, and other formats* (2nd ed.). Norwell, MA: Kluwer Academic Publishers.

Ross, K. N. (1992). *Sample design procedures for a national survey of primary schools in Zimbabwe. Issues and methodologies in educational development #8*. UNESCO: IIEP.

Royal College of Nursing. (2008). *Advanced nurse practitioners: An RCN guide to the advanced nurse practitioner role, competencies and programme accreditation*. London: Royal College of Nursing.

Rushforth, H. (2007). Objective structured clinical examination (OSCE): Review of literature and implications for nursing education. *Nurse Education Today*, 27, 481–490.

Rust, W. B. (1973). *Objective testing in education and training*. London, UK: Pitman Education Library.

Schüttpelz-Brauns, K., Narciss, E., Schneyinck, C., Böhme, K., Brüstle, P., Mau-Holzmann, U., ... Obertacke, U. (2016). Twelve tips for successfully implementing logbooks in clinical training. *Medical Teacher*, 38(6), 564–569.

Singh, K., & Singh, A. (2021). Workplace-based assessment: a real-time assessment tool. *Journal of Medical Sciences*, 7(3), 204–210.

Smith, J. D., Johnson, L., & Thompson, R. (2020). The effectiveness of assignment-based assessment in promoting student learning outcomes. *Journal of Higher Education Assessment*, 12(2), 45–62. doi:10.1080/12345678.2020.1234567

Swanwick, T., & Chana, N. (2009). Workplace-based assessment. *British Journal of Hospital Medicine*, 70(5), 290–293.

Thampy, H., Willert, E., & Ramani, S. (2019). Assessing clinical reasoning: Targeting the higher levels of the pyramid. *Journal of General Internal Medicine*, 34, 1631–1636.

The truth behind interpretative exercises about IJSSB [Internet]. [cited 2021Dec13]. https://ijssb.com/images/vol4.no.2/6.pdf

Tinkelman, S. N. (1971). Planning the objective test. In R. L. Thorndike (Ed.), *Educational measurement* (2nd ed., pp. 46–80). Washington, DC: American Council on Education.

Traynor, M., Galanouli, D., Rice, B., & Lynn, F. (2016). Evaluating the objective structured long examination record for nurse education. *British Journal of Nursing*, 25(12), 681–687.

Waldner, M., & Olson, J. (2007). Taking the patient to the classroom: Applying theoretical frameworks to simulation in nursing education. *International Journal of Nursing Education Scholarship*, 4(1), 1–14.

Ward, H., & Barratt, J. (2005). Assessment of nurse practitioner advanced clinical practice skills: Using the objective structured clinical examination (OSCE). *Primary Health Care*, 15(10), 37–41.

Wass, V., Van der Vleuten, C., Shatzer, J., & Jones, R. (2001). Assessment of clinical competence. *Lancet*, 357, 945–949.

Wilkinson, J. R., Crossley, J. G. M., Wragg, A., Mills, P., Cowan, G., & Wade, W. (2008). Implementing workplace-based assessment across the medical specialties in the United Kingdom. *Medical Education*, 42, 364–373.

Witheridge, A., Ferns, G., & Scott-Smith, W. (2019). Revisiting Miller's pyramid in medical education: the gap between traditional assessment and diagnostic reasoning. *International Journal of Medical Education*, 10, 191–192.

Withers, G. (1997). *Item writing for tests and examinations*. Paris: International Institute for Educational Planning.

CHAPTER

Guidance and counselling

8

LEARNING OBJECTIVES

This chapter is designed to enable the reader to:

- Define guidance and counselling
- Distinguish between guidance and counselling
- Describe the purposes, needs, characteristics, scope and principles of guidance and counselling
- Classify the types of guidance services
- Demonstrate knowledge and skills of organization of counselling services
- Identify types of counselling approaches
- Explore the role and needed preparation of the counsellor
- Appraise the phases of counselling process
- Explain the tools and techniques used in counselling process
- Recognize the issues of counselling in nursing
- Discuss the strategies for management of disciplinary problem and crisis management
- Understand the concept of crisis intervention

KEY TERMS

INTRODUCTION

Everyone needs assistance at some time in his life; some will need it constantly and throughout their entire lives, while others need it at rare intervals at times of great crisis.

—Arthur J. Jones

Guidance and counselling are twin concepts and have emerged as essential elements of every educational activity. The much emphasized focus on a child's holistic development demands the education system be made comprehensive enough to foster all-round development. Professional guidance personnel can help students develop skills and competencies to facilitate their personal, social and career development. For a harmonious and integrated personality development of students in an institution, a healthy climate that fosters cognitive, behavioural, developmental and emotional growth is needed. Guidance and counselling plays an important role in education in this context.

Guidance and counselling are not synonymous terms. Counselling is a part of guidance. Guidance, in the educational context, means to indicate, point out, show the way, lead out and direct. Moreover, guidance means assisting students with selecting courses of study appropriate to their needs and interests, achieving academic excellence to the best possible extent, deriving the maximum benefit from institutional resources and facilities, inculcating proper study habits and their satisfactory participation in curricular and extracurricular activities.

Counselling is a specialized service of guidance. It is the process of helping individuals learn more about themselves and their present and possible future situations to make a substantial contribution to the society. It is also a process of solving one's own problems through a face-to-face relationship with the counsellor.

DEFINITIONS OF GUIDANCE AND COUNSELLING

I. DEFINITIONS OF GUIDANCE

Guidance is defined as assistance rendered by an expert to help an individual to manage his own point of view, make his own decisions and carry his own burdens.

Guidance is that aspect of educational programme which is concerned with helping the pupil to become adjusted to his present situation and plan his future in line with his interests, abilities and social needs.

—Hamrin and Erikson

Guidance is an assistance made available by a competent counselor to an individual of any age to help him direct his own life, develop his own point of view, make his own decision and carry his own burden.

—Crow and Crow

Guidance is a process of helping every individual, through his own efforts to discover and develop his potentialities for his personal happiness and social usefulness.

—Ruth Strang

Guidance is understanding a person and making himself, so that he may bring about in himself and in his environment such change through which his proper development becomes possible.

—Knapp

Guidance is a process which helps an individual to develop his personality fully and enables him to serve the society to the best of his capabilities and talents.

—Woodworth

Guidance is a continuous process of helping the individual for development in the maximum of their capacity in the direction most beneficial to himself and to society.

—**Stoops and Wahlquist**

Guidance is a process through which an individual is able to solve their problems and pursue a path suited to their abilities and aspirations.

—**J.M. Brewer**

Guidance involves personal help given by someone; it is designed to assist a person in deciding where he wants to go, what he wants to do, how he can best accomplish his purpose; it assists him in solving problems that arise in his life. It does not solve problems for the individual, but helps him to solve them. The focus of guidance is the individual, not the problem; its purpose is to promote the growth of the individual in self-direction.

—**Jones**

II. DEFINITIONS OF COUNSELLING

According to *Webster's Dictionary*, *counselling* is mutual consultation or deliberation. It involves a minimum of two people, the *counsellor* and the *counselee*. The counselee comes to the counsellor for counselling or consultation. In other words, counselling is talking to a professionally trained individual, who can help express pent-up feelings and emotions, provide an insight into these feelings and help the patient find solutions to problems.

Counselling, in the professional sense, is helping with counselee's problems, based on empirical studies and understanding of the individual, his interests, aptitudes and emotional maturity. Essentially, counselling is a one-to-one relationship where a professionally qualified individual tries to help another individual caught up in emotional conflict and difficult decision making.

Counseling is a helping process where one person purposefully gives his/her time, attention and skills to assist a client in exploring the situation, identifying and acting upon the solutions within the limitation of their given environment.

Counseling is a series of direct contacts with the individual which aims to offer him assistance in changing his attitude and behaviors.

—**Carl Rogers**

Counseling is essentially a process in which the counselor assists the counselee to make interpretations of facts relating to a choice, plan or adjustment which he needs to make.

—**Glenn F. Smith**

Counseling is an interactive process that facilitate meaningful understanding of self and environment and results in the establishment and or clarification of goals and values for future behaviour.

—**Stone and Sherzes**

Counseling is a dynamic and purposeful relationship between two people, who approach a mutually defined problem with mutual consideration of each other to the end that the troubled one or less mature is aided to a self-determined resolution of his problem.

—**C. Gilbert Wrenn**

Counseling is a process which takes place in a one-to-one relationship between an individual beset by problems with which he cannot cope alone and a professional worker whose training and experience have qualified him to help others reach solutions to various types of personal difficulties.

—Hahu and Maclean

Counseling is a personal and dynamic relationship between two individuals (one of whom is older, or more experienced, wiser than other), who altogether approaches a more or less well-defined problem of the younger or less experienced or less wise, with mutual consideration for each other to the end that the problem may be clearly defined and that the one who has the problem may be helped to a self-determined solution of it.

—A.J. Jones

DIFFERENCE BETWEEN GUIDANCE AND COUNSELLING

Guidance and counselling are generally used interchangeably or synonymously. However, they are not synonyms. The following points are presented to illuminate the differences between the basic concepts of guidance and counselling:

- Guidance is broader and comprehensive, whereas counselling is in-depth and narrows down the problems until patients are able to understand their own problems.
- Counselling helps people understand themselves and is an inward analysis. Alternative solutions are proposed to help understand the problem at hand. The focus of counselling is not on solution but on understanding the problem. The counsellor may be able to bring about an emotional change or a change in feelings. Guidance, on the other hand, is more external, helps a person understand alternative solutions available to him and makes him understand his personality and choose the right solution. The focus here is on finding solutions. Guidance may bring about an attitude change in the patient.
- Guidance is mainly preventive and developmental, whereas counselling is remedial as well as preventive and developmental.
- Intellectual attitudes are the raw material of guidance, whereas emotional rather than pure intellectual attitude are the raw materials of the counselling process.
- Decision making is operable at an intellectual level in guidance, whereas it operates at an emotional level in counselling.
- In the educational context, counselling is among the various services offered by the guidance programme.
- Guidance is generally education and career related and may also include personal problems. It is usually impersonal, whereas counselling is mostly offered for personal and social issues.

PURPOSES OF GUIDANCE AND COUNSELLING

Guidance and counselling services are an essential part of making proper use of human capabilities. Each of us finds ourselves at crossroads at some time in life; this is why guidance and counselling are an integral part of our lives. The main purposes of guidance and counselling are discussed in detail below (Fig. 8.1):

- ***Providing the needed information and assistance:*** Guidance and counselling is directed at providing and seeking information between two individuals as well as offering the desired assistance to an individual who requires help.

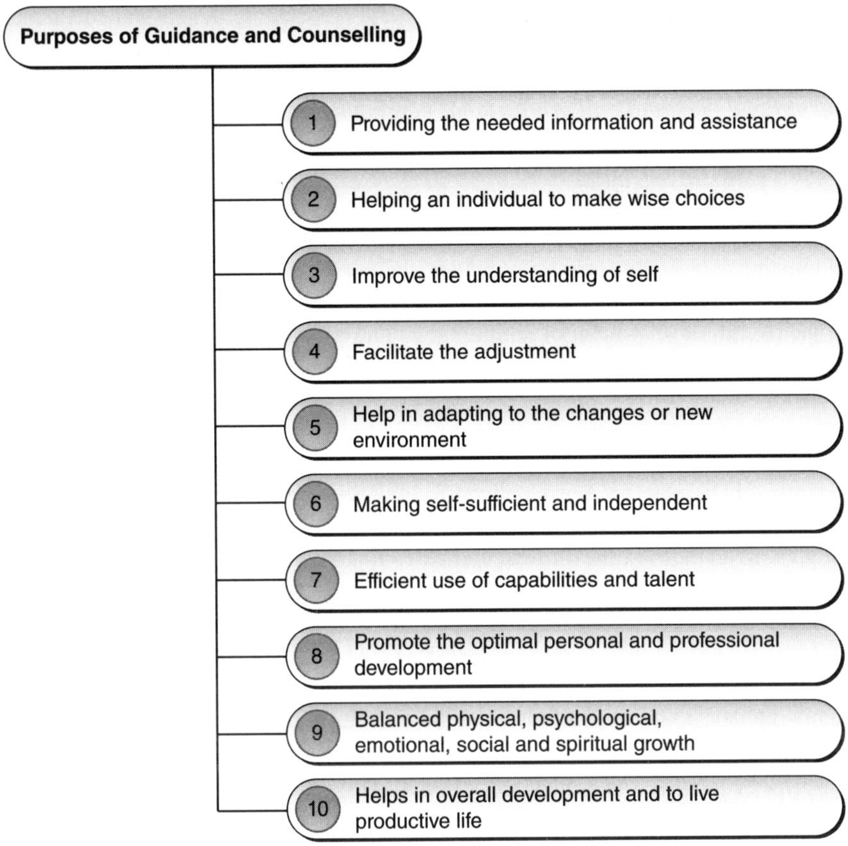

Figure 8.1

Purposes of guidance and counselling.

- ***Helping an individual make wise choices:*** Guidance and counselling is primarily offered to make an individual capable of judging each aspect (strength and weakness) of a situation and finally making a wise decision to use the available opportunities efficiently.
- ***Improve the understanding of self:*** Guidance and counselling helps the individual get a true understanding of self, where he becomes capable of evaluating each situation with full intellectual capabilities leading to holistic development.
- ***Facilitate adjustment:*** Adjustment is one of the most fundamental essentiality of an individual in personal and professional life. Guidance and counselling is the most efficient tool for facilitating the assessment and management of adjustment problems of individuals in demanding situations.
- ***Helping to adapt to changes or new environment:*** Guidance and counselling assists or helps students adapt according to tradition and the rules and regulations in a particular situation. It also helps in creating a feeling of cooperation in individuals that finally helps them adapt to new and challenging situations.
- ***Making self-sufficient and independent:*** Guidance and counselling provides opportunities for learning the essentials of self-direction with respect to educational, vocational and personal–social aspects of life. In addition, it also helps one to be self-sufficient and independent in managing demanding situations and day-to-day affairs.

- ***Efficient use of capabilities and talent:*** Guidance and counselling assists students make the maximum use of their capacities, interests and other abilities to achieve personal and academic goals.
- ***Promoting optimal personal and professional development:*** Guidance and counselling helps individuals in proper placement in all fields of their personal life and helps them in the development to their fullest capacity.
- ***Balanced physical, psychological, emotional, social and spiritual growth:*** Guidance and counselling helps individuals have balanced physical, psychological, emotional and social growth and development.
- ***Other functions of guidance and counselling:*** Some other functions of guidance and counselling helpful in the overall development of an individual and living a productive life are as follows:
    - To provide optimum development and well-being for individuals.
    - To help individuals adjust to themselves and the society.
    - To help people understand themselves in relation to the world.
    - To aid individuals in efficient decision making.
    - To help individuals plan for a productive life in their social context by focusing on their assets, skills, strengths and possibilities for further development.
    - To bring about changes in the attitude and behaviour of individuals.

CHARACTERISTICS OF GUIDANCE AND COUNSELLING

It is believed that guidance and counselling is as old as human existence and is found in each area and domain of human functioning (personal, professional, social, cultural and spiritual). Guidance and counselling is needed when people seek assistance to function optimally, both personally and professionally. Some of the most essential characteristics of guidance and counselling are as follows (Fig. 8.2):

- ***Continuous process:*** It is a continuous process starting in childhood and continuing through adolescence, adulthood and old age. Guidance and counselling is a dynamic process that helps individuals understand themselves and use their capacities, interests and other abilities to a maximum. Individuals continue to struggle for adjustment in different life situations to develop their capacity for effective decision making.
- ***Process of mutual interaction:*** Guidance and counselling is a process of mutual interaction where a trained person helps another person who needs his help for a general or specific problem.
- ***Definite purpose-oriented processes:*** Guidance and counselling is a well-planned, purpose-oriented process where two individuals, the person who is offering guidance and counselling and the person who is receiving guidance and counselling, interact keeping in mind the specific purpose to be achieved.
- ***Self-realization and self-direction:*** During the process of guidance and counselling, individuals are assisted in a way such that they are able to develop their capacities to the maximum extent. It helps individuals become familiar with their real self.
- ***Individual assistance:*** Guidance and counselling is the process of assisting individuals identify where to go, what to do and how to do, to accomplish their goals. An individual's personal development is promoted through guidance and counselling.
- ***Related with life events:*** The process of guidance and counselling is related with life events as individuals get both formal and informal guidance and counselling in their lifetime.
- ***Meant for everyone:*** All individuals need guidance and counselling to reach their maximum potential.

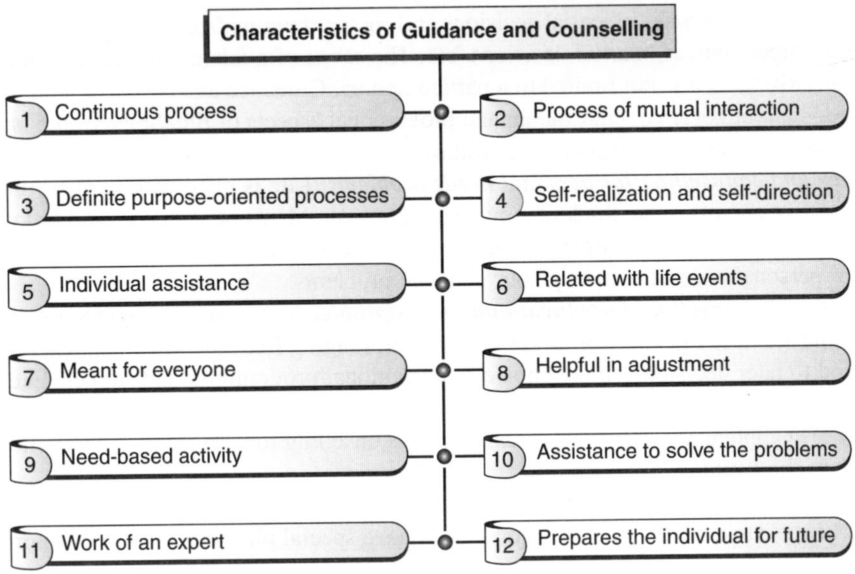

Figure 8.2

Characteristics of guidance and counselling.

- ***Helpful in adjustment:*** Guidance and counselling helps individuals adjust in different life situations.
- ***Need-based activity:*** Guidance and counselling is centred on the needs and aspirations of students. Guidance empowers individuals to discover their natural strengths so that they can use them to their best advantage making the maximum out of life.
- ***Assistance to solve problems:*** Guidance and counselling involves more than offering assistance in finding a solution to an immediate problem. Its function is to bring about changes in individuals and enabling them to deal with difficulties in a more productive and independent manner.
- ***Work of an expert:*** Providing guidance and counselling is the job of an expert. The person offering guidance and counselling services must be fully equipped with the skills to provide effective guidance and counselling services.
- ***Prepares the individual for future:*** It is well known that prevention is better than cure; therefore, individuals must be prepared and equipped to deal with future problems as quickly and efficiently as possible so that the problems can be assessed and managed before they become difficult to handle.

SCOPE OF GUIDANCE AND COUNSELLING

In ancient Indian societies, the scope of professional guidance and counselling was limited specifically because of the supportive social and joint family system. In this system, family members or people in close social proximity were considered an appropriate source of guidance and counselling. With rapid urbanization, industrialization and modernization, however, human life has become more complex. In modern Indian societies, most individuals are experiencing a strong need for professional guidance and counselling to help them make essential decisions and choices ranging from the choice of school, stream of education, career choices, marital decisions, etc. The scope of guidance and counselling is as broad as the human existence; it is not limited to a particular area. Guidance and counselling assists individuals in each domain of personal, educational and professional aspects of life. Some of the broad areas of the scope of guidance and counselling are as follows:

- ***Guidance and counselling for personal needs/problems:*** Life is filled with hurdles, obstacles and problems. Not one of us can think of someone with no problems or someone who has not needed any guidance in his or her lifetime. Therefore, guidance and counselling services are essential to meet our personal needs and manage our personal problems.
- ***Guidance and counselling for educational needs/problems:*** The scope of guidance and counselling services in education is very important; ranging from the selection of a school in childhood to later decisions on the choice of educational programmes and studies. Each teacher is, thus, provided with special training pertaining to guidance and counselling. Schools and colleges also appoint specialists in guidance and counselling to help students throughout the duration of their studies.
- ***Guidance and counselling for physical, emotional, social, moral and marital problems:*** Human beings are complex, social animals who have special physical, emotional, moral, social and marital needs and problems that need to be managed through professional guidance and counselling services. Appropriate guidance and counselling services help individuals maintain an optimal level of physical, emotional, moral, social and marital well-being and balance in his or her life.
- ***Guidance and counselling for vocational, occupational and professional needs:*** Vocational, occupational and professional guidance and counselling has a wide range of scope. Every individual has different potentialities, capabilities and abilities; through efficient guidance and counselling, individuals may be directed towards the right path at the right time so that they can achieve effective occupational and professional adjustment. Each institution imposes significantly different professional demands on individuals and has a wide scope of guidance and counselling services for their employees for better adjustment and work output.
- ***Guidance and counselling for career advancement:*** In ancient Indian societies, career options were available by chance and not by choices because individuals usually followed their family business/work. In modern societies, career is opted by choice so each one of us requires professional guidance and counselling to make a right career choice. Guidance and counselling has a very wide scope in this area.
- ***Guidance and counselling for holistic individual development:*** The main purpose of guidance and counselling is the holistic and all-round development of an individual. Guidance and counselling services have a very wide and essential scope towards optimum development of an individual.
- ***Guidance and counselling for situational problems:*** Individuals may experience adverse situations at any point in life; they may require professional assistance in the form of guidance and counselling. Some of the most critical situations that may require guidance and counselling services are given below:
  - Disease and disability
  - Discharge from hospital
  - Death of loved ones
  - Disaster and crisis
  - Divorce and marital disharmony
  - Debt and economic crisis

NEED OF GUIDANCE AND COUNSELLING

Guidance and counselling is an essential source for making effective use of human interest, values and capabilities. Problems are a part of everyone's personal and professional life and each individual needs guidance and counselling at some time in life for one reason or another. It is generally observed that individuals joining the nursing profession have several professional adjustment problems initially and they simply waste their time and energy if timely guidance and counselling services are not offered. It is evident that guidance and counselling is important in each sphere of human existence including nursing and nursing education so that its professionals and patients can benefit the most. The main needs of guidance and counselling in nursing and nursing education are discussed below (Fig. 8.3).

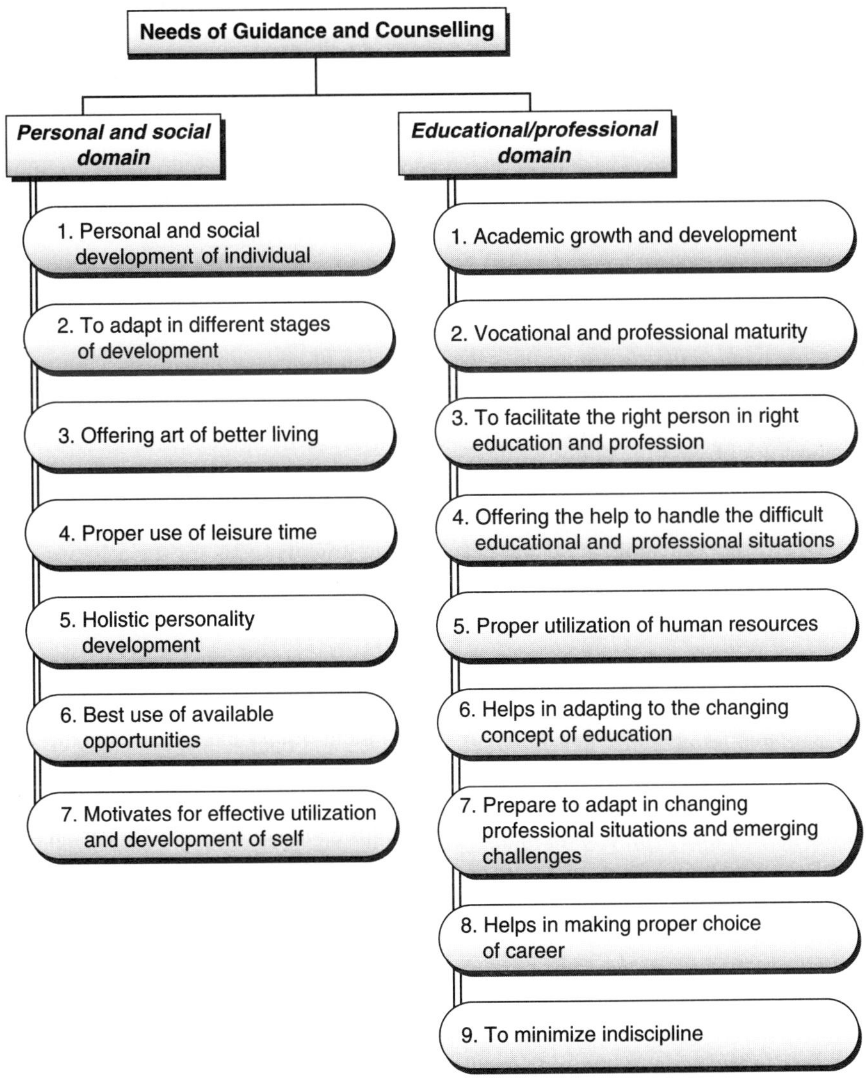

Figure 8.3

Need of guidance and counselling.

I. NEEDS FOR PERSONAL AND SOCIAL DOMAIN

- ***Personal and social development of individual:*** For the personal and social development of an individual, self-understanding and an adjustment with the self and society is necessary. It helps students adjust to their current situation at home, educational institution or community in the best possible way. Guidance and counselling helps students with their problems related to career planning and educational programming and gives them a direction in long-term personal aims and values. It is concerned with helping people achieve self-development and self-realization.
- ***To adapt in different stages of development:*** Every individual has passed through specific stages of development: infancy, childhood, preadolescence, adolescence and adulthood. On various occasions, there are interpersonal and intrapersonal clashes of interests for which guidance is needed. Without proper guidance, individuals may experience stress and strain. Guidance and counselling is essential to adapt to life's different developmental stages.
- ***Offering art of better living:*** Well-planned guidance and counselling services help individuals develop a proper attitude towards life and equip them to live a meaningful life with self-esteem and effective interpersonal relationships.
- ***Proper use of leisure time:*** These days, many people either indulge in drugs or gambling due to a lack of proper guidance. To keep them from such situations, individuals need to be guided to make use of their leisure time to enhance their education, status or adjustments in life.
- ***Holistic personality development:*** Guidance and counselling can help students understand the self and have a better understanding of their own abilities, aptitudes, intelligence and personalities so that they can choose their own path with ease and comfort.
- ***Best use of available opportunities:*** With the expansion of education, career opportunities have expanded as well. Guidance is needed to provide the youth with information regarding training, educational facilities, availability of jobs, avenues for promotion, etc. that will ultimately help him make the best use of possible opportunities.
- ***Motivates for effective utilization and development of self:*** Every individual needs a catalyst or spark to initiate movement in a particular direction. Guidance and counselling services are essential for effective self-utilization and development in individuals for the achievement of personal and professional goals.

II. NEEDS FOR EDUCATIONAL/PROFESSIONAL DOMAIN

- ***Helps in academic growth and development:*** Guidance and counselling is needed to help with the academic growth and development of individuals. It helps by eliminating problems related to the subject matter and developing abilities and skills according to changing situations.
- ***Helps in vocational and professional maturity:*** With the society getting industrialized so rapidly, young students need help with information about various jobs available to them and the requirements, responsibilities and nature of work involved in a particular job or career. Guidance and counselling services may help individuals attain the much needed vocational and professional maturity.
- ***Facilitates an individual in the right education and profession:*** Advancement in science and technology, rapid industrialization, global phenomenon and fast changing socioeconomic situations are imposing dilemmas in individuals to choose the right educational programme or professional stream choice. In such situations, guidance and counselling services can play an important role so that the individual can make the right choice of educational and professional options. This will ultimately lead to better socioeconomic growth of a country and satisfaction of the individuals.

- ***Offers help to handle difficult educational and professional situations:*** Individuals face many ups and downs in their personal and professional lives. Individuals must possess the qualities to handle positive and negative situations with the same strength and attitude. Guidance and counselling services may equip the individuals to respond positively to difficult situations in educational and professional pursuit.
- ***Helps in the proper utilization of human resources:*** With the help of guidance and counselling services, students can make the right choice of educational programmes or professions saving a lot of energy. When individuals make the right choice in education and profession at the right time, human resources may be used more efficiently without a waste of undue time and energy.
- ***Helps in adapting to the changing concept of education:*** The concept of education is changing with a rapid pace because of constant changing socioeconomic situations, science and technological development, cultural transformation and political and global interest. Efficient guidance and counselling services are needed to adapt to the changing concepts and demands of education in the current scenario.
- ***Prepares to adapt in changing professional situations and emerging challenges:*** In today's world, professions or occupations have become so varied and complex that everyone has to undergo training for adapting to the new emerging challenges of a particular profession. Hence, guidance is needed to equip individuals with the desired capabilities so that they can optimally adjust to the changing professional situations and emerging professional challenges.
- ***Helps in making proper career choice:*** Our educational system is very complex and competitive these days. Parents expect more from their children without caring for their abilities and aptitude leading to wrong career choices, which can ultimately affect their whole life. Therefore, well-planned, efficient guidance and counselling services must be offered to help individuals so that they can choose the right career option based on their abilities, interests, capabilities and aptitude.
- ***Helps to minimize indiscipline:*** Each individual has ample energy that needs to be channelized, otherwise individuals may engage themselves in nonproductive and destructive activities. Timely guidance and counselling services are needed for proper and optimum utilization of energy in productive and constructive activities.

BASIC PRINCIPLES OF GUIDANCE

Guidance is an essential and integral part of every educational programme to help students achieve the maximum self-understanding, self-insight and productive actions to be an intellectual and a useful member of the civilian society. For a better understanding of guidance, one must learn its basic principles. A few eminent educationists and philosophers gave their views on guidance which were later recognized as the principles of guidance. These principles are discussed below.

I. ACCORDING TO CROW AND CROW

Crow and Crow gave the following principles of guidance:

- ***All-round development of individuals:*** Every aspect of a person's complex personality pattern constitutes a significant factor of his or her total displayed attitudes and forms of behaviour. Guidance services aimed at bringing about desirable adjustments in a particular area of experience must take into account the all-round development of the individual.

- ***Principle of individual differences:*** No two individuals are alike. Although all human beings are similar in many respects, individual differences must be recognized and considered in any effort aimed at providing help or guidance to a particular student.
- ***Guidance is related to every aspect of life:*** The guidance programme should be related to all aspects of life, study an individual's physical and mental hygiene, his or her family and school and social and vocational needs.
- ***Cooperation among persons:*** The existing social, economic and political unrest gives rise to many maladaptive factors that require the cooperation of experienced and thoroughly trained guidance workers and the individuals with the problem.
- ***Guidance is a continuous and lifelong process:*** The guidance process is continuous and goes on lifelong from childhood to adulthood. The occurrence of problems in life and efforts for their solution are natural and, hence, the need for guidance always persists.
- ***Guidance for all:*** The main principle of guidance is that it is not for a specific person but for everyone. A person may need guidance at every step of life. Guidance services should not be limited to the few who give observable evidence of its need but should be extended to people of all ages who can be benefited either directly or indirectly.
- ***Principle of elaboration:*** Curriculum materials and teaching procedures should evidence a guidance point of view. In addition, guidance services should be as elaborative as possible so that the beneficiaries can take its best possible advantage.
- ***Responsibility of teachers and parents:*** Parents and teachers have guidance-appointed responsibilities. The responsibilities for administration of the guidance programme should be centred by a personally qualified and adequately trained person, working cooperatively with his or her assistance and other community welfare and guidance agencies.
- ***Flexibility:*** In view of the ever-changing needs of the society and community, flexibility in the guidance programme is a must. An organized guidance programme should be flexible according to individual and social needs.
- ***Principle of evaluation:*** To administer guidance intelligently and with as thorough knowledge of the individual as possible, programmes of individual evaluation should be conducted and accurate consultative records of progress should be made accessible to guidance workers.
- ***Guidance by a trained person:*** Specific guidance problems at any age should be referred to people who are trained to deal with particular areas of adjustment so that the individual seeking guidance can benefit to the maximum extent.
- ***Principle of periodic appraisal:*** Periodical appraisals should be planned for existing guidance programmes. The success of any programme can be evaluated from the outcomes reflected in the periodic appraisal.

II. ACCORDING TO HOLLIES AND HOLLIES

Hollies and Hollies gave eight principles on which any guidance programme should be based. These principles are as follows:

- The dignity of the individual is supreme.
- Each individual is different from every other individual.
- The primary concern of guidance is the individual, in his or her social setting.
- The attitude and personal perceptions of the individual are the basis on which he acts.
- The individual generally acts to enhance his or her perceived self.

- The individual has the innate ability to learn and can be helped to make choices that will lead to self-direction consistently with social improvement.
- The individual needs a continuous guidance process from early childhood through adulthood.
- Each individual may need the information and personalized assistance given by competent professional personnel at some time.

TYPES/AREAS OF GUIDANCE SERVICES

Guidance services can be used in almost every sphere of human existence. Each individual needs help and guidance in some or other phase of life to cope and adjust with personal, social and professional needs and challenges. Guidance promotes proper adjustment of students with the educational environment in which they live and learn so that the purpose of education is achieved to an optimal level. Some of the most essential types or areas of guidance that may benefit students/individuals are discussed next (Table 8.1 and Fig. 8.4). The microscopic details of guidance services can be seen in Fig. 8.5.

- ***Personal guidance:*** Each student is different in personal, physical, psychological, social, cultural, economic and spiritual dimensions of life and development. He/she may experience unique personal problems in the educational environment. Therefore, guidance services should be directed towards offering personal guidance whenever required.
- ***Social guidance:*** The main purpose of education is to make students efficient citizens. Therefore, social guidance services are essential for students to assume social leadership, conform to social norms, work as team members, develop healthy and positive attitudes, appreciate the problems of society, respect the opinions and sentiments of fellow beings and acquire traits of patience, perseverance, fraternity and friendship.
- ***Educational guidance:*** Educational guidance includes support offered to students in each and every aspect of the learning process. The purpose of educational guidance is to optimize the capabilities and satisfaction of the learner in academic work including the selection of programme, managing difficulties encountered in learning, promoting academic creativity and efficient utilization of institutional resources (classroom, faculty, library, learning material, books, etc.).
- ***Vocational guidance:*** It is generally observed that in the absence of efficient vocational counselling, individuals usually land in the wrong place. Therefore, vocational guidance is essential in making right and appropriate choice of occupation from the available options. In

Table 8.1 Description of Types/Areas of Guidance Services

Types/Areas of Guidance	Description
1. Personal guidance	This deals with a student's personal and family life, marriage, economic and emotional problems.
2. Social guidance	This helps the individual deal with social and cultural problems.
3. Educational guidance	This helps the individual adjust in institutions, in the selection of curriculum, identification of future possibilities and involves meeting the educational needs of pupils and creating favourable conditions.
4. Vocational guidance	This helps in the selection of a vocation, vocational adjustment, knowing about essential attributes and qualifications for vocations.
5. Health guidance	This helps the individual maintain positive physical development, sound health and emotional behaviour.
6. Avocational guidance	This helps to efficiently use their leisure time to enjoy life and promote creativity.

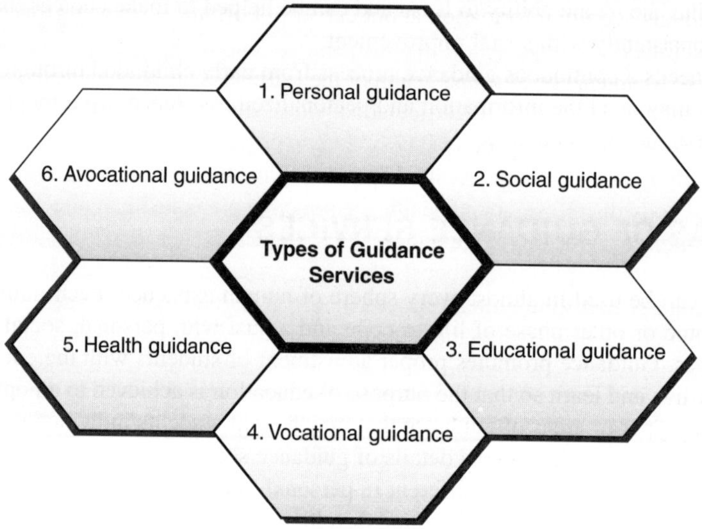

Figure 8.4

Types/areas of guidance services.

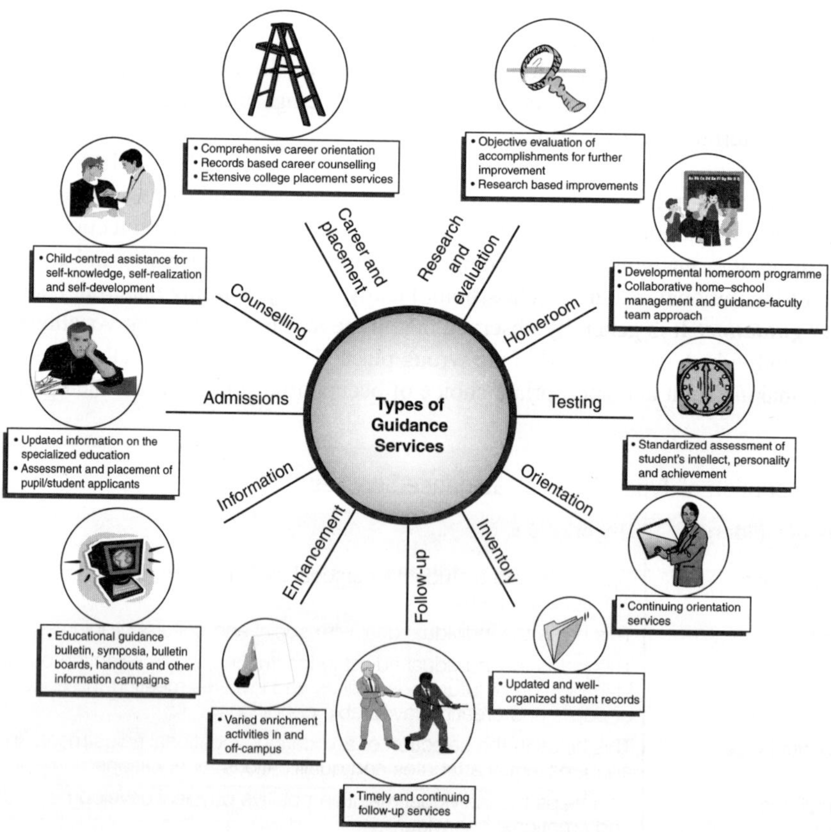

Figure 8.5

Types of guidance services.

addition, individuals acquire information about career opportunities, career growth and career advancement facilities.

- ***Health guidance:*** Maintenance of sound health of the learners is an essential responsibility of educational institutions. In addition to curricular activities, students must receive guidance on the promotion of sound health, prevention of illness, early recognition of illnesses and seeking appropriate treatment at the right time so that physical and psychological health can be ensured. A sound mind exists in a sound body; therefore, sound health is a principle prerequisite of effective learning.
- ***Avocational guidance:*** Avocational guidance refers to the efficient use of leisure time by individuals leading to refreshment. It boosts the brain for creative and innovative learning. Avocational guidance helps individuals choose the right recreational activities, such as games, photography, drama and fine arts, so that they enjoy life as well as have a holistic all-round development for the achievement of personal and professional objectives.

ORGANIZATION OF COUNSELLING SERVICES

Organization means planning, coordinating and performing certain activities systematically within the policy framework of the institution. The level and size of the educational institution, student needs, community interests, faculty attitude and budgetary provisions are some factors that determine the nature of the guidance and counselling service in any institution. The major types or forms of the organization of counselling services in an educational institution are given below:

I. ***Centralized counselling services:*** In centralized counselling, the entire responsibility of the guidance and counselling service is vested upon a group of trained personnel or the department of guidance and counselling service. Counselling activities are carried out by selected members of the teaching staff under the direction and supervision of the guidance staff. They conduct and control most of the guidance activities from the central guidance office. All teachers or faculty members also perform their duties under the supervision of the central guidance bureau and its orders.

II. ***Decentralized counselling services:*** The responsibility of the counselling service is vested upon teachers in decentralized counselling services. The teachers may give excellent and timely assistance to their students. As the teachers remain in close contact with pupils in their class, they understand the needs and problems of their pupils. Because of this reason, teachers can help students in a better way. Absence of trained personnel to give professional assistance to students is the drawback of this type of service.

III. ***Combination of centralized and decentralized counselling services:*** In this mixed form, guidance and counselling services are provided by teachers and experts collectively. Adopting the midway between centralization and decentralization is the best way to organize an effective guidance and counselling service. Crow and Crow supported the mixed form. The school guidance programme includes the coordinated services of administrators, teachers, employees and social institutions. The counselling department headed by the counsellor and the faculty cooperates with each other for students' welfare. Teachers provide counselling services and refer students who need specialized services to the counsellor.

I. PURPOSES OF ORGANIZING COUNSELLING SERVICES

The purposes of organizing counselling services in an educational institution so that optimum learning, growth and development of an individual can be achieved are discussed below:

- To help individuals with normal developmental problems.
- To help individuals through a temporary crisis during the different stages of life.

- To identify signs of disturbed/problem behaviour at the earliest possible time so that timely management can be obtained.
- To refer critical cases to specialists for the best possible management of problems.
- To facilitate communication within and between nursing institutions, homes, communities and resources.
- To support not only the tutors/nursing faculty who are helping individuals but also who themselves want guidance and reassurance at times.

II. INGREDIENTS OF GUIDANCE AND COUNSELLING SERVICES

The main ingredients of guidance and counselling services that may be offered to students in an educational institution for effective adaptation to the new educational environment and promote the best possible learning are given below:

- ***Planning service:*** It is meant to help students overcome their hostel, mess and financial problems. Help is also rendered to enable foreign students adjust to new situations. A school can organize programmes for securing scholarships for students, for getting funds from different sources and arrange different cocurricular activities, educational tours and cultural programmes with the help of the student adviser.
- ***Placement service:*** It refers to assistance offered to an individual in taking the next step, whether towards further training or a job. A strong emphasis is laid on placing students in jobs suitable for them. This can be done through coordination with employment exchanges and different employment agencies.
- ***Follow-up service:*** It involves keeping in touch with students who have graduated from the school and the school dropouts. This is done to find opportunities to help these students and to evaluate the programme. The common tools used for conducting follow-up services consist of questionnaires, interviews, letters and telephone calls.
- ***Research and evaluation:*** It is a service meant to evaluate the school counselling programme. The counsellor acts as a researcher and conducts surveys. He also carries out follow-up as well as formative and summative evaluation to assess the ultimate effect of the counselling programmes.

III. BASIC COMPONENTS OF COUNSELLING SERVICES

The principle components of counselling services (such as organizational set-up for counselling services, counselling committee, tools for counselling services and the basic requirements for counselling services) are discussed in the following section.

A. ORGANIZATIONAL SET-UP

A sound organizational set-up is required to provide effective guidance and counselling services. A different organizational set-up is recommended for different levels of educational institutions (university, constituent college of university and affiliated colleges). These set-ups are briefly discussed below:

- ***At universities:*** Deans are assisted by the head of departments (HODs) of psychology and education, the guidance committee and the counselling officer.
- ***For constituent colleges:*** A counselling officer assisted by the guidance committee in cooperation with the deputy chief and academic advisor can plan according to their needs and number of

students (<1000 students need a liaison officer while >1000 students need an assistant counselling officer).
- ***For affiliated colleges:*** A counselling officer assisted by the guidance committee and a vocational guidance officer are needed for ≥1000 students while a liaison officer only can manage the counselling services for <1000 students.

B. COUNSELLING CENTRE

All universities and large colleges should have a counselling centre headed by a trained professional, that is a counselling officer with PhD or a master's degree in psychology and counselling, with considerable experience. The counselling centre generally provides assistance, offers psychological testing, helps in training, conducts special clinics, maintains integrity and confidentiality, arranges orientation talks and gives information about the course and facilities, holds career talks and career conferences, maintains cumulative records, identifies students with problems and arranges personality counselling. In addition, it also performs the following functions:
- Selection, registration and orientation of students
- Educational and vocational counselling
- Personal adjustment counselling
- Physical and psychological services
- Remedial services
- Residence and food services
- Activities programme

C. COUNSELLING COMMITTEE

The main purpose of the guidance committee is to carry forward the total guidance programme through the united efforts of management, dean, counselling/liaison officer, deputy chief counselling officer, vocational guidance officer, peer group, librarian, warden, medical staff, principal, guidance personnel, teachers, parents and student. To this end, the committee should be a representative of all these groups, with the possible exception of parents and students. The guidance committee serves the following additional purposes:
- It establishes and maintains policies related to guidance and counselling services.
- It articulates the programme between the institution and the community.
- It acts in a planning capacity to ensure that the various functions of guidance are properly coordinated.
- It helps to clarify particular roles and offers support when these roles are challenged.
- It paves the way for the guidance personnel to function in cooperation with community agencies, such as business organizations, employer groups and voluntary agencies.
- It serves as a source of ideas and recommendations to be submitted to appropriate bodies (such as curriculum committees, professional associations of teachers and the department of education).

D. MEMBERS OF THE COUNSELLING COMMITTEE

Generally, the counselling committee constitutes the following members:
- Administrator
- Principal/Dean
- Counselling/Liaison officer

- Deputy chief of counselling section
- Counselling personnel/Counsellor
- Vocational guidance officer
- Teacher/Faculty from different departments/Specialities
- Hostel warden/Librarian (coopted members in special situations)
- Student representatives
- Parents

E. ASSIGNING RESPONSIBILITIES FOR COUNSELLING SERVICES

The guidance abilities and interests of individual members of the staff have to be assessed so that specific functions can be assigned according to their personal capacity. Establishing clear-cut lines of authority will help everyone distinguish their duties from those of others. This will prevent misguidance to the students. The following pattern may be followed for the assignment of responsibilities for counselling services:

- Formation of the guidance and counselling committee.
- The committee lists problems requiring group solution.
- Plans monthly, quarterly and yearly programme.
- Coordinates guidance activities and assesses the work done.

IV. TOOLS FOR COUNSELLING SERVICES

Counselling services impose a special need to use specific tools for collecting primary information from students. The tools for collection of information for counselling are divided into two broad categories:

A. NONTESTING TOOLS

These types of tools are usually used for individual assessment without any intention of testing the individual. These tools are generally developed by the counsellor and/or teachers themselves. Some nontesting tools are as follows:

- *Interview:* Interviews are the basic tools of counselling. An interview can be described as an interaction between the counsellor and counselee with a definite objective in mind. Interviews help the counsellor obtain desired information from students, their family members, friends or teachers, etc. or prove the same to them. This flexible tool of counselling helps the counsellor customize the interaction with a student for a specific purpose.
- *Observation:* It is the careful watching or monitoring of the counselee by the counsellor with a specific objective in mind. Observation could be participatory or nonparticipatory based on the specific purpose of counselling. Further, observation could be overt (where counselee knows he is being observed) or covert (counselee does not know he is being observed and the counsellor is concealed). Observation is a very useful tool of counselling in situations where gathering information from the counselee is not possible through an interview or other methods such as the behaviour of students in a specific situation or circumstances.
- *Anecdotal record:* It consists of recording an important incident that happened and is a carefully recorded snapshot of the incident. Anecdotal recording must be recorded with specific care so that the incident is recorded as it happened. Further, the counsellor must involve the people who directly observed the incident such as teachers, faculty and peer group.

- *Cumulative record:* It is a method of recording and providing meaningful, significant and comprehensive information about an individual over the years. It is useful in organizing and integrating information collected through the use of different tools. Besides recording attendance and achievement, it also registers students' social adjustment in school, their behaviour with other pupils and their attitude towards the school and teachers. It also records the estimate of qualities like hard work, tolerance and sociability. Cumulative records can be maintained in folders, files or in a card form.
- *Checklist:* Generally, a checklist is used to identify the presence or absence of specific attributes or skills of a particular expected behaviour in students. A checklist is a very commonly used tool to assess the skills of communication or nursing tasks in nursing students.
- *Rating scale:* Rating scales are better tools to assess the degree or extent of the performance of a particular task or the possession of a trait (truthfulness, honesty, initiative, responsibility and attitude of cooperation, etc.).
- *Sociometry:* It is used to measure sociability or the social distance between students or members of a group.
- *Autobiography and diary:* Autobiographies or diaries may also provide useful information about students. Students should be encouraged to keep diaries or a life autobiography.

B. PSYCHOLOGICAL TESTS

Psychological tests provide information about an individual's psychological characteristics such as intelligence, aptitude, interests, abilities and personality. Before the selection and use of these tests, their reliability, validity and practicability must be clearly assessed. Psychological tests are generally classified as follows:

- *Personality tests:* There are several personality tests available to assess the personality types of people. For instance, *The Rorschach* and *The Minnesota* are examples of personality measurement tests.
- *Aptitude tests:* These tests are used to estimate the extent to which an individual would profit from a specific course or training to predict the quality of his achievement in a given situation. Two types of aptitude tests usually employed are specialized aptitude test and general aptitude test.
- *Achievement tests:* These are used to assess academic performance devices rather than being used as selection instruments. Some achievement tests are cooperative test, College Board series, test of educational development, English reading test, etc.
- *Interest inventory tests:* These tests are used to assess the interests of an individual in specific disciplines such as specific vocational or occupational interests. Blank and Kuder preference inventory is one of the most commonly used tests for this purpose.
- *Study habit inventory tests:* These tests are used to assess study habits in students. The Brown–Holtzman survey of study habits is the most commonly used study habit test.

V. SPECIFIC REQUIREMENTS FOR THE ORGANIZATION OF COUNSELLING SERVICES

Some of the main requirements for organizing guidance and counselling services are discussed below:

- Presence of physical facilities, that is rooms, furniture and other equipment needed for the guidance and counselling department.
- Provision of private offices as well as general counselling rooms.
- Trained counsellors and guidance personnel.
- Planned programmes to meet objectives.

- Consultation services.
- Evaluation instruments like psychological tests, inventories, etc.
- Student data bank.
- Educational and vocational information service.
- Programmes for cooperation between home and school.
- Programmes for integrating community services with guidance services.
- Educational programmes for teachers, counsellors and other personnel to provide knowledge of current trends in guidance.
- Budgetary provisions.

VI. APPRAISAL OF COUNSELLING SERVICES

Appraisal of the guidance programme is essential to maintain its relevance. The efficiency of the programme should be tested against the changing needs of students and the society. Appropriate measures should be taken to rectify any noted defects to keep the programme student friendly.

VII. ORGANIZATION OF COUNSELLING SERVICES IN NURSING INSTITUTIONS

In recent years, a number of nursing institutes have mushroomed without proper and adequate provision for guidance and counselling services to nursing students. These institutions offer a basic diploma in doctoral nursing programmes such as Diploma in General Nursing and Midwifery, Bachelor of Science in Nursing, Master of Science in Nursing and PhD in Nursing. There is a strong need for efficient guidance and counselling services in these institutions because of reasons like rapid social changes, changing roles of nurses, more demanding patients, changes in the health care system, complexity of modern life and the global demand for qualified nurses.

A. IMPORTANCE OF COUNSELLING SERVICES IN NURSING EDUCATION

An increasing global demand for qualified nurses and the emergence of various specialties in nursing to meet the challenges of the modern health care system has given a facelift to the area of guidance in nursing education. A large number of students opt for the nursing profession without prior knowledge about the profession. Guidance and counselling services are needed to provide a clear picture of the latest trends and the emerging new specialties. The main functions of counselling services in nursing education are as follow:

- *Help students adjust in the new educational environment:* A well-planned guidance and counselling programme will help the nursing students adjust to the new educational atmosphere and make them feel more comfortable and reduce home sickness.
- *Protection from ragging:* Guidance and counselling services in the institution help students gain information about the preventive measures of ragging. An antiragging committee can be constituted in the institute in coordination with the counselling service to help newly admitted students against ragging. There should be active participation of senior students to report any ragging incident so that disciplinary action can be taken by the administration.
- *Assist students adjust with new learning experiences and overcome learning difficulties:* Personal guidance and counselling is needed to help students adjust with new learning experiences especially those provided in clinical areas.

- *Help students develop emotional maturity:* In the clinical area, nursing students have to face many situations, which may cause emotional distress especially in the newly admitted students. Helping students develop empathy rather than sympathy, teaching them to analyse events in the clinical area and to ventilate their emotions through efficient counselling services may help them develop strong emotional maturity.
- *Assist students cope with stress:* Sometimes nursing students are utilized to replace the staff nurses for patient care in situations of acute staff shortage, which create additional stress in student nurses. Teaching relaxation techniques, ensuring availability of teachers to help students in crisis situations, constituting peer groups and assigning senior students to look after juniors are some ways to deal with stress in nursing students.
- *Help students achieve balance between personal and professional life:* Students should be taught from the very beginning about how to maintain balance between personal and professional life. They should be instructed to concentrate on other responsibilities after returning from clinical areas instead of being preoccupied with matters related to patient care.
- *Help students develop a healthy interpersonal relationship with other members of the health care team:* Success of any health team is determined by how well the nurses render their services. Special attention should be given to inculcate a sense of accountability and responsibility in nursing students along with health care team cohesiveness which helps in improving the quality of patient care.
- *Train students for leadership qualities:* Leadership development programmes should be conducted under a guidance and counselling service to promote leadership qualities in nursing students.
- *Assist students acquire desirable set of values and develop a positive life philosophy:* Value-based nursing education is the need of the time. Through well-planned guidance and counselling services, emphasis must be placed on inculcating basic moral values in nursing students so they can be good human beings, citizens and nurses.
- *Motivate students contribute towards bridging the gap between nursing education and nursing service:* In the Indian scenario, there is still a large existing gap between nursing education and nursing practice, what is taught to nursing students in the classroom is not practised in organizations. Therefore, nursing students must be motivated through guidance and counselling services to practice what is taught to them in the classroom or the simulation laboratory.
- *Financial guidance:* Financial guidance can be given to help needy students determine the financial assistance they need in light of expected expenses. They need to be guided on fee concessions, scholarships and available stipends in the institution or those offered by other welfare agencies.

B. STRATEGIES TO ORGANIZE COUNSELLING SERVICES IN NURSING EDUCATION

The following strategies may be used to offer guidance and counselling services in nursing institutions:

- A combined centralization and decentralization approach of counselling may be used to organize guidance and counselling services in the nursing institution.
- The department of guidance and counselling is headed by a qualified counsellor and is assisted by one or two clerical staff.
- Faculty members are trained to provide nonspecialist guidance and counselling to students with the help of the counsellor.
- Any student in need of specialized services is referred to the counsellor, who provides counselling with the help of the faculty members.

- Many nursing institutions have successfully implemented teacher guardian programmes. In a teacher guardian programme, each faculty member is given full responsibility of a group of 10 students. In addition, the class coordinator also looks after all students in the class. Thus, a student is looked after by a teacher guardian at the ground level and the class coordinator at the next level. The teacher guardian has to conduct periodic meetings with the assigned group of students to assess their performance and send the filled *proforma* to the counselling department for further verification and filing through the principal. During the meeting, the teacher guardian also has to fix a date for the next follow-up session. Students can approach the teacher guardian as needed to seek help in academic and personal matters. Further,
    - when the teacher guardian feels that a student needs specialized help, he reports the student's details to the student's class coordinator, counsellor and principal. The counsellor then takes over the student and with the help of faculty members and other concerned personnel (like parents and peers) renders help as needed.
    - a number of student problems are solved at the teacher guardian or class coordinator level, and students who need a specialized service are referred to the counsellor.
    - the counsellor is not overloaded and can concentrate on other areas/services of guidance and counselling this way.
    - the proforma sent to the counselling department through the principal is verified by the counsellor before filing.
- To review the functioning of the guidance and counselling services, a monthly meeting is held under the chairmanship of the principal. In this meeting, teacher guardians, class coordinators and the counsellor present a brief report.

TYPES OF COUNSELLING APPROACHES

Counselling is a continuous, mutual and interactive process between the counsellor and the counselee for definite objectives. Three basic types of counselling approaches, that is directive, nondirective and eclectic, may be used based on the nature of the counselling procedure and the role of the counsellor.

I. DIRECTIVE COUNSELLING APPROACH

The directive counselling approach is also known as *prescriptive counselling* or *counsellor-centred approach of counselling*. In directive counselling, the counsellor is the central figure and plays a more active role. This approach of counselling is advocated by E.G. Williamson, a professor at University of Minnesota. In directive counselling, the counsellor plays a leading role and uses a variety of techniques to suggest appropriate solutions to the counselee's problems. This approach is also called an *authoritarian* or *psychoanalytic approach*. The counsellor is active and helps individuals in making decisions and finding solutions to their problems. The counsellor believes in the limited capacity of the patient. This approach emphasizes on the cognitive and intellectual aspects of the problem. The patient makes the decision but the counsellor does all he can to get the patient make a decision keeping with his diagnosis. The counsellor tries to direct the patient's thinking by informing, explaining, interpreting and advising. The basic assumptions related to directive counselling approach are discussed below:

- ***A need-based approach:*** It is assumed that the directive counselling approach is a need-based approach. Whenever a patient has problems and is incapable of handling them himself, the counsellor helps solve these problems.

- ***Problem-focused rather than patient-focused approach:*** The major focus is placed on the patient's existing problems rather than the patient himself. The existing problems of the individual are targeted in this approach. It is solely a remedial measure to solve an individual's acute problems.
- ***Used for patients incapable of solving their problems:*** It is assumed that directive counselling is used in situations where the individual is not capable of solving his problems and desires help from a competent person. The counsellor uses his intellectual abilities to solve these problems by offering the best possible solutions.
- ***Task of a competent counsellor:*** Directive counselling is a counsellor-centred task; it requires a competent counsellor to minutely analyse an individual's problems and offer the best possible solutions using his intellectual and counselling competence.
- ***Making the best possible use of counselee's intellectual abilities and resources:*** Although directive counselling approach is counsellor-centred, it is still assumed that the counsellor must make the best possible use of the counselee's intellectual abilities, strengths and resources.

A. STEPS OF THE DIRECTIVE COUNSELLING APPROACH

E.G. Williamson has given the following six steps in providing directive counselling to individuals:

- *Information gathering and analysis:* In this step, the counsellor tries to elicit relevant details from the counselee. The data or detailed information is gathered that helps in focusing on the current problem. Information may be collected using different tools such as interview, questioning, observation, case history and psychological tests.
- *Synthesis:* Synthesis is the process of summarizing and organizing data from the analysis to reveal the counselee's assets, liabilities, adjustments and maladjustments. Initially, collected data are retained in a nonsystematic manner. The data are organized under specific heads to establish the status of the counselee as well as his problem.
- *Diagnosis:* In this stage, the actual problem is identified, defined and focused upon. The synthesized data leads to identification of the problem. The problem is identified in terms of assets and liabilities of the counselee. It also identifies the root cause of the problem.
- *Prognosis:* This step may or may not be a part of the diagnosis step. The problem is identified and the counsellor determines what has to be offered to help the counselee mange his problem at the best possible level.
- *Counselling:* This is the most important step of the whole procedure. The counsellor asks the counselee questions and offers the best possible solutions to manage the present problems. Alternatively, the counsellor also makes the best possible use of the counselee's strengths and resources to manage the identified problems.
- *Follow-up:* In this stage, the effectiveness of the counselling process is evaluated. The counsellor assesses how far the planned objectives of the counselling session are achieved. In certain cases, follow-up may be required to give a few counselling sessions to the counselee.

B. ADVANTAGES OF THE DIRECTIVE COUNSELLING APPROACH

The advantages of the directive counselling approach are listed below:

- Directive counselling approach saves time.
- It emphasizes the problem and not the individual. The counsellor can see the patient more objectively than the patient himself.

- Directive counselling lays more emphasis on the intellectual rather than the emotional aspects of an individual's personality. The counselee is helped to solve the intellectual problem rather than emotional problems.
- The methods used in directive counselling are direct, persuasive and explanatory.

C. LIMITATIONS OF THE DIRECTIVE COUNSELLING APPROACH

The limitations of the directive counselling approach are listed below:

- The patient does not gain any liability for self-analysis or solve new problems of adjustment by counselling.
- Counselling serves to make the counselee overdependent on the counsellor. He never becomes independent of the counsellor and this kills his initiative.
- Problems regarding emotional maladjustment may be better solved by nondirective counselling.
- Sometimes the counselee lacks information regarding the counselee. This lack of information leads to wrong counselling.
- Directive counselling does not guarantee that the counselee will be able to solve the same problems on his own in future.

II. NONDIRECTIVE COUNSELLING APPROACH

The chief exponent of this counselling approach, Carp R. Rogers, originally referred to it as the *patient-centred counselling approach*. It is also known as the *permissive counselling approach* where the counsellor's role is passive and the counselee's role is active. It is a counselee-centred or patient-centred humanistic approach. The counselee makes the final decisions as individuals are thought to have full right to make final decisions for the self and solve their problems. The counsellor has to accept the counselee's capacity to make adjustments and adapt. The principles of acceptance and tolerance are extremely important in this approach.

The basic assumptions related to nondirective counselling approach are given below:

- Patient is given more importance than the counselling directions and interventions.
- Emotional aspects are more significant than intellectual aspects.
- Creation of an atmosphere where patients can work out their understanding is more important than cultivating self-understanding in the patient.
- Counselling leads to a voluntary choice of goals and a conscious selection of courses of action.

A. STEPS OF THE NONDIRECTIVE COUNSELLING APPROACH

Carp R. Rogers has given the following five steps in the nondirective counselling approach:

- *Defining the problem situation:* This is the first stage of counselling where the counselee and counsellor collectively identify and define the actual problem. So that counselling can be focused to help the individual to solve that particular problem.
- *Counselee given freedom to express his feelings:* The counselee is given freedom to express his feelings so that the counsellor can help manage his problem in this stage.
- *Identifying counselee's feelings:* The counsellor carefully records the positive as well as negative feelings of the counselee. This helps the counsellor estimate the gravity of the present problem and the counselee's available resources to manage the problem.

- *Developing counselee's insight:* The counsellor helps the counselee develop insight into problems as well as available resources to manage the problems. This insight helps the counselee set realistic goals to solve the problem.
- *Termination of counselling:* In the final stage, the counsellor and the counselee mutually agree to end the counselling relationship because either the problem is managed or the counselee is now capable of solving his problem with insight if it recurs.

B. ADVANTAGES OF NONDIRECTIVE COUNSELLING APPROACH

The advantages of the nondirective counselling approach are listed below:

- It is a slow but sure process to make an individual capable of making adjustments.
- No tests are used so one avoids all that is laborious and difficult.
- It removes emotional block and helps an individual bring repressed thoughts on a conscious level thereby reducing tension.

C. LIMITATIONS OF NONDIRECTIVE COUNSELLING APPROACH

The limitations of the nondirective counselling approach are discussed below:

- It is a slow and time-consuming process. It is not easily possible because a counsellor has to attend to many patients.
- One cannot rely upon one's resources, judgement and wisdom as the patient is immature in making the decision himself.
- It depends too much on the ability and initiative of the patient. The patient is already under stress and inexperienced.
- There are likely to arise occasions when it becomes difficult to control the pace of the interview discussion.
- As this approach to counselling is individual centric, it may not be possible for the counsellor to attend to every patient equally well.
- It requires a high degree of motivation in the patient. The counsellor's passiveness is likely to prove a hurdle in the way.

III. ECLECTIC COUNSELLING APPROACH

This approach is based on the fact that all individuals are different from one another. No single approach can, therefore, be applied to each and every problem. The counsellor makes use of both directive and nondirective counselling that may be considered useful for the purpose of modifying the patient's ideas and attitudes. The techniques are elective in nature because they have been derived from all sources of counselling. This approach is based on selecting the best and leaving out what is least required.

The assumption of this nondirective counselling approach is that every individual is capable of solving his or her own problem. The counsellor should assist the counselee in seeing the nature of the problem. The goal of this approach is independence and integration of the patient. The counsellor creates an atmosphere in which the patient can work out his own understanding. It leads to a voluntary choice of action. This counselling approach rests on fundamental respect for an individual and the belief in a person's ability to solve personal problems with the aid of a sympathetic listener. This method is useful in solving educational, vocational and marital problems. In this approach, the counsellor respects the personal autonomy of the patient. This means the patient has to make the final decision. The basic assumptions related to the eclectic counselling approach are given below:

- There is objectivity and coordination between the counsellor and the patient during the counselling experience.
- The patient is active and the counsellor remains passive in the beginning.
- The principle of low expenditure is adopted.
- The counsellor makes use of all the tools and methods in his armour. His professional skills are an important factor in the successful completion of the counselling experience.
- The counsellor enjoys the freedom to resort to directive and nondirective counselling methods.
- The counselling relationship is built during the counselling interview. This helps the patient gain reassurance and confidence.

A. STEPS OF THE ECLECTIC COUNSELLING APPROACH

The following six steps are recommended in the eclectic counselling approach:

- *Establishing rapport:* In the first stage of the eclectic counselling approach, the counsellor tries to establish intimate rapport with the counselee so that interaction between the counsellor and the counselee is smooth. Rapport establishment helps the counsellor understand the counselee's problems, strengths and weaknesses more deeply and extensively.
- *Diagnosing the problem:* After establishing rapport with the counselee, the counsellor tries to assess and diagnose the counselee's problem. During this stage, the counsellor asks the counselee a few essential questions to understand problems accurately and establish a prompt diagnosis of the problem.
- *Analysing the case:* During this stage of counselling, the counsellor obtains more information related to the counselee's problem from other sources so that he can get detailed information about the counselee's problems and resources to plan for suitable and best possible solutions so the counselee may acquire better self-understanding.
- *Preparing a tentative plan for modifying behaviour:* At this stage, the counsellor is in a position to prepare a tentative plan for the patient's modification of behaviour. This also requires emotional release and a change in the patient's perception and attitude about himself.
- *Counselling:* Eclectic counselling approach believes that effective counselling uses one-to-one interview, stimulates the counselee to develop his own resources and assumes responsibilities for finding solutions to his problems.
- *Follow-up:* This is the final stage of counselling and is carried out to either assess the effectiveness of the counselling process or to provide a few more follow-up sessions if more help is required by the counselee.

B. ADVANTAGES OF ECLECTIC COUNSELLING APPROACH

The advantages of eclectic counselling approach are as follows:

- It is a more cost-effective and practical approach of counselling as it includes features of both directive and nondirective counselling based on the needs, abilities and resources of the counselee.
- It is a more flexible approach of counselling, where the counsellor and the counselee may assume active and passive roles based on the needs and nature of the problem.
- It is a more objective and coordinated approach of counselling and is more suitable to handle complex problems of the modern era.

C. LIMITATIONS OF ECLECTIC COUNSELLING APPROACH

The disadvantages of eclectic counselling approach are as follows:

- The roles of counsellor and the counselee are not predetermined so they may experience dilemma about their roles at a particular phase of counselling.
- It requires more skilled counsellors to handle the dynamic feature of this counselling approach.

IV. OTHER TYPES OF COUNSELLING

Counselling may be further classified based on the length of the counselling session, the number of counselees involved and the purpose of counselling as follows.

A. BASED ON LENGTH OF THE COUNSELLING SESSION

- *Short-term counselling:* This type of counselling service is used in situational crisis where disruption of life occurs. It focuses mainly on concerns of the patient or family. The counsellor assists the patient and guides him in problem solving or decision making in a systematic and logical manner.
- *Long-term counselling:* It can be on a daily, weekly or monthly basis, and extends over a prolonged period of time. It is focused on patients experiencing a developmental crisis.

B. BASED ON NUMBER OF COUNSELEES INVOLVED

- *Individual counselling:* It is a process of mutual one-to-one interchange of opinions to get and give information. The counsellor tries to establish rapport and structures counselling plan so that the patient understands what to expect during counselling.
- *Group counselling:* It is a technique where a group of people are counselled by applying the group interaction method to arrive at a solution to the problem. All group members are provided with an opportunity to discuss their problems together in a free environment. In group counselling, group work helps the group members in understanding and finding solutions to their problems. Some components like knowledge of reality, self-understanding and self-realization can be achieved through the group interaction process.

C. COUNSELLING FOR EDUCATIONAL AND PROFESSIONAL PURPOSES

- *Student counselling:* Students are considered to be capable of setting goals, making decisions and generally assuming responsibility for their own behaviour and future. Student counselling is mainly concerned with helping students solve their problems pertaining to the selection of educational institution, course, method of study and adjustment.
- *Educational counselling:* This type of counselling helps the students get the maximum benefit out of education and solve their problems related to education. Students understand or orient themselves to the new purpose or philosophy of education. Educational counselling also assists the students in identifying the need of educational planning. Students develop study habits and choose specializations according to their need and interest.
- *Vocational counselling:* For any problem within a specific vocation, advice is sought to solve those problems through vocational counselling. The counsellor helps the patient improve his all-round

personality development and helps him develop skills, efficiency and mastery over the vocation so that the counselee is best among his colleagues.

- *Career counselling:* Career choice is one of the most difficult tasks. Therefore, career counselling is needed for individuals so that they can make a wise choice in choosing careers that suit them best according to their interests, abilities and capabilities.
- *Placement counselling:* The counsellor gives advice to the counselee regarding jobs and posts suitable for the patient depending on his abilities, attitude, aptitude and interest.

D. COUNSELLING FOR HEALTH-RELATED PURPOSES

- *Psychotherapeutic counselling:* Individuals trained in providing psychological counselling consciously attempt to assist the person verbally to modify his or her maladaptive behaviour. There are various methods of psychotherapy like the following:
  - Behaviour counselling
  - Transaction analysis
  - Gestalt therapy
  - Psychoanalytic psychotherapy
- *Crisis counselling:* It helps individuals overcome the effects of a crisis such as loss of a family member and family conflict. These situations may affect the normal behaviour of an individual and he/she may develop feelings of anxiety or guilt. The counsellor helps the individual understand the situation and develop a new pattern of behaviour.
- *Health counselling:* It involves helping an individual learn more about health and healthy habits. This helps the person become more aware of the role of exercise, nutrition and healthy habits to maintain good health.
- *Genetic counselling:* This is a specialized type of health counselling, where individual or families with genetics problems are guided to receive the best possible genetic diagnostic and therapeutic interventions.
- *Preventive counselling:* The preventive counselling is a relatively newer approach, which is prevention-oriented, where practitioners ensure that expected problems may be prevented by implementing the best available interventions. For example, some of the students may be having examination or test anxiety, they may be provided with preventive counselling interventions to prevent acute attacks of examination anxiety or panic episodes.

E. COUNSELLING FOR PERSONAL/SOCIAL PURPOSES

- *Personal counselling:* Student face certain problems about which they may be very anxious. They generally try to cope with these problems. The counsellor helps students understand and solve these problems. The counsellor helps students by providing advice on personal problems. The counsellor also helps students develop interpersonal skills, improve study habits and accept themselves and others.
- *Marriage counselling:* Marriage counselling is directed at improving a disturbed marital relationship. It is a centred effort to change the psychodynamics and behaviour of the partner. Two partners meet the therapist in joint sessions. Marital counselling may be conducted on a problem-solving level. It focuses on the need of each partner to understand the other's point of view and feelings.
- *Motivational counselling:* Motivational counselling involves discussing feelings and incentives with the patient. The counsellor can encourage an individual by establishing a helping relationship to avoid feelings of despair and work towards developing feelings of motivation.

- *Developmental counselling:* Different stages of development in life impose a need for specialized counselling services, such as child counselling, adolescent counselling, premarital counselling, preconception counselling, child-rearing counselling and geriatric counselling. All these stages in life require guidance and counselling, collectively known as *developmental counselling.*

ROLE AND PREPARATION OF THE COUNSELLOR

A counsellor is the key player in the counselling process. The success of the counselling process primarily depends on the vision and planning of the counsellor. A counsellor is not from another world; however, he must possess some special qualities and attributes (Table 8.2). He is one who has the right understanding of the relation between what counselee thinks, wants and do and say. The word *counsellor* is derived from *counselling* and means a 'person who performs counselling'. D.W. Lefeuer states that a counsellor will be one who devotes half or more of his time to guidance; *a teacher–counsellor* is one who has been relieved of at least one class for guidance work but who will not denote as much as half the time to counselling.

I. ROLE OF THE COUNSELLOR

The major role of a counsellor is to help all students with growth in self-understanding, developing interpersonal, problem-solving and decision-making skills and occupational awareness. This is accomplished through classroom guidance, large and small group sessions and individual counselling. The counsellor must understand and fulfil a number of his patient's needs. A counsellor is expected to perform the following main roles and responsibilities:

- Arrange orientation programmes for the other support staff to enlist their cooperation.
- Prepare an up-to-date list of resources, information, referral and energy available to him.
- Organize the guidance committee.
- Set up an educational and occupational information centre.
- Display the information collected in an attractive way.
- Disseminate information through educational and career talks, group discussions and so on.
- Arrange talks by experts from different fields.
- Organize career days, career weeks, career conferences, parents day and so on.

Table 8.2 Qualities of a Good Counsellor

G – Good technical knowledge	C – Confidentiality maintenance
O – Obtaining appropriate information from the patient	O – Observant
O – Objectively answering questions	U – Unbiased
D – Demonstrating professionalism	N – Nonjudgemental
	S – Sensitive to the needs of the patient
	E – Empathetic
	L – Listens carefully
	L – Lets the patient make decisions
	O – Open-minded
	R – Respects the rights of the patients

- Educate students regarding proper study habits and assist them in their development.
- Arrange individual discussions with students and their parents for giving them educational and occupational information.
- Arrange visits to places of work like industries, business establishments, offices, higher education institutions and other important educational places.
- Maintain an active relationship with schools, colleges, universities and other regional, national and social agencies.
- Maintain an active liaison with clubs like Lions Club and Rotary Club.
- Refer serious mental cases to clinical psychologists or psychiatrists.
- Maintain complete secrecy of the discussion between him and the patient.
- Administer psychological tests.
- Provide counselling services to students.
- Help in the student placements.
- Take up research projects relating to the fields of educational, vocational, personal and social guidance in the colleges.
- Prepare guidance leaflets, brochures and monographs and get them printed for distribution to the students.

II. PREPARATION OF COUNSELLOR

Preparation of a counsellor must include the following components so that he can impart efficient counselling services.

- ***Educational background:*** Master's or bachelor's degree in teaching and education. Counsellors should have completed basic courses in the principles and practices of guidance programmes and additional areas of training in behavioural science (such as psychology, sociality or community health). Essentially, the counsellor must be trained in the areas of counselling process, understanding individual, educational and occupational information, administrative and occupational information, and research and evaluation procedures used in counselling.
- ***Experience:*** A practising counsellor must have at least 2 years of counselling experience. Further, one year of cumulative work experience in the field of school programmes and 3–6 months of supervised counselling experience. The counsellor must have significant experience in social activities, for example working within the community, volunteer work and participating in community training programmes to reveal interest.
- ***Personal fitness and attributes:*** A good counsellor should show positive interest in working with others and indicate a leadership ability to work for the people. The characteristics or qualities of a counsellor are discussed below:
  - *Personal characteristics:* The following personal characteristics must be enhanced in a person to act as an efficient counsellor:
    - Should be imbibed with basic human qualities.
    - Should be a person with cultural values and awareness.
    - Should have a deep interest in helping people.
    - Should patiently listen to others.
    - Should be sensitive to other's attitude and reactions.
    - Should have a capability for being trusted by others.

- Should have respect for the personal autonomy of the patients.
- Should be tolerant of and accept the patient's point of view.
- Should have ability to understand himself and his emotional limitations.

- *Interpersonal relationships:* Some interpersonal qualities a counsellor must possess are as follows:
  - Friendly nature
  - Sympathetic understanding
  - Sincerity
  - Tactfulness
  - Patience
  - Ability to maintain confidentiality
  - Attentive listener
  - Show concern
- *Personal adjustment:* Some personal adjustment qualities a counsellor must possess are as follows:
  - Maintain emotional stability
  - Emotionally sound and healthy
  - Able to accept criticism
  - Knowledge of self
- *Scholastic potentialities:* Some of the scholastic potentialities a counsellor must possess are as follows:
  - Relevant knowledge and efficient skills
  - Motivated and committed
  - Aware of policies, beliefs, misconceptions and rumours in the community
  - Possess common sense and use good judgement while tackling issues
  - Experience in teaching and follow-up services
- *Health and personal appearance:* Some health and personal appearance related qualities a counsellor must possess are as follows:
  - Pleasing voice and appearance
  - Vitality and endurance
  - Free from any mannerism
- *Leadership skills:* Some leadership qualities a counsellor must possess are as follows:
  - Ability to stimulate and lead others
  - Reinforce important information
  - Direct the counselee to ways to solve the problem
- *Philosophy of life:* A counsellor must have the following ingredients in his philosophy of life:
  - Good character
  - Integrated personality
  - Faith in human values and human nature
  - Show significant human values and religious belief
- *Professional dedication:* The type of professional dedication a counsellor must possess are as follows:
  - Show enthusiasm in providing services
  - Maintain helping relationship
  - Have a high sense of morality

COUNSELLING PROCESS

The counselling process takes place through a series of phases, which are interrelated, interconnected and overlap such as the nursing process. The process is not a rigid entity; it is flexible and can be modified based on the nature of problems and person to be counselled. The basic phases of a counselling process are as discussed below (Fig. 8.6).

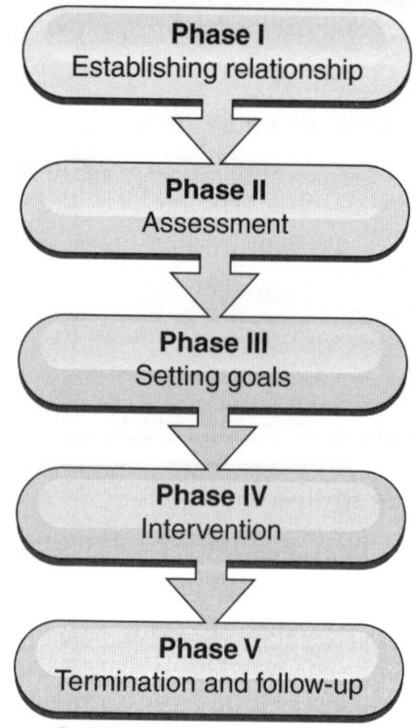

Figure 8.6
Phases of the counselling process.

I. PHASE I: ESTABLISHING RELATIONSHIP

This is the first and main phase of the counselling process and is considered as the foundation to the counselling process. It is an ice-breaking session during which the counsellor and the counselee introduce each other and establish a primary rapport that continues building further in the following phases of the counselling process. Good rapport building provides the respect, trust and sense of psychological comfort to the counsellor–counselee relationship for progression to the counselling process. Establishing a relationship may not be possible in a single session but may require multiple sessions before the next phases of counselling begin, so that the counsellor and the counselee interact with ease. The following strategies may be used by a counsellor to establish an effective relationship:

- Introduce yourself.
- Begin the phase with adequate social skills.
- Always address the individual by his or her name and remember the patient's name.
- Ensure physical comfort of the counselee and self.
- Do not interrupt the individual when he/she is talking.
- Listen attentively.
- Observe nonverbal communication.

II. PHASE II: ASSESSMENT

The second phase of counselling is basically a data collection phase, where the counsellor motivates the counselee to provide complete information about the problem. During this phase, the counsellor's job is to motivate the counselee to speak about the problems and listen to him patiently. The counselee's job is to provide all the relevant information pertaining to the present problem for which he is seeking counselling. During this phase, detailed information is collected from the counselee. The type of information collected from the counselee during this phase is depicted in Table 8.3. After the collection of information, diagnosis related to the counselee's behaviour is made. Diagnosis in a counselling situation refers to the concise statement of the patient's problems in his present condition. It tries to identify possible causes of difficulty to predict future patient behaviour. Diagnosis thus may be considered as a hypothesis of the counsellor regarding a counselee's present attitudes, thoughts and

Table 8.3 Types of Information Collected From the Counselee During the Assessment Phase

Type of Data	Description
General data	Information that is helpful in locating an individual and establishing contact.
Physical data	Information about an individual's health and physical characteristics.
Psychological data	Information about an individual's mental characteristics such as intelligence and special aptitude and personality traits.
Social/environment data	It includes social and environmental conditions and factors that influence the individual and his vocational plans.
Achievement data	It includes information of what an individual has achieved in school and outside.
Data and educational and vocational plans	It includes information about an individual's plans regarding educational and vocational progress.

Table 8.4 Types of Problems Diagnosed During Assessment Phase of Counselling

Type of Problem	Description
Personality problems	Difficulties pertaining to adjustment, family conflicts, personal problems, etc.
Educational problems	Unwise choice of courses of study, differential scholastic achievement, inadequate general scholastic aptitude, ineffective study habits, reading difficulties, lack of motivation, under achievement and the like. The patient is primarily concerned with adjustment to current academic situations rather than planning for the future.
Vocational problems	Deals with career choice and planning, choice of college and educational planning that would ultimately be implemented and lead to a career plan. It includes unwise vocational choice, differences between interest and attitudes, etc.
Financial problems	Problems related to financial support needed for school or college education.
Health problems	Inability to go about one's routine activities owing to problems of health.

Williamson and Darley (1937) proposed the above classifications.

BOX 8.1 TOOLS AND TECHNIQUES USED FOR DATA COLLECTION DURING COUNSELLING

Standardized	Nonstandardized	
Intelligence tests	Questionnaires	Rating scale
Achievement tests	Interview	Cumulative record charts
Aptitude tests	Observation	Case studies
Interest tests	Autobiography	Sociometric techniques
Personality tests	Anecdotal records	Informal collection of information
		Systematic recording

possible future behaviour (as presented in Table 8.4). Various tools may be used in the collection of information during the assessment phase as illustrated in Box 8.1.

III. PHASE III: SETTING GOALS

During this third phase of the counselling process, goals are set cooperatively by both the counsellor and the counselee. While setting goals, the counselee's strengths, weaknesses, constraints and available resources must be kept under consideration. The goal could be immediate and ultimate, which directs the counsellor and the counselee to further progress in the counselling process and finally help in evaluation of the counselling outcome. Goals set during counselling are not fixed, but are dynamic, which may change based on needs and new information. Effective and reliable goal setting requires the following skills in counsellors:

- Multifaceted knowledge related to the problems of the counselee
- Ability to think critically and inference-drawing skills
- Judgement, planning and management skills
- Skills to segregate and differentiate the provided information
- Ability to teach individuals to think critically and realistically
- Help the counselee set feasible, reliable and achievable goals

IV. PHASE IV: INTERVENTION

This stage of counselling is an operational phase where the counselee is suggested the best possible options for the management of the present problem. This phase is affected by the counsellor's own thoughts about the counselling process. The intervention will depend on the approach used by the counsellor, the problem and the individual. The choice of intervention is a process of adaptation and the counsellor should be prepared to change the intervention when the selected intervention does not work.

V. PHASE V: TERMINATION AND FOLLOW-UP

This is the final stage of the counselling process, where counselling comes to an end. Termination must be planned well ahead so that the counselee may feel comfortable at the departure and gradually able to handle the problem independently. Some follow-up sessions may be required to help the counselee further to handle the problem independently.

TOOLS AND TECHNIQUES FOR THE COUNSELLING PROCESS

A number of tools and techniques are used in a guidance and counselling programme. With the help of these tools and techniques, data pertaining to all aspects of an individual's life are collected. These tools and techniques can be divided into two categories.

I. STANDARDIZED TOOLS AND TECHNIQUES

Standardized tools are also known as *testing techniques* and are more widely used than nonstandardized techniques to collect information about an individual as they are objective and reliable. They are developed by special agencies or institutions with the help of psychologists. The various types of standardized tools/tests generally used to collect information about an individual are as follows:

- ***Intelligence tests:*** Intelligence tests are used to measure the intelligence of an individual keeping in view the different dimensions of intelligence.
- ***Achievement tests:*** These are used to evaluate the achievement of an individual in different subjects of study.

- ***Aptitude tests:*** These tests are also called *special ability tests*. They are meant to judge the capacity of an individual to be skilled in some work or some subject of study after receiving formal or informal education.
- ***Interest tests:*** These tests are used to know the tendency of an individual to become absorbed in an experience and to continue it for a long time.
- ***Personality tests:*** These tests are meant to find out the traits, aptitudes, areas of interest, potentialities and behaviour of an individual at all times.

II. NONSTANDARDIZED TESTS

There are certain nonstandardized tests/techniques for collection of information about an individual. They are used to supplement other information available concerning the patient. Some nonstandardized techniques commonly used in counselling are as follows:

- ***Autobiography:*** An autobiography is an introspective report of one's own experience. It is designed to provide answers to specific questions put up by the counsellor. Structured autobiographies are asked to be written along a suggested outline consisting of topics such as my family, my childhood, my years before school, places I have lived, trips I have taken, my experiences in high school, my teachers and my class fellows, my ambitions and my aspirations.
- ***Anecdotal records:*** Froehlich and Hoyt (1959) define anecdotal records as: 'an anecdotal record consists of an objective description of pupil behaviour in a particular environmental setting, an interpretation of the behaviour by the observer, writing the description and recommendation for future action based on the incident and its interpretation'.
- ***Questionnaire:*** A list of questions is prepared pertaining to information about the individual. He is asked to give answers. The questionnaire consists of items regarding the student's home, family, health, educational and vocational plans, out of school and in school activities, study habits, etc. They are used to obtain comprehensive information dealing with the student, employing both his idiographic and normative data and serve to supplement incomplete information available about a student and improve the collection of data in an efficient manner.
- ***Interview:*** An interview is a face-to-face contact between the individual and the counsellor. The counsellor can get direct information from the individual through this technique.
- ***Observation:*** In this technique, the counsellor observes the counselee without letting him know he is being observed. Hence, his natural behaviour is observed through this technique under natural circumstances.
- ***Cumulative record chart:*** A cumulative record chart contains a record of all the important aspects of an individual. It provides an organized, progressive record of information regarding the student which distinguishes him from all other individuals. The cumulative folder includes information such as personal data and family background, medical and health condition, date of admission, academic attendance, academic performance, grades, test results, personality and behaviour trait ratings and performance in other curricular and cocurricular activities.
- ***Case study:*** A case study is the full study of an individual about the various aspects of his life to bring about an adjustment with society and life at large. It is an analysis and documentation of data collected in the case history. It comprises the information gathered about a patient, including the family history and physical development. Educational, social and vocational history is also covered in a case study. It presents a cumulative picture of an individual's personality. The information is gathered from sources such as cumulative records, observations, interviews, autobiographies,

self-reports, tests and other school records. The case study provides an opportunity for the person to be understood and treated as an individual. It helps in the prediction of behaviour. One of the disadvantages of the case history method is that it leads to a delay in providing assistance to the individual. Another limitation is that the case study may not be sufficient as a basis for drawing conclusions and formulating diagnosis for a patient.

- ***Rating scale:*** Rating scales are used for evaluating the characteristics of an individual. The student's characteristics such as dependability, honesty, cooperativeness, self-reliance and leadership are rated by teachers and counsellors. The rating scales are subject to bias and halo effect.
- ***Sociometric technique:*** It is a technique to discover the nature of an individual's relationships within a group. It measures the interpersonal preferences among the members of the group in reference to a criterion. The purpose of this technique is to measure each individual's social worth or personal value as viewed by his peers.
- ***Informal collection of information:*** Information about an individual can be collected informally. There are social and cultural functions/events the individual may participate in. Information about his behaviour can be collected in such functions.

ISSUES OF COUNSELLING IN NURSING EDUCATION

Counselling services in nursing education are quite essential but generally neglected, especially in the Indian scenario. The several pertinent issues of counselling in nursing, which need immediate attention, are discussed below:

- **Scarcity of qualified and competent counsellors:** In our own scenario, there is great scarcity of qualified and competent counsellors, either in nursing education or nursing services. One can hardly find a qualified and competent counsellor working for nurses in educational institutions or practice settings. It is generally observed that newly selected student nurses are found in great need of guidance and counselling services for better adjustment with the new demanding and challenging environment of their college and hospital. Therefore, the Indian Nursing Council must ensure that each college has at least one part-time counsellor who is qualified and competent.
- **Lack of awareness about needs and resources of counselling:** It is generally observed that there is a lack of awareness in nursing students and nurses about the need and importance of counselling services for a better future. Most of the student nurses join nursing education without any formal preadmission counselling and face difficulties adjusting with this demanding professional education, which leads to quite a stressful time for them. In spite of all the odds, nursing students and nurses are found to be quite unaware about the need and importance of counselling services. In addition, in situations where they feel a need for counselling services, they are not aware about the available resources, which adds to their problems. Therefore, nursing institutions must be proactive in improving the awareness in nursing students about the need and importance of counselling services as well as the availability of best resources.
- **Minimal pro-counselling environment:** Nursing institutions or hospitals do not give much importance to counselling services for nursing students and practising nurses. Very few health care institutions realize the importance of counselling for nurses or students nurses. In the absence of such pro-counselling environment, one cannot expect nurses or student nurses to receive standardized counselling services. It is high time the institutions realize the importance of counselling services for nurses and nursing students so that they can adjust to the new environment or their stressful job better for better learning and job performance, which is most essential for quality patient care.

- **Lack of counselling training for nurses/nursing faculty:** The nursing faculty or teachers could act as good counselling resources in nursing institutions, but there is a lack of adequate training for the nursing faculty and nursing teachers. The same is observed in the hospital setting where nurses could act as a good counsellor for their patients. It is therefore recommended that there must be an adequate curriculum related to counselling in the basic as well as advanced level of nursing education. In addition, there must be regular continuing education related to counselling for nurses and nursing faculty so that they can be updated with new aspects of counselling to benefit their patients.
- **Poor organizational set-up for counselling services:** A good organizational set-up is required for the efficient implementation of counselling services such as infrastructure, money and manpower. There is very poor attention towards building a competent and quality organization set-up for counselling services in health care institutions of either nursing education or nursing services.
- **Lack of interest and initiatives for counselling services:** There is poor interest and initiative for establishing counselling services among the nursing faculty, nursing teachers, nurses and management in India. Interest brings about the motivation to act and one can achieve initiatives. Therefore, nursing faculty, nursing teachers and nurses must be motivated to spark an interest in establishing counselling services for their patients so that the standard and quality of nursing services and nursing education can be ensured.
- **Poor counsellor–counselee ratio:** There are few initiatives to establish counselling services in Indian institutions. There is very poor counsellor–counselee ratio that has created a poor image and outcome of the counselling services. An adequate counsellor–counselee ratio must be ensured to achieve a better counselling outcome.
- **Lack of funds for counselling services:** There is a scarcity of funds for providing counselling services (including nursing students and practising nurses) in Indian health care institutions. In the absence of adequate funds for counselling services, one cannot imagine anything positive happening in the field of counselling services for nursing students and practising nurses. Therefore, the government and management must realize the importance of counselling services and dedicate adequate funds for these services for nursing students and practising nurses, so that the actual objective of nursing services and nursing education can be achieved.
- **Noncompliance with counselling interventions:** The other most crucial issue in the field of counselling services in nursing and nursing education is the problem of noncompliance with counselling interventions. This nonadherence or noncompliance is because of several reasons such as lack of interest, incompetent counsellors, poor access to qualified counsellors, lack of time and inadequate funds.
- **Ethical and moral issues:** This is also one of the most crucial issues of counselling services in nursing because the absence or poor practice of ethical and moral principles in counselling services may cause several serious problems. There are some critically essential ethical principles in counselling services that must be followed by counsellors, such as autonomy of practice, anonymity of subjects and confidentiality of information so that ethical, moral and legal problems pertaining to counselling can be prevented.

MANAGING DISCIPLINARY/GRIEVANCES PROBLEMS

Disciplinary problems are not only observed in Indian institutions but may also be seen in institutions around the world. Common disciplinary problems seen in Indian students are absenteeism, nonsubmission or late submission of assignments, disturbing classroom atmosphere, threatening strikes, damaging or spoiling institutional property, picking quarrels over small matters, using mobile phones in the classroom and so on. Disciplinary problems have increased many folds in Indian schools, colleges and universities. According to the Indian Education Commission, 'briefly there have been many ugly strikes and demonstrations often without any justifications, leading to violence, walk out from classrooms and examination halls, ticketless travel, clashes with police, burning of buses and cinemas, houses and sometimes even manhandling of teachers'. Reports of student trouble and indefinite closure of schools, colleges and even universities are pouring in from all over the country. Naturally this state of affairs has attracted the attention of educationists, leaders, social scientists and general public to seriously manage this problem so that the image and objectives of education can be optimally achieved.

STRATEGIES FOR MANAGEMENT OF DISCIPLINARY PROBLEMS

Disciplinary problems may arise because of several factors such as complex educational system, incompetence of teachers in handling students, student's personal and professional stress, lack of adequate cocurricular and extracurricular activities, inappropriate selection and use of disciplinary standards, neglecting the importance of positive reinforcement, poor teacher–student relationship, inadequate parent–teacher–student contacts and lack of efficient guidance and counselling services. The following strategies may be quite helpful in the prevention and management of disciplinary problems in students:

- ***Appropriate training of faculty and teachers:*** Adequate education and updated training is required to maintain the effective competence of practice including disciplinary management. There must be a provision of adequate training for principals, faculty and teachers to handle the disciplinary problems of students efficiently.
- ***Adequate practice of cocurricular and extracurricular activities:*** It is sometimes observed that exclusive intense curricular activities become a source of boredom and stress and may trigger an episode of indiscipline in students. Therefore, adequate incorporation of cocurricular and extracurricular activities is required in routine academic schedule. So the boredom of the students can be minimized and academic activities made more interesting.
- ***Appropriate selection and use of disciplinary standards:*** In the selection and use of disciplinary rules and standards, the following guidelines must be followed:
    - Identify the specific behaviours that are necessary to maintain a conducive learning environment in the institution.
    - Simplify disciplinary standards to three or four general classroom rules. They should be broad enough to cover the spectrum of appropriate expected behaviour.
    - Determine the positive and negative consequences of the disciplinary standards based on inputs received from teachers, parents and students.
    - Display standards in the classroom with a list of approved consequences from which effective consequences can be selected to fit the needs of each student.
    - Review the discipline plan daily with the class during the first two weeks of admission in the institution.
    - Meet with parents individually or collectively during the first two weeks of admission in the institution. Obtain parents' written approval for the discipline plan.
    - Implement the discipline plan. Be consistent, focus on praise and encouragement. Address infractions firmly, fairly and consistently.
- ***Use reward and punishment:*** Positive reinforcement is a tool often absent in the majority of educational institutions. Often, only the negative consequences are placed on the wall; there is

no visual display for consequences for positive behaviour. Overemphasis of the negative and minimization of the positive is detrimental in maintaining strong classroom discipline. Therefore, there must be adequate use of reward and punishment so that students are inclined towards positive behaviour and refrain from negative behaviour.

- ***Promoting better teacher–student relationship:*** An intimate teacher–student relationship always helps in the early identification and management of problems related to indiscipline. In addition, because of good teacher–student relationships, disciplinary problems may be prevented in time.
- ***Cultivation of ethical, moral and spiritual values:*** Values are the foundation to discipline in life. They guide the person on right path and act as a preventive measure for indiscipline. There must be significant stress on the cultivation of ethical, moral and spiritual values in students so that indiscipline can be prevented.
- ***A close teacher–parent–student contact:*** Parents are the first teachers and teachers are the second parents for students in their life. Both parents and teachers have a significant impact and influence on a student's life. Teachers must regularly communicate to students and their parents about their progress. A close loop of contact between the teacher, parents and students must be maintained and may be very helpful in the prevention and management of disciplinary problems.
- ***Effective use of guidance and counselling programmes:*** Guidance and counselling services may help students resolve their problems and they may feel comfortable and satisfied with their stay in the institution. In addition, regular guidance and counselling programmes can be helpful in the assessment and management of disciplinary problems in time.
- ***Preventive guidance and counselling:*** It is also known as supportive guidance and counselling, which is offered to students who have issues managing some of the acute academic and life-related challenges. The aim of preventive guidance and counselling is to restrict the problems before they cause problems or offer preventive interventions for the problems before they become worse. The most common example of preventive guidance and counselling is preexamination counselling or mid-term preventive academic guidance where poor performers are invited and guidance is offered, so that their academic performance may be improved in the subsequent examinations.

ROLE OF STUDENTS' GRIEVANCE REDRESSAL CELL/COMMITTEE

University Grant Commission has mandated to have a grievance redressal cell or committee in each institute of higher education or university. The aim of this grievance redressal cell is to entertain and redress complaints lodged by students, which may be related to academic or nonacademic matters. Students' grievance redressal cell is a very important committee in any educational institute as it provides an opportunity for students to address their academic and nonacademic matters, such as assessment, victimization, attendance, charging of fees, conducting of examinations and harassment by colleagues, students or teachers. The recommended composition of the students' grievance redressal committee is as given below:

- Chairperson – principal of the college
- Members – Two (among senior faculty members of the college, who are nominated by the principal)

Generally, the tenure of this committee lasts for 2 years, and to fulfil the quorum of the committee, at least two members should be present, including the chairperson of the committee. Students' redressal committee follow natural justice while deliberating on the grievances of students, and the report is submitted to the Vice-Chancellor or Director within the period of 15 days of receiving the complaint.

REVIEW QUESTIONS

LONG-ANSWER QUESTIONS

1. List down the purpose of guidance and counselling.
2. Describe how you will organize counselling services.
3. Explain the differences between guidance and counselling.
4. What are the objectives of guidance and counselling services in a college of nursing?
5. Explain the steps of the counselling process.
6. What is the importance of guidance and counselling for nursing students?
7. Discuss the basic principles of counselling.
8. Describe the approaches of counselling and steps of the counselling process.
9. Explain the organization of counselling services for first year B.Sc. (N) students.
10. Describe the issues of counselling services in nursing.
11. What are the different types of counselling, and how will you differentiate counselling from guidance?
12. Discuss the principles of counselling. How will you organize a counselling programme for students in your college of nursing?
13. Discuss the scope of guidance and counselling in nursing education.
14. Discuss the needs and purposes of guidance and counselling.

SHORT-ANSWER QUESTIONS

1. Discuss the terms guidance and counselling.
2. List down four issues for counselling nursing students.
3. Mention four principles of counselling.

MULTIPLE-CHOICE QUESTIONS (MCQs)

1. An elder sibling helps his younger one to make the right career choice. The approach used in this situation is best called as
   (a) Guidance
   (b) Counselling
   (c) Motivation
   (d) Appreciation
2. A teacher advises a student to face the sudden death of her mother with courage. The approach used in this situation is best called as
   (a) Guidance
   (b) Counselling
   (c) Motivation
   (d) Appreciation
3. At which one of the following levels does counselling operate?
   (a) Intellectual
   (b) Cognitive
   (c) Emotional
   (d) Social

4. Guidance and counselling is offered in which of the following situation(s)?
   (a) Personal
   (b) Educational
   (c) Social
   (d) All of these

5. The ultimate purpose of guidance and counselling is
   (a) Facilitating the adjustment
   (b) All-round development of personality
   (c) Self-understanding
   (d) Adjustment of the environment

6. Following are the characteristics of counselling except
   (a) Required in childhood
   (b) Self-realization
   (c) Professional activity
   (d) Need-based assistance

7. Which of the following plays an important role in delivering guidance and counselling services?
   (a) Teachers
   (b) Parents
   (c) Counsellors
   (d) All of these

8. While counselling an individual, an important principle to follow is
   (a) Cooperation with patient
   (b) Continuity of interaction
   (c) Individual differences
   (d) Joint responsibility

9. Which of the following approaches should be used while counselling an individual?
   (a) Firm
   (b) Flexible
   (c) Manipulative
   (d) Rigid

10. Organization of counselling services can be
   (a) Centralized and decentralized
   (b) Commanding and discommending
   (c) Reciprocal and mutual
   (d) Coordination and cooperation

11. Checklist and rating scales as tools of counselling are
   (a) Testing tools
   (b) Nontesting tools
   (c) Standardized tools
   (d) Personality tools

12. For counselling services at an affiliated college of the university having more than 1000 students, there should be provision of
   (a) HOD of psychology and team
   (b) Liaison officer and team
   (c) Counselling officer and team
   (d) Team of teachers

13. Following are the types of counselling types, except
    (a) Directive
    (b) Nondirective
    (c) Eclectic
    (d) Impersonal
14. Directive counselling is also called
    (a) Patient-oriented
    (b) Problem-oriented
    (c) Goal-oriented
    (d) Counsellor-oriented
15. Who evolved the concept of nondirective counselling?
    (a) Carl Rogers
    (b) E.G. Williamson
    (c) A.J. Jones
    (d) Gilbert Wrenn

ANSWERS OF THE MULTIPLE-CHOICE QUESTIONS

1. (a), 2. (b), 3. (c), 4. (d), 5. (b), 6. (a), 7. (d), 8. (c), 9. (b), 10. (a), 11. (b), 12. (c), 13. (d), 14. (b), 15. (a)

FURTHER READING

Aguileta, D. C. (1998). *Crisis intervention: Theory and methodology* (8th ed.). St. Louis, MO: Mosby.

Bhatia, K. K. (2002). *Principles of guidance & counselling* (1st ed.). Ludhiana: Kalyani Publishers.

Blanco, P. J., & Ray, D. C. (2011). Play therapy in elementary schools: A best practice for improving academic achievement. *Journal of Counseling & Development*, 89, 235–243.

Bodenhorn, N., Wolfe, E. W., & Airen, O. E. (2010). School counselor program choice and self-efficacy: Relationship to achievement gap and equity. *Professional School Counseling*, 13, 165–174.

Brigman, G. A., & Campbell, C. (2003). Helping students improve academic achievement and school success behavior. *Professional School Counseling*, 7, 91–98.

Brigman, G. A., Webb, L. D., & Campbell, C. (2007). Building skills for school success: Improving the academic and social competence of students. *Professional School Counseling*, 10, 279–288.

Bruce, A. M., Getch, Y. Q., & Ziomek-Daigle, J. (2009). Closing the gap: A group counseling approach to improve test performance of African-American students. *Professional School Counseling*, 12, 450–457.

Buser, J. K. (2010). American Indian adolescents and disordered eating. *Professional School Counseling*, 14, 146–155.

Cholewa, B., & West-Olatunji, C. (2008). Exploring the relationship among cultural discontinuity, psychological distress, and academic achievement outcomes for low-income, culturally diverse students. *Professional School Counseling*, 12, 54–61.

Froehlich, C. P., & Hoyt, K. B. (1959). *Guidance testing* (p. 34). Chicago: Science Research Associates.

Holcomb-McCoy, C. (2007). School counseling to close the achievement gap: A social justice framework for success. Thousand Oaks, CA: Corwin Press.

Holcomb-McCoy, C. (2007). Transitioning to high school: Issues and challenges for African American students. *Professional School Counseling*, 10, 253–260.

School of Health Sciences & Indra Gandhi National Open University. *Unit-5: Guidance and counseling in nursing education*. New Delhi: Program Guide Post Basic B.Sc. Nursing.

Ivey, A. E., Ivey, M. B., & Simek, D. L. (1996). Counselling and psychotherapy: Integrating skills theory and practice (3rd ed.). New Jersey: Prentice Hall International.

Jeynes, W. (2007). The relationship between parental involvement and urban secondary school student academic achievement: A meta-analysis. *Urban Education*, 42, 82–110.

Johnson, R. S. (2002). *Using data to close the achievement gap: How to measure equity in our schools*. Thousand Oaks, CA: Corwin.

Jones, A. J. (1963). *Principles of guidance* (5th ed.). New York: McGraw Hill Company Inc.

Kochhar, S. K. (1984). *Guidance & counseling in colleges & universities*. New Delhi: Sterling Publishers Pvt. Ltd.

Miranda, A., Webb, L., Brigman, G., & Peluso, P. (2007). Student success skills: A promising program to close the academic achievement gaps of African American and Latino Students. *Professional School Counseling*, 10, 490–497.

Nanda S. K. (1985). *Educational psychology*. Jalandhar: New Academics Publishing Co.

Newman, B. M., Lohman B. J., Myers, M. C., & Newman P. R. (2000). Experiences of urban youth navigating the transition to ninth grade. *Journal of Youth and Society*, 31, 387–416.

Newman, B. M., Myers, M. C., Newman, P. R., Lohman, B. J., & Smith, V. L. (2000). The transition to high school for academically promising, urban, low-income African American youth. *Adolescence*, 35, 45–66.

Pasricha, P. (1976). *Guidance and counseling in Indian education*. New Delhi: National Council of Educational Research and Training.

Poynton, T. A., Carlson, M. W., Hopper, J. A., & Carey, J. C. (2006). Evaluating the impact of an innovative approach to integrate conflict resolution into the academic curriculum on middle school students' academic achievement. *Professional School Counseling*, 9, 190–196.

Rosatl, G., & Marianmett, M. (2001). *Introduction to guidance and counselling* (6th ed.). New York: Publishers.

Schellenberg, R. (2008). *The new school counselor: Strategies for universal academic achievement*. Lanham, MD: Rowman Littlefield Education.

Schellenberg, R., & Grothaus, T. (2009). Promoting cultural responsiveness and closing the achievement gap with standards blending. *Professional School Counseling*, 12, 440–449.

Schellenberg, R., & Grothaus, T. (2011). Using culturally competent responsive services to improve student achievement and behavior. *Professional School Counseling*, 14, 222–230.

Sciarra, D. T. (2010). Predictive factors in intensive math course-taking in high school. *Professional School Counseling*, 13, 196–207.

Shields, L. (1975). Crisis intervention: Implications for the nurses. *Journal of Psychiatric Nurses*, 13, 37.

Sink, C. A. (2009). School counselors as accountability leaders: Another call for action. *Professional School Counseling*, 13, 68–74.

Stuart, G. W. (2009). *Principles and practice of psychiatric nursing* (9th ed., pp. 184–193). St. Louis, MO: Saunders Elsevier.

Stone, C. B., & Dahir, C. A. (2011). *School counselor accountability: A measure of student success* (3rd ed.). Boston, MA: Pearson.

Suri, S. P., & Sodhi, T. S. (2006). *Guidance and counseling* (3rd ed.). Patiala: Bawa Publications Pvt. Ltd.

Trusty, J., Mellin, E. A., & Herbert, J. T. (2008). Closing achievement gaps: Roles and tasks of elementary school counselors. *Elementary School Journal*, 108, 407–421.

Tucker, C., Dixon, A., & Griddine, K. (2010). Academically successful African American male urban high school students' experiences of mattering to others at school. *Professional School Counseling*, 14, 135–145.

Villalba, J. A., Akos, P., Keeter, K., & Ames, A. (2007). Promoting Latino student achievement and development through the ASCA National Model. *Professional School Counseling*, 12, 272–279.

Walia, J. S. (1982). *Foundations of educational psychology*. Jalandhar: Paul Publishers.

Webb, L. D., & Brigman, G. A. (2006). Student success skills: Tools and strategies for improved academic and social outcomes. *Professional School Counseling*, 10, 112–120.

Weinbaum, A. T., Allen, D., Blythe, T., Simon, K., Seidel, S., & Rubin, C. (2004). Teaching as inquiry: Asking hard questions to improve student achievement. New York: Teachers College Press.

West-Olatunji, C., Shure, L., Pringle, R., Adams, T., Lewis, D., & Cholewa, B. (2010). Exploring how school counselors position low-income African American girls as mathematics and science learners. *Professional School Counseling*, 13, 184–195.

Young, A., & Kaffenberger, C. J. (2011). The beliefs and practices of school counselors who use data to implement comprehensive school counseling programs. *Professional School Counseling*, 15, 67–76.

CHAPTER 9

Ethics and evidence-based teaching in nursing education

LEARNING OBJECTIVES

This chapter is designed to enable the reader to:

- Understand the concept of ethics in nursing education and ethical standards for students
- Appreciate importance of ethical standards and value-based nursing education
- Demonstrate skills in value development strategies among nursing students
- Describe evidence-based teaching process and its application in nursing education

KEY TERMS

INTRODUCTION

Nursing education has undergone a significant transformation from hospital-based training to university-based undergraduate, postgraduate and doctoral nursing education. Today, the evidence-based nursing education is a buzz world in nursing academia. There are increasing numbers of research and latest evidence on the topics related to nursing education, ranging from innovative educational philosophies, curriculum, teaching–learning processes and assessment methods. Furthermore, it has been observed that a significant number of good quality scientific nursing education journals are being published, few to name are *Nurse Education Today, Journal of Nursing Education, Nursing Education Perspectives, International Journal of Nursing Education Scholarship* and *Nurse Educator*.

The term ethics comes from the Greek word *ethos* and reflects societal standards. Nurses and nurse academicians routinely face the ethical issues, challenges and dilemma in their practices. Thus, ethics has been always cored to the nurses, nursing and nursing education. However, recently it is becoming more popular in nursing education because of increasing echo on patient-centric care. When a nursing curriculum adequately addresses ethics and provides nurses with tools to help them reflect critically about what nursing care implies, nursing education contributes to the development of nurses as skilled collaborators in care. The application of ethical principles within the teaching profession and nursing practice forms the core of the nurse educator's professional ethics.

ETHICS IN NURSING EDUCATION

Ethics in nursing education provides a foundation for addressing ethical questions that may arise in the nurse–patient relationship. Further, knowledge and skills in the use of ethical principles in nursing practices including nursing education are paramount important for nurses, and thus it is essential to prepare them in ethics at the undergraduate as well as postgraduate levels, which helps them to work collaboratively with other team members and share their voices when ethical issues confront clinicians, patients and families. It is essential that every student nurse become a worthy and an effective member of society as a citizen and a nurse encompassing highest possible moral and ethical values. Nurse educators have the role to encourage nursing students to exercise sound clinical judgement and practice using ethical standards vis-à-vis support and respect for their colleagues.

Teaching ethics is becoming an essential requirement in nursing curriculum. Nursing students and nurses must be taught ethics and ethical decision-making in order to practice ethical nursing. Effective methods of teaching ethics are being discovered by research and documented in the literature. Teaching methods such as role-playing, case study analysis, play and problem-based learning were found to be more effective than traditional teaching methods.

ETHICAL PRINCIPLES IN NURSING EDUCATION

Ethical principles provide a foundation for ethical practice for all members of the nursing education community and are based on the core values of caring, integrity, diversity and excellence as detailed below (refer Fig. 9.1):

I. **Caring:** Caring actions lead to positive outcomes for coworkers, students and community members. Self-care turns into caring for others effectively, an approach evidenced by open, two-way communication, active efforts to understand the needs of others, and the development of an

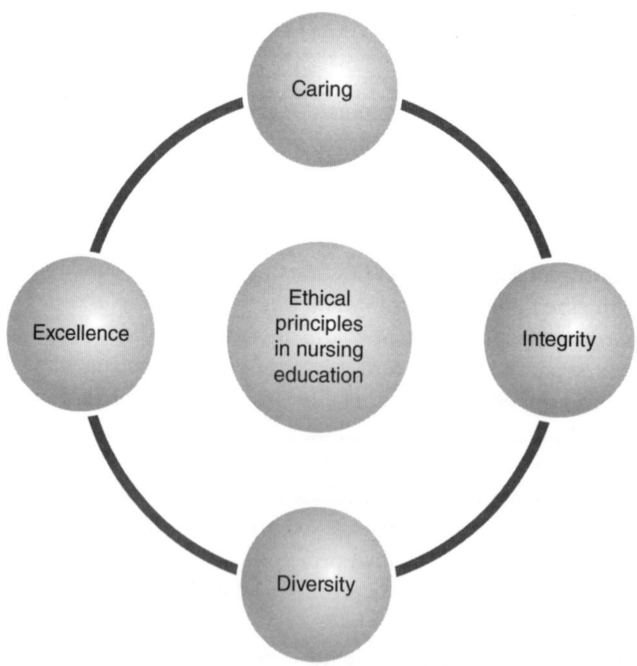

Figure 9.1

Ethical principles in nursing education.

environment that provides support to those in need of their physical and psychological needs. The learning environment should encourage freedom to explore and question. Nurse educators need to foster an educational environment that respects diverse perspectives, encourages curiosity, seeks and inquires about knowledge. To take care of others, one needs to take care of oneself. The foundation of this belief is in the concept of academic freedom, which holds that freedom of inquiry by students and faculty members is essential for excellence in nursing education. In order for students to learn caring behaviours, it is important for nurse educators to model those behaviours to peers and students by:

- Recognizing the importance of self-care is fundamental to caring for others.
- Creating an environment that acknowledges acceptance and encourages freedom of speech.
- Constructive criticisms and concerns engaging in relationship-focused conversations.

II. Integrity: Integrity involves treating others with respect – communicating with each other in a positive, courteous manner, respecting beliefs and maintaining a professional demeanour inside and outside the workplace. Communication transcends verbal communication and includes email, social networking and texting. Integrity demands taking responsibility for one's actions and advocating for professional values and beliefs. Decisions should reflect the demand for transparency, doing what is right for others, and fairness and equality by:

- Modelling professional behaviours that demonstrate honesty, respect for self and others, accountability and self-development.
- Building the trust of colleagues, students and the people we care about.
- Demonstrating the courage to challenge the status quo and advocate for professional values and beliefs.
- Making decisions that reflect ethical principles.

III. Diversity: Diversity supports environments that celebrate the uniqueness of individuals, fostering open, respectful and candid communication. It encourages innovative teaching strategies to address a variety of learning styles, taking into consideration the impact of cultural and experiential influences. Fair treatment of all is supported through nondiscriminatory practices in relation to race, ethnicity, gender, sexual orientation, socio-economic status, age, physical abilities, religious beliefs, political beliefs and other ideologies. Diversity can be achieved by:

- Creating environments that promotes open and respectful exchange and fair practices among all persons.
- Promoting autonomy and freedom of conscience.
- Developing and implementing teaching strategies that respond effectively to individual learning styles.
- Reaffirming the value and significance of contributions made by individuals of diverse backgrounds, experiences and beliefs.

IV. Excellence: Excellence requires scholarship and engagement in activities that promote professional development, improvement and understanding. A healthy nursing academic work environment includes the development and sustainability of a collegial environment, institutional support for the nursing unit, and strong leadership that guides efforts to create and implement transformative strategies with courageous ingenuity. Generate excellence by:

- Co-creating an environment that embraces collegiality, competence and support for ongoing professional development.
- Fostering a spirit of inquiry that can create a culture of innovation and creativity.
- Creating a conducive environment for transformational education through a better education system.

GAPS IN ETHICS EDUCATION IN NURSING CURRICULUM

Despite the advancement in ethics education still, the gaps in the nursing curriculum remain hidden. It is important to address the gaps in ethics education in the nursing curriculum to provide sufficient empirical data. Katelin et al. (2018) provided instruction to future generations of nurses towards ethics education in nursing, which highlighted the importance of ethics education in nursing. Following are the gaps identified which need an immediate address for safeguarding the workforce from frustration and physical or emotional worn out.

1. **Low quality of ethics pedagogy:** Ethics pedagogy is an academic discipline where educators impart knowledge and skill through the ethical context. Nurses are prepared with ethics knowledge in their bachelorette programme as a part of their nursing profession. They are obliged to follow moral principles of ethics in their daily practice. Besides this, there is a low quality of ethics pedagogy observed. A study conducted by Grady et al. highlighted that 22.7% of nurses had no knowledge of ethics and called to pay more attention to the content of ethics education. Another study conducted by Osingada et al. (2015) showed that only 15% of nurses score ≥50% and exhibit low knowledge of nursing ethics.
2. **Lack of continuous nurses' ethics education (CNEE):** Every day nurses deal with the ethical decision to protect the rights of the patient but they fail to follow the ethical vocabulary and education due to a lack of appropriate knowledge, quandaries and overwhelmed emotions. Osingada et al. (2015) addressed that 95.6% of nurses need training in nursing ethics. Abbasi et al. (2019) showed that there was a decrease in moral distress among nurses after the training.
3. **Failure to recognize the emerging ethical problems and address the micro-ethical practice:** Nurses' practice is embedded with the everyday ethical challenge. Some navigate effective interpersonal relationships by demonstrating advocacy and exquisite ethical reasoning skills while some report feeling distressed and powerless due to feelings of despair. Katelin et al. (2018) address that nurses often failed to recognize the emerging ethical problems which need a solid knowledge base of nursing ethics.

   Microethics is defined as the everyday ethical decision that practising nurses make in the context of common or routine clinical situations. Nurses often failed to address these microethics which later on becomes a habit of negligence. Krautscheid and Brown (2014) conducted a qualitative study which highlighted that those participants who were facing micro-ethical issues were struggling with recall and deliberately applying the ethical principles.
4. **Differences in ethics content delivery and actual practice:** Though the International Council of Nurses has revised the ICN Code of ethics for nurses, still there is a difference in the ethics content delivery and actual practice. Laabs (2012) survey results showed that APRNs (Advance Practice Registered Nurses) had a high level of confidence in managing ethical problems but their ethical knowledge was low. Further, it is identified that their ethics course completion percentage was 94% while their average score on tests was 55%. This difference creates an emergence to revise and reassess the teaching strategies related to ethical content. Baykara (2015) highlights that, nursing educators must reform the ethical teachings so that future nurses become more aware of the importance of nursing ethics.
5. **Lack of body for ethical curricula:** Nurses are offered ethics content during their undergraduate, graduate and doctoral programmes as a part of the nursing education domain, but they do not offer specific curricular content on ethics. Ethics itself is a broad area which requires its own body of knowledge. Studies highlighted that nurses who graduate from any nursing programme do not share the ethical vocabulary nor had sufficient knowledge to address the ethical challenge in practice. Further, it highlights the specific content issue in the ethics curriculum which creates controversy regarding theory versus skill-based approach.

Benner and colleagues identify redesigning the ethics curricula, which will not only focus on critical or ethical dilemmas but also on everyday issues related to ethical comportment. The other reason is the national shortage of faculty, and those who are present lack credibility which became a barrier to ethical education content delivery and its development (Laabs, 2015).

INNOVATIVE METHODS FOR ETHICS PEDAGOGY

1. **Undergraduate level methods:**
    - The undergraduate programme includes ethics content in the subject fundamentals of nursing and nursing education. Despite this, there is a lack of ethics knowledge among nursing students. High-quality nursing demands the ability to make an ethical judgement which brought a paradigm shift in nursing from a passive to an actual learner approach. These methods include a case-control approach in nursing education, team-based learning, readiness assurance process, simulation-based learning for more rehearsal and feedback and Refinement of teaching and evaluation methods in nursing ethics education.
    - Hickman and Wocial (2013) highlighted that at the undergraduate level, it is a must to use team-based learning (TBL) concepts in the ethical course. Further, they emphasized the need for strong undergraduate moral competence, which can be acquired by conducting small group activities on developing ethical skills based on critical thinking and problem-solving approach for active learning. Including the readiness assurance process (RAP) allows students to clarify reading concepts before a test and gets immediate feedback. The TBL is an important strategy for imbibing ethics in undergraduates. It reinforces the three ethical competence – moral perception, judgement and behaviour.
    - Krautscheid used simulation-based education micro-ethical decision-making approach. They used high-fidelity simulation for rehearsing ethical knowledge and managing conflict communication in case of micro-ethical dilemmas like unsafe medication administration and confidentiality breach. After the implementation of this approach, learners gained confidence and advocacy skill.
    - Lee used the case-control approach for enhancing the nursing ethics ability. They highlight that the teaching methodology must encourage active participation, provide an opportunity for ethical reflection in actual practice, to execute different evaluation methods in nursing ethics education.
2. **Postgraduate level or APRNs methods**
    - The postgraduation level is an advanced clinical practice specialization in a specific area. This level of students is considered to have more advocacy in managing ethical challenges. The methods include measuring and improving the existing teaching methods and provision of programmed instruction module for ethical dilemmas.
    - Laabs conducted a survey and identified that postgraduate nurses or APRNs have more confidence in managing ethical problems but exhibit less knowledge of ethics. Therefore, variety of diverse pedagogical methods are required to enhance knowledge on ethics and ethical decision-making. They recommend measuring the essential ethical education and teaching methods.
    - Pariseau-Legault and Lallier (2016) stressed to use training programme for ethics which includes a six-step decision-making framework for building moral integrity and procurement of ethical competencies. The training programme includes three pedagogy objectives: building moral integrity, clinical to ethical judgement and fostering interpersonal collaboration. This pedagogical approach has the potential to optimize the ethical, reflective and deliberate competencies among advanced practice nurses. They suggested encouraging students to find creative solutions instead of dualistic decision-making while facing ethical challenges. The decision-making process should be on problem-solving rather than exclusively on ethical dilemmas.

3. Education in a clinical setting

- Everyday ethical problems create a threat to ethical values which require more training and education on ethical principles. Often nurses while working in clinical settings become highly emotional and take things personally which leads to unethical behaviour. The methods for enhancing ethical education in the clinical setting include CNEE, simulation practice, a fellowship programme in curriculum development, Clinical Ethics Residency for nurses (CERN) programme and mentored clinical practicum.
- Robinson et al. (2014) and Grace et al. (2014) highlight the inclusion of enhancing moral agency: clinical ethics residency for nurses (CERN). CERN is a 10 months, 96-hours residency programme in clinical ethics which includes didactics learning, simulation-based practice and clinical mentorship. It is a pedagogical innovation which increased ethical knowledge, decreases moral distress and provides moral agency among adult learners. This programme includes reinforcing learning and providing peer support.

VALUE-BASED EDUCATION IN NURSING

The professional values of nurses guide the delivery of nursing care and decision-making. Modification of personal values and internalization of professional values result from the educational process and continuous professional experience. Personal values are imbibed within a person; examples are love, compassion and integrity. Professional values are truthfulness, courage and care and they are acquired through socialization, experience, teachers, peers and a code of conduct in nursing. Shahriari et al. (2013) mentioned 10 nursing ethical values related to patient care, that is human dignity, altruism, social justice, autonomy in decision-making, precision and accuracy in caring, responsibility, human relationship, individual and professional competency, sympathy and trust.

The American Association of Colleges of Nursing identifies five professional values: altruism, autonomy, human dignity, integrity and social justice. Altruism refers to the sacrificial attitude expressed by the nurses, and the autonomy of the profession means its independent functioning or self-governance. Showing self-respect and self-respect towards patients/families/colleagues reflects human dignity. Integrity also plays an important role for nurses that express honesty and ethical principles. Social justice refers to respecting the rights of all and treating all equally.

Value clarification and role modelling by teachers in the classroom as well as in the clinical area throughout their educational programme can help promote the development of appropriate values. Value-based education provides the foundation for nurses to practice value-based nursing care. Training designed to support the integrated personal and professional development of learners is called value education or vocational training and is referred to as value-based learning in nursing education. The development of values among nursing students in different types of educational programmes varies significantly. One of the research study compared the values of nursing students in an associate degree, diploma and B.Sc. Nursing degree programme, and results showed that values differed between programmes, where diploma nursing students scored significantly higher in overall value scores in most domains (Fisher, 2014).

STRATEGIES FOR VALUE DEVELOPMENT

Nurses today are faced with so many complex choices and alternative responses that they have to deal with health, illness, death, distress, family, sex, work, friendships, leisure, rules and authority, confusion about the value of physical appearance and lifestyles. The training in value development or values creation is both experiential and contemplative. Personal narratives, stories and illustrations that focus on the integration of self, presence and expertise and discussion of important events and personal experience are some of the methods used.

It is important for a teacher to model appropriate behaviour to deal with the issue of ethics and morality. The value clarification approach can give learners a conceptual framework and a set of skills for problem-solving as well as articulating and developing values, whether a teacher is present or not. The purpose of value clarification is to facilitate an awareness of individual values and the valuing process to move towards the point of choosing one's own values, rather than merely reacting to prior programming and experiences.

STEPS FOR VALUE CLARIFICATION

Value clarification is a process by which individuals identify and examine their own values and value systems. Raths et al. (1978) described a 'valuing process', including following components:

1. *Choosing (cognitive)*: beliefs are chosen freely from alternative and reflection and consideration of consequences.
2. *Prizing (affective)*: beliefs are prized and cherished.
3. *Acting (behaviour)*: chosen beliefs are confirmed to others, incorporated into behaviour consistently in one's life.

ETHICAL DECISION-MAKING

Nurses in their daily routine encounter many situations that would require them to make ethical judgement and decisions. The people who are involved in such decision-making situations are patients and their family members facilitated by doctors, nurses and other healthcare professionals. In any ethical dilemma, there is no right or wrong answer. Ethical decision-making can be taught well using situation analysis and role-play. The most vital steps in making ethical decision-making process are discussed below.

FIVE STEPS ETHICAL DECISION-MAKING PROCESS

There are five steps of decision-making process according to Ethical Decision-Making Framework (EDMF). Logical linear sequence of these five steps increases the ethical awareness, strengthen ethical decision-making capability and accountability (Fig. 9.2).

1. **Assessment:** When there is existence of any ethical dilemma, first ensure the collection of all substantial facts before moving to the next step of decision-making. Gather the data regarding magnitude of the dilemma, abide by or agree with the existing law, code of ethics and conduct and own culture's ethical values. If these all data are not enough or it does not comply the law, proceed for further collection of facts or seek professional advice.
2. **Alternatives:** List all the possible alternatives considering their pros and cons. If one of the alternatives looks most feasible and a potential solution, then move forward to the next step, i.e. analysis. If none of the identified alternatives looks to be a possible soultion, then collect more data and facts.
3. **Analysis:** After choosing an alternative, verify it again in terms of current and future impact on the organization, nursing education system, teacher, student, culture and teaching environment. While doing further analysis, be calm, take sufficient time and remain free from any influence, otherwise continue with review process of the potential decision.

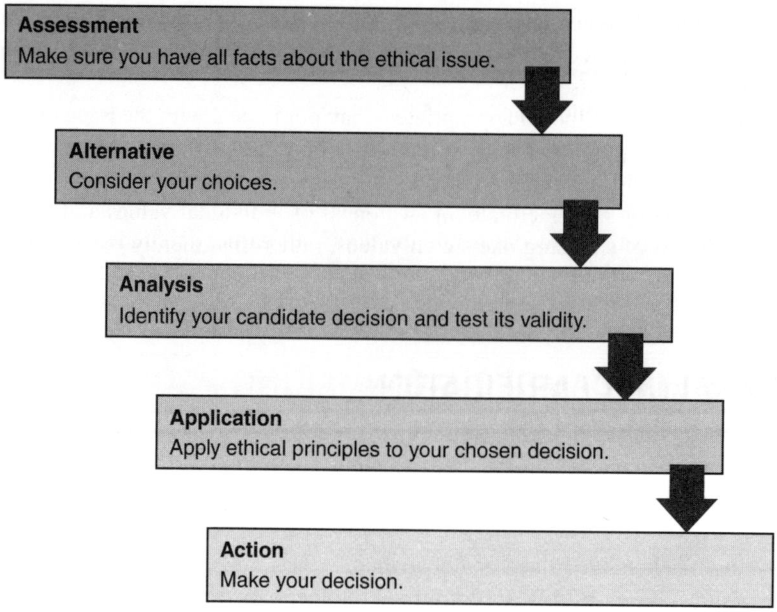

Figure 9.2

Steps of ethical decision-making process.

4. **Application:** Potential decision should be compatible with ethical principles and values (responsibility, respect, fairness, honesty). If still the decision does not look like the best, even if persist a single dilemma can continue with review process or else move for taking the action.
5. **Action:** If potential decision found as most suitable considering every aspect then make the decision. Be responsible for the decision, make it public, be consistent and happy for the decision. If dilemma exists, continue the cycle.

THE SIX STEPS FRAMEWORK FOR ETHICAL DECISION-MAKING PROCESS

This crystal clear, systematic, well-organized steps for ethical decision-making process is typically meant for practitioners and to help them deal effectively with ethical issues.

The six step processes are as follows:

Information: Gather in-depth information related to patient (medical, surgical and social history, diagnosis, prognosis, goals of care, treatment plan, consulting services).

Identification: Identify that issues are coming under ethical or legal first. The institutional or social issue needs to be addressed by dedicated departments.

Clarification: In the steps clarify about:

i) Does the practitioner himself and all other team members know and understand all the necessary and relevant medical information?
ii) Does that specific patient and their family members know and understand all the necessary and relevant medical information?

- **iii)** Are any other options easily available like: switching services, departments or transferring the patient?
- **iv)** 'Is a trial period possible?'
- **v)** 'Is it an ethical issue or dilemma?'

After detailed clarification, frame it as an ethical question.

Assessment: Do the assessment considering medical indications, patient's preferences, interests, values and their quality of life.

Recommendation: Prepare the recommendation which all parties can understand.

Documentation: Do record all recommendations in patient's record. Do follow up.

SEVEN STEPS ETHICAL DECISION-MAKING PROCESS

Davis' (1999) approach believes in identifying numerous potable options while responding to an ethical dilemma and prescribes seven steps process for the same.

1. **State the problem:** Identify the uncomfortable zone and area of conflict of interest.
2. **Check the facts:** Problems may abolish if examined promptly and intensively or may change radically. Determine the surrounded facts.
3. **Identify relevant factors:** Identify all relevant factors, that is educator, student or all involved personnel of the system, professional codes, policies and practical constraints.
4. **Develop a list of options**: Considering all relevant factors, prepare a list with possible options for solution.
5. **Test options**: Next test the options in terms of the following:
   Harm test: Find which alternative has less harms than others.
   Publicity test: Check where you want to publish your choice of this option.
   Defensibility test: Test the defensibility of the choice before teacher, student, principal, parents, peers or any related person.
   Reversibility test: Check the reversibility of the option also if any adverse consequences happen.
   Colleague test: Mind the colleague's response also for the option.
   Professional test: Test the suitability of the option according to the nursing council.
   Organization test: Test in respect of policy of the esteemed institution.
6. **Make a choice based on steps:** Choose the best option by reviewing 1–5 steps.
7. **Review steps 1–6:** Do further review of 1–6 steps and make the decision.

ETHICAL STANDARDS FOR STUDENTS

The ethical issues that arise in academic and clinical settings are many and they pertain to students and faculty. Ethical expectations for nursing students are not limited to clinical practice but also extend into other aspects of the professional role, such as academics and interprofessional relationships. Ethical issues that affect students' academic performance and student–faculty relationships are academic dishonesty (cheating, plagiarism and forgery) and clinical dishonesty. Students face many personal, family, academic and professional stresses/pressures. When these pressures intensify, values such as honesty and integrity can become challenging. It is the faculty's responsibility to serve as a role model and teach values that are vital to maintaining integrity among nursing students.

ACADEMIC DISHONESTY

Academic dishonesty is defined as dishonesty in relation to any university activities, such as fraud, plagiarism and willfully providing false information to the university. Academic dishonesty includes acts of deception and reflects a lack of commitment to truthfulness (telling the truth). Academic dishonesty is intentional complicity in the deceptive performance of one's or another's academic work. According to educational theories, poor teaching environments, lack of ethics training by the university, poor communication with peers and teachers (according to social psychologists) and certain cultural factors are associated with academic dishonesty. There are many factors that can influence academic dishonesty, which are:

1. **Psychological factors** that will result in pressure to perform well and students' own expectations for success.
2. **Ethical factors** such as valuing success at any price.
3. **Social factors** such as competitiveness and the belief that 'everyone else cheats'.
4. **Environmental factors** that encourage cheating.

CLINICAL DISHONESTY

Clinical dishonesty is a complex problem that threatens the health and safety of patients. The frequency of clinical dishonesty among nursing students is high and needs attention. Furthermore, given the positive association between dishonesty and perceived clinical stress, it is essential to teach nursing students effective strategies to empower them to cope with clinical stress. Many studies have proved that nursing students are likely to commit dishonest behaviour in both the clinical setting and the classroom.

One study had found that 66% of nursing students engage in unethical clinical behaviour. Reasons for unethical behaviour by nursing students in clinical practice include overwork, inappropriate clinical culture of nurses, poor role models, noncooperation of patients with students, fear of being rejected by the peers, faculty or hospital, lack of awareness, high volume and difficult courses, fear of failure, stress and pressure for success and competition with peers. Dishonesty is considered a major risk to learning; it harms patient care and safety, and may be a recurring pattern in future professional behaviour that puts patients at risk. Therefore, nursing faculty, tutors and clinical instructors should provide necessary training to students about the impact of ethical behaviour on patient care and teach students to use effective strategies to deal with clinical stress to ensure the health of patients.

STUDENT–FACULTY RELATIONSHIP

Effective student–faculty relationships can have an impact on students' resilience. Protective factors such as caring relationships, high expectations and opportunities to participate and contribute not only improve students' academic performance but also strengthen their resilience. Caring teachers who show concern for students and act as confidants, role models and mentors, thus, can contribute to students' ability to overcome personal weaknesses and environmental adversities. Therefore, teachers can have a positive impact not only on students' academic achievement and behaviour but also on their resilience and long-term success in life. There are three main elements that are important in the faculty–student relationship namely: (1) the teaching–learning environment, (2) the exchange of information, (3) the mentor–peer association.

In addition to the above elements, Beutel (2009) – while exploring teachers' understanding of their relationship with students – gave five main categories, namely: (1) providing information, (2) providing instructions, (3) facilitating, (4) guided participation and (5) mentoring. Resilience has been found to be an important factor in fostering positive and supportive relationships between teachers and students.

To ensure that an effective faculty–student relationship exists, a teacher must possess certain qualities. Teachers need to listen to their students, engage them as fellow human beings, recognize and understand their perspectives and views of the world and meet their relational needs.

FACULTY SUPPORT FOR STUDENTS

A teacher must ensure support for students in the mental, social, physical and academic areas. One study reported that when nursing students felt that their academic efforts were not supported by faculty, they often voluntarily or involuntarily withdrew from the nursing profession. Reported that they feel supported by faculty who portray caring qualities in their pedagogy. There are three subthemes that emerged from literature in relation to faculty support for students namely: mentorship, accessibility and approachability of faculty.

MENTORSHIP

Mentorship cannot be based only on a random system of matching students with faculty but serves the purpose of mentorship, and a student should be purposefully paired with a faculty member to ensure that both are interested in sharing their backgrounds, personal strengths, limitations and goals. It helps build the foundation for the natural progression of productive student–faculty relationships. It has been proven that mentorship empowers students and faculty, fosters their personal development and professional relationships, creates a safe learning environment and promotes the overall success of students.

ACCESSIBILITY AND APPROACHABILITY

Nonaccessibility is a hindrance to faculty–student relationships, and it has also been reported by some studies that 50% of nursing students disclosed that needed support from faculty was not available and that faculty were perceived as inaccessible either because they were unapproachable or because they failed to respond to formal communication. This condition can hinder academic relationships and success. A supportive environment means that faculty is accessible and caring, which can offer a road map to helping students succeeds in their academic careers.

MAJOR BARRIERS IN STUDENT–FACULTY RELATIONSHIP

There are several barriers related to student–faculty relationship. The major barriers along with ways to overcome these barriers are presented in Box 9.1.

STRATEGIES TO FOSTER POSITIVE AND SUPPORTIVE STUDENT–FACULTY RELATIONSHIPS

- Build authentic relationships inside and outside of the classroom to be more supportive.
- Model qualities of caring rather than simply saying that we care.

BOX 9.1 MAJOR BARRIERS IN STUDENT–FACULTY RELATIONSHIP

Barrier	Ways to Overcome
1. **Incivility:** A barrier to the development of respectful and positive relationships between nursing students and faculty. Incivility includes abusive environments (particularly verbal abuse), disruptive and irresponsible behaviours and unfair/biased treatment. Students' incivility is an impolite and disturbing behaviour in education and if ignored could lead to behavioural complexities and eventually violence and aggression in classrooms.	• Maintain a civil learning environment. • Overlooking and nonstrictness. • Appropriate decision-making. • Create workshops on communication. Techniques. • Setting strict rules. • Training through role-playing. • Friendship strategy by providing motivation and devoting enough time for students • Using appropriate apprenticeship methods. • Defining standards and norms. • Self-reflection, self-control, personal experience. • Interactive educational environment. • Acknowledging concerns and reciprocating in a fair and respectful fashion may minimize the escalation of uncivil practices.
2. **Diversity:** The greatest potential barriers to student–faculty relationships in the literature are language, cultural diversity and gender diversity.	• Use words wisely. For example, when faculty refers to nurses as 'she', this can create a division and imply that the profession lacks acceptance of male nurses, which in turn can hinder building professional relationships between male nursing students and faculty. • Be aware of all the factors such as individual's unique learning abilities, challenges and differences. • Create a learning space that is safe for students and teacher. • Be aware of the potential bias that may exist in the learning environment.

- Practice mutual respect, in words and in actions to reduce uncivil behaviour.
- Consider that diversity is not just about culture.

EVIDENCE-BASED TEACHING

Evidence-based teaching (EBT) practice in nursing is defined as 'the validation, generation, application, and perpetuation of those methods that facilitate the preparation of skilled and thoughtful nurses who function in a constantly evolving, global health care environment'. EBT is the comprehensive measurement and evaluation of faculty learning activities, with tools that capture multiple sources of evidence for accurate and complete measurement of learning outcomes. It is a dynamic, holistic system using evidence-validated educational principles to support, maintain and promote a new level of knowledge for the learners in a variety of settings.

PROCESS OF EVIDENCE-BASED TEACHING

There are many different components of the EBT process that support, interact and challenge other components within the model. Here, the learner is seen as the centre of the process within evidence-based learning. The objective of each academic session and resource is to ensure that the learner is

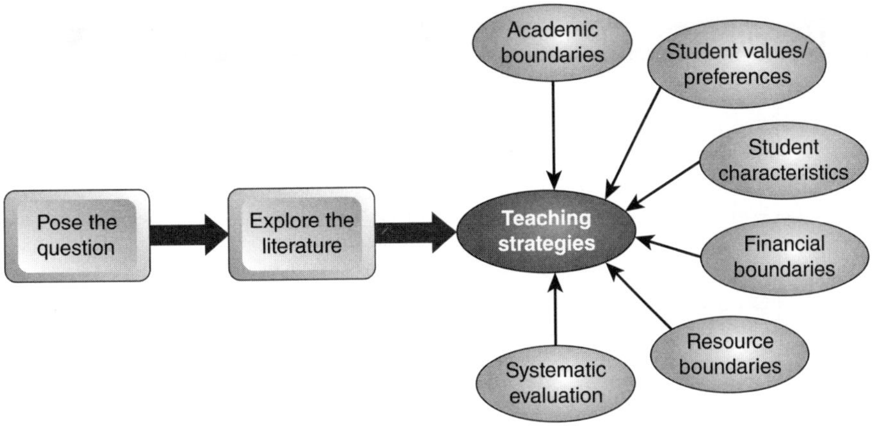

Figure 9.3

Schematic diagram for evidence-based teaching.

effectively placed in a position to gain maximum knowledge from the educational environment. The process of EBT is reflected in Fig. 9.3.

Posing a question: This is the first step in initiating an investigation into the evidence surrounding the educational process. The wording of the question must be clear and concise.

Explore the literature: A well-developed question provides keywords and concepts imperative for identifying and narrowing the selection of the articles. Evidence supporting the learning environment can be easily discovered by locating articles through a question-driven literature search.

Many factors – such as student values or preferences, student characteristics, academic limitations, systematic assessment and financial or resource limitations – affect teaching strategies. Each of these aspects within the synthesis of evidence must be carefully and systematically considered along with other aspects as the analysis of the evidence is completed. The aspects within the educational process need to be founded upon evidence. EBT poses the question using the PSCOT format: P (population), S (strategy), C (comparison), O (outcome), T (time), whereas within the process of EBP. Whereas in evidence practices, the questions are presented in PICOT format: P (population), I (intervention), C (comparison), O (outcome), T (time).

To understand the difference between evidence-based practice and evidence-based teaching, refer Table 9.1.

APPLICATION OF EVIDENCE-BASED TEACHING IN NURSING EDUCATION

EBT refers to teaching approaches that are often constructivist in nature, encouraging students to be active participants in building on and reflecting on their learning. Nurse educators have an important role in advising student nurses with regard to developing evidence-based practice (EBP) skills, accessing research products and participating in research projects. This requires more innovative learning approaches that promote active participation, creativity and critical thinking in students such as online teaching and learning, access to electronic resources, video conferencing and research-based teaching and learning. EBT practices in nursing education require sustained institutional, administrative and collegial support to promote faculty effectiveness and student learning.

Table 9.1 Difference Between Evidence-Based Practice and Evidence-Based Teaching

Category	Evidence-Based Practice	Evidence-Based Teaching
Clinical question	Poses the clinical questions using the PICOT format: P (population), I (intervention), C (comparison), O (outcome), T (time)	Poses the question using the PSCOT format: P (population), S (strategy), C (comparison), O (outcome), T (time)
Evidence	Explores available evidence to determine best practice using a clinical evaluation approach	Explores available evidence to determine best practice of teaching and assessment using a critical evaluation approach
Intervention	Consider individual clinical expertise and client preferences/values as interventions	Integrate teaching expertise with students' characteristics, priorities and values in the teaching and learning environment as solutions and ideas are created
Implementation	Fostering clinical changes as needed within the parameters of resources and stakeholders	Initiate academic revision as needed within academic, financial and resource limits
Evaluation	Evaluate change with respect to patient satisfaction, financial considerations, institutional considerations and professional considerations	Consider changes based on key performance criteria identified with systematic assessment for the academic setting

Like EBP, no model has been created in evidence-based education yet, but the teaching faculty can follow models and theories related to EBP to contribute to important aspects in nursing education and practice. The key elements of the EBP theories can be combined to address the process of EBT and requires manipulation to address the pedagogical and educational aspects of EBT.

The changes within nursing education are imperative and necessary and this reflects the need to adopt EBT in nursing education, and the recommendations for nursing programmes include changing:

- From a focus on covering nonrelevant knowledge to an emphasis on teaching for a sense of prominence, positioned cognition and action in particular situations.
- From a sharp separation of clinical and classroom teaching to an integration of the two.
- From an emphasis on critical thinking to an emphasis on clinical reasoning and multiple ways of thinking.
- From an emphasis on socialization and role-playing to an emphasis on formation.

The above recommendations strongly support the idea that educational processes used within the classroom and clinical settings should embody the process of verifying the appropriateness and effectiveness of the various teaching strategies used. Recent studies in teacher education emphasize the implementation of EBT practices as a way to bridge this gap (Bauer & Prenzel, 2012; Slavin, 2002; Wiseman, 2010).

Quality improvement (QI) is often associated with the improvement of nursing care at the point of care and has become a recognized form of EBP and is essential in the provision of nursing care. Similarly, QI also has an impact on EBT, as shown in the evaluation process of programmes, courses, faculty and students. The assessment should be considered as a parallel between EBP and EBT. Quality improvement in EBT is specific to educational institutions providing nursing education, whereas in EBP, QI is considered in relation to the improvements required by the organization providing patient care.

EBP models should be applied to nursing education. The evidence for promoting best practices in the classroom and clinical setting must incorporate the motivation and compliance of students to critically think when providing nursing care, especially to patients from diverse settings and complex healthcare needs. Research is used as a tool in developing new teaching and learning strategies. Nurse teachers are guided by EBP in teaching and research reports. EBP in learning is also research-based, meaning that students learn by using research findings. Research-based teaching and learning encourages and stimulates critical thinking for students. Traditional teaching methods and learning styles still dominate nursing education and these strategies do not encourage critical thinking among nursing students; therefore, these methods will not prepare student nurses to make sound clinical decisions in practice.

TIPS FOR APPLYING EVIDENCE-BASED PRACTICE IN NURSING EDUCATION

Following are the key elements to remember for a teacher to apply EBT in nursing education:

- Develop a clear definition of EBP and EBT.
- Incorporate an evidence-based model approach to EBT.
- Consider generational differences when trying to motivate students.
- Fostering attention, relevance, confidence and satisfaction to involve students in the learning process.
- Use feedback, listening and problem-solving/critical thinking.
- Emphasize rewards, results and success while maintaining high expectations.
- Include operant conditioning and social learning theory.

REVIEW QUESTIONS

LONG-ANSWER QUESTIONS

1. Define and discuss the ethics in nursing education.
2. Enlist ethical principles in nursing education.
3. Explain innovative methods for ethics pedagogy in nursing education.
4. Discuss decision making and decision making process with an example.
5. Elaborate the evidence-based teaching in nursing education.

SHORT-ANSWER QUESTIONS

1. Gaps in ethics education in nursing curriculum.
2. Academic and clinical dishonesty.
3. Student-faculty relationship.
4. Barriers of student-faculty relationship.
5. Application of evidence-based teaching in nursing education.
6. Value-based education in nursing.
7. Ethical standards for nursing students

MULTIPLE-CHOICE QUESTIONS (MCQs)

1. Which of the following best describes the concept of autonomy in nursing ethics?
   (a) Respecting the rights and decisions of patients
   (b) Prioritizing the needs of the healthcare system

(c) Following the instructions of the healthcare team
(d) Focusing on personal beliefs and values

2. In nursing education, the principle of beneficence refers to:
(a) Focusing on personal gain and advancement
(b) Acting in the best interest of the patient
(c) Avoiding any harm to oneself
(d) Promoting the interests of the healthcare organization

3. Which ethical principle emphasizes the duty of healthcare professionals to maintain confidentiality?
(a) Non-maleficence
(b) Veracity
(c) Justice
(d) Fidelity

4. A nurse encounters a situation where the patient's cultural beliefs conflict with the proposed medical treatment. Which ethical principle is most relevant in this scenario?
(a) Autonomy
(b) Beneficence
(c) Non-maleficence
(d) Justice

5. The principle of non-maleficence in nursing education requires nurses to:
(a) Ensure fairness and equality in patient care
(b) Maintain professional competence and integrity
(c) Avoid causing harm or injury to patients
(d) Respect the rights and dignity of patients

6. What does the principle of veracity emphasize in nursing ethics?
(a) Respecting patient confidentiality
(b) Upholding honesty and truthfulness
(c) Promoting equality in healthcare
(d) Advocating for patient rights

7. When nurses allocate resources and distribute care equitably among patients, they are following the principle of:
(a) Autonomy
(b) Fidelity
(c) Justice
(d) Non-maleficence

8. The ethical principle of fidelity in nursing education refers to:
(a) Promoting the welfare of patients
(b) Providing care without discrimination
(c) Avoiding conflicts of interest
(d) Maintaining professional boundaries and trust

9. Which ethical principle guides nurses to advocate for vulnerable populations and address health disparities?
(a) Autonomy
(b) Justice
(c) Veracity
(d) Fidelity

10. Nurses who engage in lifelong learning and continuously update their knowledge and skills are demonstrating adherence to which ethical principle?
 (a) Autonomy
 (b) Beneficence
 (c) Non-maleficence
 (d) Fidelity

11. What is the primary goal of value-based education in nursing?
 (a) Developing clinical skills
 (b) Enhancing critical thinking abilities
 (c) Instilling ethical values and professionalism
 (d) Promoting teamwork and collaboration

12. Which of the following best describes the concept of empathy in value-based nursing education?
 (a) Demonstrating sympathy towards patients' suffering
 (b) Understanding and sharing patients' feelings and experiences
 (c) Maintaining emotional distance from patients
 (d) Focusing on personal well-being over patient care

13. In value-based nursing education, the principle of integrity emphasizes:
 (a) Providing care without discrimination
 (b) Upholding honesty and ethical conduct
 (c) Respecting patients' autonomy and decisions
 (d) Advocating for vulnerable populations

14. Nurses who demonstrate accountability in value-based education:
 (a) Take responsibility for their actions and decisions
 (b) Focus on personal interests rather than patient needs
 (c) Engage in unethical behaviour without consequences
 (d) Prioritize financial gain over patient well-being

15. The principle of respect for diversity in value-based nursing education encourages nurses to:
 (a) Uphold cultural and religious beliefs of patients
 (b) Ignore individual differences and treat everyone the same
 (c) Promote their own personal beliefs and values
 (d) Prioritize their own comfort over patient preferences

ANSWERS OF THE MULTIPLE-CHOICE QUESTIONS

1. (a), 2. (b), 3. (d), 4. (a), 5. (c), 6. (b), 7. (c), 8. (d), 9. (b), 10. (d), 11. (c), 12. (b), 13. (b), 14. (a), 15. (a)

FURTHER READING

Abbasi, S., Ghafari, S., Shahriari, M., & Shahgholian, N. (2019). Effect of moral empowerment program on moral distress in intensive care unit nurses. *Nursing Ethics*, *26*, 1494–1504. doi:10.1177/0969733018766576

Allas, R., Leijen, Ä., & Toom, A. (2017). Supporting the construction of teacher's practical knowledge through different interactive formats of oral reflection and written reflection. *Scandinavian Journal of Educational Research*, *61*, 600–615. doi:10.1080/00313831.2016.1172504

Bauer, J., & Prenzel, M. (2012). European teacher training reforms. *Science*, *336*, 1642–1643. doi: 10.1126/science.1218387

Baykara, Z., Demir, S., & Yaman, S. (2015). The effect of ethics training on students recognizing ethical violations and developing moral sensitivity. *Nursing Ethics*, *22*(6), 661–675. doi:10.1177/0969733014542673

Benner, P., Sutphen, M., Leonard, V., & Day, L. (2009). *Educating nurses: A call for radical transformation*. San Francisco, CA: Jossey-Bass.

Broekkamp, H., & van Hout-Wolters, B. (2007). The gap between educational research and practice: A literature review, symposium, and questionnaire. *Educational Research and Evaluation*, *13*, 203–220. doi:10.1080/13803610701626127

Chiafery, M. C., Hopkins, P., Norton, S. A., & Shaw, M. H. (2018). Nursing ethics huddles to decrease moral distress among nurses in the Intensive Care Unit. *The Journal of Clinical Ethics*, *29*, 217–226.

Davis, M. (1999). *Ethics and the university* (pp. 166–167). New York: Routledge.

Enck, G. (2014). Six-step framework for ethical decision making. *Journal of Health Services Research & Policy*, *19*(1), 62–64. doi:10.1177/1355819613511599

Fisher M. (2014). A comparison of professional value development among pre-licensure nursing students in associate degree, diploma, and bachelor of science in nursing programs. *Nursing education perspectives*, *35*(1), 37–42. doi:10.5480/11-729.1.

Georgiou, D., Mok, S. Y., Fischer, F., Vermunt, J. D., & Seidel T. (2020). Evidence-based practice in teacher education: The mediating role of self-efficacy beliefs and practical knowledge. *Frontiers in Education*, *5*, 559192. doi:10.3389/feduc.2020.559192

Grace, P. J., Robinson, E. M., Jurchak, M., Zollfrank, A. A., & Lee, S. M. (2014). Clinical ethics residency for nurses: An education model to decrease moral distress and strengthen nurse retention in acute care. *Journal of Nursing Administration*, *44*(12), 640–646. doi:10.1097/NNA.0000000000000141

Grady, C., Danis, M., Soeken, K. L., O'Donnell, P., Taylor, C., Farrar, A., & Ulrich, C. M. (2008). Does ethics education influence the moral action of practicing nurses and social workers? *The American Journal of Bioethics*, *8*(4), 4–11. doi:10.1080/15265160802166017

Hickman, S. E., & Wocial, L. D. (2013). Team-based learning and ethics education in nursing. *The Journal of Nursing Education*, *52*(12), 696–700.

Hoskins, K., Grady, C., & Ulrich, C. M. (2018). Ethics education in nursing: Instruction for future generations of nurses. *OJIN: The Online Journal of Issues in Nursing*, *23*(1), 3.

Kunter, M., Baumert, J., & Köller, O. (2007). Effective classroom management and the development of subject-related interest. *Learning and Instruction*, *17*, 494–509. doi:10.1016/j.learninstruc.2007.09.002

Krautscheid, L., & Brown, M. (2014). Microethical decision making among baccalaureate nursing students: A qualitative investigation. *Journal of Nursing Education*, *53*(3), S19–S25. doi:10.3928/01484834-20140211-05

Laabs, C. A. (2012). Confidence and knowledge regarding ethics among advanced practice nurses. *Nursing Education Perspectives*, *33*(1), 10–14. doi:10.5480/1536-5026-33.1.10

Laabs, C. A. (2015). Toward a consensus in ethics education for the doctor of nursing practice. *Nursing Education Perspectives*, *36*(4), 249–251. doi:10.5480/13-1195

Lee, W., Choi S., Kim S., & Min, A. (2020). A case-centered approach to nursing ethics education: A qualitative study. *International Journal of Environmental Research and Public Health*, *17*(21), 7748. doi:10.3390/ijerph17217748

Molazem, Z., Tavakol, N., Sharif, F., Keshavarzi, S., & Ghadakpour, S. (2013). Effect of education based on the "4A Model" on the Iranian nurses' moral distress in CCU wards. *Journal of Medical Ethics and History of Medicine*, *6*, 5.

O'Brochta, M., Meloni, G., Raghupathy, S., Pfeiffer, P., & Taylor, M. (2012). *The leader's choice: Five steps to ethical decision making*. Paper presented at PMI® Global Congress 2012—North America, Vancouver, British Columbia, Canada. Newtown Square, PA: Project Management Institute.

Osingada, C. P., Nalwadda, G., Ngabirano, T., Wakida, J., Sewankambo, N., & Nakanjako, D. (2015). Nurses' knowledge in ethics and their perceptions regarding continuing ethics education: A cross-sectional survey among nurses at three referral hospitals in Uganda. *BMC Research Notes*, *8*, 319. https://doi.org/10.1186/s13104-015-1294-6

Pariseau-Legault, P., & Lallier, M. (2016). Constructing an ethical training for advanced nursing practice: An interactionist and competency-based approach. *The Journal of Nursing Education*, *55*(7), 399–402. doi:10.3928/01484834-20160615-08

Robinson, E. M., Lee, S. M., Zollfrank, A., Jurchak, M., Frost, D., & Grace, P. (2014). Enhancing moral agency: Clinical ethics residency for nurses. *Hastings Center Report*, *44*(5), 12–20. doi:10.1002/hast.353

Shahriari, M., Mohammadi, E., Abbaszadeh, A., & Bahrami, M. (2013). Nursing ethical values and definitions: A literature review. *Iranian Journal of Nursing and Midwifery Research*, *18*(1), 1–8.

Slavin, R. E. (2002). Evidence-based education policies: Transforming educational practice and research. *Educational Research*, *31*, 15–21. doi:10.3102/0013189X031007015

Sullivan, K. J., Wayne, C., Patey, A. M., & Nasr, A. (2017). Barriers and facilitators to the implementation of evidence-based practice by pediatric surgeons. *Journal of Pediatric Surgery*, *52*, 1666–1673. doi:10.1016/j.jpedsurg.2017.02.001

Wiseman, A. W. (2010). The uses of evidence for educational policymaking: Global contexts and international trends. *Review of Educational Research*, *34*, 1–24. doi:10.3102/0091732X09350472

Lesson plan on course equivalency, transcript and credit system

A

LESSON PLAN

Subject	:	Nursing Education
Topic	:	Course equivalency, transcript and credit system
Group of students	:	M.Sc. (N) First year
No. of students	:	25
Name of student teacher	:	Ms Kumud Kumari
Method of teaching	:	Lecture cum discussion method
Date of teaching	:	12/12/12
Time of teaching	:	10.00 am
Language	:	English
Duration	:	25 minutes
AV Aids	:	PowerPoint presentation (PPT), flannel board and flash cards
Venue	:	M.Sc. (N) First year classroom
Supervisor	:	Dr Suresh K. Sharma

Previous knowledge of the group: Students have basic knowledge regarding course equivalency, transcript and credit system in B.Sc. Nursing.
General objective: At the end of teaching, students will be able to develop knowledge about course equivalency and transcript and credit system.
Specific objective: At the end of the teaching, students will be able to

- Define course equivalency, transcript and credit system.
- Explain the steps of course equivalency.
- Elaborate the implications for implementation and assurance of standards.
- Describe the items of transcript.
- Explain the credit system.
- Explain the continuing nursing education credit system.

S. No.	Contributory Objectives	Time	Content	Teaching and Learning Activities	
				AV Aids	Evaluation
	At the end of the class students will be able to . . .				
1.		1/2 min	Good afternoon to all of you. My name is Ms Kumud Kumari. The topic of my presentation is course equivalency, transcript and credit system.	Verbally	
2.	Define course equivalency	2 min	**Course equivalency** • *Course equivalency* is the term used in higher education, describing how a course offered by one college or university relates to a course offered by another. • If a course is viewed as equal or better than the course offered by the receiving college or university, the course can be noted as an equivalent course.	LCD	What is course equivalency?
3.	Explain the steps of course equivalency	2 min	**Process** • The university/board from where the student has acquired the qualification shall duly fill up the transcript performa. • The duly filled transcript performa will be placed before the equivalency committee meeting; the recommendation with regard to equivalency status will be informed thereafter to the concerned candidates. • The equivalency process can take 2–3 months to complete.	Flannel board	What is the process of course equivalency?
4.	Explain the principles of course equivalency	1 min	**Principles of course equivalency** • Courses are regarded as equivalent if they have the same intended learning outcomes and consequently the same graduate profile. • Equivalent courses should therefore have the same overall educational aims and assess their achievement at the same standard.	LCD	What are the principles of course equivalency?

S. No.	Contributory Objectives	Time	Content	Teaching and Learning Activities	
				AV Aids	**Evaluation**
5.	Elaborate the implications for the implementation and assurance of standards	5 min	**Implications for implementation and assurance of standards** • Assurance of standards. • Course structures and subject material. • Academic programmes office • Admission standards. • Teaching standard and support. • Learning environment and support. • Transfer between equivalent courses. • Monitoring and evaluation.	LCD	List down the steps of implementation and assurance of standards.
6.	Define the transcript	2 min	**Transcript** • A nursing school/college transcript contains academic career record from the nursing school and college or university. • Transcripts are needed to confirm the equivalency of the course. • It itemizes all sorts of academic information.	LCD	What do you mean by a transcript?
7.	Describe the items of a transcript	5 min	**What is contained in a transcript?** • Name of student. • Previous school names, addresses and phone numbers. • List of courses you took—usually by year. • Dual enrollment and/or any honors—as applicable. • Your class grades (either letter or numeric). • Total GPA (grade point average). • Number of credits taken/achieved per semester and year. • Grade scale used by that school. • State proficiency exams (if any). • Graduation date and degrees achieved. • Classes you had learning experiences.	LCD	What are the items of a transcript?

Continued

S. No.	Contributory Objectives	Time	Content	Teaching and Learning Activities	
				AV Aids	Evaluation
8.	Explain the credit system	5 min	**Credit system** • A course credit (often credit hour, or just credit or 'unit') is a unit that gives weightage to the value, level or time requirements of an academic course taken at school or other educational institution. • Students in a school or university earn credits for the successful completion of each course for each academic term. • The state or the institution generally sets a minimum number of credits required to graduate. • Various systems of credits exist: one per course, one per hour/week in class, one per hour/week devoted to the course (including homework), etc. • The credit system is basically a division of hours of the whole syllabus unitwise. The credit system (total hours) are different for different courses. Also the requirement is also different in different courses.	LCD	What is the credit system?
9.	Explain the continuing nursing education credit system	2 min	**Continuing Nursing Education (CNE) credit system** • The percentage of staff fulfilling the CNE requirement, which is 15 credit points per year, has risen from 70 to 85%. • Nursing staff have also shown appreciation of an annual record of their CNE achievement as it provides a kind of recognition of their professional activities. • In general, one CNE point is allocated for an hour's learning activity, which may consist of a talk, workshop, seminar and conference, related to patient care issues and/or nursing professional development.	LCD	What is CNE credit system?
10.	Summarize the topic	1/2 min	Today in the class I have discussed the definitions, steps, principles of course equivalency, transcript and credit system. **References** **Assignment** Develop course equivalency, transcript and credit system for B.Sc. Nursing programme.	Verbally Flash cards	

APPENDIX

B

Comprehensive review: Multiple-choice questions

Chapters 1 and 2. Education and Educational Technology and Principles and Philosophies of Education

1. What is the primary aim of nursing education?
   a. To provide job opportunities for nurses
   b. To develop clinical skills in nursing students
   c. To foster professional growth and competence
   d. To enhance social interactions among nurses

2. Which of the following best describes the aim of nursing education?
   a. To prepare students for licensure and professional practice
   b. To equip students with theoretical knowledge only
   c. To provide hands-on training in healthcare facilities
   d. To focus solely on technical skills development

3. What is the overarching aim of nursing education programmes?
   a. To produce nurses with high leadership qualities
   b. To train nurses in basic patient care skills
   c. To ensure patient safety and quality care delivery
   d. To enhance nurses' administrative and managerial skills

4. The primary aim of nursing education is to
   a. Prepare students for medical school
   b. Promote evidence-based practice in nursing care
   c. Develop specialized nursing roles within the profession
   d. Focus on administrative tasks and healthcare management

5. The aim of nursing education is to
   a. Promote a standardized approach to patient care
   b. Encourage nurses to focus solely on technical skills
   c. Establish nurses as the primary decision-makers in healthcare settings
   d. Develop critical thinking and clinical reasoning abilities

6. What is the primary aim of integrating educational technology in nursing?
   a. To replace traditional teaching methods entirely
   b. To reduce the workload of nursing faculty
   c. To facilitate effective and efficient learning experiences
   d. To decrease the need for clinical practice

7. How does educational technology contribute to nursing education?
   a. By providing access to online nursing courses
   b. By improving communication between nurses and patients
   c. By enhancing critical thinking and problem-solving skills
   d. By automating nursing tasks and procedures

8. Which statement best describes the relationship between education and nursing technology?
   a. Education is essential to the effective use of nursing technology
   b. Nursing technology can replace the need for nursing education
   c. Education and nursing technology have no relationship
   d. Nursing technology can hinder the educational process

9. How does educational technology promote collaborative learning in nursing?
   a. By allowing students to interact with their peers in online forums
   b. By providing access to virtual simulations and case studies
   c. By automating group assignments and assessments
   d. By reducing the need for classroom discussions and debates

10. What role does educational technology play in nursing practice?
    a. It replaces the need for human interaction in patient care
    b. It enables nurses to access patient records more quickly
    c. It facilitates lifelong learning and professional development
    d. It reduces the need for continuous training and education

11. What is the significance of educational technology in nursing research?
    a. It eliminates the need for data analysis and interpretation
    b. It enables nurses to conduct experiments more efficiently
    c. It provides access to online databases and research resources
    d. It hinders the dissemination of research findings

12. Which of the following is NOT a potential benefit of educational technology in nursing?
    a. Increased access to educational resources
    b. Improved patient outcomes and quality of care
    c. Enhanced critical thinking and clinical reasoning skills
    d. Reduction in the need for evidence-based practice

13. How does educational technology contribute to the development of nursing skills?
    a. By replacing the need for clinical practice and hands-on experience
    b. By providing virtual simulations and scenarios for practice
    c. By reducing the need for critical thinking and decision-making
    d. By limiting the scope of nursing practice to technical skills

14. What is the primary approach of educational technology in nursing?
    a. Enhancing patient care through advanced technology
    b. Automating administrative tasks for nurses
    c. Supporting effective teaching and learning methods
    d. Minimizing the need for clinical practice

15. How does educational technology support personalized learning in nursing?
    a. By providing individualized study materials for each student
    b. By automating the grading process for assessments
    c. By reducing the need for interaction with nursing faculty
    d. By eliminating the need for group discussions and collaboration

16. Which statement best describes the role of educational technology in nursing education?
- **a.** Educational technology replaces the need for nursing faculty
- **b.** Educational technology enhances traditional teaching methods
- **c.** Educational technology limits the scope of nursing practice
- **d.** Educational technology hinders the learning process in nursing

17. What is the approach of educational technology in improving clinical skills in nursing?
- **a.** Automating clinical procedures to reduce human errors
- **b.** Enhancing communication between nurses and patients
- **c.** Providing virtual simulations and scenarios for practice
- **d.** Minimizing the need for critical thinking and decision-making

18. How does educational technology contribute to the assessment process in nursing education?
- **a.** By automating all assessment tasks for nursing faculty
- **b.** By reducing the importance of formative and summative assessments
- **c.** By eliminating the need for objective and standardized assessments
- **d.** By providing online platforms for efficient and timely evaluations

19. How does transformational education impact nursing practice?
- **a.** It limits nurses' autonomy and decision-making abilities
- **b.** It encourages nurses to conform to established norms and practices
- **c.** It promotes innovative thinking and individualized care approaches
- **d.** It discourages nurses from seeking career advancement

20. What is the role of educators in facilitating transformational education in nursing?
- **a.** To enforce strict rules and regulations in the classroom
- **b.** To discourage critical thinking and independent decision-making
- **c.** To limit students' exposure to new and emerging healthcare technologies
- **d.** To create a supportive and empowering learning environment

21. Transformational education in nursing focuses on
- **a.** Replicating traditional teaching methods from the past
- **b.** Minimizing the importance of personal growth and development
- **c.** Enhancing students' self-awareness and self-reflection
- **d.** Restricting access to evidence-based practice guidelines

22. Relationship-based education in nursing focuses on
- **a.** Building strong interpersonal connections with patients and colleagues
- **b.** Memorization of facts and information
- **c.** Rote learning and standardized assessments
- **d.** Following established protocols and procedures

23. How does relationship-based education impact nursing practice?
- **a.** It discourages nurses from forming connections with patients
- **b.** It promotes a patient-centred approach to care delivery
- **c.** It limits the importance of effective communication in nursing
- **d.** It focuses solely on technical skills and procedures

24. Relationship-based education in nursing emphasizes
   a. Passive learning and adherence to established norms
   b. Rigid and inflexible approaches to patient care
   c. Collaboration, empathy and therapeutic relationships
   d. Following a hierarchical structure within healthcare teams

25. Relationship-based education in nursing promotes
   a. Limited patient interactions to reduce workload
   b. Resistance to building connections with colleagues
   c. A supportive and trusting learning environment
   d. Reliance on standardized protocols and guidelines

26. What is the role of educators in facilitating relationship-based education in nursing?
   a. To enforce strict rules and regulations in the classroom
   b. To foster meaningful relationships and effective communication
   c. To discourage collaborative learning and teamwork
   d. To limit students' exposure to diverse patient populations

27. Relationship-based education in nursing focuses on
   a. Replicating traditional teaching methods from the past
   b. Minimizing the importance of building connections with patients
   c. Restricting access to evidence-based practice guidelines
   d. Enhancing students' understanding of ethical and professional values

28. Competency-based nursing education focuses on
   a. Memorization of facts and information
   b. Developing specific skills and abilities required for nursing practice
   c. Rote learning and standardized assessments
   d. Following established protocols and procedures

29. What role does competency-based education play in improving patient outcomes?
   a. It has no significant impact on patient outcomes
   b. It leads to standardized and uniform care delivery
   c. It ensures nurses possess the necessary skills for optimal patient care
   d. It focuses solely on technical skills rather than patient outcomes

30. What is the role of educators in facilitating competency-based nursing education?
   a. To assess and guide students' progress towards achieving competencies
   b. To enforce strict rules and regulations in the classroom
   c. To discourage collaboration and teamwork among students
   d. To limit students' exposure to diverse patient populations

31. Competency-based nursing education focuses on
   a. Replicating traditional teaching methods from the past
   b. Minimizing the importance of specific skills and abilities
   c. Restricting access to evidence-based practice guidelines
   d. Identifying and measuring specific nursing competencies

32. How does competency-based education impact the nurse–patient relationship?
   a. It limits communication and interaction with patients
   b. It promotes standardized care delivery based on competencies
   c. It emphasizes routine tasks and technical skills over patient needs
   d. It discourages nurses from developing therapeutic relationships

33. Competency-based nursing education encourages students to
   a. Rely solely on textbooks and academic literature
   b. Avoid challenging the existing health-care system
   c. Demonstrate and apply specific nursing competencies
   d. Focus solely on individual achievements rather than teamwork

Chapter 3. Teaching–Learning Process

34. What is the term used to describe the process of acquiring knowledge, skills, attitudes or values through study, experience or teaching?
   a. Learning
   b. Teaching
   c. Instruction
   d. Assessment

35. Which of the following is NOT a component of the teaching–learning process?
   a. Teacher
   b. Student
   c. Curriculum
   d. Administrator

36. Which of the following is an example of a formative assessment?
   a. Final examination
   b. Quiz during a lesson
   c. Project presentation
   d. Standardized test

37. In the teaching–learning process, what is the purpose of instructional objectives?
   a. To guide the teacher's lesson planning
   b. To assess students' performance
   c. To provide feedback to students
   d. To determine the curriculum content

38. Which of the following is an example of an informal assessment?
   a. Multiple-choice test
   b. Oral presentation
   c. Essay examination
   d. Standardized achievement test

39. Which teaching strategy involves breaking down complex tasks into smaller, more manageable steps?
   a. Differentiation
   b. Scaffolding
   c. Direct instruction
   d. Cooperative learning

40. What is the term used to describe the process of adapting instruction to meet the diverse needs of students?
   a. Differentiation
   b. Assessment
   c. Grading
   d. Collaboration

41. Which of the following is an example of an extrinsic motivator in the teaching–learning process?
   a. Intrinsic interest in the subject
   b. Personal satisfaction from learning
   c. Grades or rewards
   d. Curiosity and exploration

42. Learning can be defined as
   a. The acquisition of knowledge through teaching
   b. The process of changing behaviour based on experience
   c. The innate ability to understand concepts
   d. The transmission of information from one person to another

43. Which of the following is NOT a characteristic of learning?
   a. It is a relatively permanent change
   b. It involves a change in behaviour, knowledge or understanding
   c. It occurs only through formal education
   d. It can be intentional or unintentional

44. Which of the following is an example of implicit learning?
   a. Memorizing a poem for a recitation
   b. Solving a complex math problem
   c. Riding a bicycle without conscious effort
   d. Studying historical events for an exam

45. Learning that occurs through direct instruction, explicit teaching and structured activities is known as
   a. Formal learning
   b. Informal learning
   c. Nonformal learning
   d. Experiential learning

46. What is the term used to describe the process of learning by observing others and imitating their behaviour?
   a. Classical conditioning
   b. Operant conditioning
   c. Observational learning
   d. Reinforcement

47. Which of the following is an example of active learning?
   a. Listening to a lecture
   b. Watching a documentary
   c. Participating in a group discussion
   d. Reading a textbook silently

48. The process of organizing and connecting new information to existing knowledge or schemas is known as
   a. Assimilation
   b. Accommodation
   c. Encoding
   d. Retrieval

49. Which of the following is an example of a cognitive learning outcome?
   a. Demonstrating a physical skill
   b. Changing attitudes or beliefs
   c. Recalling facts or information
   d. Developing social skills

50. Which of the following is a principle of learning that emphasizes the importance of active participation and engagement in the learning process?
   a. Principle of readiness
   b. Principle of exercise
   c. Principle of primacy
   d. Principle of active learning

51. The principle of reinforcement suggests that
   a. Learning is more effective when individuals are ready to learn
   b. Learning is strengthened when followed by rewards or positive consequences
   c. Learning is influenced by the order in which material is presented
   d. Learning is enhanced through meaningful connections and associations

52. The principle of transfer states that learning in one context can be applied to another context. This is known as
   a. Positive transfer
   b. Negative transfer
   c. Near transfer
   d. Far transfer

53. Which principle of learning emphasizes the importance of repetition and practice for strengthening memory and skill acquisition?
   a. Principle of readiness
   b. Principle of reinforcement
   c. Principle of exercise
   d. Principle of primacy

54. Which principle of learning emphasizes the importance of creating meaningful and relevant associations between new information and existing knowledge?
    a. Principle of readiness
    b. Principle of reinforcement
    c. Principle of exercise
    d. Principle of meaningfulness

55. The principle of scaffolding suggests that
    a. Learning is more effective when individuals are motivated and ready to learn
    b. Learning is influenced by the order in which material is presented
    c. Learning is enhanced through meaningful connections and associations
    d. Learning is supported by providing appropriate guidance and support as learners progress

56. The principle of reflection emphasizes the importance of
    a. Active participation and engagement in the learning process
    b. Practice and repetition for strengthening memory and skill acquisition
    c. Creating meaningful and relevant associations between new and existing knowledge
    d. Encouraging learners to think critically and analyse their own learning experiences

57. The principle of individual differences recognizes that
    a. Learning is more effective when individuals are motivated and ready to learn
    b. Learning is influenced by the order in which material is presented
    c. Learners have unique abilities, backgrounds and learning styles
    d. Learning is strengthened when followed by rewards or positive consequences

58. According to behaviourist learning theory, learning is primarily influenced by
    a. Reinforcement and punishment
    b. Cognitive processes and mental structures
    c. Personal experiences and reflection
    d. Social interactions and observation

59. Which learning theory emphasizes the importance of self-efficacy and the role of personal beliefs in motivation and learning?
    a. Behaviourist learning theory
    b. Social cognitive learning theory
    c. Humanistic learning theory
    d. Constructivist learning theory

60. The cognitive learning theory focuses on
    a. Observable behaviours and their consequences
    b. Self-directed learning and personal growth
    c. The mental processes involved in acquiring, processing and organizing knowledge
    d. Collaborative learning and social interactions

61. According to the constructivist learning theory, learning is
    a. A process of reinforcing desired behaviours
    b. A result of internal cognitive processes and mental structures
    c. Facilitated by the teacher through direct instruction and guidance
    d. A collaborative and active process of constructing knowledge

62. The theory of adult learning, also known as andragogy, emphasizes
    a. The importance of behaviour modification techniques in teaching
    b. The role of social interactions and observation in learning
    c. Self-directed learning and the relevance of learning to the learner's life experiences
    d. The influence of cognitive processes and mental structures on learning

63. The ecological systems theory, developed by Urie Bronfenbrenner, focuses on
    a. The role of environmental factors and social interactions in learning
    b. The influence of cognitive processes and mental structures on learning
    c. The importance of behaviour modification techniques in teaching
    d. The role of self-efficacy and personal beliefs in motivation and learning

64. Which learning theory emphasizes the significance of the affective domain, including attitudes, values and emotions, in learning?
  a. Behaviourist learning theory
  b. Cognitive learning theory
  c. Humanistic learning theory
  d. Social cognitive learning theory

65. The theory of transformative learning, proposed by Jack Mezirow, focuses on
  a. The importance of behaviour modification techniques in teaching
  b. The role of social interactions and observation in learning
  c. Self-directed learning and the relevance of learning to the learner's life experiences
  d. The process of critically reflecting on and challenging existing beliefs and assumptions

66. According to the social learning theory, learning occurs through
  a. Reinforcement and punishment of behaviours
  b. The internal cognitive processes of the learner
  c. Personal reflection and self-directed learning
  d. Observation and modelling of others' behaviours

67. Experiential learning in nursing education emphasizes
  a. Memorization of theoretical concepts
  b. Passive listening to lectures
  c. Hands-on practical experiences
  d. Standardized testing

68. The experiential learning cycle typically involves the following stages
  a. Input, repetition, assessment, feedback
  b. Analysis, evaluation, synthesis, application
  c. Observation, lecture, practice, examination
  d. Experience, reflection, conceptualization, experimentation

69. Experiential learning allows students to develop
  a. Theoretical knowledge only
  b. Critical thinking and problem-solving skills
  c. Passive listening skills
  d. Rote memorization abilities

70. Which teaching strategy is commonly used in experiential learning to facilitate skill development?
  a. Lectures
  b. Demonstrations
  c. Multiple-choice quizzes
  d. Written assignments

71. The goal of experiential learning in nursing education is to
  a. Focus solely on theoretical knowledge
  b. Minimize practical experiences
  c. Integrate theory and practice
  d. Rely on passive learning methods

72. Experiential learning in nursing education enhances students'
  a. Ability to memorize facts
  b. Knowledge of textbook content
  c. Understanding of the nursing process
  d. Performance on standardized tests

73. Reflective learning is a process that involves
  a. Memorizing facts and information
  b. Engaging in critical self-reflection
  c. Following a structured curriculum
  d. Taking standardized tests

74. The primary purpose of reflective learning is to
  a. Passively receive knowledge from instructors
  b. Memorize information for later use
  c. Promote self-awareness and personal growth
  d. Achieve high scores on assessments

75. The process of reflective learning involves
  a. Avoiding feedback and evaluation
  b. Critically analysing past experiences and actions
  c. Ignoring personal experiences and emotions
  d. Focusing solely on theoretical knowledge

76. The role of a mentor or facilitator in reflective learning is to
   a. Provide all the answers and solutions
   b. Minimize self-reflection and evaluation
   c. Guide and support the reflective process
   d. Avoid sharing personal experiences

77. The reflection process in reflective learning involves
   a. Ignoring personal biases and assumptions
   b. Solely focusing on external feedback and criticism
   c. Relying on others to provide solutions
   d. Examining personal beliefs and values

78. The success of reflective learning depends on
   a. Avoiding self-assessment and evaluation
   b. Memorizing information without reflection
   c. Actively engaging in critical self-reflection
   d. Relying solely on external sources of knowledge

79. Scenario-based learning typically involves the use of
   a. Multiple-choice quizzes
   b. Group discussions and role-playing
   c. Passive listening to lectures
   d. Memorization of textbook content

80. Scenarios used in scenario-based learning are designed to
   a. Avoid real-life situations and focus on theory
   b. Minimize learner engagement and participation
   c. Simulate authentic workplace challenges and tasks
   d. Promote rote memorization of facts

81. The primary benefit of scenario-based learning is that it
   a. Reduces critical thinking and problem-solving skills
   b. Limits learner engagement and active participation
   c. Enhances transfer of learning to real-world situations
   d. Relies solely on theoretical knowledge

82. In scenario-based learning, learners are encouraged to
   a. Avoid practical application of knowledge
   b. Rely solely on theoretical concepts
   c. Apply knowledge to realistic situations
   d. Memorize information without understanding

83. Scenario-based learning is particularly effective in developing learners'
   a. Ability to memorize information
   b. Understanding of theoretical concepts
   c. Critical thinking and problem-solving skills
   d. Performance on standardized tests

84. Scenarios used in scenario-based learning are often based on
   a. Hypothetical situations
   b. Theoretical textbooks only
   c. Passive listening to instructors
   d. Real-life experiences and challenges

85. The success of scenario-based learning relies on
   a. Avoiding real-life situations
   b. Memorizing information from textbooks
   c. Reflection and active participation
   d. Passive reception of knowledge

86. Simulation-based learning in education involves
   a. Passive observation of real-life situations
   b. Rote memorization of theoretical concepts
   c. Immersive and interactive simulated experiences
   d. Traditional lecture-based instruction

87. Simulations in simulation-based learning are designed to
   a. Replicate real-life scenarios and challenges
   b. Avoid complexities and uncertainties
   c. Provide direct answers and solutions
   d. Focus solely on theoretical knowledge

88. The role of the facilitator in simulation-based learning is to
    a. Provide step-by-step instructions
    b. Minimize learner engagement and participation
    c. Guide and support the learning process
    d. Avoid realistic and challenging scenarios

89. Simulation-based learning often involves
    a. Individual learning in isolation
    b. Rote memorization of facts and figures
    c. Collaborative problem-solving and teamwork
    d. Passive reception of information

90. The feedback provided in simulation-based learning is primarily focused on
    a. Criticizing learners' mistakes and errors
    b. Discouraging active experimentation
    c. Guiding learners towards optimal performance
    d. Avoiding reflection and self-assessment

91. The complexity of simulations in simulation-based learning is designed to
    a. Simplify real-life scenarios and challenges
    b. Avoid learner engagement and critical thinking
    c. Provide direct solutions and answers
    d. Foster realistic decision-making and problem-solving

92. In a blended learning model, online learning components are typically delivered through
    a. Video lectures and multimedia resources
    b. Physical textbooks and printed materials
    c. Interactive online quizzes and assessments
    d. Live virtual classrooms with real-time interaction

93. The main advantage of blended learning is
    a. Reduced cost of education.
    b. Elimination of face-to-face interaction
    c. Increased flexibility for learners
    d. More efficient use of instructional time

94. Blended learning refers to an educational approach that combines
    a. Traditional classroom teaching with outdoor activities
    b. Online learning with in-person instruction
    c. Group discussions with individual study
    d. Lectures with practical demonstrations

95. Blended learning is suitable for nursing students who
    a. Prefer traditional classroom instruction only
    b. Have limited access to clinical settings
    c. Thrive in independent study environments
    d. Benefit from a mix of different learning modalities

96. The principle of individualization in nursing education means
    a. Treating each nursing student the same way
    b. Tailoring teaching strategies to meet students' unique needs
    c. Focusing solely on theoretical knowledge
    d. Implementing standardized assessments for all students

97. The principle of relevance in nursing education involves
    a. Teaching irrelevant content to challenge nursing students
    b. Providing real-life examples and applications of nursing concepts
    c. Ignoring the current trends and advancements in nursing practice
    d. Focusing solely on theoretical knowledge without practical relevance

98. The principle of active student engagement in nursing education promotes
    a. Passive listening and observation
    b. Memorization of nursing theories
    c. Collaboration and critical thinking
    d. Relying solely on instructor-centred instruction

99. The principle of learner-centredness in nursing education focuses on
   a. Prioritizing the needs and interests of the nursing instructor
   b. Ignoring individual learning preferences of nursing students
   c. Providing flexible and adaptable teaching strategies
   d. Rigidly adhering to a standardized curriculum

100. The principle of repetition and reinforcement in nursing education emphasizes
   a. Teaching concepts once and expecting immediate mastery
   b. Avoiding repetition to challenge nursing students
   c. Reinforcing learning through various activities and practice opportunities
   d. Overloading nursing students with excessive information

101. The principle of creating a supportive learning environment in nursing education includes
   a. Promoting competition and comparison among nursing students
   b. Ignoring the emotional well-being of nursing students
   c. Fostering a safe and inclusive learning environment
   d. Excluding collaboration and teamwork

102. The principle of lifelong learning in nursing education emphasizes
   a. Cessation of learning after completing nursing education
   b. Relying solely on initial knowledge and skills
   c. Encouraging nursing students to continuously update their knowledge
   d. Excluding professional development and growth

103. What is a characteristic of good teaching?
   a. Focusing solely on teacher-centred instruction
   b. Ignoring the use of assessment and feedback
   c. Encouraging a growth mindset and fostering resilience
   d. Following a one-size-fits-all teaching approach

104. What is the nature of teaching?
   a. A passive and one-way process
   b. A dynamic and interactive process
   c. An individualistic and isolated process
   d. A static and unchanging process

Chapter 4. Curriculum, Assessment and Planning

105. Which quality helps a nursing teacher effectively convey complex information to students?
   a. Empathy
   b. Patience
   c. Clarity
   d. Adaptability

106. Which of the following qualities is crucial for a nursing teacher to establish trust and rapport with students?
   a. Leadership skills
   b. Respect for diversity
   c. Continuous learning mindset
   d. Competence in nursing skills

107. Which quality enables a nursing teacher to motivate and inspire students?
   a. Confidence
   b. Creativity
   c. Flexibility
   d. Integrity

108. Which quality allows a nursing teacher to effectively assess and evaluate student performance?
   a. Attention to detail
   b. Objectivity
   c. Organization
   d. Critical thinking

109. Which quality helps a nursing teacher to adapt teaching strategies to meet the individual needs of students?
   a. Adaptability
   b. Cultural sensitivity
   c. Problem-solving skills
   d. Professionalism

110. Which of the following qualities is essential for a nursing teacher to provide constructive feedback to students?
   a. Analytical skills
   b. Compassion
   c. Time management
   d. Open-mindedness

111. Which quality promotes a positive learning environment in nursing education?
   a. Collaboration
   b. Technical expertise
   c. Punctuality
   d. Perseverance

112. Which of the following qualities is important for a nursing teacher to foster lifelong learning among students?
   a. Humility
   b. Organization
   c. Resourcefulness
   d. Confidence

113. Which quality allows a nursing teacher to effectively manage classroom dynamics and facilitate group discussions?
   a. Active listening
   b. Professional ethics
   c. Technological proficiency
   d. Interpersonal skills

114. Which teaching style focuses on providing information and allowing students to absorb knowledge passively?
   a. Lecture-based teaching
   b. Collaborative learning
   c. Experiential learning
   d. Problem-based learning

115. Which teaching style emphasizes active participation, group work and discussion among students?
   a. Lecture-based teaching
   b. Collaborative learning
   c. Experiential learning
   d. Problem-based learning

116. Which teaching style encourages students to learn through hands-on experiences and real-world situations?
   a. Lecture-based teaching
   b. Collaborative learning
   c. Experiential learning
   d. Problem-based learning

117. Which teaching style involves presenting students with real-life scenarios and challenging them to solve problems?
   a. Lecture-based teaching
   b. Collaborative learning
   c. Experiential learning
   d. Problem-based learning

118. In the demonstrator style, how can the nursing instructor ensure student understanding and competency?
   a. By assigning written assignments and quizzes
   b. By providing constructive feedback and evaluation
   c. By encouraging peer teaching and mentoring
   d. By organizing group presentations and debates

119. What is a potential limitation of the demonstrator style in nursing education?
   a. Limited student engagement and interaction
   b. Inability to address diverse learning needs
   c. Overemphasis on theoretical concepts
   d. Lack of opportunities for independent thinking

120. Which teaching style encourages students to develop observational skills and attention to detail?
   a. Demonstrator style
   b. Facilitator style
   c. Lecture style
   d. Collaborative style

121. Which teaching style is most suitable for teaching technical skills and procedures in nursing practice?
   a. Demonstrator style
   b. Facilitator style
   c. Lecture style
   d. Collaborative style

122. Which teaching style in nursing education focuses on modelling and providing examples for students to observe and imitate?
   a. Demonstrator style
   b. Facilitator style
   c. Lecture style
   d. Collaborative style

123. Which teaching style encourages students to develop leadership and organizational skills?
   a. Delegator style
   b. Facilitator style
   c. Lecture style
   d. Collaborative style

124. What is a potential limitation of the delegator style in nursing education?
   a. Lack of guidance and support for students
   b. Overemphasis on theoretical concepts
   c. Limited opportunities for collaboration and teamwork
   d. Inability to address diverse learning needs

125. Which teaching style in nursing education involves assigning responsibilities and tasks to students?
   a. Delegator style
   b. Facilitator style
   c. Lecture style
   d. Collaborative style

126. In the delegator style, how does the nursing instructor engage with students?
   a. By providing direct instructions and demonstrations
   b. By facilitating group discussions and problem-solving activities
   c. By assigning tasks and empowering students to take responsibility
   d. By lecturing and delivering theoretical content

127. Which teaching style in nursing education involves guiding and facilitating the learning process for students?
   a. Facilitator style
   b. Delegator style
   c. Lecture style
   d. Collaborative style

128. In the facilitator style, what is the role of the nursing instructor?
   a. Delivering lectures and providing direct instructions
   b. Assigning tasks and responsibilities to students
   c. Promoting active discussions and critical thinking
   d. Demonstrating skills and procedures to students

129. Which teaching style promotes student engagement, participation and collaboration?
   a. Facilitator style
   b. Delegator style
   c. Lecture style
   d. Collaborative style

130. In the facilitator style, how does the nursing instructor engage with students?
   a. By lecturing and providing theoretical content
   b. By assigning tasks and monitoring student progress
   c. By facilitating discussions and guiding learning activities
   d. By demonstrating skills and procedures to students

131. What is a potential limitation of the facilitator style in nursing education?
- **a.** Lack of structure and clear direction for students
- **b.** Overemphasis on theoretical concepts
- **c.** Limited opportunities for independent thinking
- **d.** Inability to address diverse learning needs

132. In the facilitator style, how can the nursing instructor assess student learning and understanding?
- **a.** By assigning written assignments and quizzes
- **b.** By providing constructive feedback and evaluation
- **c.** By encouraging peer teaching and mentoring
- **d.** By organizing group presentations and debates

133. Which type of learner prefers to learn through listening and auditory cues?
- **a.** Visual learner
- **b.** Auditory learner
- **c.** Kinesthetic learner
- **d.** Tactile learner

134. Which type of learner learns best through visual aids, such as diagrams, charts and images?
- **a.** Visual learner
- **b.** Auditory learner
- **c.** Kinesthetic learner
- **d.** Tactile learner

135. Which type of learner prefers hands-on activities and learns by doing?
- **a.** Visual learner
- **b.** Auditory learner
- **c.** Kinesthetic learner
- **d.** Tactile learner

136. Which type of learner learns best by touching and manipulating objects?
- **a.** Visual learner
- **b.** Auditory learner
- **c.** Kinesthetic learner
- **d.** Tactile learner

137. Which type of learner benefits from group discussions, verbal explanations and listening to lectures?
- **a.** Visual learner
- **b.** Auditory learner
- **c.** Kinesthetic learner
- **d.** Tactile learner

138. Which type of learner excels in activities that involve physical movement and coordination?
- **a.** Visual learner
- **b.** Auditory learner
- **c.** Kinesthetic learner
- **d.** Tactile learner

139. Which type of learner prefers to take notes and write down information for better retention?
- **a.** Visual learner
- **b.** Auditory learner
- **c.** Kinesthetic learner
- **d.** Tactile learner

140. Which type of learner benefits from using flashcards, models and manipulatives for learning?
- **a.** Visual learner
- **b.** Auditory learner
- **c.** Kinesthetic learner
- **d.** Tactile learner

141. Which type of learner finds it easier to remember information by associating it with physical sensations or movements?
- **a.** Visual learner
- **b.** Auditory learner
- **c.** Kinesthetic learner
- **d.** Tactile learner

142. Which type of learner prefers a combination of different learning methods and adapts well to various teaching styles?
- **a.** Visual learner
- **b.** Auditory learner
- **c.** Kinesthetic learner
- **d.** Tactile learner

143. Learning styles in nursing refer to
- **a.** The methods used to teach nursing concepts
- **b.** The ways in which individuals prefer to learn and process information
- **c.** The specific skills required for nursing practice
- **d.** The types of assessments used in nursing education

144. The most effective teaching approach in nursing education is to
- **a.** Focus on a single learning style for all students
- **b.** Incorporate a variety of teaching methods to cater to different learning styles
- **c.** Use only traditional lecture-based instruction
- **d.** Assign independent reading as the primary learning method

145. What are the primary determinants of learning in nursing?
- **a.** Environment, motivation and readiness to learn
- **b.** Intelligence, memory and cognitive abilities
- **c.** Teaching methods, curriculum and assessment techniques
- **d.** Learning styles, preferences and individual differences

146. In the context of nursing, which determinant of learning refers to the physical and social surroundings in which learning takes place?
- **a.** Environment
- **b.** Motivation
- **c.** Readiness to learn
- **d.** Learning style

147. What does motivation refer to as a determinant of learning in nursing?
- **a.** The ability to comprehend and retain information
- **b.** The willingness and desire to engage in the learning process related to nursing
- **c.** The availability of appropriate learning resources for nursing education
- **d.** The influence of peers and social interactions on nursing education

148. Readiness to learn as a determinant of learning in nursing refers to
- **a.** Prior knowledge and skills that serve as a foundation for new nursing knowledge
- **b.** The physical and psychological state of the nursing student during the learning process
- **c.** The use of appropriate teaching methods and instructional techniques in nursing education
- **d.** The integration of technology and multimedia in the nursing learning environment

149. Which determinant of learning in nursing focuses on the individual's unique way of processing information and acquiring nursing knowledge?
- **a.** Environment
- **b.** Motivation
- **c.** Readiness to learn
- **d.** Learning style

150. How do individual differences influence learning in nursing as a determinant?
- **a.** They determine the pace and speed of learning for each nursing student
- **b.** They influence the type of teaching methods used in nursing education
- **c.** They affect the level of motivation and engagement in the nursing learning process
- **d.** They determine the readiness of nursing students to learn new nursing concepts

151. Which determinant of learning in nursing is associated with the instructional strategies, materials and techniques used by nursing educators?
   a. Environment
   b. Motivation
   c. Readiness to learn
   d. Teaching methods

152. What is the role of assessment techniques in the determinants of learning in nursing?
   a. They measure the effectiveness of teaching methods in nursing education
   b. They determine the readiness of nursing students to engage in the learning process
   c. They provide feedback and evaluation of nursing student performance
   d. They shape the social interactions and collaboration among nursing students

153. Which determinant of learning in nursing refers to the internal cognitive processes, including attention, memory and problem-solving abilities?
   a. Environment
   b. Motivation
   c. Readiness to learn
   d. Cognitive abilities

154. How do cognitive abilities influence learning in nursing as a determinant?
   a. They determine the physical and social surroundings for effective nursing learning
   b. They shape the nursing student's motivation and willingness to engage in learning
   c. They affect the nursing student's readiness to acquire new nursing knowledge and skills
   d. They influence the nursing student's ability to process and retain nursing information

155. Which of the following is a potential challenge in developing emotional intelligence in nursing education?
   a. Lack of opportunities for patient interaction
   b. Overemphasis on technical skills in the curriculum
   c. Inadequate knowledge of medical procedures
   d. Limited access to educational resources

156. Which of the following is a characteristic of emotionally intelligent nurses?
   a. Lack of empathy towards patients
   b. Inability to adapt to changing situations
   c. Recognition and management of their own emotions
   d. Resistance to feedback and personal growth

157. How does emotional intelligence contribute to teamwork in nursing?
   a. It encourages competition among team members
   b. It fosters effective communication and collaboration
   c. It results in conflicts and misunderstandings
   d. It diminishes the importance of empathy in teamwork

158. Emotional intelligence can be developed through
   a. Avoiding interactions with patients
   b. Engaging in self-reflection and mindfulness
   c. Focusing solely on technical skills
   d. Following strict protocols without considering emotions

159. Which of the following is an example of emotional intelligence in nursing practice?
- **a.** Ignoring a patient's emotional needs
- **b.** Reacting impulsively to a difficult situation
- **c.** Offering emotional support to a distressed patient
- **d.** Expressing frustration openly to colleagues

160. Which of the following is a key component of emotional intelligence?
- **a.** Logical reasoning
- **b.** Ability to perform medical procedures
- **c.** Self-awareness
- **d.** Physical strength

161. Emotional intelligence in nursing education refers to
- **a.** The ability to control one's emotions while studying
- **b.** The capacity to understand and manage emotions in oneself and others
- **c.** The ability to memorize emotional responses
- **d.** The skill of expressing emotions openly during clinical practice

162. Which type of curriculum focuses on the knowledge and skills required for entry-level nursing practice?
- **a.** Concept-based curriculum
- **b.** Competency-based curriculum
- **c.** Integrated curriculum
- **d.** Traditional curriculum

163. A curriculum that organizes content based on key concepts and principles is known as
- **a.** Concept-based curriculum
- **b.** Competency-based curriculum
- **c.** Integrated curriculum
- **d.** Traditional curriculum

164. An approach that combines different subjects and topics into a single, cohesive curriculum is called
- **a.** Concept-based curriculum
- **b.** Competency-based curriculum
- **c.** Integrated curriculum
- **d.** Traditional curriculum

165. Which type of curriculum focuses on transmitting a specific body of knowledge and skills?
- **a.** Concept-based curriculum
- **b.** Competency-based curriculum
- **c.** Integrated curriculum
- **d.** Traditional curriculum

166. Which type of curriculum is most aligned with the current trend in nursing education?
- **a.** Concept-based curriculum
- **b.** Competency-based curriculum
- **c.** Integrated curriculum
- **d.** Traditional curriculum

167. A traditional nursing curriculum typically follows a
- **a.** Linear progression of subjects and topics
- **b.** Flexible and individualized learning path
- **c.** Project-based learning approach
- **d.** Completely clinical-focused structure

168. Which of the following is an external factor that influences curriculum development?
- **a.** Student learning styles
- **b.** Teaching methodologies
- **c.** Educational policies and standards
- **d.** Subject content

169. The availability of resources such as textbooks, technology and facilities is an example of which factor influencing curriculum development?
- **a.** Internal factors
- **b.** External factors
- **c.** Societal factors
- **d.** Individual factors

170. The cultural and ethnic backgrounds of students is an example of which factor influencing curriculum development?
- **a.** Internal factors
- **b.** External factors
- **c.** Teacher expertise
- **d.** Learning theories

171. Which factor focuses on the abilities and interests of the students?
   a. Learning theories
   b. Teacher expertise
   c. Student diversity
   d. Educational policies

172. The changing trends and advancements in a particular field can influence the content and focus of the curriculum. This is an example of which factor?
   a. Student learning styles
   b. Teacher expertise
   c. Societal needs
   d. Subject content

173. When writing a learning objective, it is important to consider
   a. The preferences of the teacher
   b. The interests of the students
   c. The standards or curriculum requirements
   d. The length of the lesson or course

174. Bloom's Taxonomy is often used to
   a. Determine the length of a learning objective
   b. Assess the quality of a learning objective
   c. Categorize different levels of cognitive skills
   d. Determine the teaching strategies to be used

175. Which of the following is an example of a poorly written learning objective?
   a. 'Students will read a chapter from the textbook'
   b. 'Students will complete a worksheet on grammar'
   c. 'Students will understand the importance of teamwork'
   d. 'Students will be able to write a persuasive essay with a clear thesis statement'

176. The condition or context component of a learning objective describes
   a. The prerequisite knowledge or skills required
   b. The materials or resources provided
   c. The time frame for completing the objective
   d. The specific learning environment or situation

177. Which of the following action verbs is most appropriate for a learning objective focused on higher-order thinking skills?
   a. Memorize
   b. Analyse
   c. Define
   d. List

178. A well-written learning objective should include all of the following components EXCEPT
   a. Action verb
   b. Assessment method
   c. Condition or context
   d. Criteria for success

179. Which of the following is an example of a well-written learning objective?
   a. 'Students will understand biology'
   b. 'Students will appreciate the value of literature'
   c. 'Students will be able to solve mathematical equations using the quadratic formula'
   d. 'Students will enjoy participating in physical education activities'

180. Learning objectives should be
   a. Measurable and specific
   b. Flexible and adaptable
   c. Broad and general
   d. Subjective and opinion-based

Chapter 5. Methods of Teaching

181. Which quality helps a nursing teacher effectively convey complex information to students?
   a. Empathy
   b. Patience
   c. Clarity
   d. Adaptability

182. Which of the following qualities is crucial for a nursing teacher to establish trust and rapport with students?
   a. Leadership skills
   b. Respect for diversity
   c. Continuous learning mindset
   d. Competence in nursing skills

183. Which quality enables a nursing teacher to motivate and inspire students?
   a. Confidence
   b. Creativity
   c. Flexibility
   d. Integrity

184. Which quality allows a nursing teacher to effectively assess and evaluate student performance?
   a. Attention to detail
   b. Objectivity
   c. Organization
   d. Critical thinking

185. Which quality helps a nursing teacher to adapt teaching strategies to meet the individual needs of students?
   a. Adaptability
   b. Cultural sensitivity
   c. Problem-solving skills
   d. Professionalism

186. Which of the following qualities is essential for a nursing teacher to provide constructive feedback to students?
   a. Analytical skills
   b. Compassion
   c. Time management
   d. Open-mindedness

187. Which quality promotes a positive learning environment in nursing education?
   a. Collaboration
   b. Technical expertise
   c. Punctuality
   d. Perseverance

188. Which of the following qualities is important for a nursing teacher to foster lifelong learning among students?
   a. Humility
   b. Organization
   c. Resourcefulness
   d. Confidence

189. Which quality allows a nursing teacher to effectively manage classroom dynamics and facilitate group discussions?
   a. Active listening
   b. Professional ethics
   c. Technological proficiency
   d. Interpersonal skills

190. Which teaching style focuses on providing information and allowing students to absorb knowledge passively?
   a. Lecture-based teaching
   b. Collaborative learning
   c. Experiential learning
   d. Problem-based learning

191. Which teaching style emphasizes active participation, group work and discussion among students?
   a. Lecture-based teaching
   b. Collaborative learning
   c. Experiential learning
   d. Problem-based learning

192. Which teaching style encourages students to learn through hands-on experiences and real-world situations?
   a. Lecture-based teaching
   b. Collaborative learning
   c. Experiential learning
   d. Problem-based learning

193. Which teaching style involves presenting students with real-life scenarios and challenging them to solve problems?
   a. Lecture-based teaching
   b. Collaborative learning
   c. Experiential learning
   d. Problem-based learning

194. In the demonstrator style, how can the nursing instructor ensure student understanding and competency?
   a. By assigning written assignments and quizzes
   b. By providing constructive feedback and evaluation
   c. By encouraging peer teaching and mentoring
   d. By organizing group presentations and debates

195. What is a potential limitation of the demonstrator style in nursing education?
   a. Limited student engagement and interaction
   b. Inability to address diverse learning needs
   c. Overemphasis on theoretical concepts
   d. Lack of opportunities for independent thinking

196. Which teaching style encourages students to develop observational skills and attention to detail?
   a. Demonstrator style
   b. Facilitator style
   c. Lecture style
   d. Collaborative style

197. Which teaching style is most suitable for teaching technical skills and procedures in nursing practice?
   a. Demonstrator style
   b. Facilitator style
   c. Lecture style
   d. Collaborative style

198. Which teaching style in nursing education focuses on modelling and providing examples for students to observe and imitate?
   a. Demonstrator style
   b. Facilitator style
   c. Lecture style
   d. Collaborative style

199. Which teaching style encourages students to develop leadership and organizational skills?
   a. Delegator style
   b. Facilitator style
   c. Lecture style
   d. Collaborative style

200. What is a potential limitation of the delegator style in nursing education?
   a. Lack of guidance and support for students
   b. Overemphasis on theoretical concepts
   c. Limited opportunities for collaboration and teamwork
   d. Inability to address diverse learning needs

201. Which teaching style in nursing education involves assigning responsibilities and tasks to students?
   a. Delegator style
   b. Facilitator style
   c. Lecture style
   d. Collaborative style

202. In the delegator style, how does the nursing instructor engage with students?
   a. By providing direct instructions and demonstrations
   b. By facilitating group discussions and problem-solving activities
   c. By assigning tasks and empowering students to take responsibility
   d. By lecturing and delivering theoretical content

203. Which teaching style in nursing education involves guiding and facilitating the learning process for students?
- **a.** Facilitator style
- **b.** Delegator style
- **c.** Lecture style
- **d.** Collaborative style

204. In the facilitator style, what is the role of the nursing instructor?
- **a.** Delivering lectures and providing direct instructions
- **b.** Assigning tasks and responsibilities to students
- **c.** Promoting active discussions and critical thinking
- **d.** Demonstrating skills and procedures to students

205. Which teaching style promotes student engagement, participation and collaboration?
- **a.** Facilitator style
- **b.** Delegator style
- **c.** Lecture style
- **d.** Collaborative style

206. In the facilitator style, how does the nursing instructor engage with students?
- **a.** By lecturing and providing theoretical content
- **b.** By assigning tasks and monitoring student progress
- **c.** By facilitating discussions and guiding learning activities
- **d.** By demonstrating skills and procedures to students

207. What is a potential limitation of the facilitator style in nursing education?
- **a.** Lack of structure and clear direction for students
- **b.** Overemphasis on theoretical concepts
- **c.** Limited opportunities for independent thinking
- **d.** Inability to address diverse learning needs

208. In the facilitator style, how can the nursing instructor assess student learning and understanding?
- **a.** By assigning written assignments and quizzes
- **b.** By providing constructive feedback and evaluation
- **c.** By encouraging peer teaching and mentoring
- **d.** By organizing group presentations and debates

209. Which type of learner prefers to learn through listening and auditory cues?
- **a.** Visual learner
- **b.** Auditory learner
- **c.** Kinesthetic learner
- **d.** Tactile learner

210. Which type of learner learns best through visual aids, such as diagrams, charts and images?
- **a.** Visual learner
- **b.** Auditory learner
- **c.** Kinesthetic learner
- **d.** Tactile learner

211. Which type of learner prefers hands-on activities and learns by doing?
- **a.** Visual learner
- **b.** Auditory learner
- **c.** Kinesthetic learner
- **d.** Tactile learner

212. Which type of learner learns best by touching and manipulating objects?
- **a.** Visual learner
- **b.** Auditory learner
- **c.** Kinesthetic learner
- **d.** Tactile learner

213. Which type of learner benefits from group discussions, verbal explanations and listening to lectures?
- **a.** Visual learner
- **b.** Auditory learner
- **c.** Kinesthetic learner
- **d.** Tactile learner

214. Which type of learner excels in activities that involve physical movement and coordination?
   a. Visual learner
   b. Auditory learner
   c. Kinesthetic learner
   d. Tactile learner

215. Which type of learner prefers to take notes and write down information for better retention?
   a. Visual learner
   b. Auditory learner
   c. Kinesthetic learner
   d. Tactile learner

216. Which type of learner benefits from using flashcards, models and manipulatives for learning?
   a. Visual learner
   b. Auditory learner
   c. Kinesthetic learner
   d. Tactile learner

217. Which type of learner finds it easier to remember information by associating it with physical sensations or movements?
   a. Visual learner
   b. Auditory learner
   c. Kinesthetic learner
   d. Tactile learner

218. Which type of learner prefers a combination of different learning methods and adapts well to various teaching styles?
   a. Visual learner
   b. Auditory learner
   c. Kinesthetic learner
   d. Tactile learner

219. Learning styles in nursing refer to
   a. The methods used to teach nursing concepts
   b. The ways in which individuals prefer to learn and process information
   c. The specific skills required for nursing practice
   d. The types of assessments used in nursing education

220. The most effective teaching approach in nursing education is to
   a. Focus on a single learning style for all students
   b. Incorporate a variety of teaching methods to cater to different learning styles
   c. Use only traditional lecture-based instruction
   d. Assign independent reading as the primary learning method

221. What are the primary determinants of learning in nursing?
   a. Environment, motivation and readiness to learn
   b. Intelligence, memory and cognitive abilities
   c. Teaching methods, curriculum and assessment techniques
   d. Learning styles, preferences and individual differences

222. In the context of nursing, which determinant of learning refers to the physical and social surroundings in which learning takes place?
   a. Environment
   b. Motivation
   c. Readiness to learn
   d. Learning style

223. What does motivation refer to as a determinant of learning in nursing?
   a. The ability to comprehend and retain information
   b. The willingness and desire to engage in the learning process related to nursing
   c. The availability of appropriate learning resources for nursing education
   d. The influence of peers and social interactions on nursing education

224. Readiness to learn as a determinant of learning in nursing refers to
- **a.** Prior knowledge and skills that serve as a foundation for new nursing knowledge
- **b.** The physical and psychological state of the nursing student during the learning process
- **c.** The use of appropriate teaching methods and instructional techniques in nursing education
- **d.** The integration of technology and multimedia in the nursing learning environment

225. Which determinant of learning in nursing focuses on the individual's unique way of processing information and acquiring nursing knowledge?
- **a.** Environment
- **b.** Motivation
- **c.** Readiness to learn
- **d.** Learning style

226. How do individual differences influence learning in nursing as a determinant?
- **a.** They determine the pace and speed of learning for each nursing student
- **b.** They influence the type of teaching methods used in nursing education
- **c.** They affect the level of motivation and engagement in the nursing learning process
- **d.** They determine the readiness of nursing students to learn new nursing concepts

227. Which determinant of learning in nursing is associated with the instructional strategies, materials and techniques used by nursing educators?
- **a.** Environment
- **b.** Motivation
- **c.** Readiness to learn
- **d.** Teaching methods

228. What is the role of assessment techniques in the determinants of learning in nursing?
- **a.** They measure the effectiveness of teaching methods in nursing education
- **b.** They determine the readiness of nursing students to engage in the learning process
- **c.** They provide feedback and evaluation of nursing student performance
- **d.** They shape the social interactions and collaboration among nursing students

229. Which determinant of learning in nursing refers to the internal cognitive processes, including attention, memory and problem-solving abilities?
- **a.** Environment
- **b.** Motivation
- **c.** Readiness to learn
- **d.** Cognitive abilities

230. How do cognitive abilities influence learning in nursing as a determinant?
- **a.** They determine the physical and social surroundings for effective nursing learning
- **b.** They shape the nursing student's motivation and willingness to engage in learning
- **c.** They affect the nursing student's readiness to acquire new nursing knowledge and skills
- **d.** They influence the nursing student's ability to process and retain nursing information

231. Which of the following is a potential challenge in developing emotional intelligence in nursing education?
- **a.** Lack of opportunities for patient interaction
- **b.** Overemphasis on technical skills in the curriculum
- **c.** Inadequate knowledge of medical procedures
- **d.** Limited access to educational resources

232. Which of the following is a characteristic of emotionally intelligent nurses?
   a. Lack of empathy towards patients
   b. Inability to adapt to changing situations
   c. Recognition and management of their own emotions
   d. Resistance to feedback and personal growth

233. How does emotional intelligence contribute to teamwork in nursing?
   a. It encourages competition among team members
   b. It fosters effective communication and collaboration
   c. It results in conflicts and misunderstandings
   d. It diminishes the importance of empathy in teamwork

234. Emotional intelligence can be developed through
   a. Avoiding interactions with patients
   b. Engaging in self-reflection and mindfulness
   c. Focusing solely on technical skills
   d. Following strict protocols without considering emotions

235. Which of the following is an example of emotional intelligence in nursing practice?
   a. Ignoring a patient's emotional needs
   b. Reacting impulsively to a difficult situation
   c. Offering emotional support to a distressed patient
   d. Expressing frustration openly to colleagues

236. Which of the following is a key component of emotional intelligence?
   a. Logical reasoning
   b. Ability to perform medical procedures
   c. Self-awareness
   d. Physical strength

237. Emotional intelligence in nursing education refers to
   a. The ability to control one's emotions while studying
   b. The capacity to understand and manage emotions in oneself and others
   c. The ability to memorize emotional responses
   d. The skill of expressing emotions openly during clinical practice

238. Which type of curriculum focuses on the knowledge and skills required for entry-level nursing practice?
   a. Concept-based curriculum
   b. Competency-based curriculum
   c. Integrated curriculum
   d. Traditional curriculum

239. A curriculum that organizes content based on key concepts and principles is known as
   a. Concept-based curriculum
   b. Competency-based curriculum
   c. Integrated curriculum
   d. Traditional curriculum

240. An approach that combines different subjects and topics into a single, cohesive curriculum is called
   a. Concept-based curriculum
   b. Competency-based curriculum
   c. Integrated curriculum
   d. Traditional curriculum

241. Which type of curriculum focuses on transmitting a specific body of knowledge and skills?
   a. Concept-based curriculum
   b. Competency-based curriculum
   c. Integrated curriculum
   d. Traditional curriculum

242. Which type of curriculum is most aligned with the current trend in nursing education?
- **a.** Concept-based curriculum
- **b.** Competency-based curriculum
- **c.** Integrated curriculum
- **d.** Traditional curriculum

243. A traditional nursing curriculum typically follows a
- **a.** Linear progression of subjects and topics
- **b.** Flexible and individualized learning path
- **c.** Project-based learning approach
- **d.** Completely clinical-focused structure

244. Which of the following is an external factor that influences curriculum development?
- **a.** Student learning styles
- **b.** Teaching methodologies
- **c.** Educational policies and standards
- **d.** Subject content

245. The availability of resources such as textbooks, technology and facilities is an example of which factor influencing curriculum development?
- **a.** Internal factors
- **b.** External factors
- **c.** Societal factors
- **d.** Individual factors

246. The cultural and ethnic backgrounds of students is an example of which factor influencing curriculum development?
- **a.** Internal factors
- **b.** External factors
- **c.** Teacher expertise
- **d.** Learning theories

247. Which factor focuses on the abilities and interests of the students?
- **a.** Learning theories
- **b.** Teacher expertise
- **c.** Student diversity
- **d.** Educational policies

248. The changing trends and advancements in a particular field can influence the content and focus of the curriculum. This is an example of which factor?
- **a.** Student learning styles
- **b.** Teacher expertise
- **c.** Societal needs
- **d.** Subject content

249. When writing a learning objective, it is important to consider
- **a.** The preferences of the teacher
- **b.** The interests of the students
- **c.** The standards or curriculum requirements
- **d.** The length of the lesson or course

250. Bloom's Taxonomy is often used to
- **a.** Determine the length of a learning objective
- **b.** Assess the quality of a learning objective
- **c.** Categorize different levels of cognitive skills
- **d.** Determine the teaching strategies to be used

251. Which of the following is an example of a poorly written learning objective?
- **a.** 'Students will read a chapter from the textbook'
- **b.** 'Students will complete a worksheet on grammar'
- **c.** 'Students will understand the importance of teamwork'
- **d.** 'Students will be able to write a persuasive essay with a clear thesis statement'

252. The condition or context component of a learning objective describes
- **a.** The prerequisite knowledge or skills required
- **b.** The materials or resources provided
- **c.** The time frame for completing the objective
- **d.** The specific learning environment or situation

253. Which of the following action verbs is most appropriate for a learning objective focused on higher-order thinking skills?
   a. Memorize
   b. Analyse
   c. Define
   d. List

254. A well-written learning objective should include all of the following components EXCEPT
   a. Action verb
   b. Assessment method
   c. Condition or context
   d. Criteria for success

255. Which of the following is an example of a well-written learning objective?
   a. 'Students will understand biology'
   b. 'Students will appreciate the value of literature'
   c. 'Students will be able to solve mathematical equations using the quadratic formula'
   d. 'Students will enjoy participating in physical education activities'

256. Learning objectives should be
   a. Measurable and specific
   b. Flexible and adaptable
   c. Broad and general
   d. Subjective and opinion-based

257. Which of the following is NOT an example of an audio-visual aid?
   a. PowerPoint presentation
   b. Flipchart
   c. Video clip
   d. Handout

258. What is the purpose of using audio-visual aids in presentations?
   a. To entertain the audience
   b. To engage the audience
   c. To confuse the audience
   d. To distract the audience

259. Which of the following is an advantage of using audio-visual aids?
   a. They require minimal preparation time
   b. They increase the chances of audience interaction
   c. They eliminate the need for verbal communication
   d. They can replace the presenter altogether

260. What should be considered when selecting audio-visual aids for a presentation?
   a. Personal preference of the presenter
   b. Availability of the latest technology
   c. Relevance to the topic and audience
   d. Cost-effectiveness of the aids

261. Which of the following is a guideline for using audio-visual aids effectively?
   a. Keep the aids simple, clear and visually appealing
   b. Make the aids the main focus of the presentation
   c. Use as many different aids as possible to cater to all learning styles
   d. Avoid using any aids that require electricity

262. Which of the following is a principle of using audio-visual aids effectively?
   a. Overloading the presentation with multiple aids
   b. Using complex and technical visuals
   c. Using small font sizes to fit more information
   d. Aligning the aids with the learning objectives

263. What is the principle of simplicity in using audio-visual aids?
   a. Including as much text as possible on the slides
   b. Using a variety of colours and fonts to make it visually appealing
   c. Presenting information in a clear and concise manner
   d. Including complex diagrams and charts

264. Which principle suggests using appropriate timing when using audio-visual aids?
   a. Principle of timing
   b. Principle of relevance
   c. Principle of engagement
   d. Principle of balance

265. What does the principle of visibility imply in using audio-visual aids?
   a. Using small visuals to avoid distractions
   b. Making sure the aids are visible to all audience members
   c. Using dim lighting to enhance the visual experience
   d. Avoiding the use of colours and graphics

266. Which principle suggests using appropriate audio levels when using audio-visual aids?
   a. Principle of aesthetics
   b. Principle of audibility
   c. Principle of complexity
   d. Principle of relevance

267. What is one advantage of using a chalkboard/blackboard as an audio-visual aid?
   a. It allows for easy erasing and modifying information
   b. It provides vibrant colours and high-resolution visuals
   c. It requires minimal preparation and setup time
   d. It can be easily shared and distributed to the audience

268. When using a chalkboard/blackboard, which of the following is recommended for better visibility?
   a. Using small and intricate handwriting
   b. Writing with different colours simultaneously
   c. Writing with a clear and bold style
   d. Filling the entire board with information

269. What should be considered when writing on a chalkboard/blackboard during a presentation?
   a. Writing everything in full sentences and paragraphs
   b. Writing in a random and unorganized manner
   c. Using simple and concise phrases or bullet points
   d. Writing only key information and omitting details

270. Which of the following is a limitation of using a chalkboard/blackboard as an audio-visual aid?
   a. It lacks the ability to incorporate multimedia elements
   b. It is not suitable for large audiences
   c. It requires technical expertise to operate
   d. It is not cost-effective compared to other aids

271. How can a presenter enhance audience engagement when using a chalkboard/blackboard?
   a. Encouraging active participation through discussions
   b. Turning their back to the audience while writing
   c. Avoiding any interaction with the audience
   d. Erasing and rewriting information frequently

272. What is one advantage of using charts as audio-visual aids?
   a. They provide dynamic and interactive content
   b. They allow for easy erasing and modifying information
   c. They can present complex data in a visual and concise manner
   d. They require minimal preparation and setup time

273. Which type of chart is best suited for comparing quantities or proportions?
- **a.** Line chart
- **b.** Pie chart
- **c.** Scatter plot
- **d.** Bar chart

274. When using a chart as an audio-visual aid, which of the following is important to consider for better visibility?
- **a.** Using a small font size to fit more information
- **b.** Choosing vibrant colours for aesthetic appeal
- **c.** Keeping the chart simple and uncluttered
- **d.** Including multiple charts on a single slide

275. What should be the source of data used in a chart as an audio-visual aid?
- **a.** Randomly generated data for demonstration purposes
- **b.** Reliable and credible sources
- **c.** Personal opinions and anecdotes
- **d.** Imaginary or fictional data

276. How can a presenter effectively explain a chart to the audience?
- **a.** Quickly skim through the chart without providing any explanations
- **b.** Rely solely on visual elements without verbal explanations
- **c.** Provide a detailed analysis of each data point
- **d.** Use clear and concise verbal explanations to highlight key points

277. Which type of graph is most suitable for showing trends over time?
- **a.** Bar graph
- **b.** Pie chart
- **c.** Line graph
- **d.** Scatter plot

278. What does the x-axis represent in a graph?
- **a.** The independent variable
- **b.** The dependent variable
- **c.** The labels or categories
- **d.** The data points

279. When using a graph as an audio-visual aid, what should be considered for better readability?
- **a.** Keeping the labels and axis titles clear and legible
- **b.** Including as much data as possible on the graph
- **c.** Using a variety of colours for visual appeal
- **d.** Adding decorative elements to enhance the graph's aesthetics

280. What is one advantage of using posters as audio-visual aids?
- **a.** They allow for easy modification and erasing of information
- **b.** They provide a dynamic and interactive presentation experience
- **c.** They can capture attention and engage the audience visually
- **d.** They require minimal preparation and setup time

281. What should be the key element of a poster as an audio-visual aid?
- **a.** Visually appealing design and layout
- **b.** Intricate and complex visuals
- **c.** Detailed paragraphs of text
- **d.** Multiple font styles and colours

282. What should be the content of a flashcard as an audio-visual aid?
- **a.** Detailed paragraphs of information
- **b.** Multiple images and illustrations
- **c.** Key points or keywords for reference
- **d.** Lengthy explanations and examples

283. How many points or pieces of information should be included on each flashcard?
- **a.** Only one point or piece of information
- **b.** As much information as possible to maximize content
- **c.** No more than three points or pieces of information
- **d.** It depends on the presenter's personal preference

284. What is the recommended size for flash-cards used as audio-visual aids?
- **a.** A5 (5.8 × 8.3 inches)
- **b.** 4 × 6 inches
- **c.** A4 (8.3 × 11.7 inches)
- **d.** 8.5 × 11 inches

285. Why is the 4 × 6-inch size commonly used for flashcards?
- **a.** It fits easily in the presenter's hand
- **b.** It allows for larger, more readable text
- **c.** It provides more space for detailed information
- **d.** It creates a visual impact during the presentation

286. What is the recommended size for a flannel board used as an audio-visual aid?
- **a.** 24 × 36 inches
- **b.** 18 × 24 inches
- **c.** 12 × 18 inches
- **d.** 8.5 × 11 inches

287. What can be the disadvantage of using a smaller flannel board as an audio-visual aid?
- **a.** It may limit the number of flannel pieces that can be displayed
- **b.** It may not be visually impactful for larger audiences
- **c.** It may require frequent adjustments to fit all the visuals
- **d.** It may be difficult to transport and handle during presentations

288. What is the recommended size for a poster used as an audio-visual aid?
- **a.** A4 (8.3 × 11.7 inches)
- **b.** A3 (11.7 × 16.5 inches)
- **c.** 18 × 24 inches
- **d.** 24 × 36 inches

289. What is the primary purpose of using cartoons as audio-visual aids?
- **a.** To add humour and entertainment to the presentation
- **b.** To engage the audience visually and emotionally
- **c.** To provide detailed information and data
- **d.** To replace verbal communication entirely

290. How can cartoons be effective in convey-ing information during a presentation?
- **a.** By using complex and detailed illustrations
- **b.** By relying solely on visual elements without any text
- **c.** By incorporating captions or speech bubbles with key messages
- **d.** By using a wide range of colours and artistic styles

291. What should be considered when selecting cartoons for an audio-visual aid?
- **a.** Relevance to the topic and audience
- **b.** The latest popular cartoon characters
- **c.** Personal preference of the presenter
- **d.** The complexity of the artwork

292. What is a potential disadvantage of using cartoons as audio-visual aids?
- **a.** They may distract the audience from the main message
- **b.** They require technical expertise to create and display
- **c.** They may not be visually appealing to all audience members
- **d.** They limit the amount of information that can be conveyed

293. What is one advantage of using models or specimens as audio-visual aids?
- **a.** They provide a hands-on and tangible experience for the audience
- **b.** They can be easily replicated and distributed to the audience
- **c.** They eliminate the need for verbal explanations during the presentation
- **d.** They require minimal preparation and setup time

294. How can a presenter enhance the effectiveness of models or specimens as audio-visual aids?
- **a.** Using multiple models or specimens simultaneously on display
- **b.** Providing detailed written explanations alongside the models or specimens
- **c.** Encouraging audience members to touch and explore the models or specimens
- **d.** Using models or specimens as the sole focus of the presentation

295. How can a presenter enhance the effectiveness of puppets as audio-visual aids?
- **a.** Using multiple puppets simultaneously for different roles
- **b.** Providing detailed explanations about the history of puppets
- **c.** Using puppets sparingly to support key points or messages
- **d.** Including complex puppet movements and acrobatics

296. How can puppets be effective in conveying information during a presentation?
- **a.** By using complex and realistic puppet designs
- **b.** By relying solely on visual elements without any speech
- **c.** By using a wide range of puppet sizes and materials
- **d.** By incorporating puppet dialogues and storytelling

297. What should be considered when selecting puppets for an audio-visual aid?
- **a.** Relevance to the topic and audience
- **b.** The popularity of specific puppet characters
- **c.** Personal preference of the presenter
- **d.** The complexity of puppet movements

298. What is a potential limitation of using exhibitions as audio-visual aids?
- **a.** They may require significant time and resources to set up
- **b.** They may not be visually appealing to all audience members
- **c.** They limit the number of people who can interact with them simultaneously
- **d.** They may distract the audience from the main message of the presentation

299. How can a presenter enhance the effectiveness of exhibitions as audio-visual aids?
- **a.** Using a wide variety of displays and artefacts simultaneously
- **b.** Providing detailed written explanations alongside the exhibits
- **c.** Encouraging audience members to explore and ask questions about the exhibits
- **d.** Using the exhibition as the sole focus of the presentation

300. What is the primary purpose of using exhibitions as audio-visual aids?
- **a.** To showcase products or artefacts related to the topic
- **b.** To provide interactive and hands-on experiences for the audience
- **c.** To entertain the audience with visually appealing displays
- **d.** To replace verbal communication entirely

Chapter 6. Educational Media

301. What is a potential limitation of using pamphlets as audio-visual aids?
- **a.** They may not be visually appealing to all audience members
- **b.** They may be difficult to distribute or handle during a presentation
- **c.** They require technical expertise to design and print
- **d.** They limit the amount of information that can be conveyed

302. How can a presenter enhance the effectiveness of pamphlets as audio-visual aids?
- **a.** Providing pamphlets to the audience before the presentation
- **b.** Reading all the text on the pamphlet aloud during the presentation
- **c.** Incorporating pamphlet content into the slide presentation
- **d.** Using the pamphlets as the sole focus of the presentation

303. Which of the following is an example of projected audio-visual aid?
- **a.** Flipchart
- **b.** Whiteboard
- **c.** PowerPoint presentation
- **d.** Model or specimen

304. What is the primary advantage of using projected audio-visual aids?
- **a.** They require minimal setup and preparation time
- **b.** They allow for dynamic and visually engaging presentations
- **c.** They eliminate the need for verbal communication
- **d.** They can be easily distributed to the audience

305. What should be considered when creating a projected audio-visual aid?
- **a.** Personal preferences of the presenter
- **b.** The availability of the latest technology
- **c.** Relevance to the topic and audience
- **d.** The number of slides in the presentation

306. What is a potential limitation of using projected audio-visual aids?
- **a.** They may require technical expertise to operate
- **b.** They may not be visually appealing to all audience members
- **c.** They limit audience interaction and engagement
- **d.** They are not suitable for large venues or audiences

307. How can a presenter enhance the effectiveness of projected audio-visual aids?
- **a.** Using excessive animations and transitions for visual appeal
- **b.** Reading all the text on the slides verbatim
- **c.** Using a consistent and legible font size and style
- **d.** Using a monotonous and low-volume voice while presenting

308. How can a presenter enhance the effectiveness of PowerPoint as an audio-visual aid?
- **a.** Reading the slides verbatim to ensure audience understanding
- **b.** Using a consistent and legible font size and style
- **c.** Incorporating excessive animations and transitions for visual appeal
- **d.** Avoiding the use of images or multimedia elements in the slides

309. What is PowerPoint primarily used for as an audio-visual aid?
- **a.** Providing background music during a presentation
- **b.** Creating and displaying visual slides with text, images and multimedia
- **c.** Generating audio recordings for audience playback
- **d.** Serving as a platform for live audience interaction

310. What is an advantage of using PowerPoint as an audio-visual aid?
  a. It allows for real-time collaboration with the audience
  b. It can be easily customized to fit the presenter's preferences
  c. It eliminates the need for verbal communication during the presentation
  d. It requires minimal technical expertise to operate

311. How can a presenter apply the principle of balance in PowerPoint presentations?
  a. Filling each slide with excessive text and visuals
  b. Using a mix of colours and fonts for a vibrant appearance
  c. Distributing content evenly across the slides for visual harmony
  d. Displaying slides with uneven amounts of content and visuals

312. How can PowerPoint slides be effectively utilized during a presentation?
  a. By overcrowding slides with excessive text and information
  b. By using a variety of font styles and colours for visual appeal
  c. By incorporating relevant visuals and concise bullet points
  d. By animating every element on the slide for entertainment purposes

313. Which principle suggests using appropriate visuals in PowerPoint slides?
  a. Principle of simplicity
  b. Principle of overload
  c. Principle of complexity
  d. Principle of relevance

314. What is a key principle of using PowerPoint as an audio-visual aid effectively?
  a. Including as much text as possible on each slide
  b. Limiting the amount of information on each slide for clarity
  c. Using a wide variety of font styles and colours for visual appeal
  d. Using complex animations and transitions for entertainment

315. How does the principle of 'one idea per slide' relate to the number of words on a PowerPoint slide?
  a. It encourages the use of complex sentences to convey multiple ideas
  b. It suggests limiting the number of words to a single word or phrase
  c. It advocates for including all related information on a single slide
  d. It recommends focusing on one main idea and using concise wording

316. How does the principle of line length in PowerPoint slides impact readability?
  a. Longer lines are preferable as they contain more information
  b. Shorter lines are easier to read and comprehend
  c. Varying line length keeps the audience engaged and attentive
  d. Line length has no impact on readability

317. What is a key component of an overhead projector used for audio-visual presentations?
  a. Transparencies or acetate sheets
  b. Interactive touchscreens
  c. Slides or film rolls
  d. Projection screens or surfaces

318. How can a presenter enhance the effectiveness of an overhead projector presentation?
  a. Using excessive animations and transitions for visual appeal
  b. Reading all the text on the transparencies verbatim
  c. Providing additional handouts or materials to the audience
  d. Adjusting the projection brightness and focus for optimum visibility

319. What type of slides are typically used with a slide projector?
- **a.** Transparencies or acetate sheets
- **b.** Digital slides created on a computer
- **c.** Printed photographs or images
- **d.** Magnetic slides for magnetic boards

320. How can a slide projector be effective in enhancing understanding during a presentation?
- **a.** By providing a high-resolution display of visuals and text
- **b.** By allowing the presenter to interact directly with the projected content
- **c.** By incorporating multimedia elements, such as audio and video
- **d.** By enabling the presenter to navigate through slides manually

321. What is a key principle when using audiotapes or compact discs as audio-visual aids?
- **a.** Providing a visual representation of the content alongside the audio
- **b.** Ensuring a high-quality sound system for optimal audio playback
- **c.** Incorporating interactive elements for audience engagement
- **d.** Using them as the sole source of information during the presentation

322. How can audiotapes or compact discs be effective in enhancing understanding during a presentation?
- **a.** By providing a visual representation of complex concepts
- **b.** By allowing the audience to interact and respond to the audio
- **c.** By presenting detailed information and data through audio alone
- **d.** By using a combination of audio and visual elements for reinforcement

323. What is a potential limitation of using audiotapes or compact discs as audio-visual aids?
- **a.** They may require technical expertise to operate and play
- **b.** They may not be visually appealing to all audience members
- **c.** They limit the amount of information that can be conveyed
- **d.** They may be difficult to transport and handle during presentations

324. How can a presenter enhance the effectiveness of audiotapes or compact discs as audio-visual aids?
- **a.** Playing the audio continuously without any pauses or breaks
- **b.** Providing written transcripts or summaries of the audio content
- **c.** Using a variety of audio sources simultaneously for impact
- **d.** Using audiotapes or compact discs as the sole focus of the presentation

325. What is the primary advantage of using web-based videoconferencing as an audio-visual aid?
- **a.** It allows for real-time communication and collaboration with remote participants
- **b.** It provides a convenient and portable solution for virtual presentations
- **c.** It eliminates the need for in-person meetings and travel
- **d.** It requires minimal technical expertise to set up and operate

326. How can web-based videoconferencing be effective in enhancing understanding during a presentation?
- **a.** By providing high-definition video and audio quality
- **b.** By incorporating interactive features, such as screen sharing and chat
- **c.** By replacing the need for visual aids altogether
- **d.** By limiting the number of participants in a video conference.

327. What is a potential limitation of using web-based videoconferencing as an audio-visual aid?
   a. It may require a stable and high-speed internet connection
   b. It may not be visually appealing to all participants
   c. It limits the amount of information that can be shared during a session
   d. It is only suitable for small audiences or one-on-one interactions

328. How can a presenter enhance the effectiveness of web-based videoconferencing as an audio-visual aid?
   a. Sharing a large number of visual materials simultaneously
   b. Ensuring clear and concise communication through video and audio
   c. Encouraging participants to mute their audio and disable their video
   d. Using videoconferencing as the sole method of content delivery

329. How can a designer enhance the effectiveness of e-learning as an audio-visual aid?
   a. Using excessive animations and effects for visual appeal
   b. Providing written transcripts for all audio content
   c. Incorporating complex technical tools and features for engagement
   d. Using e-learning as the sole method of content delivery

330. What is a key principle of e-learning as an audio-visual aid?
   a. Providing engaging and interactive multimedia content
   b. Eliminating the need for audio or visual elements in learning
   c. Restricting access to learning materials to a specific time and place
   d. Using e-learning as the sole method of content delivery

331. How can e-learning be effective in enhancing understanding and engagement?
   a. By presenting content in a static and text-heavy format
   b. By incorporating multimedia elements, such as videos and interactive quizzes
   c. By limiting the access to learning materials for select individuals
   d. By eliminating the need for learner participation and interaction

332. What is a smart classroom?
   a. A classroom with advanced technology and digital resources
   b. A classroom that focuses solely on traditional teaching methods
   c. A classroom that prohibits the use of technology during lessons
   d. A classroom specifically designed for physical education activities

333. What is a key feature of a smart classroom?
   a. Avoiding the use of multimedia and audio-visual aids
   b. Exclusively using traditional textbooks and printed materials
   c. Restricting access to digital devices and the internet
   d. Integration of interactive whiteboards or smartboards

334. How does a smart classroom enhance the learning experience?
   a. By providing access to a wide range of digital resources and educational apps
   b. By limiting student interaction and promoting individual learning
   c. By discouraging the use of multimedia and audio-visual aids
   d. By relying solely on traditional teaching methods and materials

335. What is the benefit of using interactive whiteboards in smart classrooms?
   a. They eliminate the need for teachers to interact with students
   b. They provide a platform for collaborative and interactive learning
   c. They limit the content to predetermined textbook materials
   d. They restrict student engagement and participation

336. How can a smart classroom contribute to student engagement?
- **a.** By eliminating the need for student participation and interaction
- **b.** By providing access to real-time student performance data
- **c.** By restricting access to digital devices and online resources
- **d.** By replacing traditional teaching methods with automated systems

337. What is telenursing education?
- **a.** Education focused on telecommunication technology for nurses
- **b.** Education on traditional nursing practices and techniques
- **c.** Education specific to nursing in rural areas
- **d.** Education on nursing administration and management

338. What is a key benefit of telenursing education?
- **a.** Limited opportunities for hands-on learning and clinical experiences
- **b.** Decreased need for nurses to engage in continuous professional development
- **c.** Elimination of face-to-face interaction between instructors and students
- **d.** Increased access to educational resources for nurses in remote areas

339. How does telenursing education enhance learning for nurses?
- **a.** By providing virtual simulations and case studies for clinical practice
- **b.** By replacing traditional nursing education with online courses
- **c.** By minimizing the need for ongoing education and training
- **d.** By restricting access to practical learning experiences

340. How can telenursing education contribute to professional development for nurses?
- **a.** By replacing the need for ongoing education and certifications
- **b.** By providing real-time access to expert nurse mentors and instructors
- **c.** By eliminating the need for practical clinical experiences
- **d.** By restricting access to current and updated nursing research and resources

341. How does Blackboard technology support personalized learning?
- **a.** By offering adaptive learning algorithms for individual students
- **b.** By limiting access to educational resources based on student performance
- **c.** By eliminating the need for differentiated instruction
- **d.** By replacing teachers with automated grading systems

342. How does Blackboard technology support collaborative learning?
- **a.** By providing discussion forums and group workspaces
- **b.** By limiting access to course materials and resources
- **c.** By restricting student participation in online activities
- **d.** By replacing face-to-face interaction in the classroom

343. What is Blackboard technology?
- **a.** A physical board used for teaching in classrooms
- **b.** A traditional classroom management tool
- **c.** An online learning management system
- **d.** A software used for video editing

344. What is the primary purpose of evaluation in education?
- **a.** Assigning grades to students
- **b.** Comparing students' performance
- **c.** Assessing the effectiveness of teaching and learning
- **d.** Identifying students' strengths and weaknesses

Chapter 7. Assessment and Evaluation

345. How does evaluation benefit education?
   a. It provides feedback for improvement
   b. It guides instructional decision-making
   c. It informs curriculum development
   d. It supports student growth and development

346. What is the focus of evaluation in education?
   a. Determining students' intelligence levels
   b. Ranking students based on performance
   c. Assessing the quality of teaching and learning
   d. Categorizing students into ability groups

347. Why is evaluation important in education?
   a. It helps identify areas for improvement
   b. It provides accountability and transparency
   c. It ensures the effectiveness of educational programmes
   d. It supports evidence-based decision-making

348. What is one of the purposes of evaluation in education?
   a. Measure students' physical fitness
   b. Assess students' creativity
   c. Inform policy-making decisions
   d. Determine students' career aspirations

349. Which type of evaluation in education focuses on assessing students' learning outcomes and achievements?
   a. Formative evaluation
   b. Summative evaluation
   c. Diagnostic evaluation
   d. Norm-referenced evaluation

350. What type of evaluation in education is conducted during the learning process to provide ongoing feedback for improvement?
   a. Formative evaluation
   b. Summative evaluation
   c. Diagnostic evaluation
   d. Criterion-referenced evaluation

351. Which type of evaluation in education is designed to identify students' strengths, weaknesses and learning needs?
   a. Formative evaluation
   b. Summative evaluation
   c. Ipsative evaluation
   d. Diagnostic evaluation

352. What type of evaluation in education involves comparing students' performance with predetermined standards or criteria?
   a. Formative evaluation
   b. Summative evaluation
   c. Criterion-referenced evaluation
   d. Ipsative evaluation

353. Which type of evaluation in education focuses on ranking or comparing students' performance with their peers?
   a. Norm-referenced evaluation
   b. Summative evaluation
   c. Formative evaluation
   d. Ipsative evaluation

354. What is the primary purpose of formative evaluation in education?
   a. Assigning grades to students
   b. Monitoring students' progress during the learning process
   c. Ranking students based on their performance
   d. Assessing students' intelligence levels

355. Formative evaluation in education is primarily focused on
   a. Determining students' final achievement levels
   b. Assessing students' knowledge at the end of a course
   c. Providing feedback for improvement and adjustment
   d. Comparing students' performance with predetermined criteria

356. How is formative evaluation different from summative evaluation in education?
- **a.** Formative evaluation occurs at the end of a learning unit, while summative evaluation happens during the learning process
- **b.** Formative evaluation focuses on ongoing feedback, while summative evaluation provides a final judgement of student achievement
- **c.** Formative evaluation involves assigning grades, while summative evaluation emphasizes diagnostic assessment
- **d.** Formative evaluation and summative evaluation are interchangeable terms for the same evaluation process

357. What methods are commonly used in formative evaluation in education?
- **a.** Standardized tests and examinations
- **b.** Assigning grades and rankings
- **c.** Observations, quizzes and feedback surveys
- **d.** Comparing students' performance with peers

358. What is the benefit of formative evaluation in education?
- **a.** It identifies students' final grades and rankings
- **b.** It promotes competition among students
- **c.** It provides timely feedback for instructional adjustment and student improvement
- **d.** It determines students' eligibility for further education

359. Summative evaluation in education is primarily focused on
- **a.** Providing real-time feedback to students
- **b.** Evaluating students' learning at the end of a course or programme
- **c.** Identifying areas for improvement in instructional practices
- **d.** Comparing students' performance with their peers

360. What methods are commonly used in summative evaluation in education?
- **a.** Observations, quizzes and feedback surveys
- **b.** Assigning grades and rankings
- **c.** Standardized tests and examinations
- **d.** Comparing students' performance with peers

361. What is the benefit of summative evaluation in education?
- **a.** It provides ongoing feedback for instructional adjustment
- **b.** It promotes continuous student improvement
- **c.** It assesses students' final achievement and provides accountability
- **d.** It determines students' eligibility for further education

362. Which principle should be considered when selecting an evaluation method in nursing education?
- **a.** Alignment with institutional policies
- **b.** Popularity among students
- **c.** Cost-effectiveness of the method
- **d.** Availability of resources

363. When selecting an evaluation method in nursing education, it is important to consider
- **a.** The personal preference of the instructor
- **b.** The length of time required for the evaluation
- **c.** The level of difficulty of the method
- **d.** The validity and reliability of the method

364. Which principle emphasizes the importance of selecting an evaluation method that aligns with the learning objectives?
- **a.** Authenticity of the method
- **b.** Practicality of the method
- **c.** Relevance of the method
- **d.** Flexibility of the method

365. Which principle emphasizes the need to select an evaluation method that provides a comprehensive assessment of student performance?
   a. Feasibility of the method
   b. Validity of the method
   c. Efficiency of the method
   d. Diversity of the method

366. Which guideline should be followed when developing assessments in nursing education?
   a. Use a single assessment method for all students
   b. Base assessments solely on theoretical knowledge
   c. Align assessments with learning outcomes and competencies
   d. Design assessments without considering students' prior knowledge

367. When developing assessments in nursing education, it is important to
   a. Include only closed-ended questions
   b. Focus solely on factual recall
   c. Make assessments overly complex to challenge students
   d. Include a variety of question types and assessment methods

368. What is a key guideline for developing assessments in nursing education?
   a. Assess only cognitive knowledge
   b. Ignore students' clinical skills
   c. Use authentic and realistic scenarios
   d. Avoid providing feedback to students

369. Which principle should be followed when developing assessments in nursing education?
   a. Assess only individual performance, not teamwork
   b. Avoid using assessment rubrics
   c. Use subjective assessment methods exclusively
   d. Incorporate both formative and summative assessments

370. What is a crucial guideline for developing assessments in nursing education?
   a. Ignore the use of technology in assessments
   b. Avoid assessing psychomotor skills
   c. Ensure fairness and equity in assessments
   d. Exclude critical thinking skills from assessments

371. What is the primary characteristic of an essay-type question?
   a. It requires a short, concise response
   b. It involves a lengthy and detailed response
   c. It focuses on multiple-choice options
   d. It assesses only factual knowledge

372. Essay-type questions are commonly used to assess
   a. Memory recall
   b. Problem-solving skills
   c. Multiple-choice options
   d. Factual knowledge

373. What is a benefit of using essay-type questions in assessment?
   a. They are quick and easy to grade
   b. They provide limited scope for creativity and critical thinking
   c. They allow for in-depth responses and analysis
   d. They assess only factual recall

374. Essay-type questions are particularly suitable for assessing
   a. Closed-ended knowledge
   b. Simple recall of facts
   c. Single-word answers
   d. Higher-order thinking skills

375. Which statement best describes the structure of an essay-type question?
   a. It includes a prompt or topic followed by space for a detailed response
   b. It requires a brief, one-sentence response
   c. It consists of a single question with multiple-choice options
   d. It assesses only objective knowledge

376. Multiple-choice questions (MCQ) are commonly used to assess
- **a.** Memory recall
- **b.** Problem-solving skills
- **c.** Subjective opinions
- **d.** Factual knowledge

377. What is a benefit of using MCQs in assessment?
- **a.** They allow for in-depth analysis and critical thinking
- **b.** They provide an objective and standardized format
- **c.** They require lengthy and detailed responses
- **d.** They assess only subjective knowledge

378. MCQs are particularly suitable for assessing
- **a.** Higher-order thinking skills
- **b.** Open-ended knowledge
- **c.** Creative expression
- **d.** Closed-ended knowledge

379. Which statement best describes the structure of an MCQ?
- **a.** It consists of a single question with multiple answer choices
- **b.** It requires a brief, one-word response
- **c.** It includes a prompt or topic followed by space for a detailed response
- **d.** It assesses only subjective opinions

380. What is a key guideline for creating effective MCQs?
- **a.** Include as many answer choices as possible for each question
- **b.** Use complex language and technical jargon in the question stem
- **c.** Ensure each question has only one correct answer
- **d.** Include distracting answer choices to challenge students

381. What is a crucial guideline for constructing answer choices in MCQs?
- **a.** Make all the answer choices of similar length
- **b.** Use a mix of correct and incorrect answers throughout the options
- **c.** Include only one plausible option and the rest as obviously incorrect
- **d.** Avoid using negative phrasing in any of the answer choices

382. When deciding on the number of answer choices in an MCQ, it is recommended to
- **a.** Use as few answer choices as possible to make it easier for students
- **b.** Always provide five answer choices for each question
- **c.** Select a reasonable number of options, typically three to five
- **d.** Provide an unlimited number of options to allow for flexibility

383. What is an important consideration when creating distractors for MCQs?
- **a.** Ensure that all distractors are plausible but incorrect options
- **b.** Use distracting options that are unrelated to the question
- **c.** Make the distractors longer and more detailed than the correct answer
- **d.** Avoid using distractors that are obviously incorrect or silly

384. What is item analysis in the context of assessment?
- **a.** Evaluating the difficulty level of assessment items
- **b.** Assessing students' understanding of a particular topic
- **c.** Analysing the content validity of assessment items
- **d.** Determining the reliability of assessment scores

385. Item analysis is primarily used to
- **a.** Identify the most challenging assessment items
- **b.** Determine the discriminative power of assessment items
- **c.** Calculate the average score on assessment items
- **d.** Evaluate the quality of assessment instructions

386. Which statistical method is commonly used in item analysis?
   a. Mean calculation
   b. Standard deviation estimation
   c. Item discrimination index calculation
   d. Factor analysis

387. Item difficulty in item analysis refers to
   a. The degree to which students find the item challenging
   b. The percentage of students who answer the item correctly
   c. The time it takes for students to complete the item
   d. The level of complexity of the item content

388. The purpose of item analysis is to
   a. Determine the validity of assessment items
   b. Identify the specific learning objectives covered by each item
   c. Evaluate the effectiveness of instructional practices
   d. Improve the quality of assessment items

389. According to Miller's Prism of Clinical Competence, which level represents a learner's ability to demonstrate clinical competence under direct supervision?
   a. Knows
   b. Knows How
   c. Shows How
   d. Does

390. Which level in Miller's Prism of Clinical Competence reflects a learner's ability to integrate knowledge and skills into practice without the need for conscious effort?
   a. Knows
   b. Knows How
   c. Shows How
   d. Does

391. What is an observation checklist?
   a. A list of questions to ask during an observation
   b. A document used to record observations and behaviours
   c. A tool to measure subjective opinions and attitudes
   d. A set of guidelines for conducting an observation

392. What is the primary purpose of an observation checklist?
   a. To guide the observer during the observation process
   b. To record subjective impressions and opinions
   c. To assess theoretical knowledge of the observed individual
   d. To measure physical attributes of the observed individual

393. At which level of Miller's Prism of Clinical Competence can a learner describe the underlying principles and theoretical framework of a particular clinical skill?
   a. Knows
   b. Knows How
   c. Shows How
   d. Does

394. Which level in Miller's Prism of Clinical Competence corresponds to a learner's ability to perform a clinical skill with guidance and feedback?
   a. Knows
   b. Knows How
   c. Shows How
   d. Does

395. According to Miller's Prism of Clinical Competence, which level represents a learner's ability to apply clinical knowledge and skills to solve complex patient problems independently?
   a. Knows
   b. Knows How
   c. Shows How
   d. Does

396. What is a rating scale?
- **a.** A tool used to record observations and behaviours
- **b.** A set of questions to assess subjective opinions
- **c.** A numerical scale to measure physical attributes
- **d.** A method to rate or evaluate performance or characteristics

397. What is a common format for rating scales?
- **a.** Multiple-choice questions
- **b.** Open-ended prompts for written responses
- **c.** True or false statements
- **d.** Numerical scales or Likert scales

398. How does a rating scale typically work?
- **a.** It provides a list of questions to assess subjective opinions
- **b.** It allows for qualitative descriptions of observed behaviours
- **c.** It assigns scores or ratings based on predefined criteria
- **d.** It measures physical attributes using objective measurements

399. What is the Objective Structured Clinical Examination (OSCE)?
- **a.** A written examination assessing theoretical knowledge
- **b.** An assessment method using standardized patient encounters
- **c.** A group discussion to evaluate communication skills
- **d.** A practical examination measuring physical abilities

400. What is the primary purpose of the OSCE?
- **a.** To assess theoretical knowledge in a controlled environment
- **b.** To evaluate subjective opinions and attitudes of learners
- **c.** To measure physical attributes and skills of candidates
- **d.** To objectively assess clinical competence and skills

401. How does the OSCE typically work?
- **a.** Candidates answer multiple-choice questions related to clinical scenarios
- **b.** Candidates engage in role-play with standardized patients
- **c.** Candidates complete a written essay on a clinical topic
- **d.** Candidates perform physical examinations on real patients

402. What is a key feature of the OSCE?
- **a.** It is a subjective assessment method based on personal opinions
- **b.** It focuses solely on theoretical knowledge and recall
- **c.** It uses standardized scenarios and checklists for assessment
- **d.** It is a time-limited written examination

403. What is a benefit of using the OSCE?
- **a.** It provides an opportunity for open-ended responses and interpretations
- **b.** It assesses only theoretical knowledge and recall abilities
- **c.** It allows for flexible and subjective evaluations
- **d.** It provides a standardized and structured approach to assessment

404. What is the Objective Structured Practical Examination (OSPE)?
- **a.** An assessment method using standardized patient encounters
- **b.** A written examination assessing theoretical knowledge
- **c.** A practical examination measuring physical abilities
- **d.** An assessment method using standardized practical stations

405. What is the primary purpose of the OSPE?
- **a.** To evaluate subjective opinions and attitudes of learners
- **b.** To assess theoretical knowledge in a controlled environment
- **c.** To objectively assess practical skills and abilities
- **d.** To measure physical attributes and fitness levels

406. How does the OSPE typically work?
a. Candidates answer multiple-choice questions related to practical scenarios
b. Candidates engage in role-play with standardized patients
c. Candidates perform practical tasks at different stations
d. Candidates complete a written essay on a practical topic

407. Which of the following is NOT a type of attitude assessment scale?
a. Likert scale
b. Semantic differential scale
c. Guttman scale
d. Analytical scale

408. The Likert scale is used to measure attitudes based on
a. Ratings of agreement or disagreement
b. Selection of multiple options
c. Ranking of options
d. Verbal descriptors

409. The Semantic differential scale measures attitudes based on
a. Ratings of agreement or disagreement
b. Selection of multiple options
c. Ranking of options
d. Bipolar adjectives

410. The Guttman scale is designed to
a. Measure the intensity of attitudes
b. Assess attitudes based on semantic differential
c. Determine the hierarchical ordering of attitudes
d. Evaluate attitudes through a series of questions

411. Which type of attitude assessment scale involves the respondent's selection of multiple options?
a. Likert scale
b. Semantic differential scale
c. Guttman scale
d. Analytical scale

412. Yashvi, a senior in high school, is still uncertain about her career path after attending a symposium on career choices. How can you assist her?
a. Encourage her to choose a course that aligns with her passion
b. Suggest she take an aptitude test to identify her strengths
c. Highlight your teaching profession as a model example
d. Advise her to discuss her concerns with her friends

Chapter 8. Guidance and Counselling

413. A living guidance programme includes a social information service such as a Personality Development symposium, while an educational information service can involve ______________.
a. Effective study strategies
b. Job fair
c. Parenting workshops
d. Student record profiling

414. Which aspect relates to regularly assessing the effectiveness of the guidance programme?
a. Research and evaluation
b. Follow-up
c. Counselling
d. Placement

415. If counselling service aims to foster self-awareness, follow-up service aims to __________.
a. Maintain regular contact with former students
b. Identify areas for programme improvement
c. Assist students in achieving their desired placements
d. Gain an understanding of the world of work

416. To ensure effective counselling services, the school administrator should __________.
- **a.** Evaluate the guidance office facilities
- **b.** Hire a complete counselling team
- **c.** Familiarize themselves with the nature, goals and principles of guidance
- **d.** Actively participate in all guidance activities

417. The primary responsibility of a counsellor is to _____________.
- **a.** Express their perspective to the client
- **b.** Make decisions on behalf of the client
- **c.** Collaboratively establish goals with the client
- **d.** Provide ongoing support and follow-up to the client

418. Which of the following is within the scope of guidance?
- **a.** Providing medical treatment
- **b.** Offering legal advice
- **c.** Assisting with academic planning
- **d.** None of the above

419. What is the primary focus of guidance?
- **a.** Diagnosing mental health disorders
- **b.** Providing therapy sessions
- **c.** Helping individuals make informed decisions
- **d.** Providing marriage counselling

420. Which of the following is an example of guidance in the educational context?
- **a.** Tutoring students in a specific subject
- **b.** Offering guidance on study skills and time management
- **c.** Providing career counselling
- **d.** Offering financial planning advice

421. Which of the following is a fundamental principle of guidance?
- **a.** Confidentiality
- **b.** Providing quick solutions
- **c.** Imposing decisions on individuals
- **d.** Ignorance

422. What is the principle of respect in guidance?
- **a.** Respecting the personal beliefs and values of individuals
- **b.** Dictating the choices of individuals
- **c.** Judging individuals based on their decisions
- **d.** Respecting the person according to his/her degree

423. Which principle emphasizes the importance of empathy in guidance?
- **a.** Autonomy
- **b.** Trustworthiness
- **c.** Collaboration
- **d.** None of the above

424. What does the principle of autonomy mean in guidance?
- **a.** Encouraging individuals to make their own decisions
- **b.** Forcing individuals to follow a particular path
- **c.** Ignoring the input of individuals
- **d.** Dictating the choices of individuals

425. Which principle focuses on the ongoing development and growth of individuals?
- **a.** Nondirectiveness
- **b.** Lifelong learning
- **c.** Rigidity
- **d.** Directiveness

426. What is the scope of counselling?
- **a.** Providing medical treatment
- **b.** Offering legal advice
- **c.** Assisting with personal and emotional issues
- **d.** Imposing decisions on individuals

427. Which of the following falls within the scope of counselling?
- **a.** Providing financial planning advice
- **b.** Offering career guidance and job placement
- **c.** Providing quick solutions
- **d.** Assisting with mental health disorders

428. Which of the following is an example of counselling in the educational context?
- **a.** Providing academic advice on course selection
- **b.** Offering guidance on study skills and time management
- **c.** Diagnosing and treating mental health disorders
- **d.** Offering medical advice

429. Which of the following is an appropriate scope for a counsellor?
- **a.** Providing medical diagnoses
- **b.** Assisting individuals with career exploration and decision-making
- **c.** Offering legal representation
- **d.** Diagnosing and treating mental health disorders

430. What is the principle of empathy in counselling?
- **a.** Maintaining professional boundaries
- **b.** Understanding and sharing the feelings of clients
- **c.** Providing quick solutions to problems
- **d.** Understanding cultural diversity

431. Which principle emphasizes the importance of unconditional positive regard in counselling?
- **a.** Self-disclosure
- **b.** Respect for autonomy
- **c.** Nonjudgemental acceptance
- **d.** Active listening

432. What does the principle of confidentiality mean in counselling?
- **a.** Sharing client information with others without their consent
- **b.** Ensuring that client information remains private and protected
- **c.** Disclosing client information to third parties for personal gain
- **d.** Respecting cultural norms and values

433. Which principle promotes the idea that clients are the experts in their own lives?
- **a.** Collaboration
- **b.** Directive approach
- **c.** Imposing decisions on clients
- **d.** Cultural sensitivity

434. What is the principle of self-determination in counselling?
- **a.** Forcing clients to follow a particular path
- **b.** Encouraging clients to make their own choices and decisions
- **c.** Disregarding the input and preferences of clients
- **d.** Establishing clear goals and objectives

435. What type of counselling focuses on helping individuals overcome substance abuse and addiction?
- **a.** Career counselling
- **b.** Marriage counselling
- **c.** Rehabilitation counselling
- **d.** Cognitive-behavioural therapy

436. Which type of counselling addresses conflicts and issues within a couple or marital relationship?
- **a.** Group counselling
- **b.** Family counselling
- **c.** Career counselling
- **d.** Marriage counselling

437. What type of counselling is designed to help individuals explore and make decisions about their career paths?
- **a.** Rehabilitation counselling
- **b.** Marriage counselling
- **c.** School counselling
- **d.** Career counselling

438. Which type of counselling focuses on helping individuals and families cope with grief and loss?
- **a.** Genetic counselling
- **b.** Bereavement counselling
- **c.** Marriage counselling
- **d.** Rehabilitation counselling

439. What type of counselling aims to address and resolve conflicts within a family system?
- **a.** Genetic counselling
- **b.** Family counselling
- **c.** Career counselling
- **d.** Rehabilitation counselling

440. What is the first step in the counselling process?
- **a.** Establishing rapport and building a therapeutic relationship
- **b.** Identifying the client's issues and concerns
- **c.** Setting goals and objectives for counselling
- **d.** Conducting an assessment of the client's needs

441. What is the next step after establishing rapport in the counselling process?
- **a.** Setting goals and objectives for counselling
- **b.** Identifying the client's issues and concerns
- **c.** Developing a treatment plan
- **d.** Conducting an assessment of the client's needs

442. What step comes after identifying the client's issues and concerns?
- **a.** Setting goals and objectives for counselling
- **b.** Developing a treatment plan
- **c.** Implementing interventions and strategies
- **d.** Evaluating the progress of counselling

443. What is the next step after setting goals and objectives in the counselling process?
- **a.** Developing a treatment plan
- **b.** Implementing interventions and strategies
- **c.** Evaluating the progress of counselling
- **d.** Terminating the counselling relationship

444. What is the final step in the counselling process?
- **a.** Developing a treatment plan
- **b.** Implementing interventions and strategies
- **c.** Evaluating the progress of counselling
- **d.** Terminating the counselling relationship

445. Which counselling technique involves reflecting back the client's thoughts and feelings?
- **a.** Active listening
- **b.** Cognitive restructuring
- **c.** Role-playing
- **d.** Reality testing

446. Which counselling technique helps clients explore their irrational or negative thoughts and replace them with more positive and realistic ones?
- **a.** Active listening
- **b.** Cognitive restructuring
- **c.** Role-playing
- **d.** Reality testing

447. Which counselling technique involves clients acting out certain scenarios or situations to gain insight and practice new behaviours?
- **a.** Active listening
- **b.** Cognitive restructuring
- **c.** Role-playing
- **d.** Reality testing

448. Which counselling technique helps clients examine their thoughts, feelings and behaviours in relation to their current reality?
a. Active listening
b. Cognitive restructuring
c. Role-playing
d. Reality testing

449. Which counselling technique involves asking open-ended questions to encourage clients to explore their thoughts and feelings in more depth?
a. Active listening
b. Cognitive restructuring
c. Socratic questioning
d. Reality testing

450. Which counselling technique focuses on helping clients develop problem-solving skills and strategies?
a. Active listening
b. Cognitive restructuring
c. Role-playing
d. Solution-focused brief therapy

451. Which counselling technique involves providing guidance and advice to clients based on the counsellor's expertise and knowledge?
a. Active listening
b. Cognitive restructuring
c. Directive counselling
d. Reality testing

452. Which counselling technique involves helping clients explore their past experiences and childhood to gain insight into their current issues?
a. Active listening
b. Cognitive restructuring
c. Psychodynamic therapy
d. Reality testing

453. Which counselling technique focuses on teaching clients relaxation and stress-management techniques?
a. Mindfulness-based therapy
b. Cognitive restructuring
c. Active listening
d. Reality testing

454. Which counselling technique involves guiding clients to set specific, achievable goals and develop a plan to reach them?
a. Active listening
b. Goal setting
c. Cognitive restructuring
d. Reality testing

455. What is the primary responsibility of a students' grievance redressal cell/committee in nursing education?
a. Handling disciplinary issues among students
b. Providing academic counselling to students
c. Resolving grievances and complaints raised by students
d. Assisting in career placement for students

456. The students' grievance redressal cell/committee in nursing education acts as a/an
a. Mediator between students and faculty/staff
b. Enforcer of academic policies
c. Facilitator of extracurricular activities
d. Academic advisor for students

457. What is the significance of having a students' grievance redressal cell/committee in nursing education?
a. It ensures fair treatment and justice for students
b. It supports students' academic and personal development
c. It promotes transparency and accountability in the educational system
d. It organizes social events for students

458. The students' grievance redressal cell/committee in nursing education addresses issues related to
- **a.** Academic misconduct and plagiarism
- **b.** Discrimination or harassment cases
- **c.** Unfair evaluation or grading practices
- **d.** Career counselling for students

459. How does the students' grievance redressal cell/committee contribute to the improvement of nursing education?
- **a.** By addressing concerns and issues promptly and effectively
- **b.** By advocating for students' rights and well-being
- **c.** By conducting research on nursing education practices
- **d.** By fostering a positive and supportive learning environment

Chapter 9. Ethics and Evidence-Based Teaching in Nursing Education

460. Which of the following best describes the concept of autonomy in nursing ethics?
- **a.** Respecting the rights and decisions of patients
- **b.** Prioritizing the needs of the healthcare system
- **c.** Following the instructions of the healthcare team
- **d.** Focusing on personal beliefs and values

461. In nursing education, the principle of beneficence refers to
- **a.** Focusing on personal gain and advancement
- **b.** Acting in the best interest of the patient
- **c.** Avoiding any harm to oneself
- **d.** Promoting the interests of the healthcare organization

462. Which ethical principle emphasizes the duty of healthcare professionals to maintain confidentiality?
- **a.** Nonmaleficence
- **b.** Veracity
- **c.** Justice
- **d.** Fidelity

463. A nurse encounters a situation where the patient's cultural beliefs conflict with the proposed medical treatment. Which ethical principle is most relevant in this scenario?
- **a.** Autonomy
- **b.** Beneficence
- **c.** Nonmaleficence
- **d.** Justice

464. The principle of nonmaleficence in nursing education requires nurses to
- **a.** Ensure fairness and equality in patient care
- **b.** Maintain professional competence and integrity
- **c.** Avoid causing harm or injury to patients
- **d.** Respect the rights and dignity of patients

465. What does the principle of veracity emphasize in nursing ethics?
- **a.** Respecting patient confidentiality
- **b.** Upholding honesty and truthfulness
- **c.** Promoting equality in healthcare
- **d.** Advocating for patient rights

466. When nurses allocate resources and distribute care equitably among patients, they are following the principle of
- **a.** Autonomy
- **b.** Fidelity
- **c.** Justice
- **d.** Nonmaleficence

467. The ethical principle of fidelity in nursing education refers to
- **a.** Promoting the welfare of patients
- **b.** Providing care without discrimination
- **c.** Avoiding conflicts of interest
- **d.** Maintaining professional boundaries and trust

468. Which ethical principle guides nurses to advocate for vulnerable populations and address health disparities?
- **a.** Autonomy
- **b.** Justice
- **c.** Veracity
- **d.** Fidelity

469. Nurses who engage in lifelong learning and continuously update their knowledge and skills are demonstrating adherence to which ethical principle?
- **a.** Autonomy
- **b.** Beneficence
- **c.** Nonmaleficence
- **d.** Fidelity

470. What is the primary goal of value-based education in nursing?
- **a.** Developing clinical skills
- **b.** Enhancing critical thinking abilities
- **c.** Instilling ethical values and professionalism
- **d.** Promoting teamwork and collaboration

471. Which of the following best describes the concept of empathy in value-based nursing education?
- **a.** Demonstrating sympathy towards patients' suffering
- **b.** Understanding and sharing patients' feelings and experiences
- **c.** Maintaining emotional distance from patients
- **d.** Focusing on personal well-being over patient care

472. In value-based nursing education, the principle of integrity emphasizes
- **a.** Providing care without discrimination
- **b.** Upholding honesty and ethical conduct
- **c.** Respecting patients' autonomy and decisions
- **d.** Advocating for vulnerable populations

473. Nurses who demonstrate accountability in value-based education
- **a.** Take responsibility for their actions and decisions
- **b.** Focus on personal interests rather than patient needs
- **c.** Engage in unethical behaviour without consequences
- **d.** Prioritize financial gain over patient well-being

474. The principle of respect for diversity in value-based nursing education encourages nurses to
- **a.** Uphold cultural and religious beliefs of patients
- **b.** Ignore individual differences and treat everyone the same
- **c.** Promote their own personal beliefs and values
- **d.** Prioritize their own comfort over patient preferences

475. What does the principle of compassion emphasize in value-based nursing education?
- **a.** Treating patients with kindness and empathy
- **b.** Avoiding conflicts of interest
- **c.** Maintaining professional boundaries and confidentiality
- **d.** Demonstrating competence in clinical skills

476. Nurses who practice patient-centred care in value-based education
- **a.** Focus on their own convenience and preferences
- **b.** Prioritize the needs and preferences of the healthcare system
- **c.** Advocate for patients and involve them in decision-making
- **d.** Provide care without considering patients' values and beliefs

477. The principle of lifelong learning in value-based nursing education encourages nurses to
- **a.** Focus solely on acquiring technical skills
- **b.** Avoid further professional development and growth
- **c.** Disregard advancements in healthcare technology and research
- **d.** Continuously update knowledge and skills throughout their career

478. In value-based nursing education, the principle of teamwork promotes
- **a.** Isolation and independent practice
- **b.** Collaboration and effective communication
- **c.** Ignoring the input of other healthcare professionals
- **d.** Prioritizing individual achievements over team success

479. Nurses who demonstrate advocacy in value-based education
- **a.** Prioritize their own interests over patient well-being
- **b.** Avoid engaging in difficult conversations with patients
- **c.** Speak up for patients' rights and needs
- **d.** Disregard ethical dilemmas and conflicts in healthcare

480. The ethical principle of justice in nursing decision-making refers to
- **a.** Treating patients with fairness and equality
- **b.** Maintaining professional boundaries and trust
- **c.** Advocating for vulnerable populations
- **d.** Avoiding conflicts of interest

481. Nurses faced with resource allocation decisions during a pandemic must consider which ethical principle?
- **a.** Autonomy
- **b.** Fidelity
- **c.** Justice
- **d.** Nonmaleficence

482. Evidence-based teaching in nursing is based on
- **a.** Personal opinions and experiences
- **b.** Intuition and gut feelings
- **c.** Research evidence and best practices
- **d.** Tradition and established norms

483. What is the primary goal of evidence-based teaching in nursing?
- **a.** Promoting the instructor's expertise and knowledge
- **b.** Maximizing student engagement and satisfaction
- **c.** Enhancing critical thinking and decision-making skills
- **d.** Following a standardized curriculum

484. When designing evidence-based teaching strategies, nurses should prioritize
- **a.** Use of outdated teaching materials
- **b.** Instructor-centred lectures and presentations
- **c.** Relying solely on textbooks for information
- **d.** Student-centred active learning approaches

485. Evidence-based teaching in nursing encourages educators to
- **a.** Ignore research findings and rely on personal beliefs
- **b.** Disregard the needs and preferences of students
- **c.** Stick to traditional teaching methods without adaptation
- **d.** Incorporate current research evidence into teaching practices

486. The role of research evidence in evidence-based teaching is to
- **a.** Support the effectiveness of specific teaching strategies
- **b.** Dictate rigid rules and procedures for teaching
- **c.** Validate the instructor's personal experiences
- **d.** Ignore the diverse learning needs of students

487. In evidence-based teaching, the process of critically appraising research evidence involves
- **a.** Accepting research findings at face value
- **b.** Evaluating the quality and relevance of research studies
- **c.** Ignoring research articles that challenge current practices
- **d.** Disregarding the opinions and experiences of students

488. Nurses who engage in evidence-based teaching are expected to
- **a.** Ignore feedback and suggestions from students
- **b.** Rely solely on their own expertise and knowledge
- **c.** Continuously update their teaching practices based on new evidence
- **d.** Maintain a rigid teaching style without flexibility

489. The integration of evidence-based teaching in nursing education helps to
- **a.** Limit critical thinking and independent learning
- **b.** Promote standardized and inflexible teaching methods
- **c.** Exclude the use of technology in the learning process
- **d.** Enhance the quality of education and improve student outcomes

490. When using evidence-based teaching, nurses should consider the individual
- **a.** Beliefs and values of the instructor
- **b.** Cultural and learning needs of the students
- **c.** Opinions of the most influential students
- **d.** Preferences of the healthcare organization

491. Evidence-based teaching encourages nurses to engage in
- **a.** Lifelong learning and professional development
- **b.** Ignoring advancements in nursing research
- **c.** Reproducing outdated teaching materials
- **d.** Teaching methods based solely on personal experiences

Answers

1 c, 2 a, 3 c, 4 b, 5 d, 6 c, 7 c, 8 a, 9 a, 10 c, 11 c, 12 d, 13 b, 14 c, 15 a, 16 b, 17 c, 18 d, 19 c, 20 d, 21 c, 22 a, 23 b, 24 c, 25 c, 26 b, 27 d, 28 b, 29 c, 30 a, 31 d, 32 b, 33 c, 34 a, 35 d, 36 b, 37 a, 38 b, 39 b, 40 a, 41 c, 42 b, 43 c, 44 c, 45 a, 46 c, 47 c, 48 a, 49 c, 50 d, 51 b, 52 a, 53 c, 54 d, 55 d, 56 d, 57 c, 58 a, 59 b, 60 c, 61 d, 62 c, 63 a, 64 c, 65 d, 66 d, 67 c, 68 d, 69 b, 70 b, 71 c, 72 c, 73 b, 74 c, 75 b, 76 c, 77 d, 78 c, 79 b, 80 c, 81 c, 82 c, 83 c, 84 d, 85 c, 86 c, 87 a, 88 c, 89 c, 90 c, 91 d, 92 a, 93 c, 94 b, 95 d, 96 b, 97 b, 98 c, 99 c, 100 c, 101 c,102 c, 103 c, 104 b, 105 c, 106 b, 107 d, 108 b, 109 a, 110 b, 111 a, 112 a, 113 d, 114 a, 115 b, 116 c, 117 d, 118 b, 119 a, 120 a, 121 a, 122 a, 123 a, 124 a, 125 a, 126 c, 127 a, 128 c, 129 a, 130 c, 131 a, 132 b, 133 b, 134 a, 135 c, 136 d, 137 b, 138 c, 139 a, 140 d, 141 c, 142 a, 143 b, 144 b, 145 a, 146 a, 147 b, 148 a, 149 d, 150 c, 151 d, 152 c, 153 d, 154 c, 155 b, 156 c, 157 b, 158 b, 159 c, 160 c, 161 b, 162 b, 163 a, 164 c, 165 d, 166 b, 167 a, 168 c, 169 b, 170 a, 171 c, 172 c, 173 c, 174 c, 175 c, 176 d, 177 b, 178 b, 179 c, 180 a, 181 c, 182 b, 183 d,

184 b, 185 a, 186 b, 187 a, 188 a, 189 d, 190 a, 191 b, 192 c, 193 d, 194 b, 195 a, 196 a, 197 a, 198 a, 199 a, 200 a, 201 a, 202 c, 203 a, 204 c, 205 a, 206 c, 207 a, 208 b, 209 b, 210 a, 211 c, 212 d, 213 b, 214 c, 215 a, 216 d, 217 c, 218 a, 219 b, 220 b, 221 a, 222 a, 223 b, 224 a, 225 d, 226 c, 227 d, 228 c, 229 d, 230 c, 231 b, 232 c, 233 b, 234 b, 235 c, 236 c, 237 b, 238 b, 239 a, 240 c, 241 d, 242 b, 243 a, 244 c, 245 b, 246 a,247 c, 248 c, 249 c, 250 c, 251 c, 252 d, 253 b, 254 b, 255 c, 256 a, 257 d, 258 b, 259 b, 260 c, 261 a, 262 d, 263 c, 264 a, 265 b, 266 b, 267 a, 268 c, 269 c, 270 a, 271 a, 272 c, 273 d, 274 c, 275 b, 276 d, 277 c, 278 a, 279 a, 280 c, 281 a, 282 c, 283 a, 284 b, 285 a, 286 b, 287 a, 288 d, 289 b, 290 c, 291 a, 292 a, 293 a, 294 c, 295 c, 296 d, 297 a, 298 a, 299 c, 300 a, 301 b, 302 a, 303 c, 304 b, 305 c, 306 a, 307 c, 308 b, 309 b, 310 b, 311 c, 312 c, 312 c, 313 d, 314 d, 315 d, 316 b, 317 a, 318 d, 319 c, 320 d, 321 b, 322 c, 323 c, 324 b, 325 a, 326 b, 327 a, 328 b, 329 b, 330 a, 331 b, 332 a, 333 d, 334 a, 335 b, 336 b, 337 a, 338 d, 339 a, 340 b, 341 a, 342 a, 343 c, 344 c, 345 d, 346 c, 347 b, 348 c, 349 b, 350 a, 351 d, 352 c, 353 a, 354 b, 355 c, 356 b, 357 c, 358 c, 359 b, 360 c, 361 c, 362 a, 363 d, 364 c, 365 b, 366 c, 367 d, 368 c, 369 d, 370 c, 371 b, 372 b, 373 c, 374 d, 375 a, 376 d, 377 b, 378 d, 379 a, 380 c, 381 b, 382 c, 383 a, 384 a, 385 b, 386 c, 387 b, 388 d, 389 c, 390 d, 391 b, 392 a, 393 a, 394 b, 395 d, 396 d, 397 d, 398 c, 399 b, 400 d, 401 b, 402 c, 403 d, 404 d, 405 c, 406 c, 407 d, 408 a, 409 d, 410 c, 411 b, 412 b, 413 a, 414 a, 415 a, 416 c, 417 c, 418 c, 419 c, 420 b, 421 a, 422 a, 423 b, 424 a, 425 b, 426 c, 427 d, 428 b, 429 b, 430 b, 431 c, 432 b, 433 a, 434 b, 435 c, 436 d, 437 d, 438 b, 439 b, 440 a, 441 d, 442 a, 443 b, 444 d, 445 a, 446 b, 447 c, 448 b, 449 c, 450 d, 451 c, 452 c, 453 a, 554 b, 455 c, 456 a, 457 c, 458 a, 459 d, 460 a, 461 b, 462 d, 463 a, 464 c, 465 b, 466 c, 467 d, 468 b, 469 d, 470 c, 471 b, 472 b, 473 a, 474 a, 475 a, 476 c, 477 d, 478 b, 479 c, 480 a, 481 c, 482 c, 483 c, 484 d, 485 d, 486 a, 487 b, 488 c, 489 d, 490 b, 491 a

Index

E

F

G

I

J

L

R

S

T

V

W

SYLLABUS MAPPER

Nursing Education and Educational Technology, 3e

Unit	Learning Objectives	Content	Chapter from the Book
I	Explain the definition, aims, types, approaches and scope of educational technology Compare and contrast the various educational philosophies Explain the teaching learning process, nature, characteristics and principles	**Introduction and theoretical foundations:** *Education and educational technology* • Definition, aims • Approaches and scope of educational technology *Educational philosophy:* • Definition of philosophy, education and philosophy • Comparison of educational philosophies • Philosophy of nursing education *Teaching learning process:* • Definition of teaching & learning • Teaching learning as a process • Nature and characteristics of teaching • Principles of teaching • Barriers to teaching • Nature and characteristics of learning • Characteristics of adult learners • Principles of learning • Learning theories • Barriers to learning	**Chapter 1** Education and Educational Technology **Chapter 2** Principles and Philosophies of Education **Chapter 3** Teaching–Learning Process
II	Identify essential qualities/attributes of a teacher Describe the teaching styles of faculty Explain the determinants of learning and initiates self-assessment to identify own learning style	**Assessment and Planning** *Assessment of teacher* • Essential qualities of a teacher • Teaching styles – Formal authority, demonstrator, facilitator, delegator *Assessment of learner* • Types of learners • Determinants of learning-learning needs, readiness to learn, learning styles	**Chapter 4** Curriculum, Assessment and Planning

	Identify the factors that motivate the learner Define curriculum and classify types Identify the factors influencing curriculum development Develop skill in writing learning outcomes, and lesson plan	• Emotional intelligence of the learner • Motivational factors-personal factors, environmental factors and support system **Curriculum Planning** • Curriculum – definition, types • Curriculum design – components, approaches • Curriculum development – factors influencing curriculum development, facilitators and barriers • Writing learning outcomes/behavioral objectives • Basic principles of writing course plan, unit plan and lesson plan	
III	Explain the principles and strategies of classroom management Describe different methods/ strategies of teaching and develop beginning skill in using various teaching methods	**Implementation** *Teaching in Classroom and Skill lab: Teaching Methods* • Classroom management-principles and strategies • Classroom communication o Facilitators and Barriers to classroom communication o Information communication technology (ICT) – ICT used in education *Teaching methods: Features, advantages and disadvantages* • Lecture, Group discussion, microteaching • Skill lab – simulations, demonstration & re-demonstration • Symposium, panel discussion, seminar, scientific workshop, exhibitions • Role play, project • Field trips • Self-directed learning (SDL) • Computer assisted learning • One-to-one instruction *Active learning strategies* • Team based learning • Problem based learning • Peer sharing • Case study analysis	**Chapter 5** Methods of Teaching

		• Journaling • Debate • Gaming • Inter professional education	
IV	Enumerate the factors influencing selection of clinical learning experiences Compare the advantages of different clinical education models Develop skill in using different clinical teaching strategies	**Teaching in the clinical setting: Teaching methods** • Clinical learning environment • Factors influencing selection of clinical learning experiences study, nursing rounds, concept mapping, project, debate, game, role play, clinical simulation, PBL, questioning, written assignment, process recording • Models of clinical education- traditional mode, collaborative model, preceptor model, integration of education and practice model, • Characteristics of effective clinical teacher • Writing clinical learning outcomes/practice competencies • Clinical teaching strategies- patient assignment- clinical conference, clinical presentation /bedside clinic, Case study/care study, nursing rounds, concept mapping, project, debate, game, role play, clinical simulation, PBL, questioning, written assignment, process recording	**Chapter 5** Methods of Teaching
V	Explain the purpose, principles and steps in the use of media Categorize the different types of media and describe its advantages and disadvantages Develop skill in preparing and using media	**Educational/Teaching media** • Media use – Purpose, components, principles and steps • Types of media *Still visuals* o Non projected – drawings & diagrams, charts, graphs, posters, cartoons, board devices (chalk/white board, bulletin board, flannel board, flip charts, flash cards, still pictures/photographs, printed materials- handout, leaflet, brochure, flyer o Projected – film stripes, microscope, power point slides, overhead projector	**Chapter 6** Educational Media

		Moving visuals o Video learning resources – videotapes & DVD, blu-ray, USB flash drive o Motion pictures/films *Realia and models* o Real objects & Models *Audio aids/audio media* o Audiotapes/Compact discs o Radio & Tape recorder o Public address system o Digital audio *Electronic media/computer learning resources* o Computers o Web-based videoconferencing o E-learning, Smart classroom *Telecommunication (Distance education)* o Cable TV, satellite broadcasting, videoconferencing Telephones – Telehealth/telenursing *Mobile technology*	
VI	Describe the purpose, scope, principles in selection of evaluation methods and barriers to evaluation Explain the guidelines to develop assessment tests Develop skill in construction of different tests Identify various clinical evaluation tools and demonstrate skill in selected tests	**Assessment/Evaluation Methods/strategies** • Purposes, scope and principles in selection of assessment methods and types • Barriers to evaluation • Guidelines to develop assessment tests *Assessment of knowledge*: • Essay type questions • Short answer questions (SAQ) • Multiple choice questions (MCQ – single response & multiple response) *Assessment of skills:* Clinical evaluation • Observation (checklist, rating scales, videotapes) • Written communication – progress notes, nursing	**Chapter 7** Assessment and Evaluation

		care plans, process recording, written assignments • Verbal communication (oral examination) • Simulation • Objective Structured Clinical Examination (OSCE) • Self-evaluation • Clinical portfolio, clinical logs *Assessment of Attitude:* • Attitude scales *Assessment tests for higher learning* • Interpretive questions, hot spot questions, drag and drop and ordered response questions	
VII	Explain the scope, purpose and principles of guidance Differentiate between guidance and counseling Describe the principles, types, and counseling process Develop basic skill of counseling and guidance Recognize the importance of preventive counseling and develop skill to respond to disciplinary problems and grievance among students	**Guidance/academic advising, counseling and discipline** *Guidance* • Definition, objectives, scope, purpose and principles • Roles of academic advisor/faculty in guidance *Counseling* • Difference between guidance and counseling • Definition, objectives, scope, principles, types, process and steps of counseling • Counseling skills/techniques – basics • Roles of counselor • Organization of counseling services • Issues for counseling in nursing students *Discipline and grievance in students* Managing disciplinary/grievance problems-preventive guidance & counseling • Role of students' grievance redressal cell/committee	**Chapter 8** Guidance and Counselling
VIII	Recognize the importance of value-based education	**Ethics and Evidence Based Teaching (EBT) in nursing education** *Ethics – Review*	**Chapter 9** Ethics and Evidence-Based Teaching in

	Develop skill in ethical decision making and maintain ethical standards for students Introduce knowledge of EBT and its application in nursing education	• Definition of terms • Value based education in nursing • Value development strategies • Ethical decision making • Ethical standards for students • Student-faculty Relationship *Evidence based teaching – Introduction* • Evidence based education process and its application to nursing education	Nursing Education

SYLLABUS MAPPER

Handbook of Forensic Nursing

Unit	Learning Objectives	Content	Chapter from the Book
I	Describe the nature of forensic science and discus issues concerning violence	**Forensic science** • Definition • History • Importance in medical science • Forensic science laboratory **Violence** • Definition • Epidemiology • Source of data Sexual abuse-child and women	**Unit I** Forensic Science
II	Explain concepts of forensic nursing and scope of practice for forensic nurse	**Forensic nursing** • Definition • History and development • Scope - setting of practice, areas of practice and subspecialties • Ethical issues • Roles and responsibilities of nurse • INC & SNC Acts	**Unit II** Forensic Nursing
III	Identify members of forensic team and describe role of forensic nurse	**Forensic team** • Members and their roles **Comprehensive forensic nursing care of victim and family** • Physical aspects • Psychosocial aspects • Cultural and spiritual aspects • Legal aspects • Assist forensic team in care beyond scope of her practice • Admission and discharge/referral/death of victim of violence • Responsibilities of nurse as a witness **Evidence preservation-role of nurses** • Observation • Recognition • Collection • Preservation	**Unit III** Forensic Team

		• Documentation of Biological and other evidence related to criminal/traumatic event • Forwarding biological samples for forensic examination	
	Describe fundamental rights and human rights commission	**Introduction of Indian constitution** **Fundamental rights** • Rights of victim • Rights of accused **Human rights commission**	
V	Explain Indian judicial system and laws Discuss the importance of POSCO Act	**Sources of laws and law-making powers** **Overview of Indian judicial system** • JFMC • District • State • Apex **Civil and criminal case procedures** • IPC • ICPC • IE Act **Overview of POSCO Act**	**Unit V** Indian Judicial System and Laws Related to Nursing Practice